SNAPSHOTS IN
DERMATOLOGY

SNAPSHOTS IN DERMATOLOGY

Second Edition

Editors

S Sacchidanand
MD DVD DHA FRCP
Executive Director
Siddaganga Medical College & Research Institute
Vice Chancellor, Rajiv Gandhi University of Health Sciences
(2018–2021)
Karnataka, India

Savitha AS
MD DNB FRGUHS MNAMS
Professor
Department of Dermatology
Sapthagiri Institute of Medical Sciences and Research Centre
Bengaluru, Karnataka, India

Shilpa K
MD(DVL) FRUGHS(Dermatosurgery)
Professor and Head
Department of Dermatology
Bangalore Medical College and Research Institute
Bengaluru, Karnataka, India

Associate Editor

Chaithra S
MD(Dermatology)
Assistant Professor
Sapthagiri Institute of Medical Sciences and Research Centre
Bengaluru, Karnataka, India

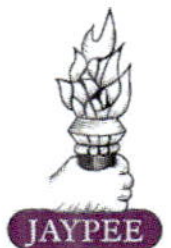

JAYPEE BROTHERS MEDICAL PUBLISHERS
The Health Sciences Publisher
New Delhi | London

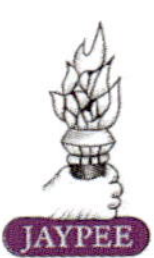

Jaypee Brothers Medical Publishers (P) Ltd

Headquarters
EMCA House, 23/23-B
Ansari Road, Daryaganj
New Delhi 110 002, India
Landline: +91-11-23272143, +91-11-23272703
+91-11-23282021, +91-11-23245672
e-mail: jaypee@jaypeebrothers.com

Corporate Office
4838/24, Ansari Road, Daryaganj
New Delhi 110 002, India
Phone: +91-11-43574357
Fax: +91-11-43574314
e-mail: jaypee@jaypeebrothers.com

Overseas Office
JP Medical Ltd.
83, Victoria Street, London
SW1H 0HW (UK)
Phone: +44-20 3170 8910
e-mail: info@jpmedpub.com

EU GPSR Authorised Representative
Logos Europe, 9 rue Nicolas Poussin
17000, La Rochelle, France
Phone: +33 (0) 6 67 93 73 78
e-mail: contact@logoseurope.eu

Website: www.jaypeebrothers.com
Website: www.jaypeedigital.com

Inquiries for bulk sales may be solicited at: jaypee@jaypeebrothers.com

Snapshots in Dermatology* / *S Sacchidanand, Savitha AS, Shilpa K

First Edition: 2013

Second Edition: **2026**

ISBN: 978-93-5696-171-5

Printed at: Samrat Offset Pvt. Ltd.

Preface to the Second Edition

Dermatology is a uniquely visual specialty. Dermatological diseases present with a wide spectrum of cutaneous manifestations. Interestingly, the same disease may appear in varied forms across different individuals, and conversely, multiple diseases can present with similar clinical patterns. The skin also frequently reflects internal systemic disorders, further adding to the complexity. Given that the number of clinical patterns is finite, significant overlap is inevitable, often making diagnosis a challenging task, particularly for undergraduates, postgraduates, and dermatology residents who are at the early stages of clinical training.

"Snapshots in Dermatology" was conceived as a quick, accessible visual guide to help beginners recognize and familiarize themselves with common skin conditions. The overwhelmingly positive response to the first edition encouraged us to expand and enrich the content in this second edition.

This updated edition includes several new clinical entities and a more extensive array of high-quality clinical photographs. A significant addition is the incorporation of dermoscopic images for many conditions, aiding in the correlation between clinical and dermoscopic features—an essential skill in modern dermatologic practice. We have also included brief insights into newer topics and updated treatment approaches in relevant sections to enhance the practical value of the book.

The layout remains compact and user-friendly, making it a convenient companion during ward rounds and outpatient clinics. While primarily designed for students and trainees, practicing dermatologists may also find it a useful refresher or a quick reference guide.

We hope this revised edition continues to serve as a helpful tool in learning, diagnosing, and appreciating the fascinating visual language of dermatology.

S Sacchidanand
Savitha AS
Shilpa K
Chaithra S

Preface to the First Edition

Dermatology is a visual field. Dermatological diseases express themselves on the skin with varied manifestations. It is likely that a single disease can present with different manifestations. It is also likely that different dermatological diseases can manifest with similar clinical presentations. Many systemic diseases also have cutaneous manifestations. Since all dermatological diseases and dermatological manifestations of systemic disease have a limited pattern of expression, overlapping features are inevitable. Hence, in a given situation on first instance, it may become difficult for undergraduates, postgraduates and residents to identify a clinical condition.

"Snapshots in Dermatology" is an attempt to orient beginners to readily acquaint with common skin conditions. This book serves the purpose as a ready reckoner during ward rounds and out-patient clinics. Practicing dermatologists may also find it useful.

S Sacchidanand
Savitha AS
Shilpa K

Acknowledgments

The completion of this book has been made possible through the dedication, ideas, time, and sincere efforts of numerous faculty members and residents, including Dr Chaithra S, Dr Shashikumar BM, Dr Hemalatha Naidu M, Dr Nagesh TS, Dr Lakshmi DV, Dr Padma Priya, Dr Roshni Goyal, Dr Soundarya Jagadeesh, Dr Mahalaxmi Khatagave, Dr Ramyasourabha CD, Dr Deepthi Upadhya, Dr Sudheer Kumar, Dr Chandan Srinivasa K, Dr Monika V, and Dr Fathima Beevi. Their invaluable contributions are deeply acknowledged and appreciated.

I remain deeply indebted to my seniors, colleagues, and residents for their unwavering support and collaboration throughout this journey. My sincere appreciation goes to the team of Jaypee Brothers Medical Publishers (P) Ltd—Ankit Vij (Managing Director), Sabyasachi Hazra (Director—Publishing), and Akhilesh Saxena (Development Editor)—for their exceptional effort in publishing this work.

Contents

1 Acquired Bilateral Nevus of Ota-like Macules

➲ SYNONYMS

Hori's nevus, nevus fusco-caeruleus zygomaticus, acquired circumscribed dermal facial melanocytosis.

➲ HISTORY

Acquired bilateral nevus of Ota-like macules (ABNOM) was first described by Hori et al. in 1984.

➲ ETIOLOGY AND PATHOGENESIS

Possible theories for the pathogenesis include the dropping off of epidermal melanocytes, migration of hair bulb melanocytes, and reactivation of preexisting latent or immature dermal melanocytes, which is triggered by dermal inflammation, ultraviolet (UV) radiation, or hormonal changes.

➲ EPIDEMIOLOGY

It is common in Asian females, particularly the Chinese and Japanese, and appears in the third to fifth decades of life.

➲ CLINICAL FEATURES

It presents clinically as asymptomatic, multiple, speckled blue-brown to slate-gray macules occurring bilaterally on malar regions or less commonly on the forehead, upper eyelids, cheeks, and nose, without ocular or mucosal involvement.

➲ HISTOPATHOLOGY

Irregularly shaped bipolar melanocytes scattered in the upper and middle dermis without disturbance of normal skin architecture.

On electron microscopy, melanocytes contain many singly dispersed melanosomes in stages II, III, and IV of melanization.

➲ DERMOSCOPY

On dermoscopy, blue-brown or gray pigmentation and a speckled homogenous pattern are seen.

➲ DIFFERENTIAL DIAGNOSIS

- Bilateral nevus of Ota—onset during infancy or adolescence, presence of ocular/mucosal involvement, and histologic studies show bipolar to stellate melanocytes widely scattered throughout the papillary and reticular dermis.

- Melasma—variable distribution; dermoscopy shows a well-defined/pseudoreticular network and brown/gray dots with perifollicular sparing.
- Riehl's melanosis—variable distribution; depending on the site of application of contactants, dermoscopy shows pseudonetwork, gray dots or granules, and telangiectatic vessels, and histology shows features of interface dermatitis.

➲ TREATMENT

Q-switched Nd: Yag laser (1,064 nm), Q-switched alexandrite laser (755 nm), and Q-switched ruby laser (694 nm) have been used in isolation or combination; complete clearance of lesion is not always possible and multiple sessions are required. Dermabrasion has been used as a cost-effective therapeutic modality.

➲ PROGNOSIS

Acquired bilateral nevus of Ota-like macules is usually gradually progressive.

➲ SUGGESTED READING

1. Rattananukrom T, Suchonwanit P, Thadanipon K, Vachiramon V. A Comparative Study of Dermatoscopic Features of Melasma and Hori's Nevus in Asian Patients. J Clin Aesthet Dermatol. 2022;15(3):16-20.

2 Acanthosis Nigricans

➲ ETIOLOGY

Acanthosis nigricans (AN) results from stimulation of tyrosine kinase growth factor receptor signaling pathways in the epidermis. Insulin resistance syndromes, insulin growth factor 1 receptor, fibroblast growth factor receptor, and tyrosine kinase receptor mutations are also associated with acanthosis nigricans.

➲ EPIDEMIOLOGY

Adults in 2nd and 3rd decades are commonly affected.

➲ CLINICAL FEATURES

Acanthosis nigricans is characterized by hyperpigmentation and thickening of the skin with papillomatous elevations. Acanthosis nigricans develops symmetrically on the neck, axillae, groins, antecubital and popliteal fossae, and umbilicus and perianal area. Involvement of hands and fingers (tripe palms) occurs in advanced cases. Acrochordons can be present along with acanthosis nigricans in many cases.

Schwartz classified AN as hereditary (autosomal dominant), benign, pseudoacanthosis nigricans (obesity), drug-induced (nicotinic acid, oral contraceptives, insulin, and steroids), malignant (gastrointestinal malignancy in 90%), acral, unilateral, and mixed. Mucosal (oral, laryngeal, vulval, nasal, and esophagus) AN can be present **(Figs. 1A and B)**.

➲ SYNDROMES ASSOCIATED

- Beare–Stevenson syndrome (FGFR2)
- Crouzon's syndrome (FGFR3)
- Cushing's syndrome
- Polycystic ovarian syndrome/Stein–Leventhal syndrome
- Rud syndrome
- Seip–Lawrence syndrome
- Hyperandrogenism and insulin resistance–acanthosis nigricans (HAIR–AN)
- Mental retardation, overgrowth, remarkable facies, and acanthosis nigricans (MORFAN)
- Severe achondroplasia, developmental delay, and acanthosis nigricans (SADDAN)

➲ DERMOSCOPY

- Linear crista cutis (elevated ridges), sulcus cutis (furrows or valleys), scattered black or brown dots and globules, and crypts

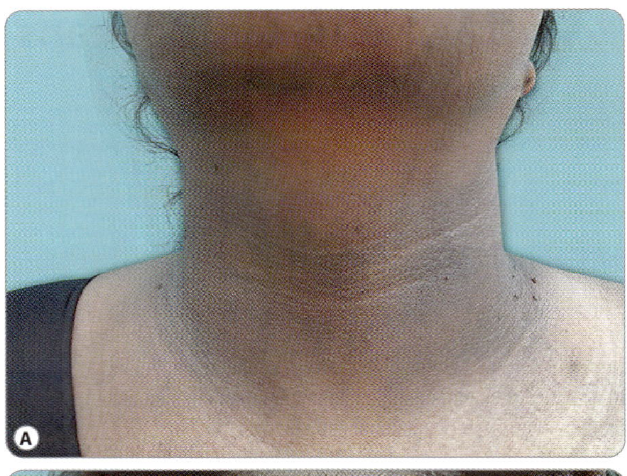

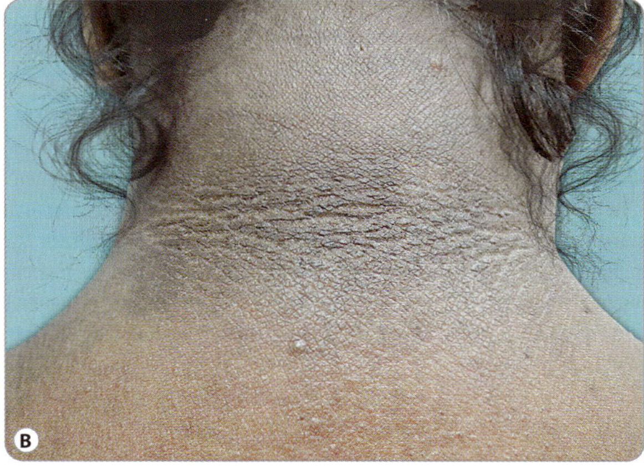

Figs. 1A and B: (A) Acanthosis nigricans with skin tags over the neck; and (B) Hyperpigmentation and thickening over the nape of the neck.

(keratin-filled invaginations that are larger than comedo-like openings)
- Barren land appearance; papillary projections in chronic cases

HISTOPATHOLOGY

Hyperkeratosis, irregular spiky papillomatosis, and minimal acanthosis.

DIFFERENTIAL DIAGNOSIS

- Intertriginous granular parakeratosis
- *Confluent and reticulate papillomatosis*: Scaly hyperpigmented patches in reticulate fashion seen over the chest and back
- *Dowling–Degos disease*: Presence of comedones over the trunk, pitting over face
- *Becker's nevus*: Hyperpigmented patch with increased hairs over it, mostly seen in adolescence
- *Pemphigus vegetans*: Macerated plaques in body folds, intra-epidermal blister with villi onhistopathology

- *Seborrheic keratosis*: Discrete hyperpigmented papules/plaques with stuck-on appearance

TREATMENT

Treatment of underlying conditions such as hyperinsulinemia, malignancy, weight loss, and discontinuation of precipitating drugs may resolve AN.

Topical agents: Keratolytics such as salicylic acid 3% ointment, tretinoin 0.025–0.05% cream, ammonium lactate 12% cream, urea, calcipotriol, podophyllin, triple combination depigmenting creams, glycolic acid, and trichloroacetic acid 15% peels.

Oral agents: Isotretinoin, etretinate, acitretin, metformin, rosigliatazone, alpha lipoic acid, and cyproheptadine in malignant AN.

Surgical: Dermabrasion, long-pulsed alexandrite laser therapy, and CO_2 laser.

SUGGESTED READING

1. Phiske MM. An approach to acanthosis nigricans. Indian Dermatol Online J. 2014;5(3):239-49.

3 Acne Keloidalis Nuchae

➲ SYNONYMS

Keloidal folliculitis, nuchal keloidal acne, folliculitis keloidalis nuchae.

➲ HISTORY

The condition was first described by Hebra in 1860, and the term was given by Bazin in 1872.

➲ ETIOLOGY

The exact etiology is unknown. It is considered to be a variant of primary cicatricial alopecia and not associated with acne vulgaris. Friction by the collar results in curling of hair and distortion or occlusion of the follicular lumen. This results in retention of the hair shaft, thereby perpetuating granulomatous inflammation and scarring.

➲ EPIDEMIOLOGY

Black, Hispanic, or Asian young men are commonly affected. The male-to-female ratio is approximately 20:1.

➲ CLINICAL FEATURES

The lesions are characterized by mildly pruritic persistent folliculitis and perifolliculitis on the occipital area and back of the neck. Initially, inflammatory papules and pustules appear on the back of the neck, followed by fibrosis at a later stage which results in papules and keloidal plaques. Broken hair and ingrown hair may be seen within the plaque **(Fig. 1)**.

➲ DERMOSCOPY

- *Early stages*: Perifollicular pustules, white halo surrounding the hair follicles corresponding to perifollicular fibrosis
- *Advanced stages*: Tufted hairs

➲ HISTOPATHOLOGY

Early lesions show perifollicular lymphocytic and plasma cell infiltrate, with lamellar fibroplasias at the level of isthmus. Later on, fibrosis and sclerotic collagen forms occur.

➲ DIFFERENTIAL DIAGNOSIS

- Dissecting cellulitis of the scalp
- Acne vulgaris

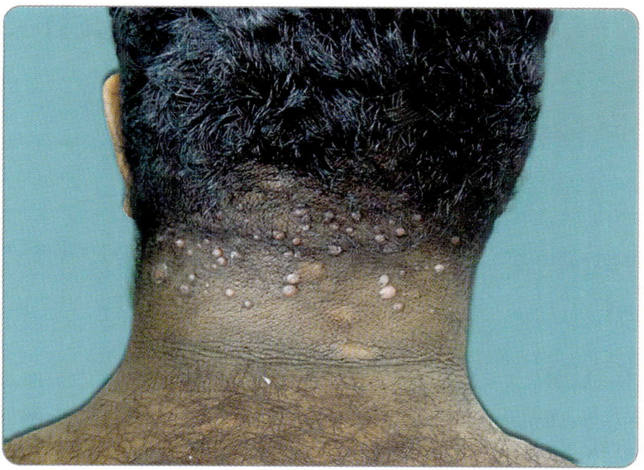

Fig. 1: Multiple papules on the nape of the neck.

- *Acne conglobata*: Multiple connecting sinuses present usually on the face.
- *Hidradenitis suppurativa*: Neck is a rare site, usually involves flexures.
- Folliculitis decalvans
- *Nevus sebaceous*: Coalescent skin colored soft papules to form plaque
- *Pseudofolliculitis*: Presence of curved ingrown hair which can be extracted

COMPLICATIONS

Abscesses and sinus tracts may develop within the lesions over time, cicatricial alopecia, and psychological morbidity due to its chronicity.

TREATMENT

Topical therapy with potent steroid ointments, tretinoin gel 0.025%, oral antibiotics of tetracycline group, isotretinoin, intralesional triamcinolone acetonide injections 10 mg/mL, primary excision and closure, CO_2 laser ablation, and cryotherapy are available options.

Close shaving of hair and tight collars should be avoided.

PROGNOSIS

Recurrences are common.

SUGGESTED READING

1. Ogunbiyi A. Acne keloidalis nuchae: prevalence, impact, and management challenges. Clin Cosmet Investig Dermatol. 2016;9: 483-9.

4 Acne Vulgaris

➲ SYNONYM

Pimples.

➲ HISTORY

Emperor Justinian's physician Aetius Amidenus used the term "acne" for the first time during the 6th century AD. It is derived from the Greek word "acme" meaning "peak".

➲ ETIOLOGY

The pathogenesis of acne is multifactorial, but four basic steps have been identified:

1. Follicular epidermal hyperproliferation
2. Excess sebum production
3. Inflammation
4. The presence and activity of *Propionibacterium acnes*

➲ EPIDEMIOLOGY

Most commonly seen in 12–25-year age group (puberty). Both sexes are equally affected.

➲ CLINICAL FEATURES

Lesions of acne vulgaris are seen on the sebaceous gland-rich body regions, mainly the face, mid-chest, back, shoulders, and upper arms. Comedones are characteristic early lesions of acne. A comedone is a plug of sebaceous and keratinous material lodged in the opening of a hair follicle. The inflammatory lesions of acne originate with comedo formation but then expand to form papules, pustules, nodules, and cysts of varying severity. Erythematous papules range from 1 to 5 mm in diameter **(Figs. 1 to 3)**.

- *Grade I (mild)*: Comedones, occasional papules
- *Grade II (moderate)*: Comedones, many papules, few pustules
- *Grade III (severe)*: Predominantly pustules, nodules and abscesses
- *Grade IV (cystic)*: Mainly cysts or abscesses, widespread scarring

Variants of acne are neonatal, infantile, juvenile acne, acne excoriee, senile acne, drug-induced, chloracne, mechanical acne, Mallorca acne, tropical acne, acne tarda, pomade acne, hippie's acne, etc. Acne conglobata, acne fulminans, pyoderma faciale, and gram-negative folliculitis are severe forms of acne.

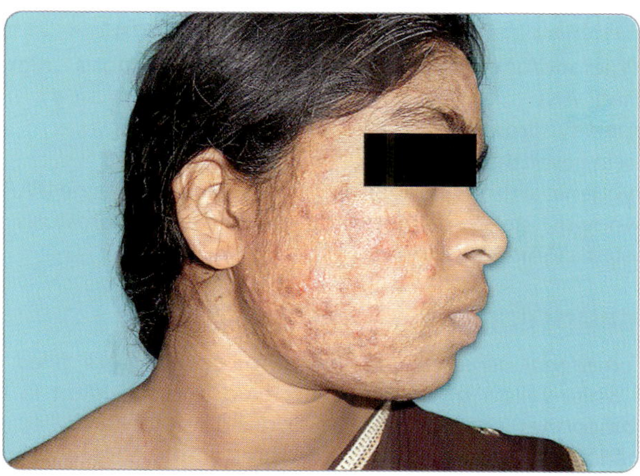

Fig. 1: Inflammatory papules and nodules over the cheek.

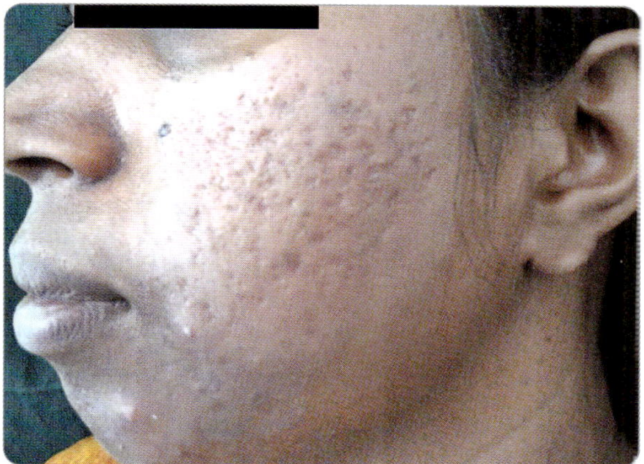

Fig. 2: Ice pick, box scars, and rolling type of acne scars.

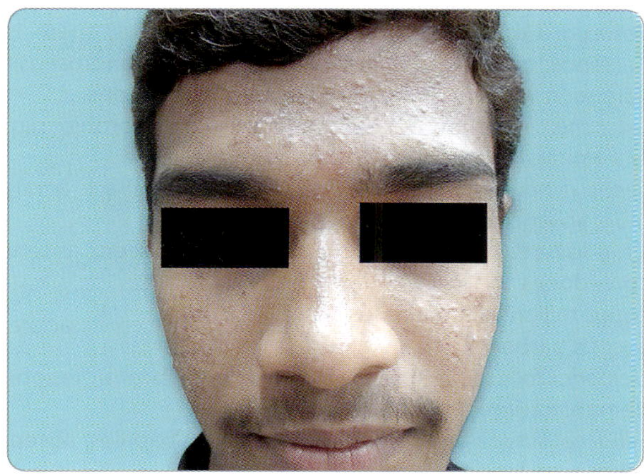

Fig. 3: Grade II acne vulgaris with multiple papules and few comedones.

SYNDROMES ASSOCIATED

- Hyperandrogenism, insulin resistance-acanthosis nigricans (HAIR-AN)
- Apert syndrome
- Stein Leventhal syndrome
- Pyogenic arthritis, pyoderma gangrenosum, and acne (PAPA)
- Synovitis, acne, palmoplantar pustulosis, hyperostosis, and osteitis (SAPHO) syndrome

DERMOSCOPY

- *Comedonal acne*: Dilated, roundish, central pore filled with a white-yellow or brown-yellow plug (more evident in open comedones) corresponding to oxidized keratin
- *Inflammatory acne*: Round structures with well-defined white center and thin brown borders and erythematous periphery
- *Pustular acne*: Well to ill-defined white-yellowish structure (corresponding to purulent material) with erythematous periphery

HISTOPATHOLOGY

In early lesions, microcomedones show a mildly distended follicle with a narrowed follicular opening impacted by shed keratinocytes. In closed comedones, the degree of follicular distension is increased, and a compact cystic structure forms. Open comedones have broad, expanded follicular ostia and greater follicular distension. The sebaceous glands are typically atrophic or absent. A mild perivascular mononuclear cell infiltrate circles the expanding follicle. As the follicular epithelium distends, the cyst (keratin, hair, and bacteria) ruptures and releases its contents into the dermis inducing a marked and brisk inflammatory response. Plenty of neutrophils appear in the pustular stage. As the lesion matures, foreign body granulomatous inflammation engulfs the follicle, and end-stage scarring results.

DIFFERENTIAL DIAGNOSIS

- *Rosacea*: Conspicuous absence of comedones, there is the presence of erythema and telangiectasias; photosensitivity, flare seen with spicy food, hot beverages, emotions
- *Oil acne*: More of hyperpigmented monomorphic papules, extremities, and trunk more commonly involved
- *Senile acne*: Large porous comedones with black keratinous plug, absence of inflammatory lesions
- *Drug-induced acne*: Monomorphic papules seen, absence of comedones
- Lupus miliaris disseminatus faciei
- Sycosis barbae
- *Demodex folliculitis*: Absence of comedones, pruritic lesions, and demonstration of mite
- *Sebaceous hyperplasia*: Yellowish to white papules, absence of other acne lesions

- *Angiofibroma*: Skin-colored papules concentrated in nasolabial folds
- *Warts*: Flat skin colored to hyperpigmented flat papules, Koebner's phenomenon seen

COMPLICATIONS

Scarring, hyperpigmentation, depression and suicidal ideation, anxiety, psychosomatic symptoms (pain and discomfort), embarrassment, body dysmorphic disorder, and social inhibition.

TREATMENT

- Comedones are treated with topical retinoids viz adapalene 0.1% gel, tazarotene 0.1% cream, tretinoin 0.1 and 0.025% at night, salicylic acid 2% wash, and benzoyl peroxide gel 2.5–5%.
- For papules and pustules, topical agents used are azelaic acid 10 and 20%, antibiotics clindamycin 1%, erythromycin 1.5, 2, and 3%, and nadifloxacin 1%.
- *Other topical agents*: Dapsone 5%, sodium sulfacetamide 10%, and sulfur 1–10%.

Systemic drugs for acne include:

- Tetracyclines—250 mg QID, erythromycin 1 g/day, minocycline 50–100 mg bd, doxycycline 100 mg, clindamycin 300–450 mg/day, lymecycline 150–300 mg/day, sulfamethoxazole + trimethoprim 800/160 mg bd (resistant acne).
- Isotretinoin 0.5 mg–1 mg/kg/day is a drug of choice for grade 4 acne.

Hormonal therapy: Hormonal agents provide effective second-line treatment in women with acne regardless of underlying hormonal abnormalities. Spironolactone 100–200 mg/day, flutamide 250 mg bd, and oral contraceptive drugs are used.

Physical modalities: Comedone extraction, chemical peeling (glycolic acid, salicylic acid, and Jessner's solution), intralesional corticosteroids (0.05–0.25 mL of triamcinolone acetonide) in nodulocystic acne, cryotherapy, lasers, and light sources.

PROGNOSIS

The disease usually runs a self-limiting course, remitting in the late twenties or early thirties. During the period of activity too, the course is variable with spontaneous flare-ups and remissions.

SUGGESTED READINGS

1. Bhat YJ, Latief I, Hassan I. Update on etiopathogenesis and treatment of Acne. Indian J Dermatol Venereol Leprol. 2017;83:298-306.
2. Arshdeep, De D. What's new in the management of acne? Indian J Dermatol Venereol Leprol. 2013;79:279-87.

5 Acrochordon

➲ SYNONYMS

Skin tags, cutaneous tags, papilloma colli, fibroma molluscum, fibroepithelial polyp, soft wart.

➲ ETIOLOGY

The exact etiology is unknown. As the number of lesions increases with weight gain and insulin resistance, acrochordons may be related to the growth hormone-like activity of insulin.

➲ EPIDEMIOLOGY

Both sexes are equally affected. It presents during the third to fourth decades and increases during pregnancy and weight gain.

➲ CLINICAL FEATURES

Small flesh-colored to dark brown, pin head-sized to larger, sessile, and pedunculated papillomas are seen commonly over the neck, axillae, and eyelids, less often on trunk and groins (pedunculated giant forms) **(Fig. 1)**. Perianal skin tags (infantile perianal pyramidal protrusion) may be congenital or acquired. It is commonly seen in girls, in the midline, anterior to the anus.

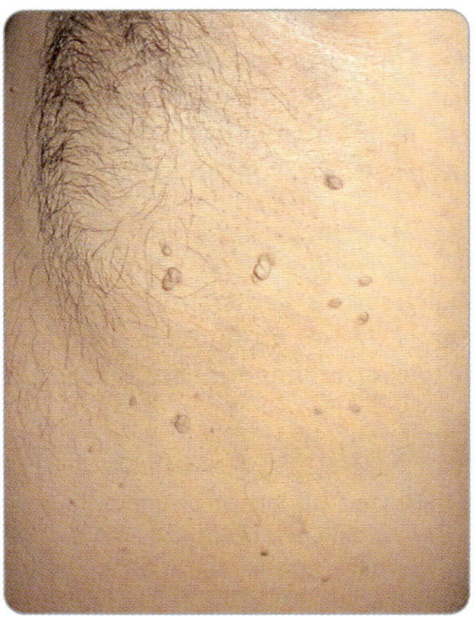

Fig. 1: Multiple sessile acrochordons over axilla.

ASSOCIATED CONDITIONS

- Birt–Hogg–Dubé syndrome
- Cowden disease
- Type 2 diabetes mellitus

HISTOPATHOLOGY

A dermal fibrovascular stalk is enclosed by the epidermis which is acanthotic and flattened.

DIFFERENTIAL DIAGNOSIS

- *Seborrhoeic keratoses*: Usually stuck on appearance, horn cysts on histopathology
- *Intradermal melanocytic nevi*: Nevoid cells in nests/sheets at various levels of the dermis
- Pedunculated neurofibroma
- *Verruca vulgaris*: Koebnerization seen, koilocytes in histopathology

COMPLICATIONS

Pedunculated tags may become inflamed, tender, and gangrenous due to twisting of the stalk.

TREATMENT

Simple scissor excision, cautery, and cryotherapy with liquid nitrogen are effective.

PROGNOSIS

Skin tags may serve as a marker of increased risk for insulin resistance, atherosclerosis, and cardiovascular disease.

SUGGESTED READING

1. Shah R, Jindal A, Patel N. Acrochordons as a cutaneous sign of metabolic syndrome: a case-control study. Ann Med Health Sci Res. 2014;4(2): 202-5.

6 Acrodermatitis Enteropathica

➲ HISTORY

Acrodermatitis enteropathica was first recognized in 1936 by the Swedish dermatologist Thore Brandt.

➲ ETIOLOGY

Acrodermatitis enteropathica is an autosomal recessive disorder due to mutations in the *SLC39A4* gene located on chromosome 8q24.3. This gene encodes a transmembrane protein that is part of the zinc/iron-regulated transporter-like protein family required for zinc uptake. This protein is highly expressed in the enterocytes of the duodenum and jejunum; therefore, affected individuals have a decreased ability to absorb zinc from dietary sources.

➲ EPIDEMIOLOGY

Acrodermatitis enteropathica typically appears in the first few weeks after birth if the child is fed bovine milk or shortly after cessation of breastfeeding.

➲ CLINICAL FEATURES

Patients have a history of refractory diarrhea, failure to thrive, irritability, dermatitis, and alopecia that gradually appeared shortly after weaning from breast milk. Occasionally, there may be a family history of similar complaints. Erythematous, dry, and scaly patches and plaques may evolve into crusted, vesiculobullous, erosive, psoriasiform, and pustular lesions predominantly distributed in a periorificial and acral pattern. Secondary infection with *Staphylococcus aureus* or *Candida albicans* occurs commonly **(Figs. 1A and B)**.

Angular cheilitis, glossitis, conjunctivitis, blepharitis, punctate keratopathy, photophobia, paronychia, nail dystrophy, loss of scalp hair, eyebrows, and eyelashes are other associated findings.

A level of plasma zinc <70 µg/L in fasting or <65 µg/dL in nonfasting individuals is considered diagnostic. Serum levels of alkaline phosphatase (a zinc-dependent enzyme) are reduced in advance disease.

➲ DIFFERENTIAL DIAGNOSIS

- Atopic dermatitis
- Epidermolysis bullosa
- Seborrheic dermatitis
- Acquired zinc deficiency
- Candidiasis

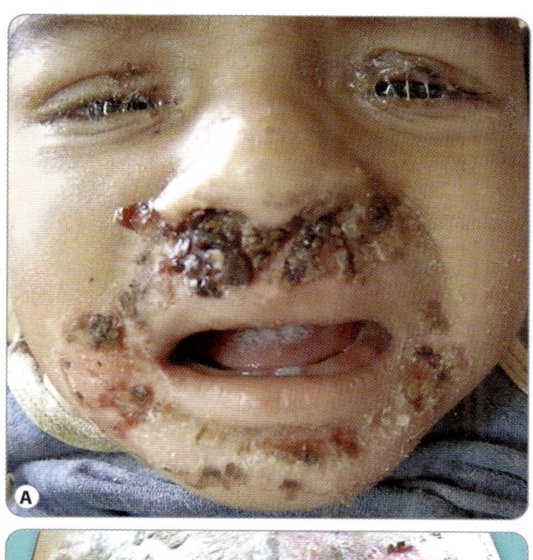

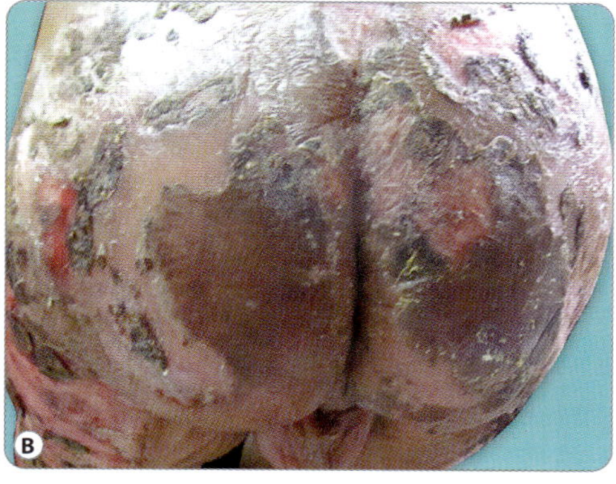

Figs. 1A and B: (A) Crusted lesions seen in the periorificial and orbital areas; and (B) Extensive crusting and erosions over the perianal and gluteal areas extending to thighs.

- Multiple carboxylase deficiency
- Necrolytic migratory erythema

COMPLICATIONS

Without appropriate zinc supplementation, acrodermatitis enteropathica usually is lethal within the first few years of life.

TREATMENT

Acrodermatitis enteropathica requires lifelong zinc supplementation. 1–3 mg/kg of zinc gluconate or sulfate is administered orally each day. Monitor serum zinc levels and alkaline phosphatase values every 3–6 months.

Warm compresses to remove the scale crust, followed by the application of white petrolatum to eroded skin lesions, may enhance re-epithelialization. Halogenated 8-hydroxyquinolines (e.g., diodoquin) have been tried to increase the absorption of zinc.

➲ PROGNOSIS

Untreated infants exhibit severe growth retardation, dermatitis, alopecia, secondary bacterial and fungal infections, and neurologic and behavioral changes; however, all symptoms are reversible with therapy.

➲ SUGGESTED READING

1. Ciampo IRLD, Sawamura R, Ciampo LAD, Fernandes MIM. Acrodermatitis Enteropathica: Clinical Manifestations and Pediatric Diagnosis. Rev Paul Pediatr. 2018;36(2):238-41.

7 Actinic Cheilitis

➲ SYNONYMS

Actinic cheilosis, solar cheilosis, sailor's lip.

➲ ETIOLOGY

Prolonged and excessive exposure to sunlight induces a chronic inflammatory reaction that is limited to the lower lip. Additional factors such as tobacco use, poor oral hygiene, and ill-fitting dentures may also play a role. Outdoor workers, sailors, and those exposed continuously to sunlight are more susceptible.

➲ EPIDEMIOLOGY

Actinic cheilitis is seen in adult elderly males with a history of chronic sun exposure.

➲ CLINICAL FEATURES

Actinic cheilitis typically affects the lower lip **(Fig. 1)**; in early stages, there may be redness or edema, later resulting in an ill-defined, atrophic, white, scaly plaque that may obliterate the vermilion border. Ulceration, induration or persistent flaking or crusting may be due to malignant transformation.

➲ DERMOSCOPY

White structureless areas, island-like areas, irregular margins with whitish projections, and tortuous and telangiectatic vessels disposed radially around ulceration are seen.

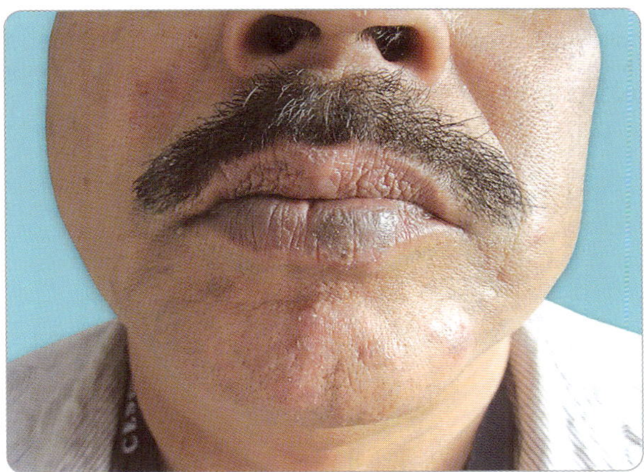

Fig. 1: Fissuring and erythema of lower lip in actinic cheilitis.

➲ HISTOPATHOLOGY

Hyperkeratosis with atypical basal keratinocytes is seen. There is irregular thickening of the spinous layer resulting in elongation of the rete ridges which have a bulbous architecture in some areas. Dysplastic changes may be seen in a few areas.

➲ DIFFERENTIAL DIAGNOSIS

- *Squamous cell carcinoma*: Ulcer is seen with indurated base, cervical lymphadenopathy
- Allergic contact dermatitis
- *Pemphigus vulgaris*: Large superficial erosions seen, acantholytic cells on Tzanck, typical HPE findings

➲ COMPLICATIONS

Malignant transformation.

➲ TREATMENT

The goal of therapy is to reduce the risk of malignant transformation while maintaining functionality and cosmesis of the lips.

- *Topical agents*: 5% fluorouracil thrice daily, imiquimod 5%, cream, ingenol mebutate, trichloroacetic acid, and diclofenac gel
- *Surgical/destructive options*: Excisional vermilionectomy which removes only the vermilion ridge of the lower lip leaving the underlying muscle intact, cryotherapy, electrocautery, and CO_2 laser ablation
- *Others*: Phototherapy, photodynamic therapy, and photo-protection

➲ PROGNOSIS

The risk of malignant transformation to squamous cell carcinoma is about 10%. Therefore, it is prudent to treat all cases of actinic cheilitis.

➲ SUGGESTED READING

1. Vasilovici A, Ungureanu L, Grigore L, Cojocaru E, Şenilă S. Actinic Cheilitis—From Risk Factors to Therapy. Front Med (Lausanne). 2022;9:805425.

8 Actinic Keratosis

➲ SYNONYMS

Solar keratosis, senile keratosis.

➲ ETIOLOGY

Actinic keratoses (AKs) occur on sun-exposed sites in fair-skinned people who have had excessive exposure to solar ultraviolet radiation (UVR). These lesions may be induced by ionizing radiation or radiant heat and in workers exposed to pitch and other products of coal distillation.

➲ EPIDEMIOLOGY

Actinic keratosis occurs usually in middle-aged or elderly subjects. The incidence is higher in men. The sides of the neck are involved in both sexes, but the ears are predominantly in men.

➲ CLINICAL FEATURES

The primary lesion is a rough erythematous papule with a white to yellow scale, varying from a few millimeters to large confluent patches of several centimeters in diameter. The diagnostic changes appear later as a dry, rough, adherent, and often yellow or brown-colored scale. The adherent scale can be picked off with difficulty, revealing a hyperemic base with punctate bleeding points. Older lesions are thicker and well defined with more visible hyperkeratosis and erythema.

Lesions typically are clustered in areas of highest sun exposure, such as the upper part of the ears, upper forehead, nasal bridge, malar eminences, dorsal hands, extensor forearms, and scalp in bald individuals. The flat, atrophic, or lichenoid variety is most commonly seen on the face.

➲ DERMOSCOPY

Nonpigmented Actinic Keratosis

- *Facial lesions*: "Strawberry pattern" composed of pink to red pseudonetwork created by erythema and wavy vessels surrounding the hair follicles, prominent white/yellowish spots (follicular openings), skin colored/white circles around a follicle opening (keratotic plug)—targetoid hair follicle and yellow-white scaling
- *Rosette sign*: A figure resembling a four-leaf clover, formed by four whitish points surrounding the follicular opening; seen only with polarized microscopy
- *Nonfacial lesions*: Erythema and superficial scales, sometimes accompanied by dotted vessels and rosette sign present

Pigmented Actinic Keratosis

Brown pseudonetwork, hyperpigmented follicular openings, annular-granular structures, brown/gray pigmentation as spots or globules, inner perifollicular gray halo, and gray rhomboidal structures.

- *Face lesions*: Pigmented pseudonetwork and granular–annular structures predominate, jelly sign—superficial pigmentation extending around follicular openings like a liquid
- *Nonfacial lesions*: Reticular pattern with a delicate pigmented network, homogeneous pigmentation, or multiple irregular dots and globules of brown to blue-gray color

HISTOPATHOLOGY

Actinic keratoses are keratinocytic dysplasias or squamous cell carcinomas in situ. Five histological types are seen: Hypertrophic, atrophic, bowenoid, acantholytic, and pigmented.

The epidermal cells have a paler cytoplasm. The epidermis shows alternating hyperkeratosis, parakeratosis, and minimal acanthosis. Some of the cells in the midportion of the epidermis show premature keratinization, resulting in dyskeratotic cells or apoptotic bodies characterized by homogeneous, eosinophilic cytoplasm with or without a nucleus. The upper dermis usually shows a fairly dense, chronic inflammatory infiltrate composed predominantly of lymphoid cells but often also containing plasma cells. The presence of an inflammatory response appears to be a warning sign of early malignant transformation.

DIFFERENTIAL DIAGNOSIS

- *Early squamous cell carcinoma*: The presence of dysplastic cells and horn pearls in histopathological examination (HPE)
- *Discoid lupus erythematosus*: Carpet-like scales seen, follicular plugging on HPE
- *Bowen's disease (Bowenoid type of AK)*: Full thickness epidermal dysplasia in HPE
- Seborrheic keratosis (pigmented type of AK)
- Lentigo maligna
- Basal cell carcinoma
- *Verruca vulgaris*: Lack of scaling, koilocytes seen in HPE
- Lichenoid keratosis
- *Porokeratosis*: Typical hyperkeratotic raised border seen, cornoid lamella seen in HPE

COMPLICATIONS

Irritation and discomfort of the skin growth, scarring from treatment, and squamous cell carcinoma.

TREATMENT

Regular use of sunscreen reduces the rate of development of new AK. The medical management includes topical 5-fluorouracil twice daily for 3–5 weeks, diclofenac in hyaluron gel, imiquimod, ingenol mebutate gel, and systemic retinoids for widespread disease.

Procedural: Cryotherapy, curettage, shave excision, electrosurgery, excision, dermabrasion, chemical destruction with trichloroacetic acid (TCA)/salicylic acid/phenol, photodynamic therapy, and ablative CO_2 laser.

➲ PROGNOSIS

An AK may regress, may persist unchanged, or it may progress to invasive squamous cell carcinoma (0.1–10%).

➲ SUGGESTED READING

1. Siegel JA, Korgavkar K, Weinstock MA. Current perspective on actinic keratosis: a review. Br J Dermatol. 2017;177(2):350-8.

9 Acute Generalized Exanthematous Pustulosis

➲ SYNONYMS

Toxic pustuloderma, exanthemic pustular psoriasis, pustular drug rash.

➲ HISTORY

Acute generalized exanthematous pustulosis (AGEP) was first recognized by Baker and Ryan in 1968.

➲ ETIOLOGY

The majority of the cases are due to an adverse drug reaction. Commonly implicated agents include antibiotics—pristinamycin, quinolones, aminopenicillins, and sulphonamides; hydroxychloroquine; antifungals—terbinafine and griseofulvin; calcium channel blockers—diltiazem. Less commonly associated drugs include corticosteroids, oxicam nonsteroidal anti-inflammatory drugs (NSAIDs), and antiepileptics.

Other triggers: Infections [*Mycoplasma pneumoniae*, coxsackie virus, parvovirus B19, and cytomegalovirus (CMV)], mercury exposure, spider bites, and contact allergens.

➲ EPIDEMIOLOGY

Rare, incidence ranging from 1 to 5 cases/million/year, adults commonly affected with female preponderance.

➲ GENETICS

IL-36 receptor antagonist *(IL36RN)* gene mutation may constitute a risk factor for the development of AGEP.

➲ CLINICAL FEATURES

The onset of lesions occurs 24–48 hours after initiation of the implicated drug. It is characterized by sheets of hundreds of small, monomorphous, nonfollicular sterile pustules on an erythematous base with minimal or no mucosal membrane involvement. Distribution favors trunk, flexures, and intertriginous regions. When mucosal involvement occurs, it is limited to a single site commonly, lips or buccal mucosa. There may be associated burning and/or pruritus. Less commonly atypical targets, purpura, vesicles, and bullae can occur.

Systemic features include fever, leukocytosis with neutrophilia or rarely; hepatic, renal, and pulmonary dysfunction can occur.

Lesions typically last from 1–2 weeks, followed by superficial desquamation.

Clinical variant: Acute localized exanthematous pustulosis is a localized form of AGEP, characterized by pustules confined to a single body area, most commonly the neck.

➲ DERMOSCOPY

Milky globules on a uniform red background, sparing the follicles.

➲ HISTOPATHOLOGY

Intracorneal, subcorneal, and/or intraepidermal pustules with papillary dermal edema and neutrophilic and eosinophilic perivascular infiltrate. Spongiform changes are seen, particularly in the intracorneal and subcorneal pustules. The epidermis may show spongiosis with exocytosis of neutrophils. Necrotic keratinocytes and leukocytoclastic vasculitis are unusual findings.

➲ DIFFERENTIAL DIAGNOSIS

- *Pustular psoriasis (von Zumbusch type)*: Personal/family history of psoriasis, slow onset, lesions overlay scaly plaques, histology shows acanthosis, pustules, papillomatosis Munro's microabscess, and tortuous, dilated dermal blood vessels
- *Subcorneal pustular dermatosis*: Less acute course, relapsing nature, and the presence of flaccid pustules which demonstrate a hypopyon sign
- *Drug reaction with eosinophilia and systemic symptoms (DRESS)*: Longer latent period, pustules less numerous, mucous membrane and internal organ involvement more common, hypereosinophilia
- *Stevens–Johnson syndrome (SJS)/toxic epidermal necrolysis (TEN)*: Epidermal sloughing, a positive Nikolsky sign, and mucous membrane involvement, histology shows full thickness keratinocyte necrosis
- *Bacterial folliculitis*: Follicular oriented lesions, gram stain, and culture positivity
- *Cutaneous candidiasis*: Potassium hydroxide (KOH) and fungal culture positivity

➲ TREATMENT

Treatment involves discontinuing the offending agent and providing supportive care such as topical ceramides, moist dressings, and antiseptic solutions to prevent secondary infection. Additional supportive treatments include topical corticosteroids, antipyretics, and antihistamines. In severe cases, systemic corticosteroids may be warranted. In cases of refractory AGEP, cyclosporine and infliximab have been tried.

PROGNOSIS

The prognosis in AGEP is excellent upon discontinuation of the offending drug, and full recovery is to be expected. The reported mortality is 5% and generally occurs as a result of multiple organ dysfunction and disseminated intravascular coagulation.

SUGGESTED READING

1. De A, Das S, Sarda A, Pal D, Biswas P. Acute generalised exanthematous pustulosis: an update. Indian J Dermatol. 2018;63(1):22-9.

10 Albinism

➲ SYNONYMS

Achromia, achromasia, achromatosis.

➲ ETIOLOGY

Oculocutaneous albinism is an autosomal recessive disease caused by the complete absence or decrease of melanin biosynthesis in melanocytes. Patients with albinism have a normal number of melanocytes in the epidermis and follicles, but the melanin pigment is totally or partially absent. The phenotypic variability of albinism is broad, ranging from the complete absence of pigmentation of the hair, skin, and eyes to mild depigmentation.

➲ EPIDEMIOLOGY

Globally, the prevalence of albinism is estimated to be 1 in 17,000 to 1 in 20,000 people.

➲ GENETICS

Seven types of nonsyndromic albinism (OCA1 to OCA7) have been described due to isolated genetic mutations.

Syndromic albinism: Hermansky–Pudlak syndrome (HPS), Chediak–Higashi syndrome (CHS), Angelman syndrome (AS), and Prader–Willi syndrome (PWS).

➲ CLINICAL FEATURES

Cutaneous findings vary widely. The most dramatic features occur in OCA1A due to a complete lack of melanin. The white hair, white eyelashes, white skin, and pink eyes are typical **(Fig. 1)**.

Ocular findings include photophobia, refractive errors, involuntary pulsatile horizontal nystagmus, strabismus, and reduced iris pigmentation.

➲ HISTOPATHOLOGY

Histopathological examination is unremarkable. Melanin staining and melanocyte-special stains (dopa oxidase or HMB45) will be slight to moderately positive since pheomelanin and melanocytes are still present in the skin.

➲ DIFFERENTIAL DIAGNOSIS

- Hermansky–Pudlak syndrome
- Chediak–Higashi syndrome
- Angelman syndrome and Prader–Willi syndrome

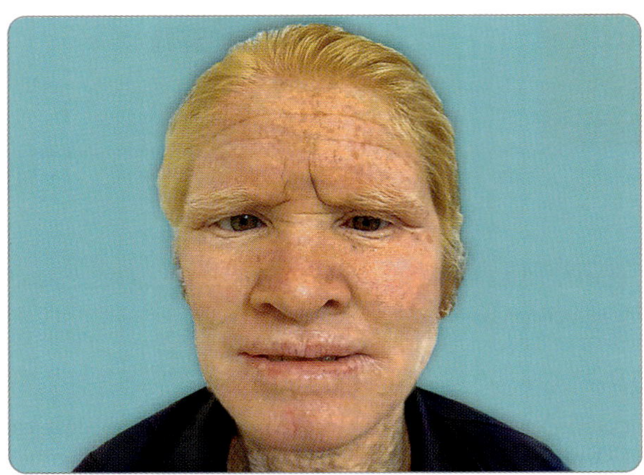

Fig. 1: Oculocutaneous albinism with fair skin, light hair, and light color iris.

- Vici syndrome
- *Waardenburg syndrome type II*: Autosomal dominant *MITF* gene mutation presenting with patchy skin hypopigmentation, white forelock or prematurely gray hair, iris heterochromia, and sensorineural hearing loss
- *Tietz albinism-deafness syndrome*: Autosomal dominant *MITF* gene mutation presenting with white eyebrows and eyelashes, iris hypopigmentation, normal visual acuity, and sensorineural hearing loss
- *Griscelli syndrome*: Present with hypopigmentation, melanin aggregation in silvery-gray hair, immunodeficiency, and decreased visual acuity with roving eye movements

TREATMENT

Treatment involves lifelong sun protection. Patients should be advised to avoid prolonged sun exposure and liberal and frequent use of sunscreens. Self-examination for melanomas and skin malignancy should be taught. Regular ophthalmologic examinations are a must.

PROGNOSIS

Life expectancy in nonsyndromic albinism is comparable to the general population. Mortality may be slightly increased due to skin malignancy.

SUGGESTED READING

1. Grønskov K, Ek J, Brondum-Nielsen K. Oculocutaneous albinism. Orphanet J Rare Dis. 2007;2:1-8.

11 Alopecia Areata

SYNONYMS

Pelade, alopecia celsi, alopecia circumscriptum, vitiligo capitis, tinea decalvans, Cazenave's vitiligo, porrigo decalvans, Jonston's alopecia.

HISTORY

It was first described about 2000 years ago by Celsus (AD 14–37).

ETIOLOGY

The etiology of alopecia areata is not known with certainty. Various proposed theories are heredity, infective, neurologic, endocrine, psychogenic, autoimmune, and atopy.

EPIDEMIOLOGY

It occurs in any age group from 5 to 35 years.

CLINICAL FEATURES

The classical lesion is an asymptomatic round or oval, smooth, well-defined patch of nonscarring alopecia. The bald patch may be slightly depressed below the surface, being deprived of the volume of hair bulbs. Short "exclamation mark" hairs (i.e., distal end broader than the proximal end and coudability hair) can often be seen, particularly at the margins of areas of alopecia. The coudability sign is the kinking of hair on compression. Paresthesia or mild erythema occasionally accompanies the onset. The scalp is the most common site affected, although any hairy area may be involved.

Other presentations include alopecia totalis (loss of all scalp hair), alopecia universalis (loss of all scalp and body hair), ophiasis pattern (band-like pattern of hair loss along the periphery of the temporal and occipital scalp), sisaipho pattern, and reticular and diffuse variant. Nonpigmented hairs may initially be spared, and, as a result, some patients with diffuse involvement note rapid or overnight graying of the hair.

Nail involvement is seen in about 10–20% of cases. Twenty-nail alopecia areata without hair changes is sine alopecia. Nail changes include superficial, uniform, minute pits arranged regularly along and across the nail giving a "scotch plaid" effect, red or mottled lunulae, nail thinning and ridging, discoloration, splitting, dystrophy, and onycholysis **(Figs. 1A to D)**.

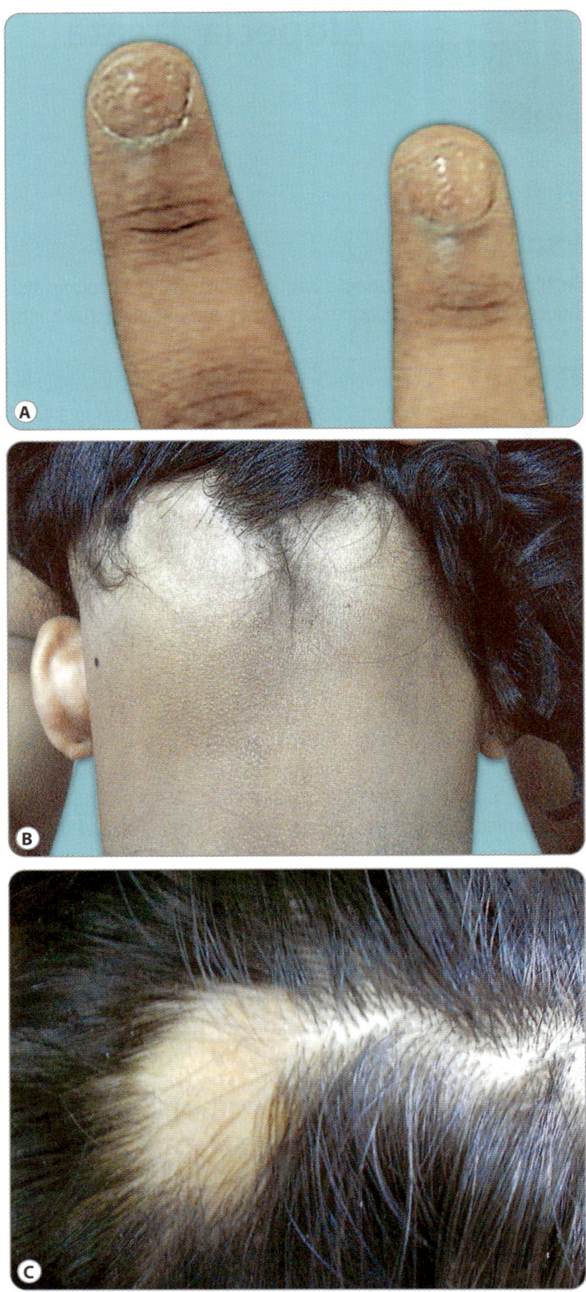

Figs. 1A to D: *Continued*

Continued

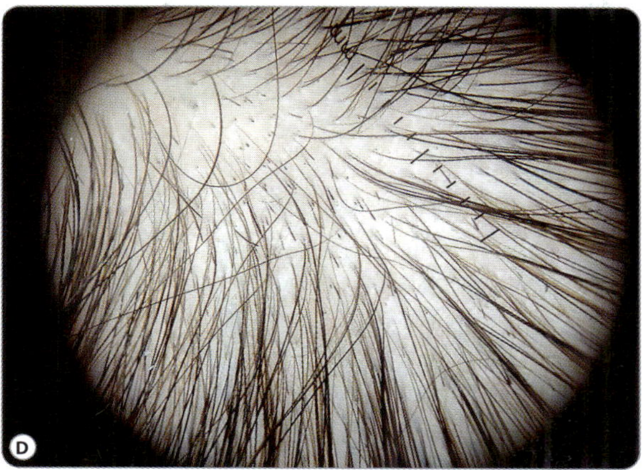

Figs. 1A to D: (A) Regular pitting of nails in a Scotch plaid pattern; (B) Loss of hair over the occipital area, i.e., ophiasis pattern; (C) Smooth patch of hair loss; and (D) Dermoscopy showing tapered hair, exclamation sign, and tulip hair.

Ikeda's classification of alopecia areata includes four types:

1. Common
2. Atopic
3. Hypertensive
4. Autoimmune

DERMOSCOPY

Dermatoscopic findings include black dots, "exclamation-mark" hairs, broken hairs, yellow dots, clustered short vellus hair, tapered hair, Pohl-Pinkus constrictions, coudability hair, pigtail hair, and tulip hair.

HISTOPATHOLOGY

A peribulbar lymphocytic infiltrate described as a "swarm of bees" appearance is the characteristic finding in the acute stage of the disease. In long-standing cases, fibrous tracts are seen in the peribulbar location.

DIFFERENTIAL DIAGNOSIS

- Traumatic alopecia
- Trichotillomania
- Tinea capitis
- Androgenetic alopecia
- Syphilis

- Neonatal alopecia
- Telogen effluvium
- Congenital triangular alopecia
- Anagen effluvium
- Folliculitis decalvans
- Alopecia mucinosa

➲ COMPLICATIONS

Alopecia areata can result in considerable psychological and social disability. Patients may not have regrowth of hair.

➲ TREATMENT

As the disease is self-limiting, treatment is not mandatory.

- *Local therapy*: Topical or intralesional corticosteroids, contact immunotherapy with squaric acid dibutyl ester or diphencyprone, topical irritants (short contact anthralin, tazarotene, and azelaic acid), topical minoxidil 5%, prostaglandin F2 alpha analogs latanoprost/bimatoprost, or phototherapy [turban psoralen plus ultraviolet A (PUVA)]
- *Systemic therapy*: Oral steroids, cyclosporine, azathioprine, methotrexate, sulfasalazine, janus kinase inhibitors—tofacitinib/ruxolitinib/baricitinib, and biologics—abatacept/dupilumumab
- *Others*: PUVA, 308 nm excimer laser, platelet-rich plasma therapy, and camouflage

➲ PROGNOSIS

Poor prognostic factors are early age of onset, nail pitting, onychodystrophy, onycholysis, anonychia, extensive scalp involvement, associated systemic disorders, atopy, hypertension, connective tissue disorders, loss of eyebrows and eyelashes, Down's syndrome, alopecia totalis, alopecia universalis, family history of alopecia areata, recurrent episodes, ophiasis, sisaipho, and reticular patterns.

➲ SUGGESTED READING

1. Zhou C, Li X, Wang C, Zhang J. Alopecia Areata: an Update on Etiopathogenesis, Diagnosis, and Management. Clin Rev Allergy Immunol. 2021;61(3):403-23.

12 Amyloidosis

ETIOLOGY

The exact etiology is unknown. There are two proposed theories for the origin of amyloid:

1. *Fibrillar body theory*: Colloid bodies are transformed by dermal macrophages into amyloid.
2. *Secretory theory*: Disrupted basal cells secrete amyloid.

Chronic scratching or rubbing of the skin, and use of nylon brushes during bathing (frictional amyloidosis) may result in the pathology.

EPIDEMIOLOGY

It is primarily a disease of adults with a more female preponderance.

CLINICAL FEATURES

Amyloid deposited in the skin and other organs are eosinophilic, homogenous, and hyaline in appearance. Amyloid deposits bind to antikeratin antibodies. The primary cutaneous amyloidosis is divided into macular, lichen, and nodular varieties.

Macular amyloidosis presents as moderately pruritic, brown, rippled macules characteristically located in the interscapular region of the back **(Fig. 1A)**. Pigmentation is not uniform, giving a salt and pepper or rippled appearance. Other sites include arms, thighs, shins, breasts, and buttocks. Lichen amyloidosis is characterized by paroxismally itchy, lichenoid papules typically appearing bilaterally on the shins. Papules group to form infiltrated large moniliform plaques. Combined macular and lichen amyloidosis is termed biphasic amyloidosis **(Fig. 1B)**.

ASSOCIATED CONDITIONS

Macular amyloidosis is associated with Sipple syndrome.

DERMOSCOPY

- *Macular amyloidosis*: Hub and spoke pattern—central hub (brown or white) surrounded by various configurations of pigmentation-like fine radiating streaks, leaf-like projections, or bulbous projections
- *Lichen amyloidosis*: Central hub is replaced by a central scar-like white area surrounded by brown/black dots, globules, or white collarette.

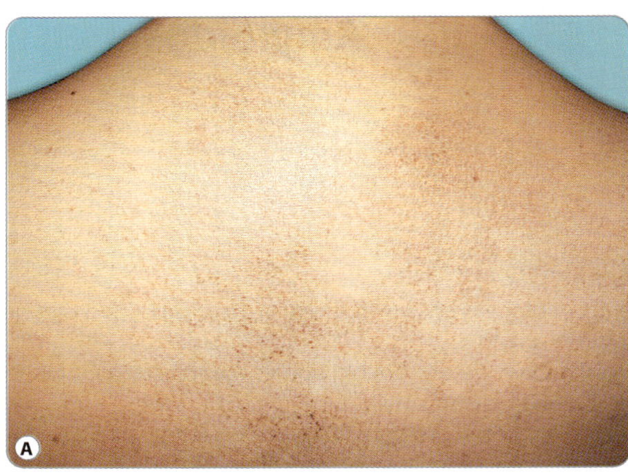

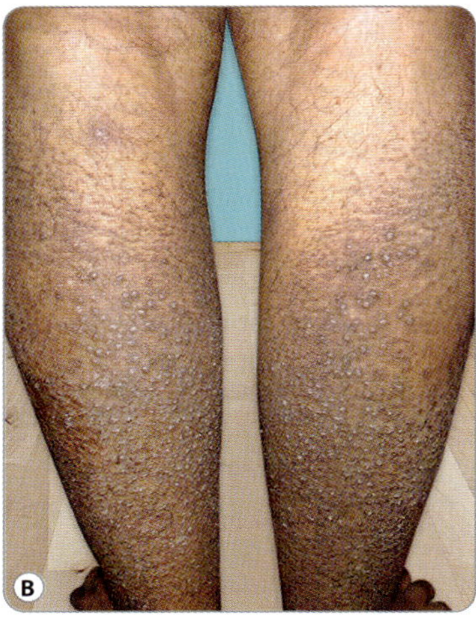

Figs. 1A and B: (A) Macular amyloidosis over the back with hyperpigmented macules giving a rippled appearance; and (B) Lichen amyloidosis, hyperkeratotic papules over both lower limbs.

HISTOPATHOLOGY

The epidermis is hyperkeratotic with focal basal keratinocyte necrosis. Dermal papillae are expanded by amorphous deposits of amyloid. Apple-green birefringence of Congo red–stained preparations is viewed under polarizing light. Pigment incontinence is seen in the dermis.

DIFFERENTIAL DIAGNOSIS

- *Lichen planus pigmentosus*: Diffuse slate grayish pigmentation, more common over the face
- *Prurigo nodularis*: Pruritic papules/nodules with hyperpigmented ring, vertically oriented collagen on HPE
- *Dermatomyositis*: Associated with other classical cutaneous features, antibody profile, and biochemistry findings

- *Postinflammatory hyperpigmentation*: Negative for birefringence on polarizing microscopy
- *Poikiloderma*: Salt and pepper pigmentation with atrophy and telangiectasia

TREATMENT

- *Localized disease*: Topical/intralesional steroid, surgery (dermabrasion, excision, and skin grafting), ablative CO_2 laser, cryotherapy, hydrocolloid dressings, and topical capsaicin
- *Widespread disease*: Phototherapy (narrowband UVB and PUVA), topical dimethyl sulfoxide (DMSO), systemic drug treatment (acitretin—0.5 mg/kg, etretinate, DMSO, cyclophosphamide, and cyclosporine)

SUGGESTED READINGS

1. Borowicz J, Gillespie M, Miller R. Cutaneous amyloidosis. Skinmed. 2011;9(2):96-100; quiz 101.
2. Aung T, Noakes R, Murrell DF, Daniel BS, Kelati A. Primary cutaneous amyloidosis: A review of the available studies and gaps in data. Australas J Dermatol. 2023;64(2):e121-4.

13 Anagen Effluvium

ETIOLOGY

Anagen hair shedding is due to the premature termination of anagen hair growth or anagen arrest, after an acute, severe metabolic insult. It is most often iatrogenic, caused by treatment with cytotoxic drugs or radiation. Antimitotic chemotherapeutic agents induce the arrest of the anagen phase and present a toxic insult to the rapidly dividing hair matrix. Other triggers of anagen hair loss include radiation, heavy-metal poisoning, and boric acid poisoning.

Alopecia areata is another case of anagen hair shedding.

CLINICAL FEATURES

Anagen hair loss presents as abrupt anagen hair shedding with severe diffuse scalp alopecia. A serious insult to the hair follicles can cause up to an 80% loss of scalp hair. The time course for anagen effluvium is usually rapid compared with telogen effluvium, occurring within days to weeks of the insult to the hair follicles. Hair loss usually begins 1–2 weeks after chemotherapy is started and is most noticeable by 1–2 months. The scalp hair is usually the most affected, but all body hair including eyelashes and eyebrows can be affected. The hair-pull test is positive for dystrophic anagen hairs with tapered ends.

DERMOSCOPY

Black dots, yellow dots, tapered hair, Pohl-Pinkus constrictions, circle hair, tulipoid hair, and peripilar sign.

DIFFERENTIAL DIAGNOSIS

- *Chronic telogen effluvium*: Hair pull test shows most hairs in the telogen phase.
- *Trichotillomania*: Patchy areas of alopecia with hairs of different lengths at accessible sites
- *Androgenetic alopecia*: Absence of triggering factors and presence of family history
- *Traction alopecia*: More loss over the anterior hairline

TREATMENT

No treatment is needed. In most cases, hair growth is reversible when chemotherapy is ceased. Some methods employed to prevent chemotherapy-induced anagen effluvium include scalp cooling using ice packs/custom-designed cooling caps or the usage of a scalp tourniquet during chemotherapy.

➲ PROGNOSIS

If the insult ceases, hair growth restarts again within weeks.

➲ SUGGESTED READINGS

1. Kanwar AJ, Narang T. Anagen effluvium. Indian J Dermatol Venereol Leprol. 2013;79(5):604-12.
2. Saleh D, Nassereddin A, Saleh HM, Cook C. Anagen Effluvium. In: StatPearls. Treasure Island (FL): StatPearls Publishing; 2024.

14 Androgenetic Alopecia

➲ SYNONYMS

Male pattern baldness, common baldness.

➲ ETIOLOGY

Two factors that lead to susceptibility to androgenetic alopecia (AGA) are androgens and genetic factors. Male balding is an androgen-dependent trait. Dihydrotestosterone, a 5-alpha-reduced metabolite of testosterone is considered to be the main culprit. Androgen is also implicated in women with patterned hair loss. AGA is inherited by a polygenic trait. No associations are found with 5α-reductase genes or insulin genes. In AGA, the duration of anagen decreases with each successive cycle, whereas the length of telogen remains constant or is prolonged. Prolongation of "the latent phase" also known as kenogen occurs that follows the release of the club hair (exogen). This leads to a reduction of the anagen:telogen ratio and corresponds to periods of excessive hair shedding, most noticeable while combing or washing.

➲ CLINICAL FEATURES

Among men, susceptibility to AGA is near universal, and variations in baldness are largely explained by age of onset and rate of progression. Patterned balding occurs in women, but the susceptibility, age of onset, rate of progression, and pattern are different from men. The most common pattern of hair loss seen in women is a diffuse reduction of hair density over the crown, with complete or nearly complete preservation of the frontal hairline. Widening of the central parting line most noticeably in the mid-frontal scalp is also sometimes seen. The female patterned hair loss is classified into three stages, given by the Ludwig scale.

Male AGA starts at any age after puberty. Male balding has two major components: Frontotemporal recession and loss of hair over the vertex. Hairs become shorter and finer in caliber **(Fig. 1)**. Ultimately, this may lead to complete hair loss except at the lateral and posterior margins of the scalp. Hamilton–Norwood classification describes the several stages of AGA.

➲ DERMOSCOPY

Hair thickness heterogeneity >20% (anisotrichosis), increased proportion of vellus hair, single hair-pilosebaceous units, yellow dots, wavy hair, honeycomb scalp pigmentation, pinpoint white dots, and brown perifollicular pigmentation (peripilar sign).

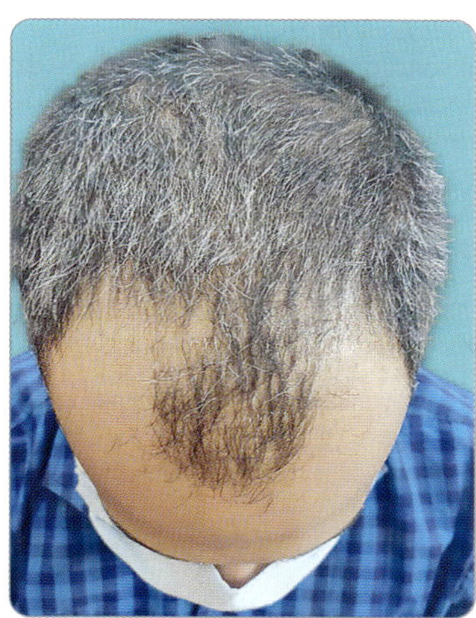

Fig. 1: Male pattern baldness. There is a loss of hair over the vertex and frontal area.

HISTOPATHOLOGY

Hair follicle miniaturization leads to finer hair that is often lighter in color. On the balding scalp, transitional indeterminate hairs represent the bridge between full-sized and miniaturized terminal hairs. Miniaturization may eventually lead to the deletion of hair follicles. A modest amount of chronic inflammation around the upper part of hair follicles, sometimes associated with perifollicular fibrosis, is seen.

DIFFERENTIAL DIAGNOSIS

- *Telogen effluvium*: Absence of miniaturization of hair follicle
- Anagen effluvium
- *Trichotillomania*: Irregular bizarre patterned hair loss, presence of underlying psychiatric illness, and perifollicular hemorrhages on biopsy
- *Tinea capitis*: Scaling, and demonstration of fungal hyphae in hair mount

TREATMENT

In men with mild/moderate vertex balding:

- Minoxidil 5%, 10%, minoxidil with finasteride for local application with gentle massaging
- Finasteride 1 mg daily/dutasteride 0.5 mg/day
- Oral minoxidil 0.5–2.5 mg

Mild/moderate frontal balding:

- Finasteride 1 mg daily.

Advanced frontal and/or vertex balding:

- Surgery—hair transplantation
- Prosthesis

In women with mild/moderate hair loss:
- 2% minoxidil solution twice daily or 5% once daily
- If clinical/biochemical signs of androgen excess, consider oral antiandrogen, e.g., spironolactone 100–200 mg daily/cyproterone acetate/flutamide
- Finasteride 2.5–5 mg/day
- Oral minoxidil 0.5–2.5 mg

For severe hair loss: Medical management as mentioned above prevents progression along with surgery and prosthesis.

Adjuvant therapy: Lower-level laser therapy, platelet-rich plasma therapy, microneedling topical caffeine, melatonin, aminexil, oral supplementation of amino acids, biotin, zinc, and other micronutrients.

SUGGESTED READINGS

1. Nestor MS, Ablon G, Gade A, Han H, Fischer DL. Treatment options for androgenetic alopecia: Efficacy, side effects, compliance, financial considerations, and ethics. J Cosmet Dermatol. 2021;20(12):3759-81.
2. Martinez-Jacobo L, Villarreal-Villarreal CD, Ortiz-López R, Ocampo-Candiani J, Rojas-Martínez A. Genetic and molecular aspects of androgenetic alopecia. Indian J Dermatol Venereol Leprol. 2018;84(3):263-8.

15 Anetoderma

➲ SYNONYM

Macular atrophy.

➲ HISTORY

Jadassohn first described anetoderma in 1892, and the term is derived from the Greek words "anetos", meaning slack, and "derma," meaning skin.

➲ ETIOLOGY

Anetoderma has been classified into primary (idiopathic) anetoderma, secondary anetoderma, drug-induced anetoderma, familial anetoderma, and prematurity-associated anetoderma.

- *Primary anetoderma*: Lesions arise on clinically normal skin and is historically subdivided into the Jadassohn–Pellizzari type (lesions develop with preceding inflammation) and the Schweninger–Buzzi type (lesions develop without preceding inflammation), strongly associated with antiphospholipid syndrome.
- *Secondary anetoderma*: Lesions arise from a preceding dermatosis; most commonly associated dermatosis are acne and varicella. It has also been reported with syphilis, sarcoidosis, tuberculosis, leprosy, mastocytosis, granuloma annulare, Lyme disease, B- and T-cell lymphoma, discoid lupus erythematosus (DLE), human immunodeficiency virus (HIV), and insect bites.
- *Drug induced*: Penicillamine
- *Familial anetoderma*: Rare, autosomal inheritance pattern develops in the first decade of life and might present as a purely skin manifestation or can also be associated with bony, neurological, and ocular anomalies.
- *Prematurity-associated anetoderma*: It occurs in premature neonates with a gestational age of 24–29 weeks due to hypoxemia or pressure effects at sites of monitoring leads or adhesives.

➲ EPIDEMIOLOGY

Young adults between the ages of 20 and 40 years are commonly affected by female preponderance.

➲ CLINICAL FEATURES

Asymptomatic skin-colored to blue–white flaccid, well-circumscribed areas of slack skin appear as depressions, wrinkling, or sac-like protrusions. These lesions vary in number from a few to hundreds and typically measure 0.5–3 cm in diameter.

The examining finger sinks without resistance into a distinct pit with sharp borders as if into a hernia ring. The bulge reappears when the pressure from the finger is released (buttonhole sign).

Common sites include chest, back, neck, and upper extremities. The scalp, mucous membranes, palms, and soles are usually spared.

➲ HISTOPATHOLOGY

Partial or complete loss of elastic fibers in the papillary and/or reticular dermis. A periadnexal and perivascular lymphocytic dermal infiltrate consisting of plasma cells and histiocytes can be present in the lesional skin.

On electron microscopy, the elastic fibers appear irregular in shape, fragmented, and occasionally engulfed within macrophages.

Direct immunofluorescence (DIF) of lesional skin may demonstrate nonspecific immunoreactant deposition along the dermal–epidermal junction or around the dermal blood vessels.

➲ DIFFERENTIAL DIAGNOSIS

- *Middermal elastolysis*: Larger areas with diffuse wrinkling without herniation and elastolysis limited to the middermis
- *Papular elastorrhexis*: Firm, noncompressible lesions
- *Atrophoderma of Pasini and Pierini*: Brown, gray, or violaceous macules/patches with a distinct drop-off sloping border on palpation
- *Nevus lipomatosus superficialis of Hoffman and Zurhelle*: Clustered group of soft, skin-colored to yellow nodules, present since birth
- *Focal dermal hypoplasia (Goltz syndrome)*: Telangiectasias, vermiculate dermal atrophy, hypopigmentation, hyperpigmentation, and fatty herniations/hamartomas
- *Glucocorticoid-induced atrophy*: Injection sites
- Acquired cutis laxa
- Post-traumatic scars
- Lichen sclerosus et atrophicus

➲ TREATMENT

No effective treatment modality exists for established lesions. Various treatment modalities tried include: Colchicine (to prevent new lesions), intralesional injections of triamcinolone and systemic administration of aspirin, dapsone, phenytoin, penicillin G, vitamin E, inositol niacinate, hydroxychloroquine, soft tissue fillers, ablative and nonablative fractionated lasers.

For limited lesions, excision is the only definitive treatment.

In the case of secondary anetoderma, the underlying disease has to be treated to prevent new lesions.

➲ PROGNOSIS

Lesions remain unchanged throughout life and do not resolve with time; new lesions often continue to form for many years.

➲ SUGGESTED READING

1. Cook JC, Puckett Y. Anetoderma. StatPearls. Treasure Island (FL): StatPearls Publishing; 2024.

16 Angioedema

➲ SYNONYMS

Angioneurotic edema, Quincke's edema.

➲ HISTORY

Hereditary angioedema (HAE) was originally described and named by Osler in 1888.

➲ ETIOLOGY

It is classified into three broad categories:

1. *Angioedema with wheals*: Due to food (fish, shellfish, and nuts) and drugs [beta-lactam antibiotics, aspirin, and nonsteroidal anti-inflammatory drugs (NSAIDs)] which is IgE-mediated type I hypersensitivity reaction
2. *Angioedema without wheals*: Encompassing C1 esterase inhibitor (C1INH) deficiency angioedema (both hereditary and acquired varieties) and angiotensin-converting enzyme inhibitor (ACE inhibitor)-induced angioedema
3. Idiopathic angioedema

➲ EPIDEMIOLOGY

Hereditary angioedema characteristically appears in the second to fourth decade.

➲ CLINICAL FEATURES

Angioedema is characterized by well-circumscribed areas of edema caused by increased vascular permeability. This condition affects mostly the skin, gastrointestinal, and respiratory tracts. Patients typically present with acute subcutaneous swelling, usually of the face, extremities, or genitalia. Urticaria may be associated with angioedema in 50% of cases. Angioedema is usually nonpruritic, but a burning sensation may be experienced **(Fig. 1)**.

➲ HISTOPATHOLOGY

Edema is the predominant finding which involves the deeper dermis and subcutaneous tissue with dilatation of venules. The dermal infiltrating inflammatory cells may be sparse or dense and include more CD4 than CD8 T lymphocytes, neutrophils, eosinophils, and basophils without B lymphocytes or natural killer cells.

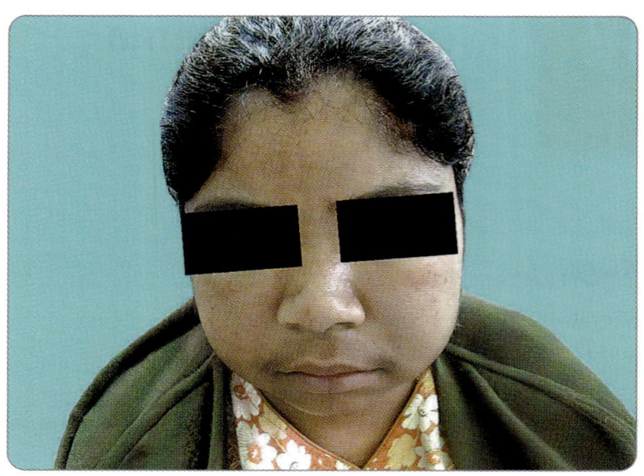

Fig. 1: Swelling of the face due to angioedema.

DIFFERENTIAL DIAGNOSIS

- Systemic capillary leak syndrome (Clarkson's syndrome)
- Schnitzler's syndrome
- Muckle–Wells syndrome
- Familial Mediterranean fever

COMPLICATIONS

A generalized anaphylactic reaction may occur, which is potentially fatal if the upper airway is compromised.

TREATMENT

Treatment is largely supportive. Acute allergic angioedema is treated with corticosteroids, antihistamines, and adrenaline.

Acute attacks of HAE can be treated with fresh-frozen plasma or C1 inhibitor concentrate—20 units/kg or bradykinin 2 receptor antagonist icatibant, or kallikrein inhibitor ecallantide. Intubation or tracheostomy is done when severe laryngeal edema is encountered. Cool, moist compresses and antihistamines can be used to control local burning.

Avoidance of known triggers, such as associated medications, is paramount. ACE inhibitors and oral contraceptives are contraindicated in patients with C1INH deficiency. Attenuated androgens danazol and stanozolol, tranexamic acid, plasma-derived C1INH, and epsilon aminocaproic acid can be used for the long-term prophylaxis of HAE.

SUGGESTED READINGS

1. Patel G, Pongracic JA. Hereditary and acquired angioedema. Allergy Asthma Proc. 2019;40(6):441-5.
2. Kazandjieva J, Christoff G. Angioedema as a systemic disease. Clin Dermatol. 2019;37(6):636-43.

17 Angiokeratoma

➲ SYNONYMS

Angiokeratoma of scrotum—angiokeratoma of Fordyce, angiokeratoma corporis diffusum—Fabry's disease.

➲ HISTORY

John Addison Fordyce described angiokeratomas of the scrotum in 1896.

➲ ETIOLOGY

Angiokeratomas are hyperkeratotic vascular cutaneous lesions which may be localized or diffuse. The diffuse variant, angiokeratoma corporis diffusum is found in Fabry's disease which is a X-linked metabolic disorder caused by the partial or complete deficiency of α-galactosidase A. Localized angiokeratoma occurs secondary to vessel ectasia caused by various entities.

➲ EPIDEMIOLOGY

Angiokeratomas are more common in males. Angiokeratoma circumscriptum presents at birth; solitary papular angiokeratoma presents between second and fourth decades; angiokeratoma of scrotum presents in middle age or older age group; and angiokeratoma corporis diffusum presents between ages of 5 and adolescence.

➲ CLINICAL FEATURES

There are two types viz. diffuse and localized.

Angiokeratoma corporis diffusum: It presents as clustered red to black papules that measure up to 1 cm in diameter, do not blanch with pressure, and show a verrucous appearance. They typically localize symmetrically in the bathing trunk area (buttocks, lower abdomen, groin, umbilicus, and upper thighs), elbows, waist, and extensor surfaces of arms, as well as along the spine.

The localized forms are:

- *Angiokeratoma circumscriptum naviforme* presents as a hyperkeratotic vascular plaque at birth. It is seen commonly over the lower leg and has a blue-black color with a segmental distribution. With time lesions develop warty papules and bleed on traumatization.
- *Angiokeratoma of Mibelli* is seen more in females with acrocyanosis and chilblains. It presents as tiny red papules which later increase in size and become warty. Lesions occur bilaterally on the dorsum of fingers and toes, hands, feet, calves, and rarely buttocks.

- *Solitary papular angiokeratomas*: The patient often presents with a history of sudden enlargement, darkening, or bleeding in a long-standing warty papule, between 2 and 10 mm in diameter, and dark red to blue–black in color.
- *Angiokeratoma of the scrotum (Fordyce)*: It is the most common type. It presents as small red papules on the scrotum and other genital areas or thighs. The lesions can become larger and darker. Symptoms include itching, soreness, or bleeding **(Fig. 1A)**.
- *Angiokeratoma of the vulva*: Lesions are analogous to scrotal angiokeratomas and may occur on the labia majora in older women or in younger women due to oral contraceptive pills.

➲ ASSOCIATED SYNDROMES

Klippel–Trenaunay syndrome.

➲ DERMOSCOPY

Well-demarcated red or dark red-blue round lacunae with a whitish veil (ill-defined structureless area). Other less frequent features—peripheral erythema and hemorrhagic crust **(Fig. 1B)**.

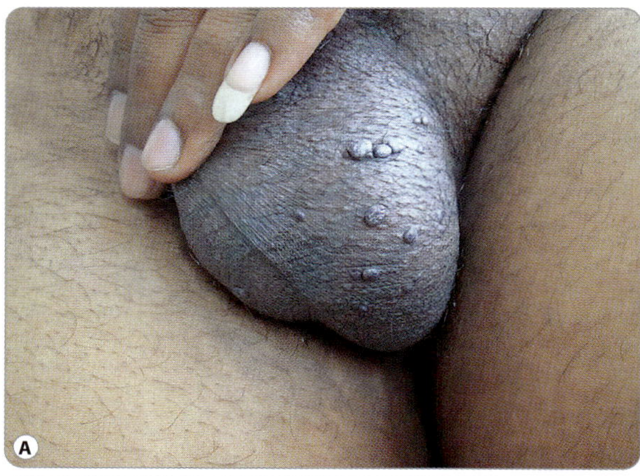

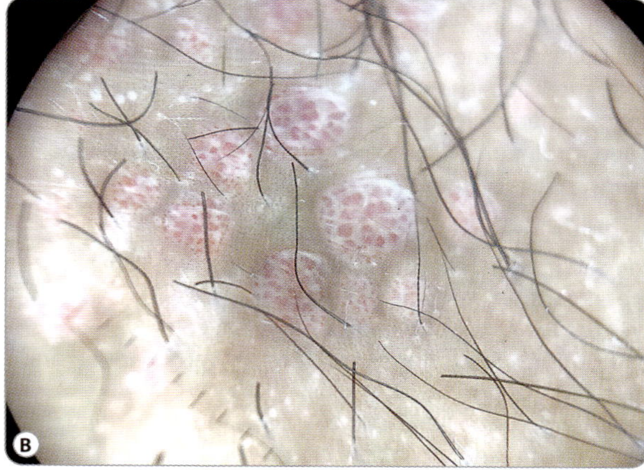

Figs. 1A and B: Angiokeratoma of the scrotum—multiple dark warty papules over the scrotum; and (B) Dermoscopy showing red lacunae with a whitish veil.

HISTOPATHOLOGY

It is similar in all kinds of angiokeratomas. There is epidermal hyperkeratosis, acanthosis and papillomatosis. Elongated rete ridges tend to encircle and enclose the vascular lacunae. There is marked ectasia of vessels within the papillary dermis.

DIFFERENTIAL DIAGNOSIS

Angiokeratoma circumscriptum:

- *Verrucous hemangioma*: Soft, compressible plaque with verrucous surface seen
- *Lymphangioma circumscriptum*: Grouped translucent vesicles present in a "frog spawn" appearance, dilated lymphatics with vertical channels connecting deeper lymph vessels on histopathological examination (HPE)

Solitary papular angiokeratomas:

- *Warts*: Koebnerization seen, presence of acanthosis, papillomatosis, and koilocytes on biopsy
- Melanocytic nevi and melanomas
- *Angiokeratoma of the scrotum*: Varicocele.

COMPLICATIONS

Necrosis due to secondary infection.

TREATMENT

- *Angiokeratoma circumscriptum*: Small lesions can be treated with curettage and cautery, and larger lesions treated with laser removal (pulsed dye/Nd:YAG/KTP) or even excision.
- *Angiokeratoma of Mibelli*: The lesions can be treated, with liquid nitrogen, electrodessication, laser ablation, or by local excision.
- *Solitary papular angiokeratomas*: Local excision can be done.
- *Angiokeratoma of the scrotum*: Liquid nitrogen cryotherapy, diathermy, or laser ablation can be used to treat symptomatic lesions. Associated conditions such as varicocele should be treated.

SUGGESTED READINGS

1. Guillen-Climent S, García-Vázquez A, Silva Díaz E, Pinazo I. Angiokeratoma circumscriptum. Dermatol Online J. 2020;26(11):13030/qt8v6170qz.
2. Chhabra G, Verma P. Angiokeratoma Circumscriptum Naeviforme on Trunk. J Cutan Med Surg. 2022;26(3):311.

18 Angioma

➲ SYNONYMS

Campbell de Morgan spots, senile hemangioma, cherry hemangioma.

➲ HISTORY

Campbell Greig De Morgan, a British surgeon, made the first note of these lesions in medical literature.

➲ ETIOLOGY

It is an acquired, well-circumscribed vascular lesion, occurring in adulthood and increasing in number with age. The exact pathogenesis is unknown. Eruptive lesions occur in association with pregnancy, high prolactin level, and following exposure to sulfur, mustard gas, bromide compounds, cyclosporine, and 2-butoxyethanol solvent. The sudden appearance of multiple lesions may herald the development of an internal malignancy.

➲ EPIDEMIOLOGY

Both sexes are affected equally. Most people over 60 years of age have one or more of these lesions.

➲ CLINICAL FEATURES

Cherry angiomas are round to oval, bright red, dome-shaped papules ranging in size from barely visible to several millimeters in diameter, most commonly on the trunk and proximal extremities **(Fig. 1)**. They are rare on the hands, feet, and face. The lesions increase in number and size with age and in diabetics. It is not unusual for elderly adults to have 50–100 cherry angiomas on their trunk. They are generally asymptomatic but may bleed when traumatized.

➲ ASSOCIATED SYNDROME

POEMS syndrome (polyneuropathy, organomegaly, endocrinopathy, monoclonal gammopathy, and skin changes).

➲ DERMOSCOPIC FEATURES

Multiple, well-demarcated, red to blue-red or blue-black to maroon, round to oval structures (lacunae/lagoons) situated on a background of bluish-red pigmentation, white lines, and irregular dilated vessels.

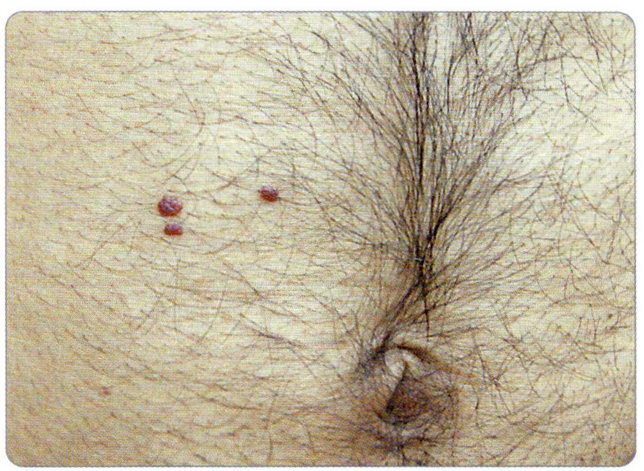

Fig. 1: Cherry red papules over the trunk.

HISTOPATHOLOGY

Histologically, these lesions consist of congested, ectatic capillaries, and postcapillary venules in the papillary dermis. Early lesions are characterized by small lumina and plump endothelial cells. With maturation, the vessels dilate and endothelial cells flatten. The epidermis shows central loss of rete ridges with peripherally placed adnexal epithelial collarettes. There is increased number of mast cells.

DIFFERENTIAL DIAGNOSIS

- *Angiokeratoma*: Hyperkeratotic blackish colored papules which bleed on touch
- Glomeruloid hemangioma
- *Petechiae*: Multiple flat lesions, underlying bleeding/coagulation disorder
- *Bacillary angiomatosis*: Demonstration of organism on Warthin-Starry stain
- *Infantile hemangioma*: Larger lesions which are compressible and spontaneously involute with age
- Malignant melanoma
- Milia
- *Miliaria*: Diffuse lesions (miliaria rubra), no vascular pathology on biopsy

COMPLICATIONS

Bleeding, secondary infection.

TREATMENT

Treatment is not mandatory. Shave excision, electrodessication or CO_2 laser ablation, cryotherapy can be done for cosmetic purposes. Pulsed dye laser or intense pulsed light has been used with success.

PROGNOSIS

Sudden appearance of numerous lesions may be an indicator for internal malignancy.

SUGGESTED READINGS

1. Nazer RI, Bashihab RH, Al-Madani WH, Omair AA, AlJasser MI. Cherry angioma: A case-control study. J Family Community Med. 2020;27(2):109-13.
2. Pastor-Tomás N, Bañuls J, Nagore E. Clinical Relevance of Cherry Angiomas. Actas Dermosifiliogr. 2023;114(3):240-6.

19 Angular Cheilitis

➲ SYNONYMS

Angular stomatitis, perleche.

➲ ETIOLOGY

Angular cheilitis is an acute or chronic inflammation of the skin and contiguous labial mucosa at the angles of the mouth. The main causes are infective agents (*Candida albicans* and *Staphylococci*), mechanical factors (edentulous patient, recurrent trauma of flossing, persistent salivation, or licking the lips), immunosuppression (HIV infection, diabetes mellitus, post-transplant, and radiotherapy patients), nutritional deficiencies (riboflavin, folic acid, iron, and protein-energy malnutrition), and skin diseases (atopic or seborrheic dermatitis). Patients with Down's syndrome are more prone, due to an increased carriage of *S. aureus* and *C. albicans*.

➲ EPIDEMIOLOGY

It is usually seen in old, immunosuppressed, and debilitated patients.

➲ CLINICAL FEATURES

Angular cheilitis presents as a roughly triangular area of erythema and edema at one or more commonly both angles of the mouth. Linear furrows or fissures radiating from the angle of the mouth (rhagades) are seen in the more severe forms, especially in denture wearers **(Fig. 1)**.

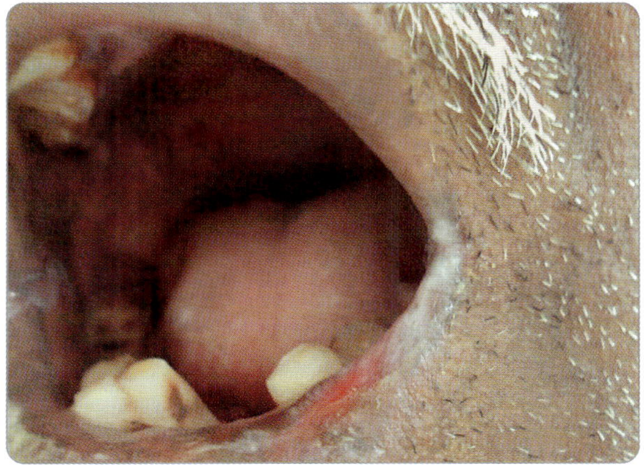

Fig. 1: Maceration, fissuring, and crusting at the angle of the mouth in angular cheilitis.

➲ ASSOCIATED CONDITIONS

Anorexia nervosa, Bulimia nervosa, Down's syndrome, and Plummer–Vinson syndrome.

➲ DIFFERENTIAL DIAGNOSIS

- Contact dermatitis
- *Lip smacking dermatitis*: Erythema, papules, and scaling present all around the mouth sparing the vermillion border
- *Impetigo*: Vesicles, pustules, and lesions with honey-colored crusts

➲ COMPLICATIONS

Acquired linear anetoderma.

➲ TREATMENT

Correction of predisposing factors yields good clinical improvement. Specific treatment depends on the etiology.

Fungal etiology: Topical-miconazole 2% cream, clotrimazole 1% cream, nystatin ointment, gentian violet, iodoquinol 1% cream, systemic–fluconazole, itraconazole.

Bacterial etiology: Topical mupirocin 2% or fusidic acid 2%.

Mechanical factors: Dentures should be removed from the mouth at night and stored in a candidacidal solution such as hypochlorite, collagen injection to the commissures.

Nutritional deficiency: Supplementation in cases of avitaminosis, mineral deficiencies, or general malnutrition.

➲ SUGGESTED READINGS

1. Cabras M, Gambino A, Broccoletti R, Lodi G, Arduino PG. Treatment of angular cheilitis: A narrative review and authors' clinical experience. Oral Dis. 2020;26(6):1107-15.
2. Lugović-Mihić L, Pilipović K, Crnarić I, Šitum M, Duvančić T. Differential Diagnosis of Cheilitis - How to Classify Cheilitis? Acta Clin Croat. 2018;57(2):342-51.

20 Antiphospholipid Syndrome

➲ SYNONYM

Lupus anticoagulant syndrome.

➲ HISTORY

Harris et al. coined the term "antiphospholipid syndrome". It was Asherson who introduced the term "primary antiphospholipid syndrome (APS)" to describe patients with APS without an underlying disorder, as opposed to secondary APS, which occurs in the context of another autoimmune disorder.

➲ ETIOLOGY

Antiphospholipid antibodies (aPL) constitute a heterogeneous group of autoantibodies that share the ability to bind phospholipid alone, protein-phospholipid complexes, or phospholipid-binding proteins. APS is the association of aPL with hypercoagulability resulting in arterial and/or venous thrombosis and pregnancy morbidity/obstetric complications. These antibodies include lupus anticoagulant antibodies, anticardiolipin antibodies (aCL), and antibodies against β2-glycoprotein I (anti-2GPI).

The exact mechanism involved in the pathogenesis of thrombotic events in APS is not clear. But the probable mechanisms are suggested:

- The antibodies directed against phospholipids may act on endothelial and/or thrombocyte membranes and interfere with the release of prostacyclin or endothelial plasminogen activator.
- The antibodies may affect clotting proteins (e.g., thrombomodulin of protein C or protein S) present on the surface of cell membranes with the help of a cofactor called apolipoprotein H.
- Inhibition of the protein C activator (thus accelerating the clotting process), inhibition of fibrinolysis, or inhibition of antithrombin III activity may be responsible for thrombosis.

➲ EPIDEMIOLOGY

Primary antiphospholipid syndrome occurs commonly in young to middle-aged females.

➲ CLINICAL FEATURES

The clinical manifestations of APS involve different organs and systems, such as blood vessels, the central nervous system, skin, kidneys, gastrointestinal tract, heart, and placenta. The unifying mechanism of all these manifestations is thrombosis, either arterial or venous.

Cutaneous manifestations include livedo reticularis (lace-like pattern of cyanosis) in the dorsum of hands and lower extremities in association with painful ulceration and purpuric spots or occasionally frank gangrene of extremities can occur. Recurrent skin ulcers or necrotizing purpura may also be present. Livedo reticularis is due to the involvement of dermal vessels.

ASSOCIATED SYNDROMES

Sneddon's syndrome.

DIAGNOSIS

The most commonly detected subgroups of aPL are lupus anti-coagulant antibodies, aCL, and anti-β2GPI. Lupus anticoagulant antibodies are identified by coagulation assays in which they prolong clotting time. In contrast, aCL and anti-β2GPI are detected by immunoassays that measure immunologic reactivity to phospholipids or phospholipids-binding protein (cardiolipin and β2GPI, respectively). In general, lupus anticoagulant antibodies are more specific for APS and aCLs are more sensitive.

For diagnosis at least one of the following clinical and one laboratory criteria should be present:

Clinical:

- A documented episode of arterial, venous, or small vessel thrombosis
- 1 or more unexplained deaths of a morphologically normal fetus (documented by ultrasound or direct examination of the fetus) at or beyond the 10th week of gestation and/or three or more unexplained consecutive spontaneous abortions before the 10th week of gestation.

Laboratory:

- Anticardiolipin immunoglobulin G (IgG) and/or immuno-globulin M (IgM) positive
- Anti-β2 glycoprotein I IgG and/or IgM positive
- Lupus anticoagulant

HISTOPATHOLOGY

Early lesions typically reveal noninflammatory thrombosis of small dermal vessels; later lesions may show inflammation following necrosis.

DIFFERENTIAL DIAGNOSIS

- Cholesterol emboli
- Hyperhomocysteinemia
- Thrombotic thrombocytopenic purpura
- Hypercoagulable states such as protein C and S deficiency and prothrombin gene mutation.

TREATMENT

Primary thromboprophylaxis with low-dose aspirin is instituted in patients with aPL and no thrombotic events. Secondary thromboprophylaxis refers to the treatment initiated after the occurrence of thrombotic events to prevent further attacks. Low molecular weight heparin has been used in the initial phase followed by warfarin in the management of APS.

Other drugs used are antiplatelet agents such as dipyridamole, ticlopidine or clopidogrel bisulfate, high-dose corticosteroids, cyclophosphamide, intravenous immunoglobulin (IVIg), plasmapheresis and recently, rituximab.

➲ SUGGESTED READING

1. Chi HS. Recent advances in the diagnosis of antiphospholipid syndrome. Int J Hematol. 2002;76(Suppl 2):47-51.

21 Aphthous Stomatitis

➲ SYNONYMS

Oral aphthae, aphthous ulcers, canker sores, simple or complex aphthosis.

➲ ETIOLOGY

Stomatitis is the inflammation of the oral mucus membrane. Etiology of aphthous stomatitis remains obscure; it is likely to be a multifactorial disorder influenced by a host of predisposing factors. It may be the result of a dysfunction of the immune system, resulting in immunologically mediated damage to epithelial cells. This abnormal immune response may be triggered or influenced by trauma, iron, folate or vitamin B12 deficiencies, hormonal fluctuations, psychological stress, infectious agents, food hypersensitivities, genetic factors, human immunodeficiency virus (HIV) infection, and gluten-sensitive enteropathy.

➲ EPIDEMIOLOGY

Women may be afflicted more commonly than men, and the peak prevalence occurs during the second decade.

➲ CLINICAL FEATURES

There are three categories of simple aphthous ulcers.

1. *Minor aphthae (Mikulicz ulcers)* are the most common form and are characterized by round to ovoid, shallow, painful ulcers that are usually <5 mm in diameter. Individual lesions are covered by a creamy white pseudomembrane and have an erythematous halo. The ulcers are typically limited to the nonkeratinized oral mucosa, viz labial and buccal mucosa, floor of the mouth, ventral surface of the tongue, soft palate, and oropharyngeal mucosa **(Fig. 1)**.
2. *Major aphthae (Sutton's ulcers)* are characterized by larger ulcerations, typically >1 cm. Lesions are deeper, persist up to 6 weeks, and may heal with scarring.
3. *Herpetiform aphthae* are very uncommon, consisting of multiple small, painful ulcerations that superficially resemble primary herpes simplex virus (HSV) infection. Up to 100 ulcers are possible at one time.

The almost constant presence of more than three oral aphthae or oral and genital aphthae is complex aphthosis.

➲ ASSOCIATED SYNDROMES

Behçet's syndrome and Sweet's syndrome.

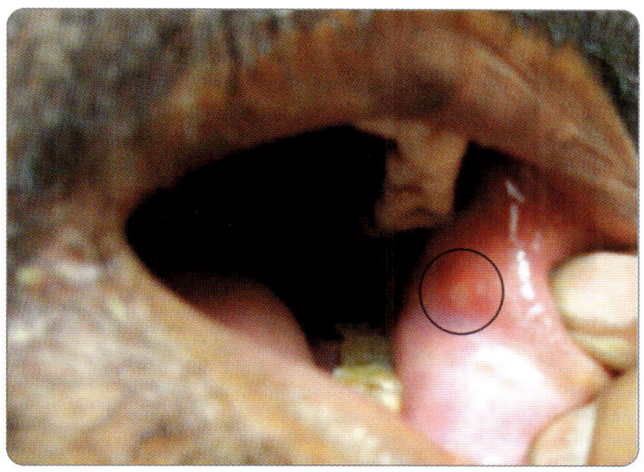

Fig. 1: Shallow ulcer surrounded by an erythematous halo on the buccal mucosa.

DERMOSCOPY

Dermoscopy reveals three zones: A central yellowish-red area surrounded by a whitish structureless region and a rim of erythema.

HISTOPATHOLOGY

Histopathologic features are relatively nonspecific. Early lesions may show a neutrophilic vessel-based submucosal infiltrate.

DIFFERENTIAL DIAGNOSIS

- Erythema multiforme
- Pemphigus vulgaris
- Herpes simplex
- Oral candidiasis
- Geographic tongue
- Hemangiomas
- Erythroplakia
- Hand, foot, and mouth disease
- Traumatic ulcers
- Primary syphilis
- Traumatic ulcer
- Reiter's syndrome

TREATMENT

Local therapy consists of local anesthetics, topical corticosteroids (triamcinolone acetonide 0.1% in ora base), intralesional corticosteroids, topical tacrolimus, and topical analgesics (diclofenac 3% with hyaluronic acid 2.5% gel).

Systemic therapy includes oral steroids, colchicine 50 µg/kg, dapsone 100 mg, and clofazimine and thalidomide 100 mg/day. Others include carbenoxolone, benzydamine, cromoglycate, levamisole, pentoxifylline, montelukast 10 mg, azathioprine, and tumor necrosis factor (TNF) alpha inhibitors.

Adjuvant therapy includes chlorhexidine rinse, antimicrobial (tetracycline) mouth rinses, folate, vitamin B12, zinc and iron supplementation, sucralfate, ascorbic acid, and low-level laser therapy (658 nm).

➲ PROGNOSIS

Minor aphthae heal in 7–14 days without scarring. Major form lasts for few weeks and heals with scarring.

➲ SUGGESTED READING

1. Elias ML, Fatahzadeh M, Schwartz RA. Recurrent Aphthous Stomatitis: An Enigmatic Entity and Sign of Systemic Disease. Indian J Dermatol. 2022;67(6):834.

22 Ashy Dermatosis

➲ SYNONYMS

Erythema dyschromicum perstans, ashy dermatosis of Ramirez, lichen pigmentosus, Cinderella dermatoses.

➲ HISTORY

In 1957, Ramirez referred to these patients as los cenicientos (the ash-colored ones) and named the condition "dermatitis cenicienta." Sulzberger then proposed the term, "erythema dyschromicum perstans."

➲ ETIOLOGY

The exact etiology of the disease is unknown. Unidentified set of pollutants in our environment, either contactants or inhaled or ingested substances, may be the cause of erythema dyschromicum perstans in certain predisposed individuals. There have been sporadic case reports of temporal associations with the ingestion of ammonium nitrate, whipworm infestation, and HIV seroconversion. Some authors consider erythema dyschromicum perstans as a variant of macular lichen planus.

➲ EPIDEMIOLOGY

It can affect any age group, but characteristically, it starts in the first or second decade of life, with a higher incidence among females.

➲ CLINICAL FEATURES

Most patients present with slowly progressing gray, gray-brown, or gray-blue macules and patches with a slightly raised palpable border like "a thin piece of string." The lesions initially have an erythematous hue but become slate-gray-colored later. Most lesions measure between 0.5 and 2.5 cm but can be larger. Although the lesions may vary in shape, many are oval with their long axes following skin cleavage lines, thus assuming a pattern similar to that of pityriasis rosea. The most common sites of involvement are the neck, trunk, and proximal arms, and the distribution is usually symmetric. The mucosa is spared **(Fig. 1)**.

➲ DERMOSCOPY

Small gray-blue or brown dots and globules in a linear/circular or speckled pattern over a bluish background.

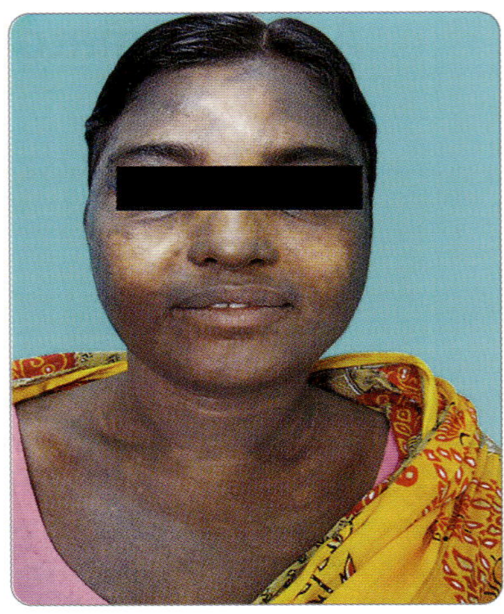

Fig. 1: Diffuse macular slate-gray pigmentation of ashy dermatosis.

HISTOPATHOLOGY

Biopsy taken from the active border of the macule reveals vacuolar degeneration of the basal cells. The central pigmented portion shows increased epidermal pigmentation, pigmentary incontinence, melanophages, and perivascular lymphohistiocytic infiltration.

Immunoglobulin M (IgM) cytoid bodies are found on direct immunofluorescence study.

DIFFERENTIAL DIAGNOSIS

- Fixed drug eruption with multiple lesions—hyperpigmented patches with erythematous ring
- Postinflammatory hyperpigmentation—lack of red border
- Pityriasis rosea—presence of herald patch, scaly lesions in Christmas tree pattern, and lack of pigmentation
- Small plaque parapsoriasis
- Lichen planus pigmentosus—lack of erythematous border
- Inverse lichen planus
- Idiopathic eruptive macular pigmentation
- Addison's disease—involvement of palmar creases and buccal mucosal pigmentation
- Hemochromatosis
- Erythema multiforme

TREATMENT

Most of the proposed treatments for erythema dyschromicum perstans are unsuccessful:

- *Topical agents*: Corticosteroids, tacrolimus, vitamin C, hydroquinone, and tretinoin
- *Oral agents*: Corticosteroids, dapsone, clofazimine, hydroxychloroquine, isoniazid, and isotretinoin
- *Others*: Narrowband ultraviolet B (NB-UVB) lasers—Q-switched/erbium, chemical peels, camouflage creams, and sun protection

➲ PROGNOSIS

Spontaneous remission can occur, but unfortunately, most patients have the disease for years.

➲ SUGGESTED READING

1. Nguyen K, Khachemoune A. Ashy dermatosis: a review. Dermatol Online J. 2019;25(5):1.

23 Atopic Dermatitis

➲ SYNONYMS

Eczema rubrum, eczema rimosum, prurigo of Hebra, Besnier's prurigo, disseminated neurodermatitis, Spatexudativ eczema.

➲ HISTORY

In 1892, Besnier first described the association between atopic eczema, rhinitis, and asthma. In 1923, Coca and associates introduced the term atopy [no (a) place (top) ness (y)]. Professors Jon Hanifin and Georg Rajka are considered as pioneers of a modern conception of atopic dermatitis (AD).

➲ ETIOLOGY

Heredity and two independent losses of functional genetic mutation in the gene encoding filaggrin (FLG) are strong predisposing factors for AD. Other factors include maternal, pregnancy, intrauterine, environmental, impairment of skin barrier function, immune dysregulation, systemic T helper 2 (Th2) disbalance, diet, infection, psychological stress, and neuropeptides.

➲ EPIDEMIOLOGY

Atopic dermatitis may start at any age but usually begins between 2 and 6 months.

➲ CLINICAL FEATURES

Common manifestations include itching, macular erythema, papules or papulovesicles, eczematous area with crusting, lichenification, excoriation, dryness of skin, secondary infection, hyperlinearity of palms and soles, infraorbital fold (Dennie–Morgan), facial pallor, and orbital darkening.

There are three stages:

1. Infantile stage lasts up to 2 years; lesions begin over the face, particularly the cheeks, and extend to the scalp and extensor surfaces of extremities. Nasolabial and napkin areas are often spared **(Fig. 1)**.
2. Childhood stage is from 2 years to puberty. The sites affected are the elbows, knee flexures, sides of the neck, wrist, and ankles. Sides of the neck show striking reticulate pigmentation called the atopy dirty neck sign.
3. Adulthood stage is from puberty onward and presents with flexural lichenification and excoriated skin lesions **(Fig. 2)**.

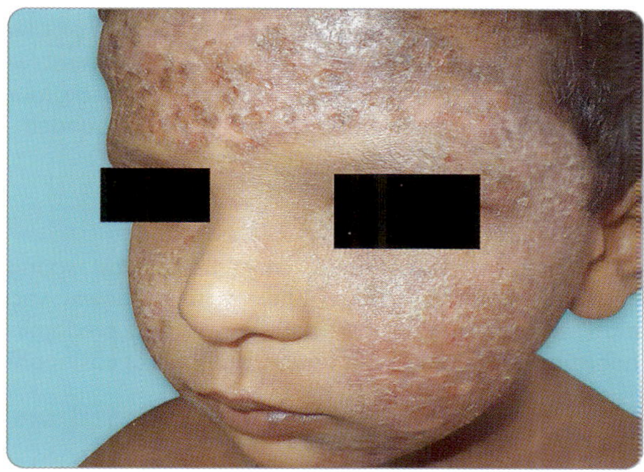

Fig. 1: Crusting and eczematous lesions over the face of the child.

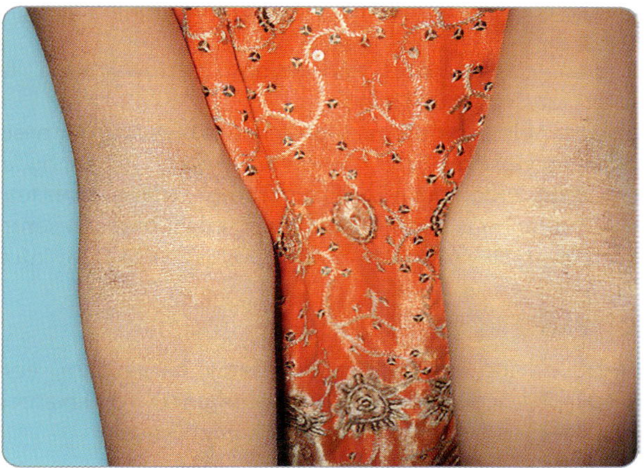

Fig. 2: Flexural lichenification in a 12-year-old girl.

Diagnostic criteria for atopic eczema (refinement of Hanifin and Rajka criteria) or UK Working Party's diagnostic criteria include:

- Itchy skin condition
- Plus three or more of the following criteria include:
  1. History of (H/o) flexural dermatitis
  2. Personal H/o asthma or hay fever or a H/o atopy in a first-degree relative and in children <4 years
  3. History of generalized dry skin in the past year
  4. Visible flexural eczema or eczema of the cheeks/forehead and outer limbs in children <4 years
  5. Onset in the first 2 years of life if the child is >4 years **(Fig. 2)**.

➲ ASSOCIATED CONDITIONS

Down's syndrome, alopecia areata, ichthyosis vulgaris, and keratosis pilaris.

➲ DERMOSCOPY

- *Acute phase*—yellow/white serocrusts and dotted vessels distributed in patchy distribution with a dull red background
- *Chronic phase*—clusters of dotted vessels surrounded by a white halo

➲ HISTOPATHOLOGY

Acute eczematous dermatitis is characterized by spongiosis, acanthosis, and parakeratosis. The dermis shows vacuolar dilatation, edema, and a superficial, perivascular, predominantly lymphohistiocytic infiltrate with varying numbers of eosinophils.

➲ DIFFERENTIAL DIAGNOSIS

- Seborrheic dermatitis—typical involvement of seborrheic areas (scalp, chest, nasolabial folds, and retroauricular area) and greasy scales
- Allergic contact dermatitis—H/o exposure to allergen and no H/o atopy
- Scabies—classical sites and lesions (burrows) seen, family history, and nocturnal itch
- Wiskott–Aldrich syndrome—presence of bleeding diathesis and thrombocytopenia
- Hyperimmunoglobulin E (IgE) syndrome—exaggerated features of AD, cutaneous and sinopulmonary infections, and serum IgE levels drastically elevated

➲ COMPLICATIONS

Complications include infections, eczema herpeticum, erythroderma, blepharoconjunctivitis, keratoconjunctivitis, keratoconus, cataract, sleep disturbances, and growth impairment.

➲ TREATMENT

- General measures include avoiding trigger factors like contact with wool and synthetic apparels, use of dust mite-proof encasings, and removal of bedroom carpets; decreasing the indoor humidity levels; and keeping furry pets.
- *First-line therapy*: Bathing should be short; soaps used should be less alkaline, and immediate lubrication of the skin should occur within 3 minutes of bath.
- Other treatments—wet wrap technique for acute eczema, topical corticosteroids, topical immunomodulators like tacrolimus 0.03% and 0.1% ointments, and pimecrolimus 1% cream.
- Systemic therapy—antihistamines, antimicrobial therapy if there is secondary infection, phototherapy, and narrowband ultraviolet B (NB-UVB). Oral prednisolone 0.5–1 mg/kg body weight, cyclosporine 3–5 mg/kg, methotrexate, azathioprine, mycophenolate mofetil, and apremilast
- Biologics—omalizumab, dupilumab, and tumor necrosis factor (TNF) alpha inhibitors

PROGNOSIS

Prognosis is variable, as the disease is characterized by exacerbations and remissions. Many cases resolve before 2 years, and some patients improve at puberty.

SUGGESTED READING

1. Lee JH, Son SW, Cho SH. A Comprehensive Review of the Treatment of Atopic Eczema. Allergy Asthma Immunol Res. 2016;8(3):181-90.

24 Bacillary Angiomatosis

➲ SYNONYMS

Epitheloid angiomatosis, disseminated cat scratch disease.

➲ HISTORY

Bacillary angiomatosis was first described in 1983 by Stoler as subcutaneous vascular proliferation in individuals having acquired immunodeficiency syndrome (AIDS). In 1989, LeBoit and colleagues coined the name "bacillary angiomatosis."

➲ ETIOLOGY

Bacillary angiomatosis is an uncommon disease found in AIDS patients with CD4 count <200 cells/μL and occasionally other patients with severe immunosuppression. Two *Bartonella* species have been associated with this infection: *B. henselae* (transmitted by cat scratch, ticks, or fleas) and *B. quintana* (transmitted via lice). About 20% of cases give a history of recent cat scratch or bite. The associated vascular proliferation may be due to an angiogenic factor produced by *Bartonella* species.

➲ CLINICAL FEATURES

There are two types of skin lesions, viz. dermal and subcutaneous. In the dermal form, the lesions are asymptomatic, single or multiple, violaceous or red, firm, nonblanching vascular papules, and nodules occurring on any part of the skin **(Fig. 1)**. The lesions clinically resemble Kaposi's sarcoma, but the oral cavity is often spared. They may ulcerate and discharge serosanguinous fluid in the late stages. Subcutaneous lesions are nodules or masses several centimeters in diameter. The overlying skin is often inflamed, and the underlying bone may have osteolytic lesions.

➲ DERMOSCOPY

Bright red oval and globular structures with grayish background. Arborizing telangiectasias in the periphery.

➲ HISTOPATHOLOGY

There is a lobular proliferation of capillaries and venules, plump and protuberant endothelial cells, and a marked neutrophilic infiltrate with leukocytoclasis throughout the interstitium with granular clumps of purplish material composed of gram-negative bacteria, which can be readily identified by Warthin–Starry stain.

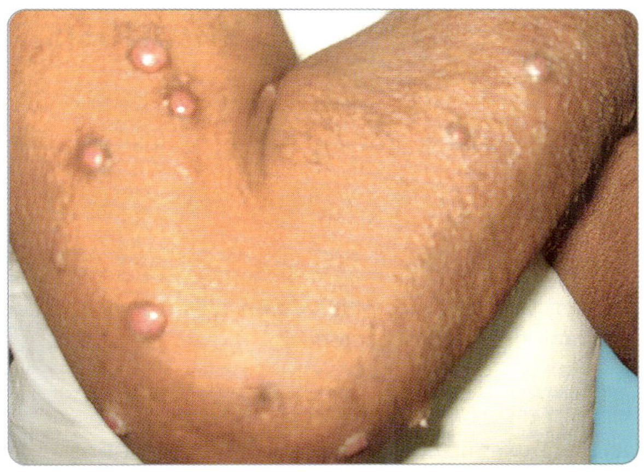

Fig. 1: Vascular nodules of bacillary angiomatosis over the forearm of an immunocompromised male.

Polymerase chain reaction is a rapid, sensitive, and simple method to identify *Bartonella* species in tissue specimens.

DIFFERENTIAL DIAGNOSIS

- Pyogenic granulomas—lesions are smaller and fewer in number and bleed on trauma.
- Molluscum contagiosum—pearly white lesions with classical umbilication can be seen; virus inclusions can be seen on crush smear of the extruded material.
- Kaposi's sarcoma—oral mucosa can be involved.
- Cherry angioma—smaller lesions and proliferation of normal-looking vessels
- Angiokeratomas
- Deep fungal infections disseminated to skin

COMPLICATIONS

Bacillary peliosis, where cyst-like inflammatory structures may develop in internal organs such as the liver.

TREATMENT

Correct diagnosis may be lifesaving. The disease is easily treated with erythromycin 500 mg given four times a day for a minimum of 4 weeks. Doxycycline and clarithromycin have also been shown to be effective. It may be necessary to use long periods of treatment for 8 weeks or longer. Relapses are common.

Cryotherapy, electrodesiccation with curettage, and surgical excision can be done for solitary cutaneous lesions.

SUGGESTED READING

1. Chian CA, Arrese JE, Piérard GE. Skin manifestations of *Bartonella* infections. Int J Dermatol. 2002;41:461-6.

25 Bacterial Vaginosis

➲ SYNONYMS

Hemophilus vaginalis vaginitis, *Gardnerella vaginalis* vaginitis, anerobic vaginosis, vaginal bacteriosis.

➲ HISTORY

Gardner and Dukes first described the condition in 1955.

➲ ETIOLOGY

Bacterial vaginosis (BV) is a dysbiosis, resulting from the replacement of normal hydrogen peroxide and lactic acid-producing *Lactobacillus* species in the vagina with overgrowth of anaerobic bacteria, including *G. vaginalis*, *Mycoplasma hominis*, *Prevotella* species, *Mobiluncus* species, *Fusobacterium*, *Peptostreptococcus*, coagulase-negative staphylococci, and other bacteria.

➲ EPIDEMIOLOGY

It is common in females of reproductive age group.

Risk factors include multiple sexual partners, intercourse at a young age, commercial sex workers, concurrent or prior sexually transmitted infection (STI), douching, and intrauterine contraceptive use.

➲ CLINICAL FEATURES

Most females present with complaints of malodorous gray-white vaginal discharge that may become more pronounced after sexual intercourse. Additional symptoms include dysuria, dyspareunia, and vaginal pruritus; however, many affected individuals may be asymptomatic.

➲ DIAGNOSIS

Amsel criteria—presence of at least three of the following criteria:

1. Thin, homogenous, uniformly adherent vaginal discharge
2. Vaginal pH > 4.5
3. Positive whiff test
4. Presence of "clue cells" (20%)

Nugent scoring—microscopic examination and gram-stain technique to evaluate the presence of different vaginal bacteria morphotypes and assigning a numerical score ranging from 0 to 10. A score of ≥7 indicates the presence of BV, 4–6 intermediate, and 0–3 normal.

DIFFERENTIAL DIAGNOSIS

- *Trichomonas vaginalis*—copious, malodorous, yellow-green, frothy vaginal discharge with pruritus and soreness, vulvitis, and vaginitis—"strawberry" appearance, and wet mount shows trichomonad.
- *Vulvovaginal candidiasis*—scanty to moderate curdy white discharge with vulvar pruritus, soreness, dysuria, erythema, edema, and/or erosions of vagina or external genitalia, budding yeast or pseudohyphae on KOH mount, and positive fungal culture
- Cervicitis due to chlamydia/gonococcal infection
- Ulcerative vaginitis due to *Staphylococcus aureus*
- Vaginitis due to the use of vaginal tampons/cervical caps/spermicide/douches/intravaginal foreign body
- Postmenopausal atrophic vaginitis
- Contact dermatitis

COMPLICATIONS

Adverse pregnancy outcomes include premature rupture of membranes, preterm labor, preterm birth, postpartum endometritis and intra-amniotic infections, pelvic inflammatory disease, increased risk of acquiring other STIs, and postsurgical infections.

TREATMENT

- As per the Centers for Disease Control and Prevention (CDC), metronidazole 500 mg orally twice daily for 7 days or metronidazole 0.75% gel (5 g) intravaginally once a day for 5 days or clindamycin cream 2% (5 g) intravaginally at bedtime for 7 days
- Alternative regimen—clindamycin 300 mg orally twice daily for 7 days or clindamycin ovules 100 mg intravaginally once at bedtime for 3 days, secnidazole 2 g oral granules in a single dose or tinidazole 2 g orally once daily for 2 days, or 1 g orally once daily for 5 days
- During pregnancy—oral metronidazole 250 mg thrice a day for 7 days or 2 g single dose or clindamycin 300 mg orally twice a day for 7 days or metronidazole 0.75% gel (5 g) intravaginally twice a day for 7 days

PROGNOSIS

Most uncomplicated cases of BV resolve with treatment. However, recurrences are not uncommon.

SUGGESTED READING

1. Coudray MS, Madhivanan P. Bacterial vaginosis-A brief synopsis of the literature. Eur J Obstet Gynecol Reprod Biol. 2020;245:143-8.

26 Balanitis Xerotica Obliterans

➲ SYNONYMS

Lichen sclerosis in the male.

➲ HISTORY

The condition was first described by Stuhmer in 1928.

➲ EPIDEMIOLOGY

The condition is most common between the ages of 15 and 50 years. It may be overlooked unless the prepuce is examined histologically in cases of circumcision for acquired phimosis.

➲ ETIOLOGY

Balanitis xerotica obliterans (BXO) is commonly used to the lesions due to lichen sclerosis. It may be a consequence of other scarring dermatoses such as lichen planus and cicatricial pemphigoid. Exact etiology is not known. Human papillomavirus (HPV) (types 6, 16, and 18), anatomical abnormality, and trauma are the contributing factors.

➲ CLINICAL FEATURES

The presenting features are acquired phimosis, recurrent balanitis, itching, soreness, painful erections, burning, bleeding, tearing, splitting, hemorrhagic blisters, discomfort with urination and narrowing of the urinary stream, changing anatomy of the genitalia, paraphimosis, urinary retention, or even renal failure. The prepuce becomes sclerotic; there is meatal "pin hole" narrowing, with ulceration of the foreskin. The glans and undersurface of the prepuce are shiny and bluish white, and there can be considerable telangiectasia **(Fig. 1)**.

➲ ASSOCIATED CONDITIONS

Morphea and vitiligo.

➲ DERMOSCOPY

Yellowish structureless areas with comedone-like openings.

➲ DIFFERENTIAL DIAGNOSIS

- Lichen planus
- Cicatricial pemphigoid
- Zoon's balanitis
- Contact dermatitis
- Fixed drug eruption

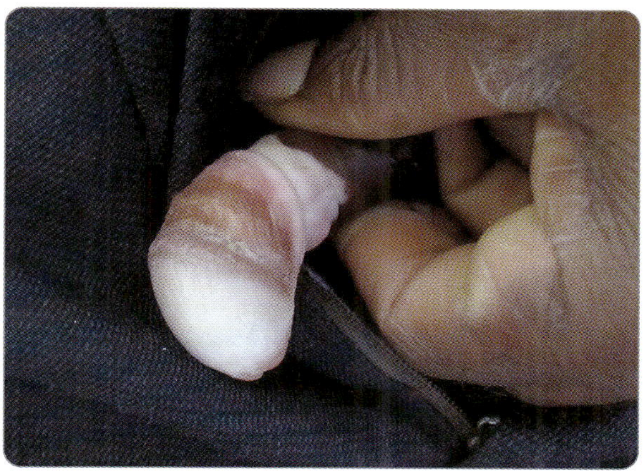

Fig. 1: Acquired phimosis with depigmentation due to balanitis xerotica obliterans.

TREATMENT

Contact with soap and urine should be avoided. Asymptomatic cases need not be treated. A very potent topical corticosteroid is effective. Secondary candidal and bacterial infection should be treated. Testosterone propionate ointment, topical calcineurin inhibitors, oral stanozolol, freezing with ethyl chloride, liquid nitrogen cryotherapy, carbon dioxide laser, and adrenocorticotropic hormone (ACTH) have been used. There is no role of systemic steroids.

Surgical modalities include circumcision, frenuloplasty, meatotomy, and sophisticated plastic repair, depending upon the clinical presentation. Foreskin preputioplasty with intralesional triamcinolone can be a good alternative therapy instead of circumcision. Buccal mucosal graft for urethral stricture caused by BXO can be done.

PROGNOSIS

The risk of developing squamous cell carcinoma is around 2–9.5%. The disease is chronic and progressive.

SUGGESTED READING

1. Fergus KB, Lee AW, Baradaran N, Cohen AJ, Stohr BA, Erickson BA, et al. Pathophysiology, Clinical Manifestations, and Treatment of Lichen Sclerosus: A Systematic Review. Urology. 2020;135:11-9.

27 Balanoposthitis

INTRODUCTION

Balanoposthitis means inflammation of the glans and prepuce and can be regarded as a special form of intertrigo. Balanitis refers to the inflammation of the glans penis, while posthitis refers to the inflammation of the prepuce.

EPIDEMIOLOGY

It is a common condition seen in both children and adults, with a prevalence of 12–20%. In pediatric age group, it mainly affects males between 2 and 5 years. In adults, diabetes and uncircumcised penis are the most common risk factors, with a prevalence of 35% in them. Circumcision is known to decrease the prevalence of balanoposthitis by 68%.

ETIOLOGY

Infection is the most common cause of balanoposthitis in India. The preputial sac of a healthy adult man harbors both aerobic and anaerobic bacteria and yeasts. Poor hygiene and systemic diseases such as diabetes mellitus, malignancy, prolonged antibiotics, and immunosuppressive drugs promote infection. *Candida albicans* is the most common organism, and others include group B streptococci, *Bacteroides*, and anaerobes such as *Fusospirochetes*, *Gardnerella vaginalis*, *Trichomonas vaginalis*, and *Gonococci*. Ulcerative venereal diseases such as syphilis, chancroid, donovanosis, lymphogranuloma venereum, and herpes genitalis may also cause erosions or ulcers on the prepuce and glans penis.

Noninfective causes include contact dermatitis, lichen sclerosus et atrophicus, Zoon's balanitis, trauma, and Crohn's disease.

CLINICAL FEATURES

Candidal balanoposthitis (CBP) is characterized by either a smooth erythematous balanitis with peeling of the skin or discrete punctate rash consisting of eroded papules on the glans. A glazed, nonpurulent surface with scaling edge and eroded satellite pustules are the distinguishing features of CBP. Maceration, fissuring, and ulceration of the prepuce may occur. A foul-smelling, purulent, subpreputial discharge may be associated with anaerobic infection **(Fig. 1)**.

Nonspecific balanoposthitis is a manifestation of a dysfunctional foreskin. Patients generally present with dyspareunia and may have variable signs, including eczematous, lichenoid, and Zoon-like inflammation and even scarring. *Candida* and other organisms represent secondary opportunistic infection. Diabetes should be excluded.

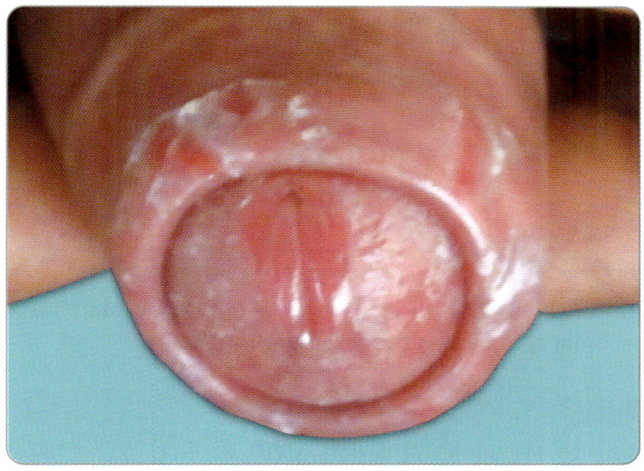

Fig. 1: Candidal balanoposthitis with erythema, edema, and curd-like material deposition.

Recalcitrant cases may represent precancerous or cancerous lesions, including lichen sclerosis and squamous cell carcinoma.

DERMOSCOPY

Linear irregular blurry nonspecific vessels.

DIFFERENTIAL DIAGNOSIS

- Psoriasis
- Fixed drug eruption
- Circinate balanitis
- Nummular eczema
- Diaper rash
- Lichen planus

TREATMENT

Proper washing and drying of the prepuce are the essential preventive measures. The recommended treatment for candidal balanitis is topical clotrimazole cream or a single 150-mg dose of fluconazole. Avoidance of contact with soap and urine and other irritants, treatment for other infections, and medical treatment for lichen sclerosus and lichen planus may be tried. The patient is cured by circumcision; however, this should be defeered till preputial edema is subsided.

PROGNOSIS

Majority of the patients respond to empirical therapy and good hygiene practices; however, 10% of patients may show recurrence and might require detailed evaluation.

SUGGESTED READING

1. Pandya I, Shinojia M, Vadukul D, Marfatia YS. Approach to balanitis/balanoposthitis: Current guidelines. Indian J Sex Transm Dis AIDS. 2014;35(2):155-7.

28 Basal Cell Carcinoma

➲ SYNONYMS

Rodent ulcer, Jacobi ulcer, trichoblastic carcinoma, basal cell epithelioma, epithelioma basocellulare, basalioma.

➲ ETIOLOGY

Exposure to ultraviolet radiation (UVR), arsenic, grenz ray, X-ray, and immunosuppression may induce basal cell carcinoma (BCC). Xeroderma pigmentosa, epidermodysplasia verruciformis, nevus sebaceous, Bazex syndrome, Rombo syndrome, and Gorlin's syndrome are the predisposing conditions. Several genes are known to be involved including *PTCH1*, *MC1R*, *ASIP*, *TYR*, *SMO*, TP53, GLI1/2, etc.

➲ EPIDEMIOLOGY

Basal cell carcinoma is the most common of the skin cancers, with a male:female ratio of 2:1. It is rarely seen below 40 years of age.

➲ CLINICAL FEATURES

Basal cell carcinomas may be divided into the following types:

- Nodular BCC (classic BCC) is the most common type and accounts for more than 60% of cases. It is characterized by raised, translucent papule or nodule with telangiectasias, and has a propensity for the face **(Fig. 1)**.

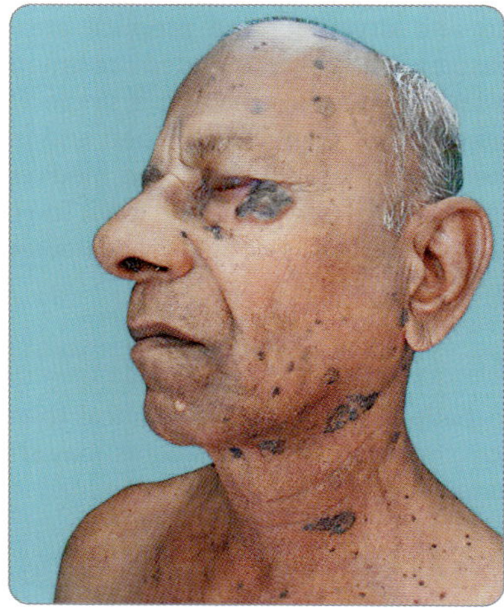

Fig. 1: Multiple basal cell carcinomas (BCCs) with rolled out borders.

- Superficial BCC presents as an erythematous macule or thin plaque, and has to be differentiated clinically from actinic keratosis. This variant of BCC is more often found on the trunk and extremities.
- Morphea form BCC (cicatricial) lesion is indurated and red or whitish in color, and there may be overlying telangiectasia.

Other types include cystic, infiltrative, micronodular, superficial multicentric, fibroepithelioma of Pinkus, polypoid, pore-like, and aberrant.

DERMOSCOPY

Blue-gray ovoid nests, maple leaf-like areas, a spoke wheel pattern, ulceration, arborising telangiectasias, blue-black globules, and absence of pigment network.

HISTOPATHOLOGY

Usually, BCCs are well differentiated, and cells appear histolog cally similar to basal cells of the epidermis. Tumor cells of nodular BCC have large, hyperchromatic, oval nuclei and little cytoplasm, and lack intercellular bridges. A mitotic figure is very rarely observed. Nodular aggregates of basalioma cells are present in the dermis and exhibit peripheral palisading and retraction artifact because of shrinkage of mucin during tissue fixation and staining **(Fig. 2)**.

DIFFERENTIAL DIAGNOSIS

- Actinic keratosis
- Angiofibroma—proliferation of vessels on histopathological examination (HPE)
- Psoriasis—scaly plaques with classical psoriasiform pattern on HPE
- Bowen's disease
- Fibrous papule of the face
- Malignant melanoma—presence of dysplastic melanocytes and absence of basaloid cells

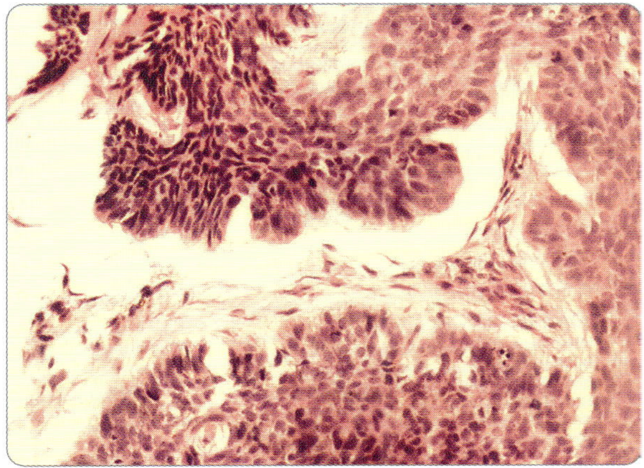

Fig. 2: Peripheral palisading of tumor cells with retraction cleft.

- Molluscum contagiosum
- Nevi
- Sebaceous hyperplasia
- Squamous cell carcinoma—presence of multiple horn pearls

COMPLICATIONS

The disease can cause severe disfigurement if not treated early due to local invasion.

TREATMENT

Topical and local destructive modalities are used for low risk and superficial lesions. The use of a chemotherapeutic agent such as 5-fluorouracil or imiquimod on premalignant lesions and severely sun exposed skin can prevent development of skin cancer.

The following methods are employed in the treatment of basal cell carcinoma: Standard surgical excision, Mohs surgery, 5-fluorouracil, topical treatment with 5% imiquimod cream, radiation therapy, photodynamic therapy, cryosurgery, electrodesiccation and curettage, vismodegib, sonidegib, patidegib, taladegib [cyclopamine—competitive antagonist of the smoothened receptor (SMO), which is part of the hedgehog signaling pathway]. Immunotherapy with checkpoint inhibitors such as pembrolizumab, nivolumab, ipilimumab, and cemiplimab (PD-1 antibody) is being tried.

PROGNOSIS

The prognosis is good. Metastasis is very rare (0.028–0.55%).

SUGGESTED READING

1. Cameron MC, Lee E, Hibler BP, Barker CA, Mori S, Cordova M, et al. Basal cell carcinoma: Epidemiology; pathophysiology; clinical and histological subtypes; and disease associations. J Am Acad Dermatol. 2019;80(2):303-17.

29 Becker's Nevus

➲ SYNONYMS

Becker hamartoma, Becker's melanosis, pigmented hairy epidermal nevus.

➲ HISTORY

The condition was first described by William Becker in 1949.

➲ ETIOLOGY

Becker's nevus is an acquired hyperpigmented epidermal nevus.

➲ EPIDEMIOLOGY

The lesion is androgen-dependent and becomes more prominent in adolescence, especially in the male population in which hypertrichosis is often associated.

➲ CLINICAL FEATURES

Becker's nevus presents as an area of increased pigmentation, often associated with increased hair growth, which is usually seen on the scapular region, although it has been described in other areas of the body **(Fig. 1)**. The hairiness always appears after the pigmentation. Acne lesions may also develop. Associated anomalies, such as ipsilateral breast hypoplasia, musculoskeletal abnormalities (scoliosis, ipsilateral limb hypoplasia, etc.), maxillofacial abnormalities, multiple leiomyomas, and additional cutaneous hypoplasias, occur in the rare Becker's nevus syndrome.

➲ DERMOSCOPY

Well-defined pigment network, perifollicular and focal hypopigmentation, hypertrophic hair follicles, skin furrow, and blood vessels are the characteristics.

➲ HISTOPATHOLOGY

Normal numbers of melanocytes, with increased levels of melanin, are seen in the basal epidermal layer (epidermal melanotic hypermelanosis). The epidermis is acanthotic with variable hyperkeratosis and elongation of the rete ridges. In the dermis, the number of arrector pili muscles are increased, making it difficult to differentiate from the related smooth muscle hamartoma.

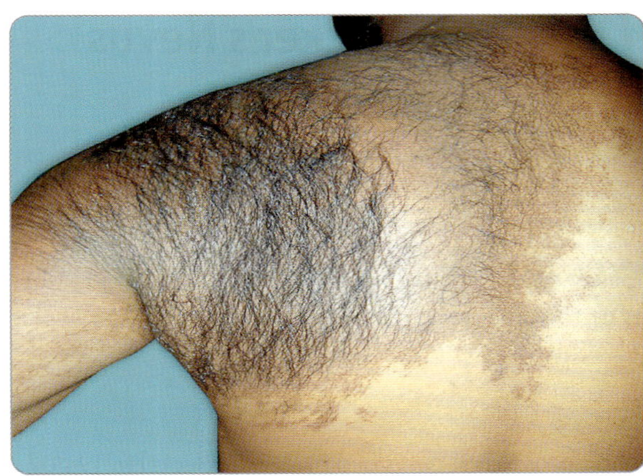

Fig. 1: Hyperpigmented patch with excessive hair over scapular region extending on to the arm.

DIFFERENTIAL DIAGNOSIS

- Melanoma
- Congenital melanocytic nevus
- Café au lait macule
- Nevus spilus—hyperpigmented patch with dark macules giving a typical spotted appearance, absence of increased hair
- Postinflammatory hyperpigmentation—can occur at any site following trauma/inflammation

TREATMENT

No treatment is required as it is a benign condition, although various lasers such as Q-switched lasers such as 694-nm Ruby laser, 1064-nm Nd:YAG laser, 755-nm alexandrite laser, and ablative lasers such as 2940-nm erbium:YAG lasers have been used for cosmetic benefit. Electrolysis and laser hair reduction using diode, Nd:YAG laser, etc., can be done for excessive hair.

PROGNOSIS

Once present, these nevi stabilize after several months or years. Spontaneous regression is not known. Becker nevus is a benign condition and malignant transformation is extremely rare, although association with malignant melanoma has been reported.

SUGGESTED READING

1. Patel P, Malik K, Khachemoune A. Sebaceus and Becker's Nevus: Overview of Their Presentation, Pathogenesis, Associations, and Treatment. Am J Clin Dermatol. 2015;16(3):197-204.

30 Behçet's Disease

➲ SYNONYMS

Adamantiades–Behçet's disease, Behçet's syndrome, Morbus Behçet, Silk road disease.

➲ HISTORY

It is named after the Turkish dermatologist Hulusi Behçet, who first described the clinical features.

➲ EPIDEMIOLOGY

Behçet's disease typically affects young adults, common in Middle Eastern and Japanese (i.e., "silk route") populations. The disease is more common and severe in men. Onset is common in age group 20–35 years.

➲ ETIOLOGY

Although the exact cause of Behçet's disease is unknown, a genetic component of the disease is suggested by its association with human leukocyte antigen B51 (HLA-B51). The possibility that infections may stimulate an abnormal immune response in persons susceptible to Behçet's disease has some support. Other genes include *MICA-A6* and *TNF-1031C* genes. Parvovirus B19 DNA was detected significantly in few patients. Other organisms such as *Borrelia burgdorferi*, *Helicobactor pylori*, *Streptococcus sanguinis*, *Staphylococcus aureus*, and *Mycoplasma* are also implicated. Increased platelet activation has also been suggested as an explanation for the thrombotic component of the disease.

➲ CLINICAL FEATURES

Patients typically have oral aphthae and genital aphthae (90%), cutaneous pustular vasculitis, ocular lesions, or arthritis.

International Study Group criteria for the diagnosis of Behcet's disease include:

- Oral aphthae that recurred at least 3 times in one 12-month period

Plus two of the following criteria:

1. Recurrent genital ulceration
2. *Eye lesions*: Anterior uveitis, posterior uveitis, or cells in vitreous on slit-lamp examination; or retinal vasculitis
3. *Skin lesions*: Erythema nodosum, pseudofolliculitis or papulopustular lesions; acneiform nodules
4. Positive pathergy test

Other systems such as gastrointestinal, lung, and central nervous system (CNS) are also involved.

ASSOCIATED CONDITIONS

Behçet's disease is associated with leukocytoclastic vasculitis, thrombotic arterial or venous disease, pyoderma gangrenosum, and Sweet's syndrome.

DERMOSCOPY

It is nonspecific. Vascular component is more common in oral apthae, and dots were the most common form of vessels in both skin and oral lesions. Oral lesions had a central white structureless area with an erythematous or pink background.

HISTOPATHOLOGY

Large vessel involvement tends to be thrombotic or aneurysmal. The mucosal lesions have neutrophilic vascular reaction initially, later lesions are lymphocytic, and primary lymphocytic vasculitis occurs in erythema nodosum-like lesions. Pustular lesions are sterile. Three main types of reactions have been described in Behçet's disease: Vascular, extravascular with or without vasculopathy, suppurative or mixed suppurative/granulomatous folliculitis comprising acneiform lesions.

DIFFERENTIAL DIAGNOSIS

- Herpes simplex infection—tender erosions/ulcers preceded by vesicles, tender inguinal lymphadenopathy, recurrent lesions, multinucleated giant cells on Tzanck smear
- Ulcerative colitis
- Crohn's disease
- Lichen planus—superficial erosions, no halo, lack of pathergy, and typical histopathological examination (HPE) picture
- Pemphigoid
- Benign aphthous stomatitis—absence of pathergy and absence of cutaneous lesions
- Systemic lupus erythematosus (SLE)—absence of other features of SLE
- Reiter's disease—presence of circinate balanitis and keratoderma blenorrhagicum
- Hypereosinophilic syndrome
- Sweet's syndrome

TREATMENT

Oral or genital ulcers may be treated symptomatically with topical or intralesional corticosteroids, sucralfate gel, tacrolimus, viscous lidocaine, and betamethasone/triamcinolone mouthwashes, chlorhexidine, tetracyclin, or triclosan mouthwashes.

Patients who have manifestations other than mucocutaneous involvement may be treated with systemic corticosteroids, azathioprine, methotrexate, ciclosporin, intravenous immunoglobulin, aspirin, infliximab or etanercerpt, colchicine (0.6 mg two to three times daily), dapsone 100 mg PO daily, apremilast, thalidomide 100–300 mg PO, or pentoxifylline 300 mg/day. Cyclophosphamide and interleukin 1 blockers (anakinra and canakinumab) are also being used.

➲ PROGNOSIS

Behçet's disease is a chronic recurrent condition and approximately 25% of patients with eye lesions become blind.

➲ SUGGESTED READING

1. McCarty MA, Garton RA, Jorizzo JL. Complex aphthosis and Behçet's disease. Dermatol Clin. 2003;21:418.

31 Blastomycosis

➲ SYNONYMS

North American blastomycosis, Gilchrist's disease, and blastomycetic dermatitis.

➲ HISTORY

Blastomycosis was first described in 1939 by Martin and Smith (based on previous work by Thomas Casper Gilchrist).

➲ ETIOLOGY

Blastomycosis is caused by the dimorphic fungi *Blastomyces dermatitidis*. It exists in warm moist soil that is rich in organic matter, such as riverbanks, lakeshores, along streams, and in swamps. When these microfoci are disturbed, the aerosolized spores or conidia are inhaled into the lungs.

➲ EPIDEMIOLOGY

Adult males between 30 and 50 years are commonly affected. Most cases are seen in states that are near the Mississippi, Ohio, and Tennessee Rivers and the Great Lakes, where growth conditions are favorable.

➲ CLINICAL FEATURES

The chief site of involvement is the lungs, but disseminated forms may involve bones, the central nervous system (CNS), the adrenal, the epididymis, and other sites.

- *Primary cutaneous form*: After inoculation, an erythematous, indurated area with a chancre appears in 1–2 weeks with associated lymphangitis and lymphadenopathy.
- *Pulmonary blastomycosis:* There may be no symptoms, or there may be low-grade fever, chest pain, cough, and hemoptysis. Occasionally, erythema nodosum develops. The pulmonary lesion may resolve, or there may be cavity formation with a lung abscess.
- *Disseminated blastomycosis:* Skin lesions are common presenting features. Lesions are symmetric and usually affect the face and extremities. The early lesion is a papule or nodule, which may ulcerate and discharge pus, or enlarge to form a hyperkeratotic lesion, often with central ulceration and/or scarring. Oral lesions are less common.

Other forms include genitourinary, osseous, and central nervous system blastomycosis.

HISTOPATHOLOGY

The skin lesions follow the bloodstream and show marked epidermal hyperplasia, which may be pseudoepitheliomatous. Intra and subepidermal polymorphonuclear abscesses and granulomatous infiltrates are found in the dermis. These include giant cells of Langhans' type, which contain round or oval organisms with thick, refractile walls.

KOH mount shows thick-walled, rounded refractile spherical cells with broad-based buds.

On dermoscopy overlapping papillomatous structures, and hemorrhagic crusting with irregular vessels are seen.

DIFFERENTIAL DIAGNOSIS

Tuberculosis: The presence of granulomas with a cuff of lymphocytes, Langhan's giant cells, and AFB on HPE:

- *Syphilis*: The presence of other lesions, history of the chancre, venereal disease research laboratory (VDRL) positivity
- Other deep mycosis—demonstration of the causative fungi
- Nonmelanoma skin cancers
- Pyoderma gangrenosum—ulcers with necrotic slough and violaceous border, healing with cribriform scarring
- Drug reactions due to bromides and iodides.

COMPLICATIONS

Dissemination and multiple organ involvement.

TREATMENT

Itraconazole 200–400 mg daily for 6 months, fluconazole 400–800 mg/day, or ketoconazole 400 mg/day for 6 months is effective. Amphotericin B 1 mg/kg/day is used for widespread disseminated forms. Other drugs include fluconazole (400–800 mg daily), voriconazole, posaconazole, and isavuconazole. Surgical debridement may be needed in a few cases.

PROGNOSIS

The prognosis is good. Most lesions resolve within 4 weeks of treatment. Disseminated and pulmonary forms require a longer duration of treatment.

SUGGESTED READING

1. Wang S, Martini MC, Groth JV, Hernandez C. Dermatoscopic and clinicopathologic findings of cutaneous blastomycosis. J Am Acad Dermatol. 2015;73(5):e169-70.

32 Botryomycosis

SYNONYMS

Bacterial pseudomycosis, staphylococcal actinophytosis, granular bacteriosis, and actinobacillosis.

INTRODUCTION

Botryomycosis is a chronic, granulomatous, suppurative bacterial infection involving the skin and subcutaneous tissues. The skin lesion is characterized by multiple fistulae draining purulent secretion with white-yellowish grains periodic acid–Schiff (PAS) positive.

HISTORY

Bollinger discovered the disease in a horse in 1870, and in 1884 Rivolta, under the impression that it is caused by fungus, named it Botryomycosis. In 1913, Opie reported the first case in humans. Magrou, in 1919, reported four cases and the isolated agent was *Staphylococcus aureus*. Winslow, in 1959, reviewed the disease and assessed 46 cases in humans, classifying it as cutaneous and visceral forms. The term "botryomycosis" is derived from the Greek word "botrys" (meaning "bunch of grapes") and "mycosis" (a misnomer, due to the presumed fungal etiology in early descriptions).

ETIOLOGY

The main etiologic agent is *Staphylococcus aureus* and other less frequent pathogens are *Pseudomonas aeruginosa*, actinophytosis, staphylococcal actinophytosis, bacterial pseudomycosis, granular bacteriosis and *Escherichia coli*, isolated or associated.

CLINICAL FEATURES

The skin lesions are single or multiple and pleomorphic, with multiple cysts, abscesses, fistulas, nodules, plaques, or ulcers. They are usually located in areas exposed to traumas (head, arms, and legs) and genital regions. Muscles, aponeuroses, tendons, and bones may also be affected. The general swollen and suppurative aspect of the lesion suggests local inoculation of a foreign body as the initial cause of infection and perpetuation of the disease.

HISTOPATHOLOGY

There is a rim of an eosinophilic matrix composed of antigen-antibody complex, tissue debris and fibrin around the bacterial granules and colonies called the Splendore–Hoeppli phenomenon (SHP).

The grains in botryomycosis are large and lobulated which are clusters of bacteria that do not have a filamentous structure.

➲ ASSOCIATED CONDITIONS/RISK FACTORS

- Altered immune function
- Diabetes mellitus
- Liver disease
- Alcoholism
- Lupus, cystic fibrosis, and asthma
- Malnutrition
- Immunoglobulin deficiency, hyperglobulinemia E (Job syndrome)
- Glomerulonephritis
- Long-term treatment with corticosteroids
- Human immunodeficiency virus/acquired immunodeficiency syndrome

➲ DIFFERENTIAL DIAGNOSIS

- Actinomycetoma
- Eumycetoma
- Scrofuloderma
- Nocardiosis

➲ TREATMENT

The treatment with a prolonged course of antibiotics depending upon pus culture and sensitivity is recommended for botryomycosis. However, appropriate antibiotics in combination with surgical excision are the most effective therapy for botryomycosis.

➲ SUGGESTED READING

1. Devi B, Behera B, Dash ML, Puhan MR, Pattnaik SS, Patro S. Botryomycosis. Indian J Dermatol. 2013;58(5):406.

33 Bowen's Disease

➲ SYNONYMS

Squamous cell carcinoma in situ.

➲ HISTORY

Bowen's disease was named after American dermatologist John T Bowen who first described the condition in 1912.

➲ ETIOLOGY

Exposure to solar radiation, radiotherapy, photochemotherapy, arsenic, human papillomavirus infection, immunosuppression, and chronic injury are predisposing causes.

➲ EPIDEMIOLOGY

Occurs mostly in elderly women (70–80%), and is rare before the age of 30 years.

➲ CLINICAL FEATURES

Bowen's disease is a form of intraepidermal squamous cell carcinoma (SCC) characterized by a persistent, scaly, or crusted plaque that is symptomless and gradually enlarges in a somewhat irregular fashion with a small potential for invasive malignancy. Progressive growth is usual but spontaneous partial regression occurs occasionally. Ulceration is usually a sign of the development of invasive carcinoma. Persistent superficial ulceration may, however, be the early clinical evidence of Bowen's disease of palmar skin without invasion. The risk of progression into invasive carcinoma is 3–5% in extragenital and 10% in genital lesions **(Fig. 1)**.

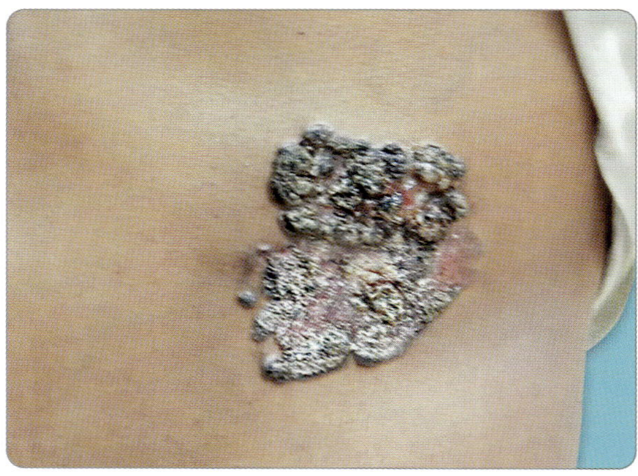

Fig. 1: Hyperkeratotic plaque with crusting of Bowen's disease.

DERMOSCOPY

Glomerular vessels, scales, small brown pigmented globules which are regularly packed and patchy, structureless gray to brown pigmentation.

HISTOPATHOLOGY

The normal epidermis is replaced by abnormal keratinocytes (windblown appearance) with acanthosis. The atypical cells have hyperchromatic nuclei. Giant, multinucleate cells and mitotic figures are frequently seen. The surface is formed by a thickened, loose, parakeratotic scale. Proliferating cells may be surrounded by relatively normal epidermal cells to give a "Borst–Jadassohn" appearance. There is retention of a distinct dermal–epidermal junction.

DIFFERENTIAL DIAGNOSIS

- Lichen simplex—presence of lesions at characteristic sites (nape of neck and ankles), absence of atypical cells on histopathological examination (HPE).
- Psoriasis—classical involvement of extensors, scalp, and nails; psoriasiform pattern on HPE.
- Superficial (pagetoid)—type of basal cell carcinoma (BCC).
- Actinic keratosis—lesions only on sun-exposed areas, crusted papules, absence of atypical keratinocytes.
- Lupus vulgaris—tubercular granulomas on HPE, Mantoux positivity.
- Tinea corporis—demonstration of fungal hyphae on potassium hydroxide (KOH) mount.
- Nummular eczema—absence of dysplasia of epidermis.
- Paget's disease

TREATMENT

Treatment options include cryotherapy, curettage and cautery, photodynamic therapy, laser destruction, excision, 5-fluorouracil cream, imiquimod cream, and radiotherapy. Other treatment options include local hyperthermia, ultrasonic surgical aspiration, diclofenac gel, 1% tribulation ointment, carbon ion therapy, etc.

PROGNOSIS

The prognosis is favorable. The risk of malignancy is about 10% in genital lesions (erythroplasia of Queyrat).

SUGGESTED READING

1. Maria Wozniak-Rito A, Rudnicka L. Bowen's disease in dermoscopy. Acta Dermatovenerol Croat. 2018;26(2):157-61.

34 Bowenoid Papulosis

➲ HISTORY

Bowenoid papulosis was described in 1977 by Kopf and Bart as papules on the penis and named after the dermatologist John Templeton Bowen.

➲ ETIOLOGY

Bowenoid papulosis is associated with human papillomavirus (HPV) infection; commonly HPV-16. Other genotypes include HPV-18, -31, -33, -34, -35, -39, -42, -48, -51, -52, 53, and -54. Smoking and immunosuppression are known to increase the rate of occurrence.

➲ EPIDEMIOLOGY

Lesions are seen in both men and women of sexually active age group, can aapear at any age but more predominantly in their third to the mid-fifth decade.

➲ CLINICAL FEATURES

Bowenoid papulosis appears as asymptomatic papules commonly on genitalia of males and extragenital sites in females. The lesions are pigmented, solitary to multiple, well-demarcated papules with a flat or verrucous surface. Bowenoid papulosis lesions are less papillomatous, smooth topped, more polymorphic and more coalescent than condylomata acuminata **(Fig. 1)**. Transformation to malignancy is rare and occurs in <1% of patients. Females affected or who have partners with Bowenoid papulosis are at high risk of developing cervical carcinoma.

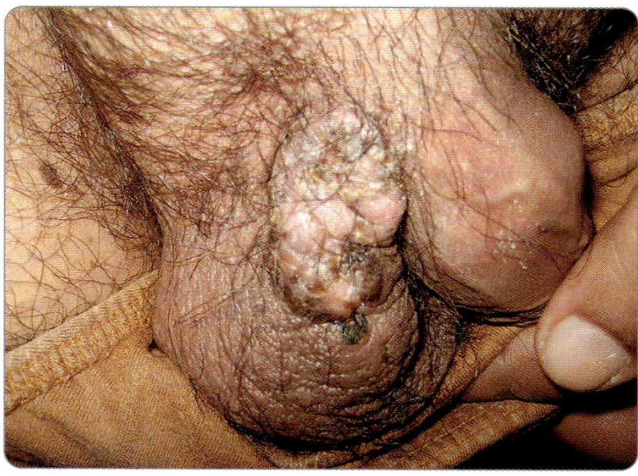

Figs. 1: Grouped papules over the scrotum in bowenoid papulosis.

➲ DERMOSCOPY

Brown-gray dots with a linear arrangement, located at the periphery of the lesion with widespread dotted vessels.

➲ HISTOPATHOLOGY

Full-thickness epidermal dysplasia resembling wind blown appearance of Bowen's disease may be seen. Koilocytes are present in epidermis. The dermoepidermal junction is intact and a few abnormal mitotic figures may be present.

➲ DIFFERENTIAL DIAGNOSIS

- *Bowen's disease*: Lesions are usually plaques with crusting, scaling more than papules; no relation to HPV and hence absence of koilocytes.
- Melanocytic nevus—presence of nevus cells on histopathological examination (HPE), rarely occur on genital area
- Lichen planus—presence of violaceous papules, which are typically pruritic, lichenoid band-like infiltrate, and basal cell degeneration on HPE
- Molluscum contagiosum—pearly white lesions with umbilication
- Seborrheic keratosis—dermoscopic findings and squamous eddies on HPE
- Angiolymphoid hyperplasia—reddish looking lesions, rarely on genitalia; proliferation of vessels with plump endothelial calls
- Squamous cell carcinoma—multiple horn pearls on biopsy
- Genital warts—history of (H/o) lesions after exposure and lack of epidermal dysplasia

➲ TREATMENT

The treatment modalities include local excision, electrodesiccation, cryosurgery, topical retinoic acid, ablation with carbon dioxide (CO_2) laser, imiquimod 5%, 5-fluorouracil, 5-aminolevulinic, acid-mediated photodynamic therapy.

➲ PROGNOSIS

It has a variable course. Recurrences after treatment are common, and rate of malignant transformation is around 2.5%.

➲ SUGGESTED READING

1. Guo J, Chang JM, Liu W. Bowenoid papulosis. Int J Dermatol Venereol. 2020;3(1):58-9.

35 Bullous Pemphigoid

➲ HISTORY

Lever in 1953, based on histopathological findings, recognized bullous pemphigoid (BP) as a distinct disorder. Jordon, Beutner, and colleagues demonstrated tissue-bound and circulating autoantibodies directed against the cutaneous basement membrane zone (BMZ) in 1950s.

➲ ETIOLOGY

The risk of developing pemphigoid increases with age. It is an immune-mediated disease that is associated with a humoral and cellular response directed against two well-characterized self-antigens: The BP antigen 180 and the BP antigen 230. These two antigens are the components of the hemidesmosomes, which are adhesion complexes promoting epithelial–stromal adhesion in stratified and other complex epithelia, such as the skin and mucous membranes. Genetic predisposition with human leukocyte antigen (HLA)-DQB1*0301 is seen in a few cases. BP appears to be triggered by trauma, burns, radiotherapy, ultraviolet (UV) irradiation, vaccination, viruses [cytomegalovirus (CMV), Epstein–Barr Virus (EBV), human herpesvirus 6 (HHV-6), HHV-8, hepatitis B, and hepatis C)], *H. pylori*, *Toxoplasma gondii,* and drugs (penicillamine, furosemide, captopril, penicillin, and sulfasalazine).

➲ EPIDEMIOLOGY

It is a disease of elderly people, with an onset usually after 60 years of age. However, it can be seen at any age.

➲ CLINICAL FEATURES

In the prodromal phase, signs and symptoms are frequently nonspecific, with mild to severe intractable pruritus alone or with excoriated, eczematous, papular and/or urticarial lesions that may persist for several weeks or months. The bullous stage of BP is characterized by the development of vesicles and bullae on apparently normal or erythematous skin together with urticarial and infiltrated papules and plaques that occasionally assume an annular or figurate pattern. The blisters are tense, up to 1–4 cm in diameter, contain a clear fluid, and may persist for several days, leaving eroded and crusted lesion **(Fig. 1)**. The lesions frequently have a symmetrical distribution, and they predominate on the flexural aspects of the limbs and the lower trunk, including the abdomen. Within intertriginous zones, vegetating plaques can be observed. Residual postinflammatory hyper- and hypopigmentation

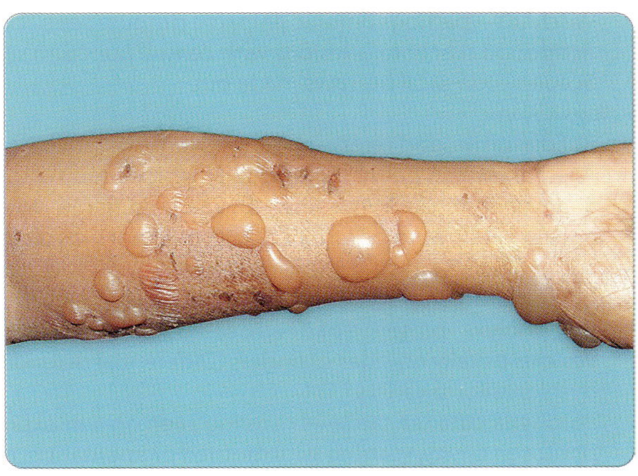

Fig. 1: Tense bulla over the forearm in bullous pemphigoid.

may be seen. Involvement of the oral cavity is observed in 10–30% of patients. In approximately 50% of patients, a peripheral blood eosinophilia is noted.

Variants of BP are nonbullous, erythrodermic, subacute prurigo, pemphigoid vegetans, localized, pemphigoid gestationis, cicatricial pemphigoid, urticarial, vesicular, dyshidrosiform, and seborrheic.

➲ ASSOCIATED CONDITIONS

Associated conditions include internal malignancies, autoimmune disorders such as rheumatoid arthritis, Hashimoto's thyroiditis, dermatomyositis, lupus erythematosus, and autoimmune thrombocytopenia.

➲ HISTOPATHOLOGY

In the nonbullous phase, less specific changes, such as subepidermal clefts and eosinophilic spongiosis, may be found. An early bulla shows a subepidermal blister at the level of lamina lucida accompanied by a dermal inflammatory infiltrate composed of eosinophils and mononuclear cells. The infiltrate favors the uppermost dermis, and the cavity of the bulla contains a net of fibrin with a variable inflammatory infiltrate. Direct immunofluorescence (DIF) microscopy studies of perilesional, uninvolved skin will characteristically demonstrate the presence of fine, linear, continuous deposits of IgG, and/or C3 along the epidermal basement membrane.

➲ DIFFERENTIAL DIAGNOSIS

- *Nonbullous phase*:
  - Drug reactions
  - Contact dermatitis—lesions present at site of contact only, history of (H/o) trigger
  - Prurigo—lack of erythematous patches, only excoriations/erosions seen
  - Urticaria—lesions are evanescent

    - Vasculitis—pathognomonic palpable purpura seen
    - Arthropod reactions—lesions with central punctum seen
    - Scabies—classical burrows made out
- *Bullous lesions*:
    - Bullous arthropod bites—negative DIF
    - Allergic contact dermatitis—smaller vesicles seen
    - Stevens–Johnson syndrome—bullae and large erosions appear following drug intake, mucosal involvement common
    - Bullous drug eruptions—negative DIF
    - Pompholyx—presence of deep-seated itchy sago grain-like vesicles usually on sides of fingers (Differential diagnosis for dyshidrosiform variety)
    - Porphyria cutanea tarda—blistering seen on sun exposure, photosensitivity, scarring with mottled pigmentation, raised porphyrin levels
    - Epidermolysis bullosa acquisita—lesions seen mostly at trauma prone sites; salt split skin immunofluorescence shows deposition only on the floor.
    - Linear immunoglobulin A (IgA) dermatosis—presence of clustered "string of pearls" like bullae; IgA linear deposits on DIF instead of IgG, C3

TREATMENT

Since most of the patients are elderly, aim is to suppress disease activity with minimum usage of drugs. Topical and systemic steroids are the mainstay of therapy. Prednisolone 0.3 mg/kg/day in mild and localized disease to 1 mg/kg/day in severe disease can be started. Other drugs include tetracycline 500 mg QID along with nicotinamide 500 mg QID, or azathioprine 2.5 mg/kg/day, dapsone, methotrexate, cyclophosphamide, mycophenolate mofetil (MMF), leflunomide, chlorambucil, intravenous immunoglobulin (IVIg), plasmapheresis, rituximab, and omalizumab.

PROGNOSIS

Blood pressure is a chronic disease characterized by spontaneous exacerbations and remissions. Because of the intractable pruritus, and the presence of bullous, eroded or impetiginized lesions, the disease is often accompanied by a significant morbidity with a profound impact on the quality of life.

Indicators of poor prognosis are age, generalized disease, low Karnofsky's score, low albumin, and high dosage of steroids used.

SUGGESTED READING

1. Bernard P, Antonicelli F. Bullous pemphigoid: a review of its diagnosis, associations and treatment. Am J Clinical Dermatol. 2017;18:513-28.

36 Café-au-lait Macule

➲ SYNONYMS

Pigmented birthmarks, giraffe spots, Coffee in milk (French) appearance.

➲ HISTORY

Marie and Bernard (1896) and Chauffard (1896) described the association of certain type of pigmentation with genodermatoses.

➲ ETIOLOGY

Café-au-lait macules (CALMs) are caused by increase in melanin content, often with presence of giant melanosomes.

➲ EPIDEMIOLOGY

Lesions may appear at or soon after birth, increase in number and size with age. It is present in 10–20% of normal children. There is no sex predilection.

➲ CLINICAL FEATURES

Discrete well-circumscribed, uniformly pale brown, oval macules that vary in size from 0.5 to 20 cm and can be found on any cutaneous surface. Borders may be smooth or irregular. It may occur as an isolated phenomenon or as a marker of multisystem disease. Isolated CALMs are less than 3 in number, measuring 0.5–1.5 cm, and occurs in 10–20% of normal population **(Fig. 1)**.

➲ DERMOSCOPY

Homogenous or accentuated reticular brown pigmentation with perifollicular halo, sparing of perieccrine and perifollicular areas.

➲ ASSOCIATED SYNDROMES

Multiple CALMs are associated with underlying syndromes:

- *Neurofibromatosis (NF-1)*: Six or more spots >5 mm in children <10 years or 15 mm in adults. Borders are smooth, compared with "Coast of California".
- Tuberous sclerosis
- *McCune–Albright syndrome*: Lesions have irregular border-shaped like the "Coast of Maine"
- Silver–Russell syndrome
- Watson syndrome
- Legius syndrome
- Noonan syndrome

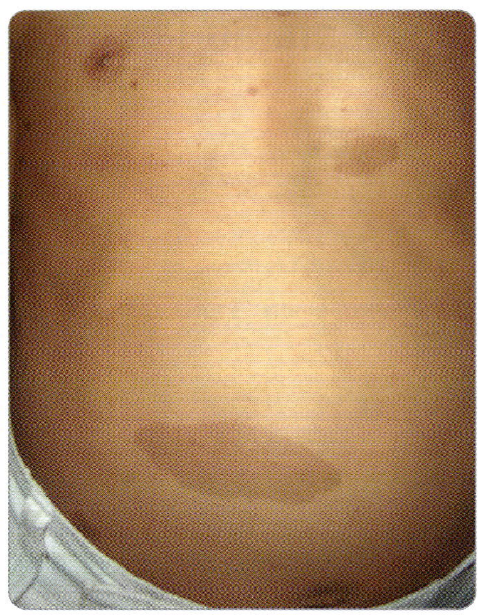

Fig. 1: Well-circumscribed, hyperpigmented macules of café-au-lait macules (CALMs) with irregular borders.

- Bloom syndrome
- Gastrocutaneous syndrome
- Multiple Lentigines syndrome
- MEN 2B syndrome
- Bannayan–Riley–Ruvalcaba syndrome
- Maffucci syndrome

HISTOPATHOLOGY

Increase in melanin pigment with macromelanosomes.

DIFFERENTIAL DIAGNOSIS

- Melanocytic nevi—melanocytic activity is present at junction of epidermis and dermis or dermis only or both; lesions are more blackish in color.
- Lentigines—can involve mucosa also
- Becker's nevus—development at puberty, increased hair growth
- Nevus spilus—presence of hyperpigmented spots over the macule/patch
- Tinea versicolor—presence of fine bran-like scales, lesions in seborrheic distribution, and "spaghetti and meatball" appearance on KOH mount
- Seborrheic keratosis—multiple raised lesions with a stuck-on appearance

COMPLICATIONS

Benign condition with no complications unless associated with other conditions.

➲ TREATMENT

No treatment is necessary. Q-switched laser (1064 nm) and erbium YAG laser treatments and hydroquinone 4% cream can be tried. Others include 532 nm Nd-YAG laser, ruby laser (694 nm), and alexandrite laser (755 nm).

➲ PROGNOSIS

Prognosis depends on the underlying disorders.

➲ SUGGESTED READING

1. Lalor L, Davies OM, Basel D, Siegel DH. Café au lait spots: when and how to pursue their genetic origins. Clin Dermatol. 2020;38(4): 421-31.

37 Calcinosis Cutis

INTRODUCTION

Calcinosis cutis is a condition in which calcium salts are deposited in the skin and subcutaneous tissue.

HISTORY

Virchow described calcinosis cutis initially in 1855.

ETIOLOGY

Calcinosis may be caused by trauma, inflammation, varicose veins, tumors, infections, connective tissue disease, hyperphosphatemia, and hypercalcemia. Calcification or calcinosis cutis results due to deposition of calcium and phosphate in collagen and elastic tissue. If the arrangement is like that seen in the bone, it is termed ossification and if the deposition is not organized, it is calcification. In pathological ectopic calcification, the matrix is altered and contains acid proteins. The calcified tissue is made up of hydroxyapatite and amorphous calcium phosphate.

EPIDEMIOLOGY

Calcinosis cutis commonly occurs in patients with systemic sclerosis, especially with limited form. About 25–40% of these patients present with calcinosis cutis.

TYPES

Aberrant calcium deposition in the skin may be divided into:
- Dystrophic
- Idiopathic
- Metastatic
- Iatrogenic

Dystrophic Calcification

The calcinosis is confined to the areas of tissue damage without any metabolic abnormality.

It may be due to dermatomyositis, generalized scleroderma, lupus erythematosus, electrical injury, fibrodysplasia ossificans, traumatic, subcutaneous injection with calcium-containing heparin, radiotherapy, foreign-body, hematoma, fat cell necrosis, acne, varicose veins, tuberculous granuloma, venous stasis, parasitic cysts, sebaceous cysts, lipomas, angiomas, liposarcomas, pseudo-xanthoma elasticum, and Ehlers–Danlos syndrome.

Idiopathic Calcification

The deposition of calcium is unrelated to any recognizable tissue injury or metabolic disorder.

- *Calcinosis universalis*: Nodules or plaques 0.5–5.0 cm are distributed over the extremities and trunk. The lesions may ulcerate, discharging chalk-like creamy material consisting mainly of calcium phosphate. The disease is eventually fatal.
- *Calcinosis circumscripta*: There may be only a few calcium deposits in the skin **(Fig. 1)**.
- *Idiopathic calcinosis of the scrotum*: Calcinosis scrotalis is a rare, benign disorder consisting of multiple asymptomatic firm nodules 0.2–1.0 cm in diameter.
- Tumoral calcinosis
- *Pinnal calcification*: Calcified ear cartilage has been observed in Addison's disease, ochronosis, acromegaly, diabetes mellitus, hyperthyroidism, and systemic chondromalacia.

Metastatic Calcification

In metastatic calcification, calcinosis occurs due to precipitation of calcium salts in normal skin, subcutaneous tissue, muscles, and internal organs. Hypercalcemia may be due to hyperparathyroidism, vitamin D intoxication, milk–alkali syndrome, or destructive bone disease with excessive osteoclastic activity, viz. metastatic carcinoma, multiple myeloma, leukemia, and Paget's disease of bone.

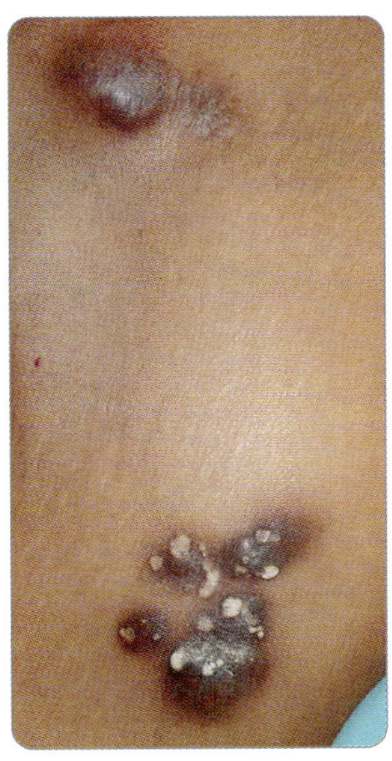

Fig. 1: Multiple nodules discharging chalk-like material.

DERMOSCOPY

Structureless whitish areas, yellowish crust, and accentuation of pigment network.

DIFFERENTIAL DIAGNOSIS

- Milia—soft papules are seen usually on face in the infraorbital area
- Molluscum contagiosum—presence of umbilication
- Osteoma cutis—absence of calcium deposits, negative Von Kossa stain
- Tuberous xanthomas—absence of foamy macrophages and Touton cells
- Mycetoma—classical triad of tumescent swelling, discharging sinuses, and grains having colony of organisms (fungi).

TREATMENT

Medical therapy of calcinosis cutis is of limited benefit. When identified, the underlying problem should be corrected. Intralesional corticosteroids, sodium etidronate and diphosphonates, topical sodium thiosulfate, probenecid, colchicines, warfarin, minocycline, ceftriaxone, diltiazem, magnesium, or aluminum antacids are the phosphate binders in patients with hyperphosphatemia. Myo-inositol hexaphosphonate is a dietary substance, which inhibits the crystallization of calcium salts. Extracorporeal shock wave lithotripsy, carbon dioxide laser, and surgical excision can be done for painful lesions, but the recurrence rate is high.

SUGGESTED READING

1. Róbert L, Kiss N, Medvecz M, Kuroli E, Sárdy M, Hidvégi B. Epidemiology and treatment of calcinosis cutis: 13 years of experience. Indian J Dermatol. 2020;65(2):105-11.

38 Calciphylaxis

INTRODUCTION

Calciphylaxis is a life-threatening disorder characterized by occlusion of microvessels in the subcutaneous adipose tissue and dermis. Calciphylaxis is a rare condition with high morbidity. Calciphylaxis predominantly affects patients with chronic kidney failure treated by dialysis. However, calciphylaxis is not limited to patients treated by dialysis and also occurs in patients with normal kidney function and those with earlier stages of chronic kidney disease (CKD; referred to as nonuremic calciphylaxis).

HISTORY

Hans Selye and his colleagues coined the term calciphylaxis in 1961. Within a few years after these experimental descriptions of calciphylaxis by Selye, two case reports were published that described patients with kidney failure who developed widespread subcutaneous calcifications.

EPIDEMIOLOGY

Calciphylaxis, although rare, has been reported worldwide, with an estimated annualized incidence of 35 cases per 10,000 patients. Calciphylaxis is more commonly seen in women compared with men, with a 2:1 female predominance. It occurs most commonly in the age group 50–70 years. Patients treated with peritoneal dialysis have a higher incidence of calciphylaxis than those treated with hemodialysis.

ETIOLOGY

The risk factors include end-stage renal disease, female sex, obesity, diabetes mellitus, hypercalcemia, hyperphosphatemia, hyperparathyroidism (both primary and secondary), oversuppressed parathyroid hormone (PTH) with adynamic bone disease (low bone turnover), elevated alkaline phosphatase, vitamin K deficiency, hepatobiliary disease, thrombophilia (e.g., antithrombin deficiency, protein C, deficiency, or lupus anticoagulant), and autoimmune disorders (e.g., systemic lupus erythematosus). The microvascular calcifications in patients with calciphylaxis may be an active, cell-mediated process that depends on the balance between the promoters and inhibitors of calcification.

CLINICAL FEATURES

Calciphylaxis causes painful skin lesions. The initial skin manifestations may include induration, plaques, nodules, livedo, or purpura. Dusky discoloration of the skin indicates an area of imminent necrosis. Patients typically have multiple, bilateral lesions, with surrounding skin showing a leather-like texture. The later lesions are stellate, malodorous ulcers with black eschars.

HISTOPATHOLOGY

The characteristic histologic features of calciphylaxis include calcification, microthrombosis, and fibrointimal hyperplasia of small dermal and subcutaneous arteries and arterioles, leading to cutaneous ischemia and intense septal panniculitis.

DERMOSCOPY

Star-like purpuric violaceous-bluish patches with angulated borders and whitish-grayish center.

ASSOCIATED CONDITIONS

Extracutaneous vascular calcifications lead to skeletal myopathy, intestinal bleeding, or visual impairment.

DIFFERENTIAL DIAGNOSIS

- Warfarin-induced skin necrosis
- Atherosclerotic vascular disease
- Venous stasis ulcer
- Cellulitis
- Cholesterol embolization
- Dystrophic calcinosis cutis
- Livedoid vasculopathy
- Nephrogenic systemic fibrosis
- Oxalosis
- Pyoderma gangrenosum
- Purpura fulminans
- Necrotizing vasculitis
- Martorell's ulcer

TREATMENT

Supportive treatment includes opioid analgesia, hyperbaric oxygen therapy, surgical debribement and elimination of risk factors. Treatment also includes sodium thiosulfate (25 g in 100 mL of solution given intravenously three times a week during the last 30–60 minutes of hemodialysis), bisphosphonates, and vitamin K1 supplementation (phylloquinone at a dose of 500 μg/day).

PROGNOSIS

High morbidity is seen with calciphylaxis.

SUGGESTED READING

1. Nigwekar SU, Thadhani R, Brandenburg VM. Calciphylaxis. New Engl J Med. 2018;378(18):1704-14.

39 Corns and Calluses

➲ SYNONYMS

Clavi, heliomata (corn), tylomata, intractable plantar keratosis (calluses).

➲ ETIOLOGY

Corns and calluses are acquired areas of thickened skin that appear over sites of repeated and prolonged trauma to the epithelium.

➲ EPIDEMIOLOGY

Corns and callosity are more common in females than males. Mentally ill health, family history of bony abnormalities or ligamentous laxity, abnormal foot biomechanics, or poor fitting shoes are the risk factors.

➲ CLINICAL FEATURES

Corns are dull aching, sharply demarcated, hyperkeratotic, small areas with a central translucent core (radix/nucleus) and intact skin markings. Direct pressure over corn produces pain, in contrast to warts where lateral pressure elicits pain. Callosities are large, diffuse areas of thickened skin with indefinite margins commonly seen over metacarpophalangeal and interphalangeal joints.

Common sites for callus are as follows:
- *Tree climbers*: Forearms and instep of foot
- Carpenters, black smith, gardeners, farmers: Palms
- *Violinists*: Fingertips/neck
- Taxi drivers: Buttocks
- *Desk workers*: Elbows
- Leprosy and diabetic patients: Callosities may precede perforating ulcers
- *Prayer callus*: Forehead and knees
- *Pinch callus*: In patients with bunions, callus forms at medioplantar aspect of the hallux, during gait, individual rolls off that portion of greater toe, and skin is subsequently pinched off.
- *Durlacher's corn*: It occurs over lateral side of small toe.

Clinical types of corn:
- *Hard corns (heloma durum)*: They are painful with a dry smooth convex surface seen over dorsa of the toes **(Fig. 1)**.
- *Soft corns (clavus molle)*: They are soft, soggy, and macerated seen in interdigital spaces.
- *Vascular corns (clavus vasculare)*: They are painful, modified hard corn in which superficial capillaries have involved epidermis due to repeated trauma.

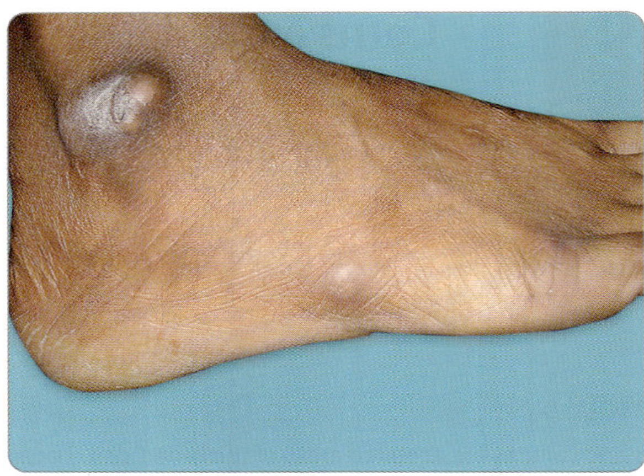

Fig. 1: Diffuse thickening of skin over bony prominences due to sitting cross legged.

- *Neurofibrous corns*: It is an advanced type of painful, hard corn with underlying fibrosis and hypertrophy of nerve filaments.
- *Seed corns (heloma miliare)*: They are multiple asymptomatic, 1–3 mm, yellowish white papules on the plantar surface of heal and 5th toe joint.

HISTOPATHOLOGY

In corns, epidermis shows parakeratotic plug in stratum corneum, loss of stratum granulosum, and atrophy of stratum malphigii. Dermis shows fibrosis, dilated eccrine ducts and blood vessels, and hypertrophied nerves; scar tissue replaces the subcutaneous fat. In callus, stratum granulosum is intact.

DIFFERENTIAL DIAGNOSIS

- Warts—presence not necessarily on pressure areas, interrupted skin markings on the surface, very painful, tender more on lateral pressure, presence of thrombosed vessels/pinpoint bleeding on paring
- Arsenic keratosis—painless, widely distributed over palms and soles, nontender
- Porokeratosis—punctuate variety restricts itself to the creases, nontender; classical cornoid lamella on histopathological examination (HPE)
- Punctuate keratoderma—nontender, located on sites other than weight bearing zones

Warts and corns interrupt dermatoglyphics, while calluses often demonstrate accentuated lines. Paring of a corn reveals a central translucent whitish yellow core, as opposed to the thrombosed capillaries and multiple bleeding points seen in a wart. Paring of a callus reveals layers of yellowish keratin, without the multiple punctate thrombosed capillaries.

DERMOSCOPY

Dermoscopy shows homogenous yellowish area, which is imminent and opaque, focal white scales, and white areas are noted. Physiological lines are preserved, and no red dots are seen.

COMPLICATIONS

Complications include painful ambulation, subhelomal bursitis, blistering, septic arthritis, osteomyelitis, and hemorrhage in keratotic tissue.

TREATMENT

Precipitating factors like ill-fitting shoes should be avoided. Physical modalities such as paring and padding should be employed. Padding includes application of keratolytics, like 40% salicylic acid plaster, after 48 hours rub off the macerated area and reapply the plaster till the corn is gone. 17% salicylic acid and 17% lactic acid in flexible collodion can be applied for 7 days and then, foot is soaked for ½ hour till collodion is peeled off. Surgical correction of bony/ muscular defects should be done.

SUGGESTED READING

1. Murahashi Y, Iba K, Teramoto A, Takahashi K, Okada Y, Kamiya T, et al. Relationship between plantar callosity and foot deformity in hallux valgus using weightbearing computed tomography. J Foot Ankle Surg. 2021;60(6):1207-11.

40 Candidiasis

➲ SYNONYMS

Candidosis, moniliasis, thrush, oidiomycosis, bronchomycosis.

➲ HISTORY

Candida infection in humans was first described by Hippocrates in the fourth century BC in his book "Epidemics". Castellani suggested that yeast species other than *Monilia albicans* might be involved in candidiasis and made the first description of the species currently known *Candida guilliermondii*, *C. krusei*, *C. pseudotropicalis,* and *C. tropicalis*.

➲ ETIOLOGY

Candidiasis is caused by any species of the genus *Candida* most commonly *C. albicans* but other species such as *tropicalis*, *krusei*, *glabrata*, and *parapsilosis*.

➲ EPIDEMIOLOGY

Any age group can be affected, but the very young, very old, and the very ill are prone to it.

➲ CLINICAL FEATURES

Cutaneous candidiasis can present as intertrigo **(Fig. 1)**, diaper candidiasis, nodular candidiasis of diaper area, candidal miliaria, nail candidiasis (paronychia and onychomycosis), and congenital and neonatal candidiasis. Oral candidiasis presents most commonly as thrush (acute pseudomembranous candidiasis). Other presentations include acute and chronic erythematous candidiasis, chronic pseudomembranous candidiasis, angular cheilitis, chronic hyperplastic candidiasis, and median rhomboid glossitis. Genital candidiasis presents as vulvovaginitis **(Fig. 2)** in female and balanoposthitis in male. Chronic mucocutaneous candidiasis consists of many clinical syndromes characterized by chronic treatment resistant superficial candidal infections of the skin, nails, and oropharnyx.

Potassium hydroxide (KOH) mount shows budding yeast cells with pseudohyphae. In gram staining, the organism is visible as gram-positive budding yeast cells with pseudohyphae. Culture on Sabouraud's Dextrose Agar shows cream colored, smooth, pasty, dry and wrinkled colonies. Speciation of *Candida* requires chromogenic media like CHROMagar, which enable species identification of *Candida*.

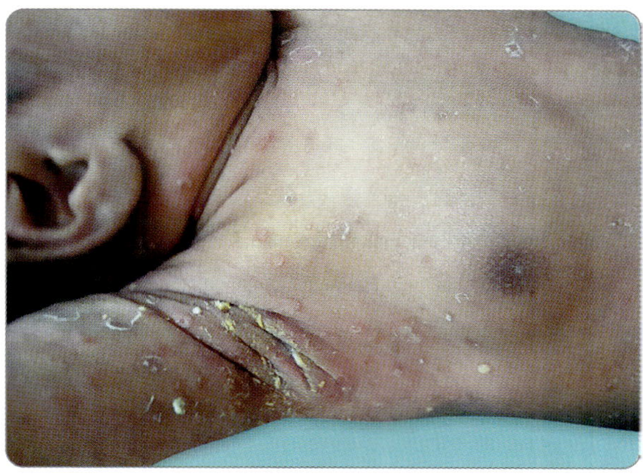

Fig. 1: Erythematous papules with pustules over the neck and axilla in neonatal candidiasis.

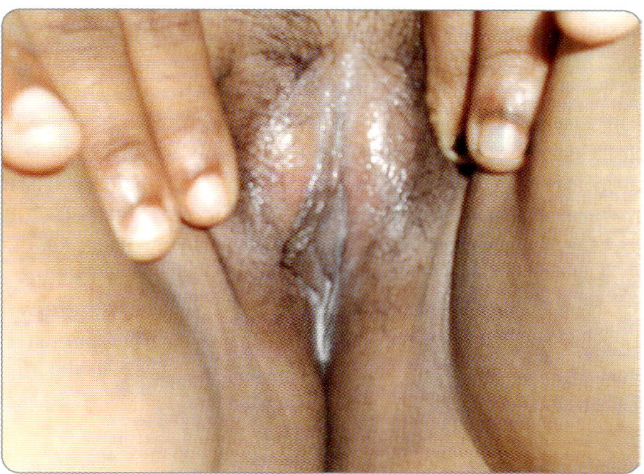

Fig. 2: Curdy white vaginal discharge.

➲ DIFFERENTIAL DIAGNOSIS

Candidal intertigo should be differentiated from tinea infections (lack of peripheral scaling and central clearing), seborrheic dermatitis (presence of budding yeast cells on KOH mount), bacterial intertrigo (presence of pustules, fringed borders, and satellite lesions), flexural psoriasis (positive KOH mount), Hailey–Hailey disease (absence of incomplete acantholysis), and flexural Darier's disease (absence of dyskeratotic corps ronds and grains).

Diaper candidiasis should be differentiated from acrodermatitis enteropathica [more psoriasiform lesions, history of (H/o) diarrhea, negative KOH mount, and response to oral zinc], seborrheic dermatitis, and inverse psoriasis.

Oral thrush should be distinguished from leukoplakia (easily scrapable curd-like precipitates showing budding yeast cells on KOH and absence of atypical keratinocytes).

COMPLICATIONS

Secondary bacterial infection may occur in cutaneous candidiasis. Candidal balanoposthitis can lead to secondary phimosis.

DERMOSCOPY

Presents as white scales with yellowish white areas on whitish pink background. Red dots and globules are seen in the center. Yellow and white band-like structures are also appreciated.

TREATMENT

Local and general predisposing factors must be addressed. In the mouth, this involves frequent toilet in the seriously ill and denture hygiene in other patients. In candidal intertrigo, careful drying of affected sites is important. *Candida* intertrigo requires topical therapy usually azole antifungals like clotrimazole 2%, given for about 2 weeks along with drying the affected area. In diaper candidiasis, the antifungal treatment should be combined with a general measure for napkin dermatitis like frequent diaper changes and avoidance of irritants in the area. In oral candidiasis, topical antifungals are the first line of treatment. These include nystatin suspensions (4–6 lakh U QID), clotrimazole troches 10 mg, 1 tablet dissolved in mouth 5 times per day, gentian violet 12%, and amphotericin gel applied several times a day. For treatment of unresponsive and chronic oral cases, fluconazole (100–200 mg/day for 1 week), itraconazole (100–200 mg/day for 3 weeks), or ketoconazole (200 mg /day for 1–2 weeks) are more effective.

For vulvovaginal candidosis, single-day oral therapy with fluconazole 150 mg or itraconazole 600 mg can be given. Topical preparations such as clotrimazole pessaries are also equally effective in uncomplicated cases.

SUGGESTED READING

1. Akpan A, Morgan R. Oral candidiasis. Postgrad Med J. 2002;78(922): 455-9.

41 Canities

SYNONYMS

Graying of hair.

Canities, or hair graying, is a process of chronological aging and occurs in all races and both genders. If the graying occurs before the age of 20 years in Whites and before 25 years in Asians, it is known as premature canities.

ETIOLOGY

Reduced melanocytic activity with a decrease and eventual cessation of tyrosinase activity in the lower bulb with progressing age, mutations in gene *Pax3* and *MITF* that play an important role in melanocyte stem cell maintenance and differentiation and autoimmunity are proposed causes.

Premature canities is mainly considered a genetic condition with the interplay of various environmental factors. It can be associated with hyperthyroidism, hypothyroidism, osteopenia, syndromes such as progeria and pangeria, drugs such as chloroquine mephenesin, imatinib, HIV, and smoking.

EPIDEMIOLOGY

Graying begins around the fourth decade, the average age for Whites is mid-30s, for Asians late 30s, and for Africans mid-40s. Both sexes are equally affected.

CLINICAL FEATURES

The beard and moustache hair may be affected earlier. Graying process starts from the temporal to the vertical area and finally culminates in the occipital area. Gray hairs are thicker and longer than normally pigmented hairs **(Fig. 1)**.

"Overnight graying" (canities subita) and migratory poliosis occur in alopecia areata, due to preferential loss of pigmented hair.

HISTOPATHOLOGY

There is a normal number of melanocytes but incompletely melanized melanosomes in gray hairs, whereas white hairs show reduced or absent melanocytes.

TREATMENT

Treatment options are very limited. Oral calcium pantothenate 200 mg/day, para-aminobenzoic acid 100 mg TID, PUVASOL therapy. Supplementation with biotin, zinc, copper, and selenium.

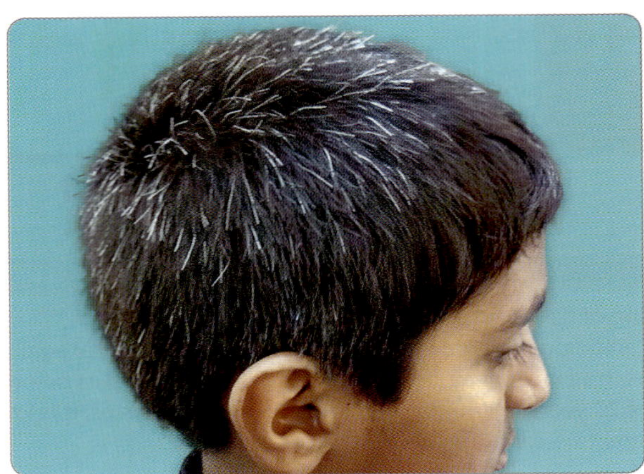

Fig. 1: Premature graying of hair in a 10-year-old boy.

Topical latanoprost (PGF2), temporary hair colorants, L-methionine, green tea polyphenols, melatonin, and phytoestrogens are being used in recent times.

➲ SUGGESTED READING

1. Poonia K, Bhalla M. Premature Graying of Hair: A Comprehensive Review and Recent Insights. Indian Dermatology Online J. 2024;15(5):721-31.

42 Carbuncle

➲ HISTORY

The word is believed to have originated from the Latin word "carbunculus", meaning a small piece of coal.

➲ ETIOLOGY

A carbuncle is a deep infection of a group of contiguous follicles caused by *Staphylococcus aureus*, accompanied by intense inflammatory changes in the surrounding and underlying connective tissues, including the subcutaneous fat. They may be seen in apparently healthy individuals but are more common in the presence of diabetes, malnutrition, chronic *S. aureus* carriage, poor hygiene, cardiac failure, drug addiction, or severe generalized dermatoses, such as exfoliative dermatitis or pemphigus, and during prolonged steroid therapy or any other immunocompromised state.

➲ EPIDEMIOLOGY

Carbuncles occur predominantly in men, and usually in middle or old age.

➲ CLINICAL FEATURES

The infection spreads from one follicle to the other through the subcutaneous tissue. More than one carbuncle is called carbunculosis. They may develop anywhere but are most common on areas of thicker skin such as the back, nape of the neck, and thigh. The lesion starts as a painful, tender, firm to hard indurated lump associated with intense inflammatory changes in the surrounding and underlying tissues. It increases in size for a few days, to reach a diameter of 3–10 cm. After about 5–7 days, suppuration begins and pus is discharged from the multiple follicular and nonfollicular orifices **(Fig. 1)**. The surface usually displays multiple draining sinus tracts and occasionally ulcerates. Constitutional symptoms such as fever, malaise, and prostration may be present. If the underlying conditions are controlled and appropriate therapy instituted, healing occurs slowly leaving a cribriform scar. Death may occur from toxemia or from metastatic infection in very ill or immunocompromised patients.

➲ HISTOPATHOLOGY

The biopsy specimen shows a dense neutrophilic infiltrate in the subcutaneous tissue. Suppurative reactions involving multiple follicles and perifollicular necrosis with fibrinoid debris can be seen.

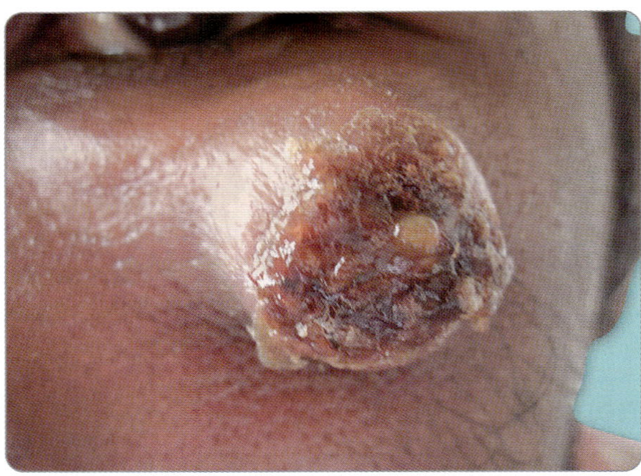

Fig. 1: Carbuncle—pus discharge noted from the swelling on the cheek.

DIFFERENTIAL DIAGNOSIS

- Ruptured epidermoid or pilar cyst
- Hidradenitis suppurativa ("acne inversa")—the presence of polyporous comedones, typical sites are axillae, groin, and other flexures

COMPLICATIONS

Spread of infection to other areas may lead to abscess formation in the brain, spinal cord, or other organs such as the kidney, endocarditis, osteomyelitis, permanent scarring of the skin, and sepsis.

TREATMENT

Treatment of underlying predisposing conditions like diabetes mellitus. Placing a warm moist cloth on the carbuncle helps it to drain, which speeds healing. Gently soak the area with a warm, moist cloth several times each day. Systemic antibiotics such as flucloxacillin 250 mg QID in adults or another penicillinase-resistant antibiotics should be given. Most common surgical approaches are saucerization, incision, and drainage.

PROGNOSIS

Carbuncles may heal on their own. Others usually respond well to treatment. However, a carbuncle can recur for months or years following the first infection.

SUGGESTED READING

1. Stulberg DL, Penrod MA, Blatny RA. Common bacterial skin infections. Am Fam Physician. 2002;66(1):119-24.

43 Cellulitis

➲ ETIOLOGY

In immunocompetent adults, cellulitis is commonly caused by *Streptococcus pyogenes* or *Staphylococcus aureus* and in children by *S. aureus*, and less commonly by *Haemophilus influenzae*. A mixture of gram-positive cocci and gram-negative aerobes and anaerobes such as *Serratia*, *Enterobacter*, *Proteus*, and *Pseudomonas* species are associated with cellulitis surrounding diabetic ulcers and decubitus ulcers. The organisms gain access to the skin via an external or a hematogenous route. Usually, in immunocompetent patients, a break in the skin barrier is responsible. In immunocompromised patients, a bloodborne route is most common. Predisposing factors are lymphedema, venous stasis, alcoholism, diabetes mellitus, intravenous drug abuse, and peripheral vascular disease.

➲ EPIDEMIOLOGY

It affects all racial and ethnic groups. No sex and age predilection is described. But higher incidence has been reported among individuals >45 years.

➲ CLINICAL FEATURES

Cellulitis is an infection of the deep dermis and subcutaneous tissue. Cellulitis is usually preceded by systemic symptoms, such as fever, chills and malaise. The affected area displays all four of the cardinal signs of inflammation: Erythema, heat, swelling, and pain or tenderness. The lesion has an ill-defined, nonpalpable border. Severe cellulitis may show vesicles and bullae and can progress to dermal necrosis, and uncommonly to fasciitis or myositis **(Fig. 1)**. Lymphangitis and lymphadenopathy are commonly present. Children usually have cellulitis of the head and neck region, whereas in adults the extremities are most often affected. In intravenous drug abusers, the upper extremities are often involved.

The diagnosis of cellulitis is usually clinical. The leukocyte count is usually normal or only slightly elevated. The causative organisms can be identified by gram staining and culture of the specimen taken from vesicle fluid or eroded or ulcerated surfaces, in addition to blood cultures.

➲ HISTOPATHOLOGY

The dermis shows a mild-to-moderate inflammatory infiltrate composed mostly of lymphocytes and neutrophils. There is also edema and dilation of lymphatics and small blood vessels. With special stains, the causative organism may be identified. Severe cases may show subepidermal bullae.

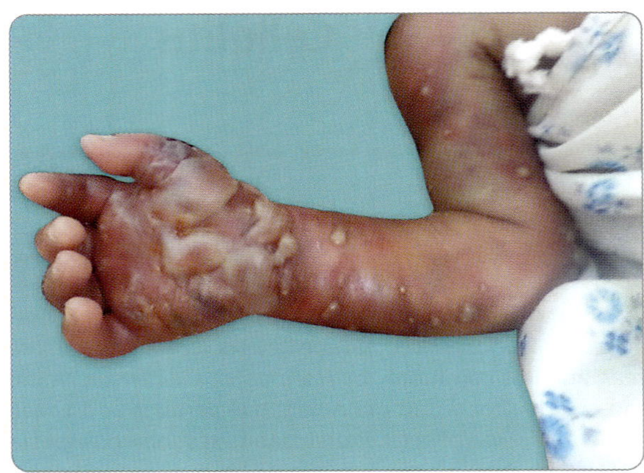

Fig. 1: Erythema, edema, and bullae over the forearm in a child with bullous cellulitis.

DIFFERENTIAL DIAGNOSIS

- *Deep vein thrombosis*: Positive Moses sign
- *Stasis dermatitis*: Typical skin changes such as hyperpigmentation, thickening, pigmented purpuras, and venous ulcers; more commonly over the lower medial aspect of the legs
- *Superficial thrombophlebitis*: Presence of red streaks along vessels
- *Panniculitis*: Presence of tender deep-seated nodules instead of diffuse swelling
- *Erysipelas*: Presence of well-demarcated erythematous border

COMPLICATIONS

Complications are rare with effective treatment. If the treatment is delayed, the following complications are common: Fasciitis, myositis, subcutaneous abscesses, septicemia, infective endocarditis, and, in some streptococcal cases, nephritis. More severe infections may be fatal, especially in infants and in the debilitated or immunocompromised.

TREATMENT

As cellulitis is commonly caused by *S. pyogenes* and *S. aureus*, treatment is empirically started against these organisms without waiting for laboratory confirmation. Flucloxacillin exerts a bactericidal effect on streptococci as well as staphylococci, started at a dose of 250 mg four times daily; clarithromycin 500 mg twice daily may be substituted in case of penicillin allergy. Mild cases require a 10-day course of treatment. Hospitalization and parenteral antibiotics should be reserved for patients who are seriously ill and those who have facial cellulitis. Immobilization and elevation, as well as the application of wet dressings to areas with bullae or exudate, are recommended. Once culture reports are available, treatment should be changed accordingly. Glycerin and magnesium sulfate dressing helps resolve swelling and responds better than normal saline dressing.

PROGNOSIS

With proper treatment, the infection clears in 7–10 days. It may recur if the underlying predisposing condition is not addressed.

SUGGESTED READING

1. Raff AB, Kroshinsky D. Cellulitis: A Review. JAMA. 2016;316(3): 325-37.

44 Chancroid

➲ SYNONYMS

Soft sore, soft chancre, ulcus molle.

➲ HISTORY

Leon Bassereau gave the first clear description of chancroid in 1852.

➲ ETIOLOGY

Chancroid is a sexually transmitted disease caused by *Haemophilus ducreyi*, a gram-negative bacillus, forming short chains, arranged in "schools of fish", "railroad tracks", or "fingerprint" manner.

➲ EPIDEMIOLOGY

It occurs in the sexually active age group.

➲ CLINICAL FEATURES

After an incubation period of 5–8 days, a small red papule develops and rapidly becomes pustular and then ulcerated. The ulcer is rounded or oval, has a ragged, undermined edge, surrounded by a red, very vascular areola. It is tender and sometimes painful, but not indurated, enlarges slowly and often gives rise to satellite lesions and kissing ulcers. Multiple ulcers are more common in women than men **(Figs. 1A and B)**.

In males, the prepuce, the balanopreputial fold or the shaft of the penis, and in females, the labia majora, the posterior commissure, and the perianal region, are the most common sites of infection. Extragenital lesions, although rare, do occur.

In about 50% of cases, inguinal adenitis develops about a week after the appearance of the ulcer. The glands on one or both sides are enlarged and tender and may suppurate, leading to chronic draining lesions.

The variants of chancroid include giant, phagedenic, mixed, transient, dwarf, papular, follicular, serpiginous, and granulomatous.

In immunocompromised patients due to HIV infection, very severe and atypical presentations are seen. The lesions heal slowly with an increased incidence of treatment failure.

Haemophilus ducreyi may be identified in the form of chains of coccobacilli in smears from the ulcer, or preferably of pus from a bubo. Culture is done a selective media which contains hemin (factor X) at 33°C in an atmosphere of high humidity.

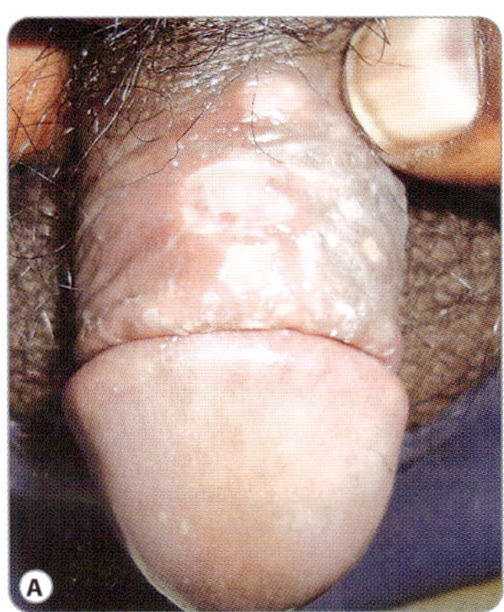

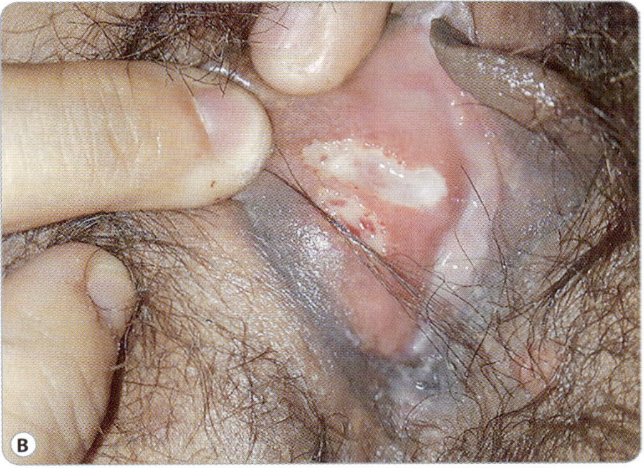

Figs. 1A and B: (A) Chancroid, round to oval ulcers with purulent discharge over the shaft of the penis; and (B) Ragged borders of the ulcer.

➲ HISTOPATHOLOGY

There are three vertical zones: The surface zone is narrow and consists of neutrophils, fibrin, erythrocytes, and necrotic tissue. The wide middle zone has newly formed blood vessels, and the deep zone is composed of a dense infiltrate of plasma cells and lymphoid cells.

➲ DIFFERENTIAL DIAGNOSIS

- *Syphilitic chancre*: Painless, usually single, clean-looking ulcer, painless inguinal lymphadenopathy
- *Herpes simplex*: Multiple tender shallow erosions/ulcers with erythematous halo, history of recurrent lesions, and multinucleate giant cells on Tzanck smear
- Secondarily infected traumatic ulcer
- *Fixed drug eruption*: Characteristic superficial erosion with erythematous-violaceous border, temporal association to drug intake, lesions elsewhere on the body

- *Granuloma inguinale*: Exuberant fleshy ulcer which bleeds on touch, pseudobubo, and demonstration of Donovan bodies on crush smear
- *Lymphogranuloma venereum*: Very transient ulcers and prominent clinical presentation with inguinal bubo
- *Candida balanitis*: Shallow erosions, fissures, and pustules
- *Behçet's disease*: Shallow ulcers with oral aphthae, cutaneous lesions, and positive pathergy test
- *Extracutaneous Crohn's disease*: Knife cut such as linear ulcers more in the perineum, presence of noncaseating granulomas, and absence of bacteria on biopsy

COMPLICATIONS

Severe phimosis, gangrene, destructive ulceration from secondary fusospirochetal infection, rupture of bubo, and balanitis.

TREATMENT

The treatment for chancroid is azithromycin 1 g single dose or injection ceftriaxone 250 mg IM single dose or ciprofloxacin 500 mg BID for 3 days or erythromycin 500 mg QID for 7 days.

Regardless of whether disease symptoms are present, partners should be examined and treated, if they had sexual contact during the 10 days preceding the patient's symptom onset.

SUGGESTED READING

1. Lewis DA. Chancroid: clinical manifestations, diagnosis, and management. Sex Transm Infect. 2003;79(1):68-71.

45 Chromoblastomycosis

➲ SYNONYMS

Chromomycosis, verrucous dermatitis, cladosporiosis, Fonsecaea's disease, Pedroso's disease, pheosporotrichosis.

➲ HISTORY

Pedroso first recognized chromoblastomycosis in 1911 and was later described by Lane and Medlar in 1915.

➲ ETIOLOGY

Chromoblastomycosis is caused by a vast variety of fungi, most commonly by *Phialophora verrucosa*, *Fonsecaea pedrosoi*, and *Cladosporium carrionii*.

➲ EPIDEMIOLOGY

Adult male agricultural workers are most affected.

➲ CLINICAL FEATURES

The initial site of infection is usually on the feet, legs, arms, or upper trunk. The initial lesion is often a warty papule that expands slowly over months or years. Alternatively, lesions may be plaque-like with an atrophic center. Eventually, hyperkeratotic masses are formed. Lesions are usually painless **(Figs. 1A to C)**.

➲ HISTOPATHOLOGY

The histology shows a mixed granulomatous response with small neutrophilic abscesses and exuberant epidermal hyperplasia. The organisms that are often seen either in giant cells or in neutrophil abscesses appear singly or in small groups of brown-pigmented cells, often with a single or double septum and thick cell wall (Medlar bodies and copper penny bodies).

Potassium hydroxide (KOH) mount: Sclerotic or muriform fungal cells are seen in scrapings.

➲ DERMOSCOPY

The most characteristic feature is multiple black dots. Pink and white areas seen on dermoscopy are said to represent rough uneven areas of the lesion. Brownish ovoid globular structures may be seen.

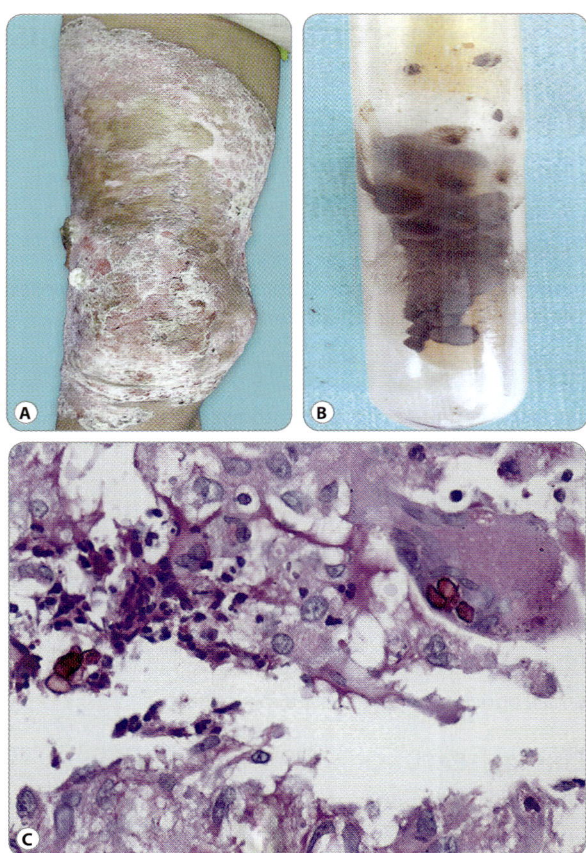

Figs. 1A to C: (A) Hyperkeratotic plaque with well-defined borders over the thigh; (B) Culture of chromoblastomycosis; and (C) Pigmented spores resembling copper pennies.

DIFFERENTIAL DIAGNOSIS

- *Cutaneous tuberculosis*: Presence of granulomas with AFB
- Chronic tropical lymphedema with hyperplasia (mossy foot)
- Blastomycosis
- *Leishmaniasis*: Presence of LD bodies in tissue samples
- *Sporotrichosis*: Presence of linear lesions with associated lymphangitis, demonstration of *Sporothrix schenckii*
- *Squamous cell carcinoma*: Chronic ulcerated lesions with indurated base, lymphadenopathy, and presence of horn pearls on histopathological examination (HPE)
- Syphilis and yaws

COMPLICATIONS

Local lymphedema may lead to elephantiasis, hematogenous spread may lead to brain abscess, and there is a risk of malignant transformation to squamous cell carcinomas in some chronic lesions.

➲ TREATMENT

Itraconazole 200 mg daily, with or without flucytosine 30 mg/kg QID or terbinafine 250 mg daily, is given till lesions resolve. Intravenous amphotericin B up to 1 mg/kg/day is given in extensive lesions. Local application of heat also helps as heat inhibits fungal growth. Severe disease is often refractory to treatment. Limited lesions are usually treated surgically. Other therapies include posaconazole, voriconazole, ravuconazole, topical imiquimod, 5-flucytosine, cryotherapy, and photodynamic therapy.

➲ PROGNOSIS

The lesion spreads very slowly and is rarely fatal. Extensive lesions often respond poorly to treatment.

➲ SUGGESTED READING

1. Ameen M. Chromoblastomycosis: Clinical presentation and management. Clin Exp Dermatol. 2009;34:849-54.

46 Cicatricial Alopecia

➲ INTRODUCTION

The term "cicatricial" or "scarring" implies that follicular epithelium has been replaced by connective tissue. This includes all forms of alopecia, in which the hair follicules are permanently lost.

➲ EPIDEMIOLOGY

The epidemiology of primary cicatricial alopecia in the general population is unknown.

➲ ETIOLOGY

In primary cicatricial alopecia, the hair follicle is the main target for destruction, evident microscopically as preferential destruction of follicular epithelium and/or its associated adventitial dermis with relative sparing of the interfollicular reticular dermis. In secondary cicatricial alopecia, nonfollicular disease indirectly causes follicular destruction.

Primary and secondary cicatricial alopecias are mentioned in **Table 1**.

➲ CLINICAL FEATURES

The features of underlying disease are seen along with permanent loss of hair. Single or multiple patches of hair loss can be seen. Acute inflammatory changes are seen in early lesions, while later have a burnt-out appearance, with a smooth surface.

➲ HISTOPATHOLOGY

Primary scarring alopecias are those in which the target structure is the pilosebaceous unit but not the associated reticular dermis. After the destruction of the follicle, the follicular remnant is vertically oriented as a linear fibrous scar including the adventitial collagen of the preexisting follicle. The adjacent reticular dermis is largely unaltered. The histology of secondary scarring alopecias is dominated by scarring of the reticular dermis and secondarily includes the pilosebaceous units.

➲ DIFFERENTIAL DIAGNOSIS

- Alopecia areata
- Tinea capitis
- Trichotillomania

Table 1: Primary and secondary cicatricial alopecias.

Primary cicatricial alopecia	*Secondary cicatricial alopecia*
Lymphocytic: • Chronic cutaneous lupus erythematosus • Lichen planopilaris • Classic lichen planopilaris • Frontal fibrosing alopecia • Graham–Little syndrome • Classic pseudopelade (Brocq) • Central centrifugal cicatricial alopecia • Alopecia mucinosa • Keratosis follicularis spinulosa decalvans *Neutrophilic*: • Folliculitis decalvans • Dissecting cellulitis/ folliculitis (perifolliculitis capitis abscedens et suffodiens) *Mixed*: • Folliculitis (acne) keloidalis • Folliculitis (acne) necrotica • Erosive pustular dermatosis *Nonspecific*	*Inherited and congenital disorders*: Aplasia cutis, chondrodysplasia punctata, cutis verticis gyrata, Darier's diseases, eccrine hamartoma, epidermal nevi, epidermolysis bullosa, hair follicle hamartoma, hypotrichosis congenita, ichthyosis (sex-linked recessive), incontinentia pigmenti, keratosis pilaris spinulosa decalvans, neurofibromatosis, polyostotic fibrous dysplasia, porokeratosis of Mibelli, and scarring follicular keratosis *Physical/chemical agents*: Chemical burns, insect bites, mechanical trauma or laceration, radiation dermatitis, anc thermal burns *Sclerosing disorders*: Lichen sclerosis et atrophicus, morphea, scleroderma, scleroderma en coup de sabre and facial hemiatrophy, and hemiatrophy porphyria cutanea tarda *Dermal granulomatous infiltrations*: Actinic granuloma, amyloidosis, infections due to fungi, protozoa, syphilis, tuberculosis, viruses, etc., Miescher's granuloma, necrobiosis lipoidica, sarcoidosis. Dermal neoplastic infiltrations Adnexal tumors, basal cell carcinoma, dermatofibrosarcoma protuberans, lymphoma, melanoma, metastatic carcinoma, squamous cell carcinoma, etc.

➲ TREATMENT

Active: Topical or intralesional steroids, tacrolimus, hydroxychloroquine (200–400 mg/dL/day), isotretinoin, prednisolone, thalidomide, dapsone, mycophenolate mofetil, methotrexate, azathioprine, vitamin E and derivatives, clofazimine, gold, salicylate bismuth, systemic (and intralesional) interferon- alpha-2, psoralen plus ultraviolet A (PUVA), and monoclonal anti-CD4 antibodies. When scarring is seen, surgical excision, micropigmentation, and hair transplantation can be done.

➲ PROGNOSIS

Scarring alopecias may be difficult to diagnose. Biopsies should be done early to attempt to establish a diagnosis. Alopecias are permanent and nonreversible.

➲ SUGGESTED READING

1. Jain N, Doshi B, Khopkar U. Trichoscopy in alopecias: diagnosis simplified. Int J Trichology. 2013;5(4):170-8.

47 Cicatricial Pemphigoid

SYNONYMS

Mucous membrane pemphigoid, desquamative gingivitis, benign mucous membrane pemphigoid, ocular pemphigus, scarring pemphigoid.

HISTORY

In 1949, Civatte separated this disorder from pemphigus, and Lever named it as benign mucous membrane pemphigoid, which was a misnomer.

ETIOLOGY

Cicatricial pemphigoid (CP) is caused by tissue-bound and less often, circulating autoantibodies directed against distinct structural components of basement membranes in stratified and some complex epithelia, e.g., the bullous pemphigoid antigen 180 or laminin 5.

EPIDEMIOLOGY

Cicatricial pemphigoid is a disease of late middle to old age, but can affect children and teenagers as well, and is more common in females. Incidence is one per million population. HLA-DQB1*0301, HLA-DQB1*02, and HLA-DRB1*11 are associated with the disease.

CLINICAL FEATURES

The condition should not be regarded as a clinical entity, but as a "disease phenotype" shared by a heterogeneous group of diseases with lesions that favor the mucosal surfaces and, less frequently, the skin. The striking features are recurrent blisters on either the mucus membrane or areas of skin near to one of the orifices such as anus, nose, larynx, esophagus, vulva, vagina, and penis.

Mucosal lesions: The most common oral presentation is erosive (desquamative) gingivitis, accompanied by bleeding erosions and paresthesias; small intact blisters are rarely observed. Chronic inflammation may lead to periodontal ligament damage and loss of teeth. In other areas of the mouth, transient vesicles give rise to chronic erosions, especially on the palate, with variable associated pain. Conjunctival involvement is common and may result in blindness. Conjunctival fibrosis can also lead to trichiasis and entropion **(Fig. 1)**. Nasopharyngeal involvement is chronic and results in crusted ulcerations, epistaxis, fibrous adhesions between adjacent mucosal surfaces, and airway obstruction. Similar lesions can occur in esophagus, genital, and anal mucosae.

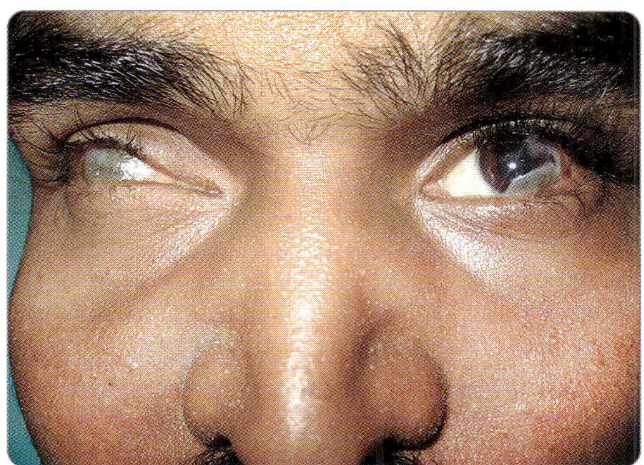

Fig. 1: Corneal opacity in cicatricial pemphigoid.

Cutaneous lesions: The skin is involved in 25–30% of patients with CP. The most frequently involved sites are the scalp, face, neck, and upper trunk. Lesions typically present as erythematous plaques, which become sites for recurrent blister formation and erosions, with subsequent atrophic scarring.

➲ HISTOPATHOLOGY

Examination of an intact vesicle demonstrates subepidermal or subepithelial blister formation (without acantholysis) and a mixed infiltrate of variable intensity, composed primarily of mononuclear cells. Older lesions tend to demonstrate fibrosis in the upper dermis. In oral lesions, the inflammatory infiltrate typically contains some plasma cells as well. By direct immunofluorescence (IF) microscopy, 80–95% of patients have in vivo-bound autoantibodies directed against the basement membrane zone (BMZ) of mucosae and/or skin. Most patients exhibit continuous, fine, linear deposits of IgG and/or C3 along the epithelial BMZ in perilesional biopsy specimens. In indirect IF, anti-BMZ antibodies can be detected in serum samples from 20 to 30% of patients.

➲ DIFFERENTIAL DIAGNOSIS

- *Bullous pemphigoid*: Presence of tense bullae on normal or erythematous skin, mucosa less commonly involved, linear immunoglobulin G (IgG), C3 deposits on direct immunofluorescence (DIF)
- *Epidermolysis bullosa acquisita*: Lesions are provoked by trauma, less severe mucosal involvement, absence of scarring
- IgA bullous dermatosis
- *Pemphigus vulgaris*: Acantholytic cells on Tzanck smear, intraepidermal blister and fishnet pattern of IgG, immunoglobulin M (IgM), C3 deposits on DIF
- *Herpes zoster*: Localized dermatomal distribution of vesicles associated with neuralgia, multinucleate giant cells on Tzanck smear

Oral lesions can be confused with erosive lichen planus and pemphigus vulgaris.

Scarring conjunctival lesions may mimic severe chronic infectious conjunctivitis and ocular pseudopemphigoid due to ophthalmologic preparations, e.g., pilocarpine, beta-blockers.

COMPLICATIONS

Frequent complications are impairment of vision due to ocular involvement, weight loss, and respiratory, sexual, or urinary complications. Even with localized disease, CP can have a major negative impact on quality of life. Life-threatening complications, due to severe laryngeal, tracheal, or esophageal disease, are rare. Patients with antilaminin 5 CP have an increased relative risk for solid-organ carcinomas, especially adenocarcinomas.

TREATMENT

- *Local therapy*: Mild-to-moderate disease activity may be successfully treated with potent topical corticosteroids fluocinonide 0.05% gel QID. Oral lesions respond to topical corticosteroids in conjunction with tetracycline mouthwashes and good hygiene.
- *Systemic therapy*: Dapsone is a first-line therapy for controlling oral and cutaneous lesions, and it may also be used for mild ocular disease. Cyclophosphamide is the treatment of choice for rapidly progressive or severe ocular disease alone, in combination with oral corticosteroids, or as pulse therapy. Other therapies include sulfapyridine, minocycline, a combination of tetracycline and niacinamide, topical tacrolimus, topical or systemic cyclosporine, thalidomide, and subconjunctival mitomycin. Etanercept may be an effective treatment option for ocular and oral mucous membranes.

PROGNOSIS

Cicatricial pemphigoid is a particularly chronic, potentially devastating, but rarely fatal disease. Rare cases may die from complications such as laryngeal stenosis or treatment complications. Unlike bullous pemphigoid, it is not self-limiting; prolonged remissions are rare except in localized lesions. Very rarely, carcinomas have arisen from chronic oral lesions and esophageal lesions.

SUGGESTED READING

1. Fleming TE, Korman NJ. Cicatricial pemphigoid. J Am Acad Dermatol. 2000;43(4):571-91.

48 Condyloma Acuminatum

➲ SYNONYMS

Anogenital warts (condyloma = knuckle, acuminatum = pointed), venereal warts.

➲ HISTORY

Greeks introduced the term "condyloma". In 1949, Strauss et al. isolated the human papillomavirus (HPV).

➲ ETIOLOGY

Anogenital warts are caused by HPV 6 (75%). The remainder are caused by HPV-11 or more unusual, low-risk HPVs. These have no malignant potential. Predisposing factors include diabetes, pregnancy, trauma, and immunosuppression.

➲ EPIDEMIOLOGY

Condyloma acuminata is seen commonly in young adults, with the mean age of onset being 16–25 years.

➲ CLINICAL FEATURES

The incubation period ranges from 1 to 8 months. They are often asymptomatic but may cause discomfort, discharge, or bleeding if secondarily infected. The typical anogenital wart is soft, pink, elongated, and sometimes filiform or pedunculated. The lesions are multiple, especially on moist surfaces, and their growth can be enhanced during pregnancy, or in the presence of other local infections. Large malodorous masses may form on the vulvar and perianal skin. This classical "acuminate" (sometimes called papillomatous, or hyperplastic) form constitutes about two-thirds of anogenital warts. The most common sites are the area of the frenulum, corona, and glans in men, and the posterior fourchette in women **(Fig. 1)**.

Other types of genital warts are papular, verruca vulgaris type or keratotic warts, flat warts, sessile warts, and giant condyloma.

In children, warts in the anogenital area are often more hyperkeratotic than in adults and may be caused by HPV types associated with cutaneous disease as well as HPV types 6 and 11.

Human papillomavirus DNA can be demonstrated in the lesions and normal skin adjacent to warts and intraepithelial neoplasia, and this latent infection correlates well with recurrence after a clinical cure. HPV typing is done by fluorescent in situ hybridization. Application of 3–5% acetic acid helps in better visualization of the lesions.

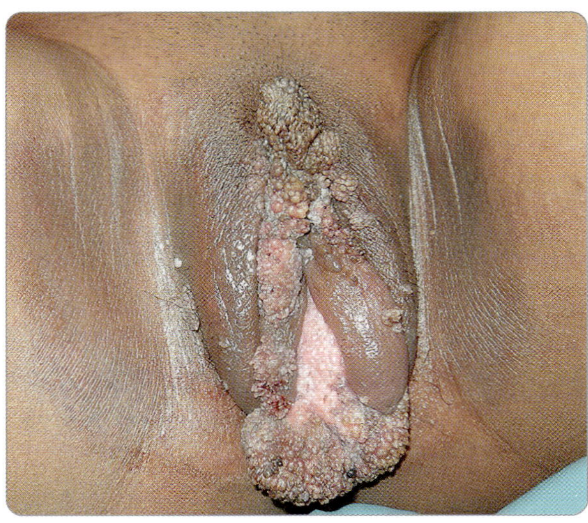

Fig. 1: Multiple pointed filiform warts over the genitalia.

HISTOPATHOLOGY

Parakeratotic types of hyperkeratosis, acanthosis, papillomatosis, moderate granulomatosis, and mitotic figures may be present in the epidermis along with koilocytes.

DIFFERENTIAL DIAGNOSIS

- *Condyloma lata*: Lesions seen in secondary syphilis, highly infectious and teeming with treponema
- Nonvenereal treponematosis
- *Verrucous type of granuloma inguinale*: Demonstration of Donovan bodies
- *Cutaneous tuberculosis*: Presence of granulomas
- *Skin tags*: Skin-colored papilliferous outgrowths with fibrous stalks
- Malignancy
- Vulval papillomatosis
- *Pearly penile papules*: Usually in the preputial cavity, the absence of koilocytes
- Seborrheic keratosis
- Erythroplasia of Queyrat
- *Bowenoid papulosis*: Multiple black popular lesions, dysplastic cells seen in histopathological examination (HPE)
- *Molluscum contagiosum*: Umbilication seen, lack of verrucous surface

COMPLICATIONS

The development of large protuberant masses with pain or serosanguinous discharge should arouse suspicion of malignant change (including Buschke–Löwenstein tumor), requiring prompt excision or biopsy.

➲ TREATMENT

Podophyllotoxin 0.5% solution or 0.15% cream is applied twice daily for 3 days followed by 4 days of no therapy; podophyllin 10–25% dissolved in tincture of benzoin; Imiquimod cream (5%), three times per week (every other night); surgical excision, cryotherapy, electrosurgery, trichloroacetic acid (TCA) 80–90% solution can be used safely during pregnancy; IFNs, 5-fluorouracil, cidofovir, or retinoids. The application of 5 aminolevulinic acid with photodynamic therapy is an emerging treatment modality and may be used as an adjuvant along with other treatment modalities.

➲ PROGNOSIS

The duration of anogenital warts varies from a few weeks to many years. Recurrences can be expected in about 25% of cases, the interval varying from 2 months to 23 years.

➲ SUGGESTED READING

1. O'Mahony C, Gomberg M, Skerlev M, Alraddadi A, de Las Heras-Alonso ME, Majewski S, et al. Position statement for the diagnosis and management of anogenital warts. J Eur Acad Dermatol Venereol. 2019;33(6):1006-19.

49 Confluent and Reticulated Papillomatosis

➲ SYNONYMS

Familial cutaneous papillomatosis, confluent and reticulated papillomatosis of Gougerot and Carteaud.

➲ HISTORY

Henri Gougerot and Alexandre Carteaud originally described confluent and reticulated papillomatosis (CRP) in 1927.

➲ ETIOLOGY

The exact etiology is not known. CRP may represent an endocrine disturbance, a disorder of keratinization, an abnormal host reaction to fungi (pityrosporum) or bacteria, a hereditary disorder, or a variant of amyloidosis.

➲ EPIDEMIOLOGY

The ratio of women to men affected by confluent and CRP has been reported to be 2.8:1. The condition appears during the second to third decade.

➲ CLINICAL FEATURES

Confluent and reticulated papillomatosis usually begins on the skin of the intermammary or epigastric region, spreading over a period of weeks or months to the breasts, the lower abdomen, the flanks, and the pubic area. It is characterized by grayish-blue hyperkeratotic papules, which coalesce to form confluent plaques centrally and a reticular pattern peripherally **(Fig. 1)**. The eruption is chronic with exacerbations and remissions. Skin markings are preserved and sometimes exaggerated, especially in the neck and the axillae, where the skin may be thickened. Scraping of lesions produces a fine powdery scale. Scattered comedone-like papules (dark dot follicles); and pitted acneiform scars may be present.

The mucous membranes are spared.

➲ DERMOSCOPY

Fine white scaling and brownish areas in a "cobblestone" or "sulci and gyri" pattern.

➲ HISTOPATHOLOGY

The epidermis shows compact hyperkeratosis, often associated with the presence of pityrosporum yeast, decreased or absent granular cell layer, papillomatosis, and a stratum spinosum that varies from acanthotic to atrophic.

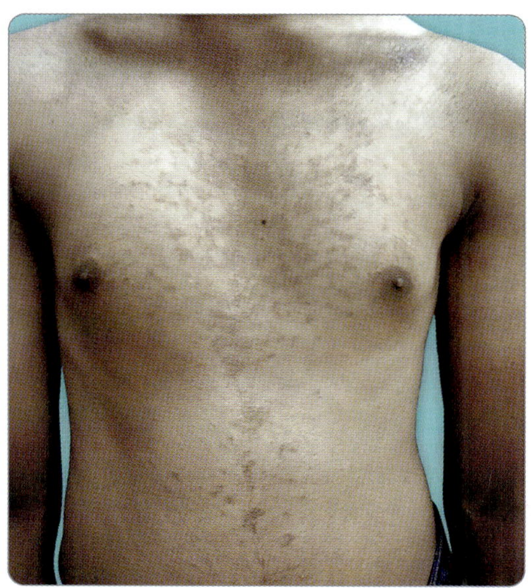

Fig. 1: Reticulated pigmentation over the trunk.

DIFFERENTIAL DIAGNOSIS

- Tinea versicolor
- *Acanthosis nigricans*: Thickened, velvety plaque seen, absence of scaling, typical sites such as nape of neck, axillae, cubital and popliteal fossae, and groin involved
- *Amyloidosis*: Homogenous deposition in dermal papillae, apple green birefringence on polarized microscopy of Congo red stained specimen
- *Dermatosis papulosa nigra*: Discrete hyperpigmented papules not in reticulate fashion and absence of scaling
- *Epidermodysplasia verruciformis*: Presence of plane wart-like lesions, seborrhoeic keratosis-like lesions, extremities also involved
- *Darier disease*: Dirty, warty, greasy, scaly papules seen in seborrhoeic areas with other features such as cobblestoning of mucosa and nail changes; corps ronds and grains on HPE
- *Pityriasis rubra pilaris (PRP)*: Orange hue of lesions, islands of normal skin seen, and keratotic (PRP) sandal seen
- Seborrheic keratosis

TREATMENT

The first line is oral minocycline, minocycline 50 mg twice a day for 6 weeks erythromycin, low-dose isotretinoin, topical retinoic acid, antifungals such as clotrimazole, miconazole, and ciclopirox olamine can be tried. Oral clarithromycin 500 mg once a day for 5 weeks and erythromycin 100 mg daily for 6 weeks have shown to produce good responses; recurrences are common with antifungals.

➲ PROGNOSIS

The condition responds to treatment but may recur.

➲ SUGGESTED READING

1. Lim JH, Tey HL, Chong WS. Confluent and reticulated papillomatosis: diagnostic and treatment challenges. Clin Cosmet Investig Dermatol. 2016;9:217-23.

50 Congenital Syphilis

ETIOLOGY

Congenital syphilis is defined as an infant born to a mother who was inadequately treated or had untreated syphilis at delivery or any infant with a reactive treponemal test and any symptoms or signs of syphilis on physical examination. The infection is acquired in utero by transplacental passage of *Treponema pallidum* or by contact with an infectious lesion during passage through the birth canal.

Kassowitz's law: The longer the interval between infection and pregnancy, the more benign the outcome in the infant.

Colles's law: The syphilitic infant does not infect its mother. It is because the mother is suffering from latent syphilis and has a degree of immunity from her child.

Profeta's law: At birth, an infected infant may appear healthy and may not develop signs till it is some weeks old.

CLINICAL FEATURES

Early Congenital Syphilis

Within the first 2 years of life, lesions are infectious and resemble those of the secondary stage of acquired form. The child presents with pemphigus syphiliticus (vesicular bullous eruptions of palms and soles) **(Figs. 1A and B)**, maculopapular rash, rhinitis (highly infectious), "snuffles", mucous patches, condylomata lata, weight loss which causes wrinkling of the skin giving an old man look, "the cafe au lait" tint (brownish yellow tint of the skin), syphilitic alopecia, syphilitic wig, syphilitic onychia, petechial lesions, hepatosplenomegaly, jaundice, generalized lymphadenopathy, hemolytic anemia, thrombocytopenia, leukopenia, leukocytosis, hydrops fetalis, desquamation, osteochondritis, periostitis, pseudo-paralysis of Parrot, syphilitic dactylitis, syphilitic leptomeningitis, chorioretinitis, salt and pepper fundus, glaucoma, pancreatitis, white pneumonia, and orchitis.

Late Congenital Syphilis

These occur from the beginning of the third year of life onward and include gummata which are identical to those of the tertiary stage. Other features are interstitial keratitis, 8th nerve deafness, neurosyphilis (asymptomatic, convulsions, meningitis, cranial nerve palsies, cerebrovascular lesions, and juvenile general paralysis), Clutton's joints, gummatous osteoperiostitis, "Parrot's nodes" (localized osteoperiostitis of the bones of the vault), aneurysm and aortic incompetence, paroxysmal cold hemoglobinuria.

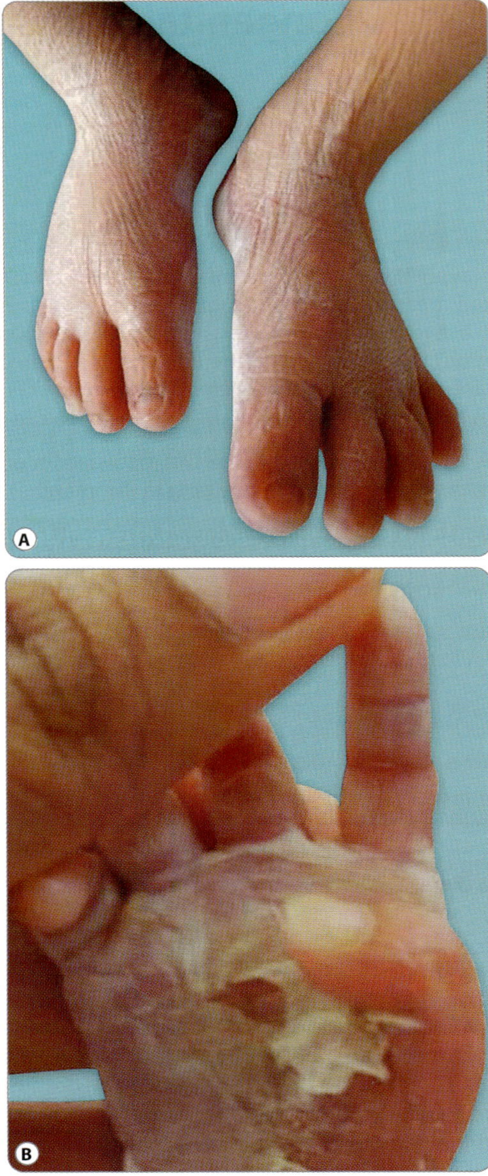

Figs. 1A and B: (A) Desquamation and wrinkling over the feet of a neonate with congenital syphilis giving an old man appearance; and (B) Bulla and peeling of skin over the palms.

The Stigmata

These are the scars and deformities of early or late lesions which are no longer active. Hutchinson's triad (notched upper incisors, interstitial keratitis, and 8th nerve deafness), mulberry molars, flaring scapulas, hydrocephalus, mental retardation, frontal bossing, saddle nose, protruding mandible, high arched palate, perioral fissures, Higoumenaki's sign (periosteal reaction of the clavicle, sternocleidomastoid), saber shins, and rhagades.

Radiological Findings

Wimberger's sign is a loss of density on the medial side of the upper end of the tibia. Thin, regular, lines of new bone formation on the surface of the cortex (earliest finding), saw tooth metaphysis, and "onion-peel periosteum" are the other findings.

Diagnosis is by dark ground examination of serum from lesions, especially the moist lesions of skin and mucous membranes. Serological tests both specific and nonspecific treponemal tests such as venereal disease research laboratory (VDRL), fluorescent treponemal antibody-absorption immunoglobulin M (FTA-ABS IgM) test, and treponema pallidum hemagglutination (TPHA) should be done.

➲ TREATMENT

In infants less than a month old aqueous crystalline penicillin G, 100,000–150,000 U/kg/day is administered as 50,000 U/kg/dose intravenously (IV) every 12th hourly for the first 7 days of life and every 8th hour thereafter for a total of 10 days or procaine penicillin, 50,000 U/kg/dose intramuscular injection (IM) daily in a single dose for 10 days.

In infants more than a month old aqueous crystalline penicillin G, 200,000–300,000 U/kg/day IV is administered as 50,000 U/kg every 4–6 hours for 10 days.

Neurosyphilis is treated with aqueous penicillin G 50,000 U/kg is given 4–6th hourly IV for 10–14 days. Any neonate at risk for congenital syphilis should receive full evaluation and testing for human immunodeficiency virus (HIV).

➲ SUGGESTED READING

1. Sankaran D, Partridge E, Lakshminrusimha S. Congenital Syphilis-An Illustrative Review. Children (Basel). 2023;10(8):1310.

51 Contact Dermatitis

➲ SYNONYM

Contact eczema.

➲ HISTORY

The term "allergie" was coined by Von Pirquet in 1906. Jadassohn has been credited with describing the technique of patch testing over 100 years ago.

➲ ETIOLOGY

Allergic contact dermatitis (ACD) is an inflammatory eczematous disease due to a delayed-type of hypersensitivity (type IV) response. It is an allergen-specific reaction that requires prior sensitization of the individual to the chemical in question. It is a T-cell-mediated inflammation of the skin caused by repeated skin exposure. The common allergens are nickel, paraphenylene diamine, balsam of Peru, chromium, neomycin, formaldehyde, thiomersal, fragrance mix, cobalt, and parthenium.

➲ EPIDEMIOLOGY

All age groups including children to elderly are affected.

➲ CLINICAL FEATURES

The typical appearance is often a well-demarcated pruritic eczematous eruption, which may be acute (blistering and weeping), or chronic (lichenified or scaly plaques). This reaction is typically localized to the area of skin that comes in contact with the allergen **(Fig. 1)**. Patchy or diffuse distribution can also be seen, depending on the nature of the causative agent. Systemic reactions and photosensitive reactions are less common.

Patch test is useful in the diagnosis of ACD.

➲ HISTOPATHOLOGY

Pathology is most useful in acute lesions as subacute and chronic lesions cause nonspecific changes. ACD is the prototype of spongiotic dermatitis. In the acute stage, there is a variable degree of spongiosis, with a mixed dermal inflammatory infiltrate containing lymphocytes, histiocytes, and a variable number of eosinophils. In moderate-to-severe reactions, marked spongiosis results in intraepidermal vesiculation.

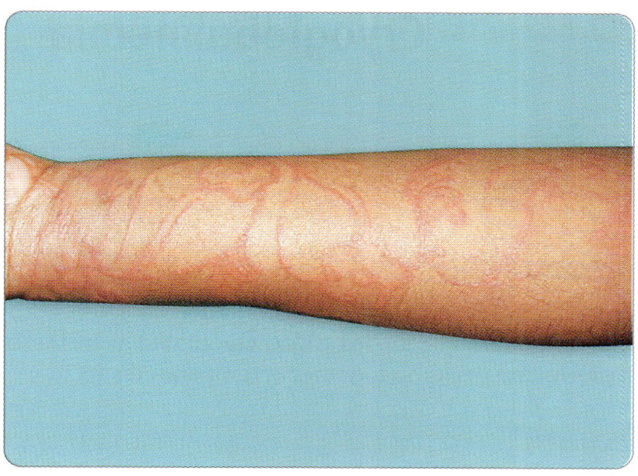

Fig. 1: Allergic contact dermatitis to Mehendi.

DIFFERENTIAL DIAGNOSIS

- Irritant contact dermatitis
- Atopic dermatitis
- Stasis dermatitis
- Seborrheic dermatitis
- Erythematous form of acne rosacea
- Scabies
- Insect bites
- Candidiasis

Hand and foot lesions need to be distinguished from psoriasis and tinea.

Widespread involvement needs to be differentiated from erythroderma and Sezary syndrome.

TREATMENT

Fundamental management of patients lies in both treatment of symptoms and avoidance of allergens. Once allergens are positively identified, the patient should be given written information on all of these chemicals. The information sheets should contain data regarding the name of the chemical, possible synonyms, typical uses for the chemical, how to avoid exposure, and, when appropriate substitutions should be made.

Acute weeping lesions can be treated with topical aluminum sulfate, and chronic lichenified lesions with emollients. Oral antihistamines can be given for pruritis.

Despite their drawbacks and long-term use, corticosteroids remain the gold standard of treatment for alleviating symptoms and hastening recovery from ACD. Phototherapy is used for resistant patients.

SUGGESTED READING

1. Nassau S, Fonacier L. Allergic contact dermatitis. Medical Clinics. 2020;104(1):61-76.

52 Cryoglobulinemia

➲ INTRODUCTION

Cryoglobulinemia is a rare medical condition characterized by the presence of abnormal proteins called cryoglobulins in the blood, which precipitate or clump together at temperatures <37°.

➲ HISTORY

Meltzer triad, i.e., purpura, arthralgia, and weakness, was first described in 1966 by Meltzer and Franklin in cases of essential mixed cryoglobulinemia.

➲ ETIOLOGY

Cryoglobulins are immunoglobulins that precipitate at low temperatures and resolve with rewarming.

Brouet classification of cryoglobulins is as follows:

- *Type I (10–15%)*: Isolated monoclonal immunoglobulins, associated with lymphoproliferative diseases (predominantly B cell).
- *Type II (50–60%)*: Mixed cryoglobulins, immunocomplexes formed by monoclonal immunoglobulin M (IgM).
- *Type III (25–30%)*: Mixed, polyclonal immunoglobulin, immunocomplexes of both immunoglobulin (IgG) and IgM.

➲ EPIDEMIOLOGY

M:F ratio is 1:3, more common in the fifth to sixth decade.

➲ PATHOPHYSIOLOGY

There is increased production of higher levels of the mono-, oligo- or polyclonal immunoglobulins due to chronic immune stimulation and lymphoproliferation, leading to the formation of cryoglobulins. These cryoglobulins are composed of immunoglobulins and complement components, deposit in small- to medium-sized blood vessels throughout the body, causing endothelial injury and end-organ damage. Cryoglobulins can cause a range of symptoms, including joint pain, skin rashes, and kidney problems, due to their tendency to obstruct blood vessels and trigger inflammatory reactions. Later there is the formation of the antigen-antibody complexes. Insufficient or poor clearance of the formed immune complexes leads to accumulation.

➲ CLINICAL FEATURES

Meltzer's triad comprises purpura, weakness, and arthralgia which are the common features. Type I has mainly cutaneous lesions in the form of inflammatory macules, papules, purpura and ulceration in nondependent areas. Mixed cryoglobulinemia has arthritis, Raynaud's phenomenon, purpura, renal involvement, hepatomegaly, and cold urticaria.

Associated conditions are hepatitis B, C, systemic lupus erythematosus (SLE), Sjögren syndrome, multiple myeloma, mycoplasma pneumonia, vaccines, and infective endocarditis. Nailfold capillary abnormalities are common and include dilatation, altered orientation, capillary shortening, and neoangiogenesis.

Diagnosis is by serum cryoglobulin level estimation.

➲ HISTOPATHOLOGY

Histopathology includes features of small-vessel leukocytoclastic vasculitis, endothelial cell swelling, fibrinoid necrosis of the vessel walls, and perivascular infiltrates of lymphocytes, macrophages, and neutrophils.

➲ DIFFERENTIAL DIAGNOSIS

- *Serum sickness*: Normal cryoglobulin levels
- *Antiphospholipid antibody syndrome*: Presence of antiphospholipid antibodies
- *Sarcoidosis*: Raised angiotensin-converting enzyme (ACE) levels, naked granulomas on biopsy, and other systemic involvement
- *Waldenstrom's hyperglobulinemia*: IgM spike on serum protein electrophoresis, normal cryoglobulin levels
- *Polyarteritis nodosa*: Necrotizing vasculitis on biopsy, normal cryoglobulin levels, other systemic involvement, and absence of renal involvement

➲ COMPLICATIONS

Glomerulonephritis.

➲ TREATMENT

The treatment of cryoglobulinemia depends on the underlying primary disorder, severity, and nature of organ involvement. Treatment options include systemic corticosteroids, nonsteroidal anti-inflammatory drugs (NSAIDs), azathioprine, mycophenolate mofetil, dapsone, methotrexate, and cyclophosphamide.

➲ PROGNOSIS

The prognosis is variable. Renal involvement is associated with increased mortality.

➲ SUGGESTED READING

1. Muchtar E, Magen H, Gertz MA. How I treat cryoglobulinemia. Blood. 2017;129(3):289-98.

53 Cryptococcosis

➲ SYNONYMS

Torulosis, European blastomycosis.

➲ HISTORY

In 1894, Busse, a pathologist, first described the yeast. In 1976, Kwon–Chung described the perfect (i.e., sexual and teleomorphic) form of *Cryptococcus neoformans*, which was named *Filobasidiella neoformans*.

➲ ETIOLOGY

Cryptococcosis is caused by a single species of fungus *C. neoformans*, which comprises two variants: *C. neoformans* var. *neoformans* and *C. neoformans* var. *gattii*. Predisposing factors include immunodeficiency state such as AIDS, Hodgkin's disease, malignant lymphomas, sarcoidosis, collagen vascular disease, systemic corticosteroid therapy, and renal transplantation.

➲ EPIDEMIOLOGY

The disease usually occurs between the ages of 30 and 60 years and is uncommon in childhood. Cryptococcal meningitis preferentially occurs in persons with impaired cell-mediated immunity and is a major AIDS-related opportunistic infection as the CD4+ cell count falls <100 cells/μL. Cryptococcal disease is reportedly more common in men than in women.

➲ CLINICAL FEATURES

The respiratory tract is the usual portal of entry by inhalation of the infectious propagules, but primary cutaneous lesions may occur. There is a marked predilection for the brain and meninges, although the lungs and occasionally the skin and other parts of the body may be involved.

Systemic involvement is usual, and the central nervous system (CNS) manifestations often predominate, presenting as chronic meningitis or as focal brain lesions simulating a tumor. Pulmonary or urinary tract cryptococcosis may occur. Other systemic manifestations include myocarditis, chorioretinitis, hepatitis, peritonitis, renal abscess, prostatitis, myositis, and adrenal gland involvement.

Cutaneous cryptococcosis is the third most common clinical manifestation of cryptococcosis. The cutaneous and mucous membrane lesions occur in about 10% and 3% of cases, respectively. The lesions are firm or cystic, slow-growing, subcutaneous, erythema nodosum-like swellings. Other presentations include molluscum contagiosum-like, acneiform, nodular, herpetiform lesions, cellulitis, keloidal or warty crusted plaques.

Any of these lesions may ulcerate or ulcers may develop in primarily unaffected skin, when they are often punched out with a rather distinctive rolled edge **(Figs. 1A and B)**.

➲ DIAGNOSIS

Definitive diagnosis is made by isolation of the organism from the clinical specimen or direct detection of fungus using Indian ink preparation **(Fig. 1C)**.

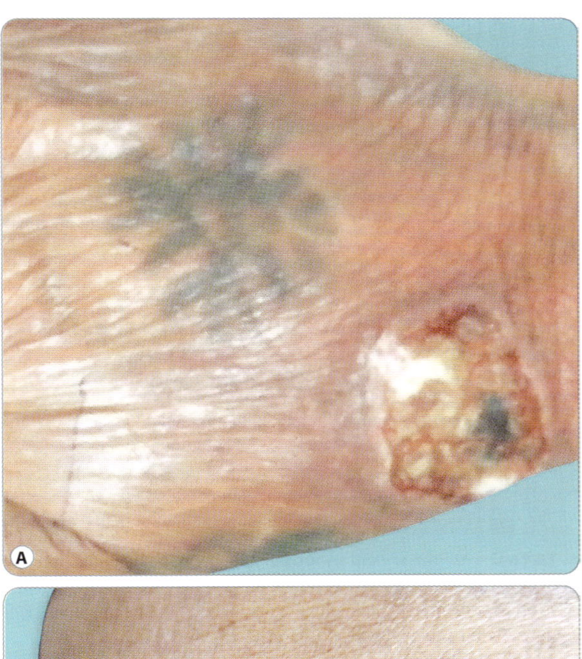

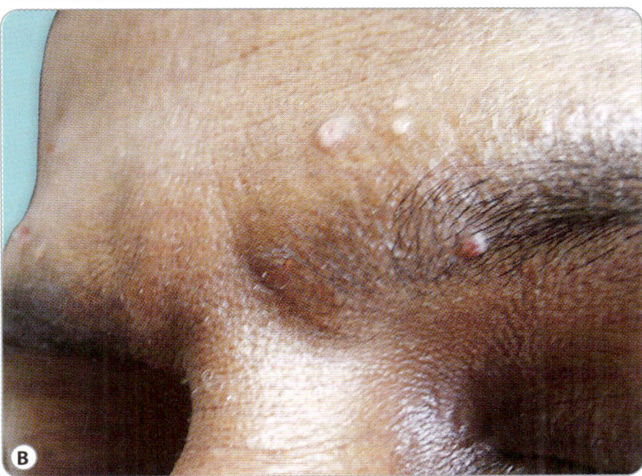

Figs. 1A to D: *Continued*

Continued

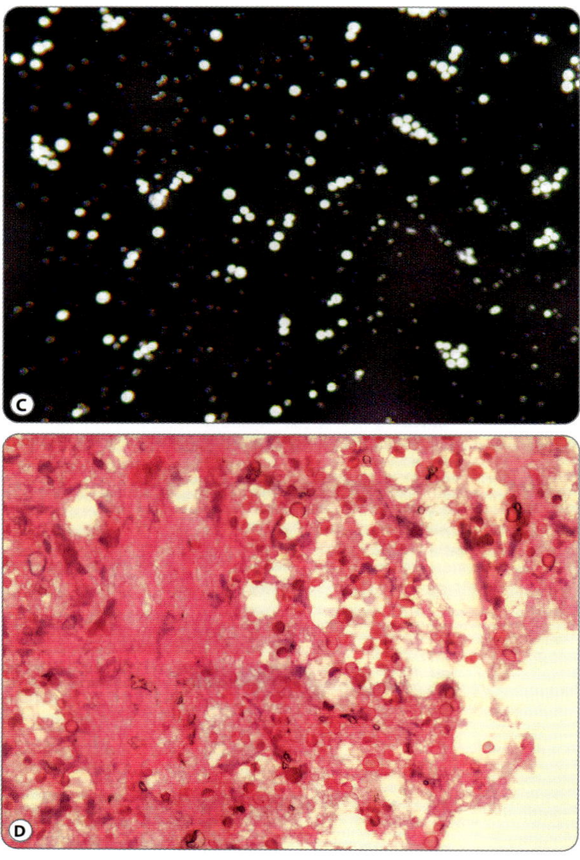

Figs. 1A to D: (A) Primary cutaneous cryptococcosis; (B) Molluscum-like lesions of cryptococcosis in an immunocompromised patient; (C) Indian ink preparation for cryptococcosis showing budding yeast cells; and (D) Spore stains with the periodic acid–Schiff (PAS) stain.

HISTOPATHOLOGY

There may be a minimal inflammatory reaction. The characteristic lesion consists of encapsulated budding cells mixed with a network of connective tissue, which enlarges and compresses the surrounding tissues. The specific stain for the capsule is mucicarmine **(Fig. 1D)**. Alternatively, a granulomatous reaction without caseation may be seen.

DIFFERENTIAL DIAGNOSIS

- *Histoplasmosis*: Absence of capsulated organisms
- *Penicilliosis*: Presence of septate broomstick-like appearance of fungi
- *Cutaneous tuberculosis*: Presence of granulomas
- Acanthamoeba
- Basal cell carcinoma

- *Molluscum contagiosum*: Demonstration of molluscum bodies on Giemsa stain of the crush smear
- *Pneumocystis (carinii) jirovecii* pneumonia
- Syphilis
- Toxoplasmosis

➲ TREATMENT

Initially administer amphotericin B at 0.7–1 mg/kg/day for 2 weeks, with or without flucytosine at 100 mg/kg/day in four divided doses, followed by fluconazole at 400 mg/day for a minimum of 8–10 weeks. For single skin lesions in non-HIV patients, fluconazole 400–600 mg/day may be used. Itraconazole is an alternative for long-term therapy.

➲ PROGNOSIS

Without treatment in CNS involvement, there is a general decline in health, ending in coma and death, usually within a year but prognosis is good for pulmonary and cutaneous forms.

➲ SUGGESTED READING

1. Noguchi H, Matsumoto T, Kimura U, Hiruma M, Kusuhara M, Ihn H. Cutaneous cryptococcosis. Med Mycol J. 2019;60(4):101-7.

54 Cutis Laxa

➲ SYNONYM

Generalized elastolysis.

➲ ETIOLOGY

Cutis laxa is a disease of connective tissue characterized by redundant skin with loss of elasticity and premature aging. Cutis laxa can be acquired or congenital. Congenital forms may be autosomal dominant or recessive, of which recessive forms are more severe. An X-linked form is now classified as copper transport disease caused by lysyl oxidase deficiency. Most of the dominant forms of cutis laxa result from a mutation in the gene encoding elastin, the recessive form results from a mutation in fibulin 5/DANCE, a newly discovered protein critical for the organization and stabilization of elastic fibers in skin, lung, and blood vessels. Hence, the disease can affect the skin as well as internal organs.

➲ CLINICAL FEATURES

Patients present with striking picture of loose, inelastic, redundant skin that sags and hangs in pendulous folds as if it were too large for the body **(Figs. 1A and B)**. The drooping and ectropion of eyelids, together with sagging of facial skin and accentuation of nasal, labial, and other facial folds produce the bloodhound or aged appearance. Systemic manifestations include aortic dilatation, pulmonary aortic stenosis, pulmonary emphysema, urinary or gastrointestinal diverticula, uterine or rectal prolapse, ventral, hiatal, or inguinal hernias because of the weakened supportive tissue. The life expectancy is almost the same as the general population.

The autosomal dominant form may occur at any age and presents mainly as cosmetic problems, with few systemic changes. The skin in cutis laxa is extensible, but in contrast to Ehlers–Danlos syndrome, does not spring back to place on release of tension.

Cutis laxa can also be acquired. In type 1 acquired cutis laxa, ill-defined areas of loose skin appear insidiously and progressively, initially on the face, progressing in a cephalocaudal direction. Lax skin may be preceded by urticarial eruption. Emphysema, aortic aneurysm, and urinary or gastrointestinal diverticula may be associated. Children may develop lesions after drug exposure to penicillin, D-penicillamine, and isoniazid.

Type 2 acquired cutis laxa is post-inflammatory elastolysis characterized by well-demarcated, nonpruritic erythematous plaques appearing in crops, in association with fever, malaise, and peripheral eosinophilia. Acquired cutis laxa occur at the sites of previous inflammation.

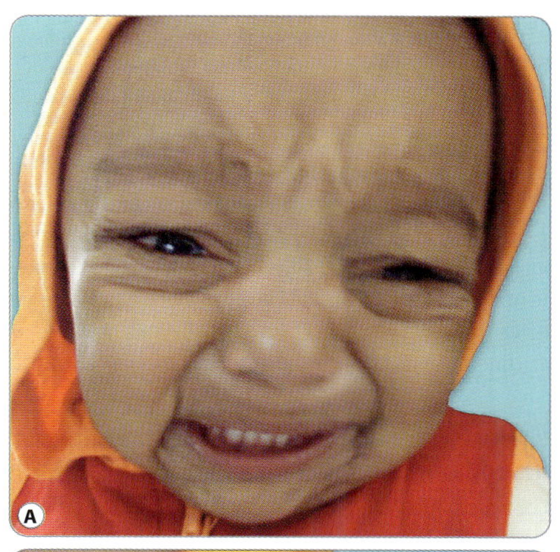

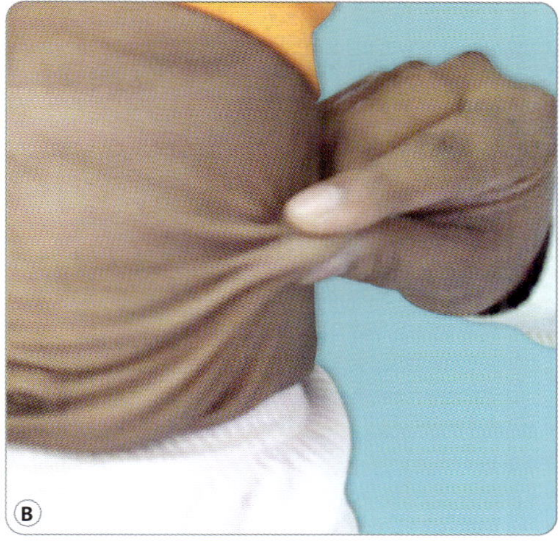

Figs. 1A and B: (A) Cutis laxa; and (B) Loose inelastic skin in folds.

ASSOCIATED SYNDROMES

Costello syndrome, De Barsy syndrome, Lens–Majewski-hyperostotic dwarfism.

HISTOPATHOLOGY

Biopsy on staining with special stains (Verhoff Van Gieson) shows significantly reduced or absent dermal elastic tissue.

DIFFERENTIAL DIAGNOSIS

- *Ehler–Danlos syndrome*: The skin is highly extensible but still retains its elastic recoil.
- *Pseudoxanthoma elasticum*: Calcification of elastic fibers in the skin, eyes, and blood vessels
- Atrophoderma

- Morphea
- Anetoderma
- Marfan's syndrome

TREATMENT

Treatment options are limited. The skin manifestations do not improve spontaneously. Surgery can be done to correct diverticula, rectal prolapse, and hernias. Plastic surgery can make dramatic improvements. Unlike in Ehlers–Danlos, patients have no vascular fragility, hence, healing well, enabling facelift procedures. Pulmonary function studies may aid in early detection of emphysema.

PROGNOSIS

In patients with aortic regurgitation (AR) disease, the disorder is gradually progressive. Death can occur in early infancy due to emphysema or pulmonary complications.

SUGGESTED READING

1. Berk DR, Bentley DD, Bayliss SJ, Lind A, Urban Z. Cutis laxa: a review. J Am Acad Dermatol. 2012;66(5):842-e1-17.

55 Cylindroma

➲ SYNONYMS

Turban tumor, Spiegler's tumor, tomato tumor.

➲ ETIOLOGY

Cutaneous cylindromas are benign adnexal neoplasms, describing a dual lineage proliferation of cells within the dermis. In cross-section, the cells have a round morphology that is likened to cylinders, hence, the name. Cylindroma may be sporadic or familial, with an autosomal dominant inheritance. Loss of CYLD (cylindromatosis gene) has been implicated. It is also found to occur after radiotherapy epilation of the scalp.

➲ EPIDEMIOLOGY

It occurs commonly in the early adult age group but may occur in adolescence or children. Females are more commonly affected.

➲ CLINICAL FEATURES

Cylindromas present as slow-growing, painless, and round nodular lesions and can sometimes be pedunculated. The tumors are frequently multiple, smooth, firm, pink to red in color, and often pedunculated. Multiple cylindromas will usually occur in cases of a familial syndrome and start earlier in life. Most are small in size but some may be as large as 5 cm. Pain may be a symptom. The most common site is the scalp and adjacent skin, followed by the face, neck, and rarely trunk and limbs. Scalp lesions are hairless when pedunculated, but smaller dermal lesions may have no loss of overlying hair. It is believed to be related to the apocrine gland **(Fig. 1)**.

➲ ASSOCIATED SYNDROMES

Brooke–Spiegler syndrome, multiple familial trichoepitheliomas, probably due to involvement of the same gene.

➲ DERMOSCOPY

Dermoscopy shows a white to light pink background, structureless light pink areas surrounded by white linear structures, fine arborizing telangiectatic vessels on the surface, and white structureless areas.

➲ HISTOPATHOLOGY

The tumor cells are closely aggregated in mosaic-like masses, as opposed to each other like pieces of a jigsaw puzzle. It is lined

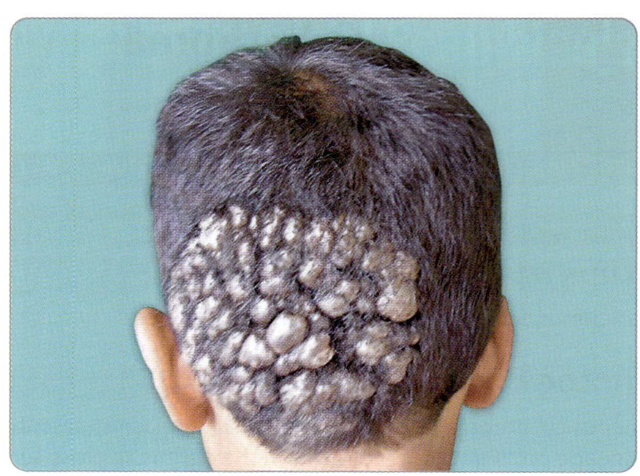

Fig. 1: Multiple nodules on the scalp of cylindroma.

by a thick, hyaline, periodic acid–Schiff (PAS)-positive basement membrane. Similar hyaline material is present within the tumor lobule. Thin bands of stroma separate the tumor lobules. Two types of cells are present, small cells with scanty cytoplasm and compact nucleus at the periphery, and large cells with moderate cytoplasm and vesicular nucleus toward the center. Within the basaloid islands interspersed small round pink globules, or "hyaline droplets," can be seen.

DIFFERENTIAL DIAGNOSIS

- *Trichilemmal cyst*: Usually discrete, thick capsule seen
- *Trichoepithelioma*: Usually smaller in size, have tumoral cells around the hair follicle
- *Steatocystoma*: Cystic lesion with whitish discharge, can get calcified
- Pilar cyst
- *Pilomatricoma*: Presence of ghost cells on histopathologic examination (HPE)
- *Eccrine spiradenoma*: Painful tumor, shows eccrine glands on section
- *Basal cell carcinoma*: Tumoral islands separated by lacunae but lack the PAS-positive deposition

COMPLICATIONS

Rarely malignant transformation may occur in the setting of Spiegler–Brooke syndrome.

TREATMENT

Excision of the nodule. CO_2 laser ablation or cryotherapy can be done. Extensive lesions on the scalp may require wide excision and replacement by a graft.

➲ PROGNOSIS

Cylindromas are usually benign lesions; however, malignant transformations can rarely occur. Malignant changes are commonly associated with Brooke–Spiegler syndrome.

➲ SUGGESTED READING

1. Jordão C, de Magalhães TC, Cuzzi T, Ramos-e-Silva M. Cylindroma: an update. Int J Dermatol. 2015;54(3):275-8.

56 Cydnidae Pigmentation

SYNONYM

Burrowing bug pigmentation.

ETIOLOGY

Cydnidae insects (family, Cydnidae; order, Hemiptera; suborder, Heteroptera; superfamily, Pentatomoidea), also known as burrowing (or burrower) bugs are commonly seen in rural areas and during rainy season. These are winged low-flying insects. They generally live in soil or sand and feed on roots or other underground parts of plants. They produce an odorous substance from special glands for self-defense, which stains the skin in oval to bizarre pigmented patterns over exposed areas.

CLINICAL FEATURES

Asymptomatic brown macules appear suddenly on the feet commonly. Lesions may be also seen over the hands and neck **(Fig. 1)**.

DERMOSCOPY

Dermoscopy shows brownish orange lesions, with superimposed irregular darker streaks; dark brown linear pigmentation along the dermatoglyphics; enhanced pigmentation around the sweat pores, and light brown pigmentation dispersed in between the lines.

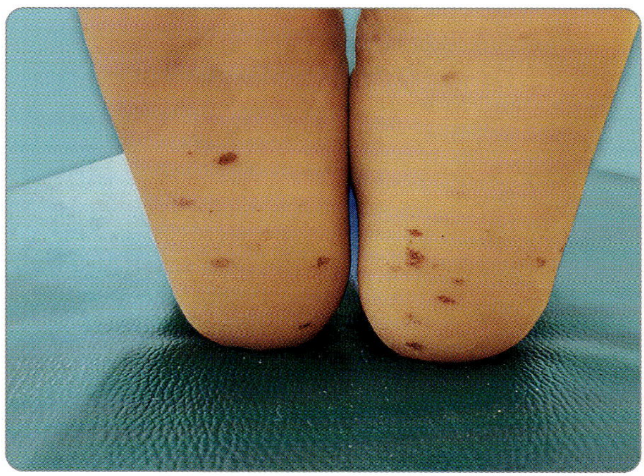

Fig. 1: Asymptomatic brown macules on the feet.

HISTOPATHOLOGY

Histopathology shows brownish-orange discoloration of stratum corneum and of keratin within the follicular ostium. Isolated necrotic keratinocytes and focal confluent necrosis are seen. Mild perivascular lymphocytic infiltrate may be seen in papillary dermis. No dermal pigment is seen, and periodic acid–Schiff, Masson–Fontana, and Perl's stains are negative.

DIFFERENTIAL DIAGNOSIS

- Lentigenes—seen commonly over the face, gradual onset
- Petechiae—erythematous
- Dermatitis neglecta—can be cleaned with soap and water
- Postinflammatory hyperpigmentation
- Junctional nevi—no abrupt onset

TREATMENT

No treatment is needed. The lesions will heal spontaneously over 2–3 weeks. They can be rubbed off with acetone, but not soap and water.

SUGGESTED READING

1. Kumar BS, Savitha AS. Cydnidae pigmentation–dermoscopic features. Pigment Int. 2021;8(2):115-6.

57 Darier's Disease

➲ SYNONYMS

Keratosis follicularis, Darier-White disease, Dyskeratosis follicularis.

➲ HISTORY

In 1889, the French dermatologist Jean Darier reported a skin disease characterized by brown, crusted, malodorous lesions with a follicular distribution.

➲ ETIOLOGY

Darier's disease (DD) is a rare autosomal dominant genodermatoses affecting both sexes and all ethnic groups. The mutations in the *ATP2A2* gene on chromosome 12q23-24 result in dysfunction of an endoplasmic reticulum Ca^{2+} ATPase (SERCA2), thus interfering with intracellular Ca^{2+} signaling. This calcium dysregulation leads to impaired control of cell-cycle checkpoints, leading to increased epidermal sensitivity to skin trauma, abnormality in epidermal cell-cell adhesion, and premature and faulty keratinization.

➲ EPIDEMIOLOGY

Darier's disease most commonly manifests between the ages 6 and 20 years; however, patients have presented as early as age 4 and as late as 70 years.

➲ CLINICAL FEATURES

The first skin lesions typically occur in the teenage years and are frequently associated with pruritus. The lesions may first appear as skin-colored or yellow-brown papules with a greasy, warty texture. These lesions are common in seborrheic areas such as the forehead, scalp, margin of the scalp, nasolabial folds, ears, chest, and back **(Figs. 1 and 2)**. 80% of patients have mild flexural involvement and 10% can have large, warty, vegetative plaques in the axillae, groin, or perineum. Lesions on the palms include punctate keratoses (80%), palmar pits (80%), and hemorrhagic macules (<10%). Acrokeratosis verruciformis–like lesions (warty flat-topped papules on the dorsal hands) are present in approximately half the patients.

Nail changes include white and red longitudinal bands, longitudinal nail ridges, longitudinal splitting, and subungual hyperkeratosis. A sandwich of red and white longitudinal bands, often with a V-shaped nick at the free margin of the nail, is the most pathognomonic nail finding **(Fig. 3)**.

Mucosal lesions (15%) appear as white papules with a central depression. These pebbly cobblestone lesions are most commonly found in the mouth, but they also may occur on the anogenital mucosa.

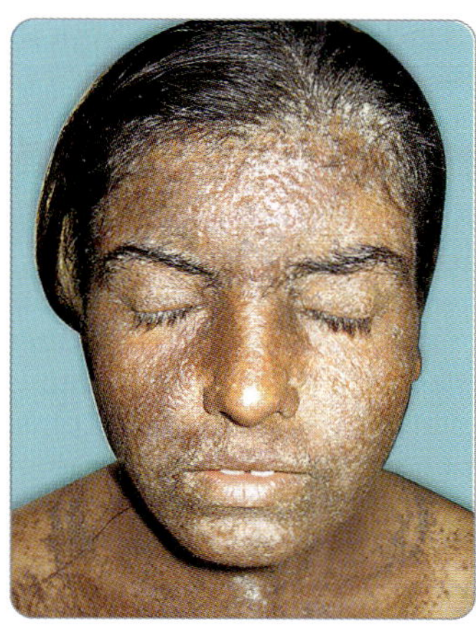

Fig. 1: Multiple dirty warty papules over the face and neck.

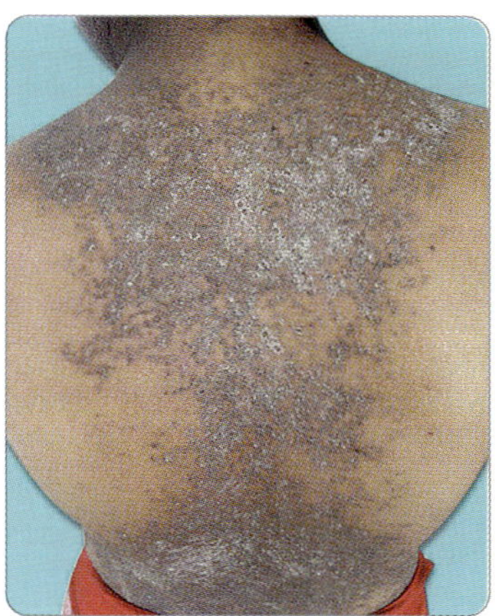

Fig. 2: Darier's disease with lesions over the back in seborrheic distribution.

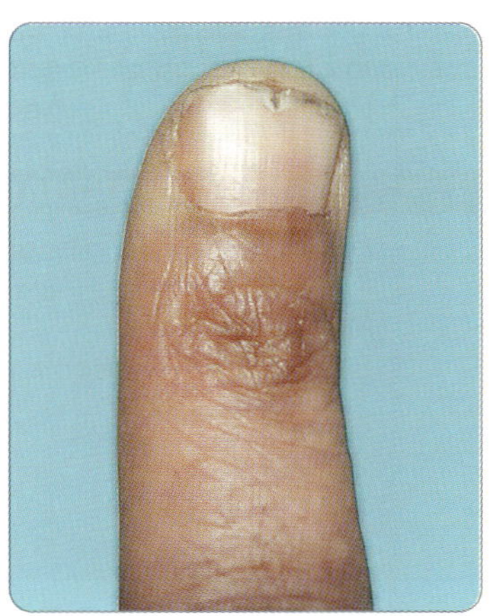

Fig. 3: V nicking.

Clinical variants include hypertrophic, vesicobullous, and linear or segmental types.

➲ HISTOPATHOLOGY

Acantholysis (loss of epidermal adhesions) and dyskeratosis (abnormal premature keratinization) are the two main features of DD. Acantholysis frequently results in the formation of characteristic suprabasal clefts. A large keratin plug, often showing focal parakeratosis, overlies each lesion. Hyperkeratosis is also common. Two types of dyskeratotic cells are present: Corps ronds and grains. Corps ronds are round keratinocytes with basophilic nuclei. Corps ronds are predominantly located in the stratum spinosum and the stratum granulosum. Corps ronds are characterized by an irregular eccentric and sometimes pyknotic nucleus, a clear perinuclear halo, and a brightly eosinophilic cytoplasm. Grains are mostly located in the stratum corneum, and they consist of oval cells with elongated cigar-shaped nuclei and abundant keratohyalin granules **(Figs. 4 and 5)**.

➲ DIFFERENTIAL DIAGNOSIS

- *Seborrheic dermatitis*: Absence of mucosal and nail changes, no dyskeratosis on histopathological examination (HPE)
- *Hailey-Hailey disease*: Erosions, fissures seen in intertriginous areas with partial acantholysis on HPE (dilapidated brickwall appearance)
- *Pemphigus vegetans*: Vegetating plaques seen in folds, suprabasal clefts with villi seen, absence of dyskeratosis, and positive direct immunofluorescence (DIF)
- *Pemphigus foliaceus*: Superficial erosion and crusted lesions in seborrhoeic areas, acantholytic cells on Tzanck smear, subcorneal blister, and positive DIF
- *Grover's disease*: Self-limiting transient vesicles mainly on the trunk

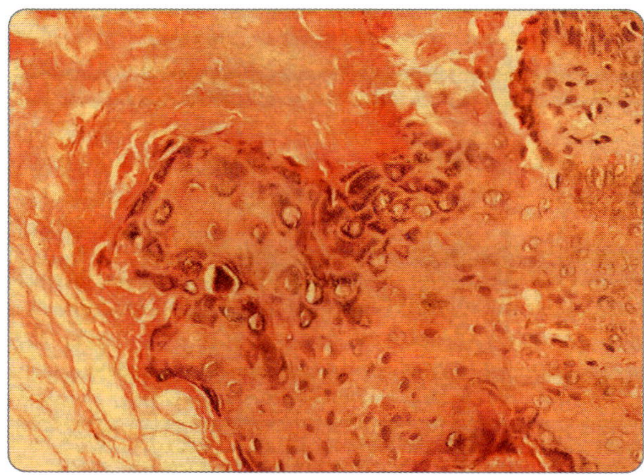

Fig. 4: Corps ronds with a central homogeneous, basophilic, pyknotic nucleus surrounded by a clear halo.

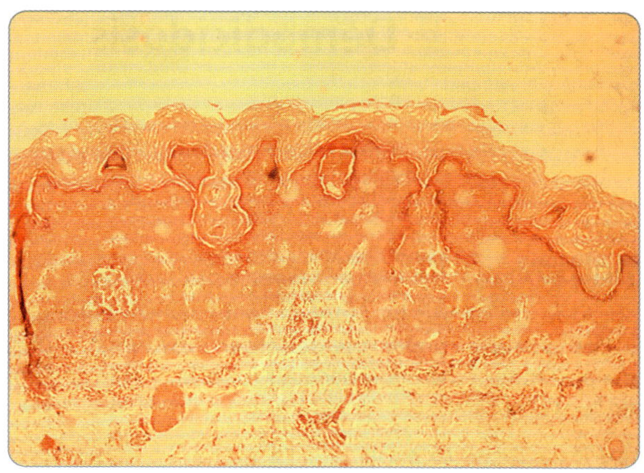

Fig. 5: Hyperkeratosis and papillomatosis with keratotic plugs, suprabasal acantholysis leading to the formation of lacunae.

- Localized form of epidermal nevus
- *Histologic D/D*: Epidermal nevus, warty dyskeratoma, and actinic keratosis

COMPLICATIONS

Bacterial sepsis and Kaposi's varicelliform eruption.

TREATMENT

Basic measures are sunscreen, cool cotton clothing, and avoidance of hot environments to prevent flares, especially during the summer. Moisturizers with urea or lactic acid can reduce scaling and hyperkeratosis. Topical medications such as adapalene, tazarotene gel 0.01%, and tretinoin can reduce hyperkeratosis in 3 months. However, irritation is a limiting factor. Emollients and topical corticosteroids can be used in combination with topical retinoids to reduce irritation. Topical 5-fluorouracil (5-FU) has been used effectively in some patients.

Acitretin at 0.6 mg/kg/day and isotretinoin at 0.5–1 mg/kg/day are effective. Oral antibiotics clear secondary bacterial superinfection, and oral acyclovir is used to treat or suppress herpes simplex virus infection. Oral contraceptives have been reported to help with perimenstrual flares.

Surgical treatments include dermabrasion, electrosurgery, shave excision, and laser ablation of recalcitrant plaques. Surgical excision can be done for hypertrophic intertriginous lesions.

PROGNOSIS

Darier's disease runs a life-long course.

SUGGESTED READING

1. Takagi A, Kamijo M, Ikeda S. Darier disease. J Dermatol. 2016;43(3): 275-9.

58 Demodicidosis

➲ ETIOLOGY

Demodicidosis is caused by *Demodex* mites which belong to the family Demodicidae, under the suborder Prostigmata. They are obligate parasites of the pilosebaceous follicles of man and animals such as dogs and cats.

Two species of *Demodex* exist:

1. *Demodex folliculorum*, the more elongated species (0.2–0.4 mm) which inhabits the hair follicles
2. *Demodex brevis*, a squatter species (0.1–0.2 mm) that mainly lives in the sebaceous and meibomian glands

Both species have a striated body and four pairs of very short stubby legs with an elongated abdomen and have altogether a worm-like appearance. Usually, only one species is seen in one person, rarely both.

➲ LIFE CYCLE

The life cycle from eggs through larvae and several nymphal stages to adults lasts about 10 days. The adult may live for another 10 days. Fertilization occurs at the pilosebaceous orifice, after which the female burrows down the hair follicle to the sebaceous gland where the eggs are laid. The eggs hatch and undergo molting within the sebaceous glands. The final nymphal stage emerges from the gland and enters another follicle where fertilization takes place to initiate a new life cycle. *Demodex* mites probably feed on cellular debris but certainly ingest bacteria.

➲ EPIDEMIOLOGY

Demodex folliculorum is uncommon in children under 5 but is almost universal in older children and adults.

➲ CLINICAL FEATURES

Two related disorders are usually considered to be the result of demodicidosis in man.

The first consists of a burning and itching sensation associated with diffuse erythema of the face with dryness, follicular scales, and "nutmeg grater-like" appearance. A skin scraping shows large numbers of *Demodex* mites. The condition is more frequently seen in women who use large quantities of make-up creams. The second type presents with the same features with the addition of rosacea-like lesions **(Fig. 1)**. The rosacea-like eruption is considered to be of external origin, in contrast to true rosacea, and hence is responsive to external treatment.

The role of *Demodex* in the pathogenesis of rosacea has been controversial for many years. The consistent demonstration of

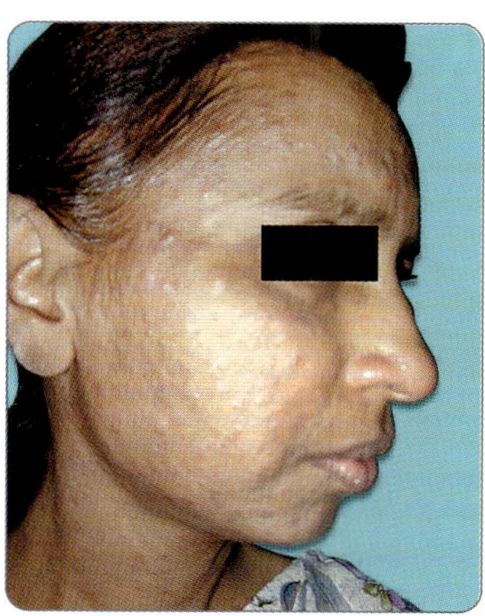

Fig. 1: Demodex folliculitis in an immunocompromised patient.

numerous mites in the inflamed pustules of acute rosacea is suggestive of its pathogenetic role and recent studies or skin surface biopsy have shown statistically significant increases in the density of *Demodex* in the facial skin of patients with rosacea compared with controls. Improvement of the condition after local application of miticides like 1% lindane also substantiates this view. Interestingly, in pustular acne vulgaris, it is usually not possible to demonstrate demodicosis.

Other types of lesions attributed to *Demodex* are pustular eruptions around the angles of the mouth, perioral dermatitis, blepharitis, and a papulonodular eruption in AIDS patients.

DERMOSCOPY

Nonfollicular and perifollicular gelatinous threads or filaments protruding out of follicular openings can be seen as "*Demodex* tails." They account for the presence of the mite itself. Dilated follicular openings containing round, amorphic, grayish/light brown plugs surrounded by an erythematous halo may be seen.

DIFFERENTIAL DIAGNOSIS

- *Rosacea*: Presence of papulopustules, telangiectasias, and photoaggravation
- *Perioral dermatitis*: Sparing of the vermilion border

TREATMENT

Cleaning with soap and water and application of miticides such as benzyl benzoate or gamma-benzene hexachloride clears the mites in about 3 days. A combination of 5% precipitated sulfur with 5% benzoyl peroxide is also effective. Topical permethrin has also been tried.

SUGGESTED READING

1. Chudzicka-Strugała I, Gołębiewska I, Brudecki G, Elamin W, Zwoździak B. Demodicosis in Different Age Groups and Alternative Treatment Options-A Review. J Clin Med. 2023;12(4):1649.

59 Dermatitis Herpetiformis

➲ SYNONYM

Duhring–Brocq disease.

➲ HISTORY

The disease was described and named in 1884 by Dr Louis Duhring at the University of Pennsylvania.

➲ ETIOLOGY

The leading theory for dermatitis herpetiformis (DH) is that of a genetic predisposition for gluten sensitivity, coupled with a diet high in gluten, leading to the formation of immunoglobulin A (IgA) antibodies to gluten-tissue transglutaminase (t-TG), which is found in the gut. Patients have an increased expression of the HLA-A1, HLA-B8, HLA-DR3, and HLA-DQ2 haplotypes. Deposition of IgA and epidermal TG complexes in the papillary dermis cause the lesions of DH. Androgen-deficient states, oral contraceptives, and leuprolide acetate, a gonadotropin-releasing hormone analog, may be a potential trigger for DH exacerbation.

➲ EPIDEMIOLOGY

Dermatitis herpetiformis presents mainly between the ages of 20 and 55 years but can present both in childhood and old age.

➲ CLINICAL FEATURES

Dermatitis herpetiformis is an exquisitely pruritic disease, characterized by grouped vesicles that are often excoriated to erosions, erythematous papules, and urticarial plaques. Eczematous changes that may be lichenified and progressive pigmentation are sometimes seen. The classic location for DH lesions is on the extensor surfaces of the elbows, knees, buttocks, and back. The axillary folds, shoulders, trunk, face, and scalp are all frequently involved. Punctate purpura may be seen on the palms and soles. Oral lesions are common but asymptomatic. Mucosal change may occur, and dental abnormalities such as enamel pits have been reported. They may have associated worsening of disease with dietary intake of gluten. The patient may experience bouts of abdominal pain, constipation, and diarrhea.

➲ ASSOCIATED CONDITIONS

Dermatomyositis, type 1 diabetes mellitus, myasthenia gravis, rheumatoid arthritis, Sjögren syndrome, systemic lupus erythematosus, and thyroid abnormalities.

➲ HISTOPATHOLOGY

Neutrophils and eosinophils accumulate within the dermal papillae and form microabscesses. The surrounding collagen is degraded, resulting in detachment of the epidermis and a subepidermal vesicle. Multilocular vesicles may coalesce to form blisters.

Direct immunofluorescence of a skin biopsy specimen shows deposition of IgA in a granular pattern in the upper papillary dermis (Picket fence appearance).

➲ DIFFERENTIAL DIAGNOSIS

- *Bullous pemphigoid*: Tense bullae seen on extremities first followed by trunk, subepidermal blister having eosinophilic infiltrate, linear immunoglobulin G (IgG), and C3 on direct immunofluorescence (DIF)
- *Erythema multiforme*: Presence of target lesions, negative DIF
- *Linear IgA dermatosis*: Cluster of jewels pattern of bullae, IgA deposits at basement membrane zone
- Neurotic excoriations
- *Scabies*: Classical involvement of circle of Hebra, nocturnal itching, family history, and burrows
- Transient acantholytic dermatosis
- Eczema
- *Papular urticaria*: Lesions only on exposed area

➲ COMPLICATIONS

Complications are related to gluten-sensitive enteropathy, there is a risk of developing gastrointestinal lymphomas.

➲ TREATMENT

Treatment includes avoidance of gluten by consuming a gluten-free diet. Dapsone is the most widely used treatment for DH. It acts by inhibiting neutrophil migration and function. The dose needed for the average case is 100–200 mg/day. New lesion formation is suppressed for up to 2 days after a single dose of dapsone. Topical steroids may be helpful in lessening symptoms. For patients unable to tolerate dapsone, sulfapyridine may be substituted. Heparin, with or without tetracyclines, in combination with nicotinamide/niacinamide is advocated for patients who cannot tolerate dapsone or sulfonamides. Other, less effective treatments include colchicine, cyclosporine, azathioprine, and prednisone. Ultraviolet light may provide some symptomatic relief.

➲ PROGNOSIS

Dermatitis herpetiformis is a lifelong disease. The prognosis is good for patients who can tolerate dapsone and the few who can maintain a gluten-free diet (which may decrease the risk of lymphoma). 10% of patients experience remissions.

➲ SUGGESTED READING

1. Salmi TT. Dermatitis herpetiformis. Clin Exp Dermatol. 2019:44(7): 728-31.

60 Dermatofibroma

SYNONYM

Fibrous histiocytoma.

ETIOLOGY

The exact etiology is not known. History of trauma, insect bite, and thorn injury may be present. They usually develop spontaneously. Dermatofibroma lesions consist of proliferating fibroblasts, along with histiocytes.

CLINICAL FEATURES

Dermatofibromas are slow-growing asymptomatic lesions that can develop on any part of the body. Clinically, they present as firm, nontender cutaneous nodules with or without accompanying skin changes, such as tan-pink to reddish-brown discoloration. The lesions measure 1 cm or less in diameter usually.

The lateral inward digital pressure on the skin produces central dimpling over the lesion due to its fixation to the subcutaneous tissue known as the dimple sign. Metastasis is rare.

Multiple eruptive dermatofibromas have been reported in patients with autoimmune diseases receiving immunosuppressive therapies, human immunodeficiency virus (HIV) infection, and pregnant women.

HISTOPATHOLOGY

There is a localized proliferation of spindle-shaped fibrous cells mixed with histiocytoid cells within the dermis. The spindle cells form a focal storiform pattern characterized by a multicentric whorling appearance of elongated nuclei. Intermixed capillaries, lymphocytes, or multinucleated giant cells may also be present. Trapped collagen bundles are seen within and in between fascicles of spindle cells. A delineated and unaffected grenz zone typically separates the overlying epidermis. The epidermis displays elongated rete ridges extending into the dermis, with hyperpigmented basal keratinocytes—dirty-feet sign.

Histological variants:

- Atypical dermatofibroma
- Cellular benign dermatofibroma
- Epithelioid dermatofibroma
- Aneurysmal dermatofibroma
- Hemosiderotic dermatofibroma

DERMOSCOPY

A central white patch surrounded by a peripheral pigmented network.

DIFFERENTIAL DIAGNOSIS

- *Dermatofibrosarcoma protuberans*: Lesions are typically more cellular, exhibiting pronounced storiform patterns and deep invasion into the subcutis, often entangling fat as it proliferates along subcutaneous septae. Dermatofibroma stains positive for factor XIIIa and vimentin but is negative for CD34.
- *Kaposi sarcoma*: Stain positive for CD31, CD34, and D2-40.
- *Intradermal nevi*: Softer consistency, the dimpling sign is negative.

TREATMENT

Treatment is not necessary as the lesions are asymptomatic. Excision is indicated when lesions show signs of malignancy. Atypical variants are prone to recurrence, so complete excision with clear margins is indicated.

PROGNOSIS

The prognosis is good, and the risk of malignancy is very low.

SUGGESTED READING

1. Myers DJ, Fillman EP. Dermatofibroma. InStatPearls [internet]. StatPearls Publishing; 2024.

61 Dermatomyositis

SYNONYM

Idiopathic inflammatory myopathy.

HISTORY

In 1975, Bohan and Peter first suggested a set of five criteria to aid in the diagnosis and classification of dermatomyositis and polymyositis. The following five subsets of myositis were suggested by them:

1. Dermatomyositis
2. Polymyositis
3. Myositis with malignancy
4. Childhood dermatomyositis/polymyositis
5. Myositis overlapping with another collagen-vascular disorder

ETIOLOGY

Dermatomyositis is one of the idiopathic inflammatory myopathies. It is considered to be the result of a humoral attack against the muscle capillaries and small arterioles (endothelium of the endomysial blood vessels). The initial event is the activation of completer factor-3 (C3), followed by the formation of the neoantigen C3bNEO and the C5b-C9 membrane attack complex (MAC). The MAC deposits on vascular walls and causes inflammation. The cause of dermatomyositis is unknown; however, the following factors have been implicated:

- A genetic component may predispose to dermatomyositis; there is a link to certain human leukocyte antigen (HLA) types, e.g., HLA-A*68, HLA-DRB1, DR5, and DR7.
- Abnormal T-cell activity may be involved in the pathogenesis.
- Infectious agents, including viruses (e.g., coxsackie virus, parvovirus, echovirus, human T-cell lymphotropic virus type 1, HIV) and *Toxoplasma* and *Borrelia* species, have been suggested as possible triggers.
- Other agents that may trigger the disease include hydroxyurea, penicillamine, statins, quinidine, phenylbutazone, silicone breast implants, or collagen injections.
- *Association with malignancy*: The primary tumor most commonly occurs in the lung, breast, female genital tract, stomach, rectum, kidney, or testis.
- Dermatomyositis has been observed to occur more frequently among women exposed to high-intensity ultraviolet radiation.

➲ EPIDEMIOLOGY

Dermatomyositis can occur in people of any age. In adults, the peak age of onset is approximately 50 years, whereas in children, the peak age is approximately 5–10 years.

➲ PATHOPHYSIOLOGY

- Humoral-mediated attack directed against the muscle capillaries and the endothelium of arterioles
- Activation of completer factor-3 (C3), which forms C3b and C4b
- Formation of the neoantigen C3bNEO and the C5b-C9 MAC
- MAC deposits on vascular walls and causes inflammation. And hypoxic injury to the muscle fibers ensues, leading to atrophy of muscle fibers.

➲ CLINICAL FEATURES

Dermatomyositis is a disease that primarily affects the skin and the muscles, but it might also affect other organ systems.

The characteristic cutaneous features of dermatomyositis are a heliotrope rash (blue-purple discoloration) that occurs on the face, especially involving the eyelids, the upper cheeks, forehead, and temples and a raised, violaceous, scaly eruption on the knuckles called Gottron papules. Other features include malar erythema, poikiloderma, violaceous erythema on the extensor surfaces, and periungual and cuticular changes. The rash may involve other body surfaces, including knees, elbows (Gottron's sign), neck, anterior chest (V sign), or back and shoulders (shawl sign). Poikiloderma involving the lateral aspects of the thigh is called a Holster sign. Dilated capillary loops at the base of the fingernails are characteristic of dermatomyositis. The cuticles may be irregular and thickened, and the palmar and lateral surfaces of the fingers may become rough and cracked (mechanic's hand).

Muscle disease commonly manifests as proximal symmetrical muscle weakness. Other systemic features include joint swelling, Raynaud phenomenon, calcinosis, panniculitis, and abnormal findings on cardiopulmonary examination. The small joints of the hands are the most frequently involved. The arthritis associated with dermatomyositis is nondeforming.

➲ HISTOPATHOLOGY

Skin biopsy reveals an interface dermatitis that is difficult to differentiate from lupus erythematosus. Vacuolar degeneration and lymphocytic inflammatory infiltrates at the dermal-epidermal junction can occur. Muscle biopsy in patients with dermatomyositis reveals perivascular and interfascicular inflammatory infiltrates with adjoining groups of muscle fiber degeneration/regeneration. Although inflammation is the histological hallmark of dermatomyositis, polymyositis, and inclusion-body myositis, dermatomyositis is the only condition that shows perifascicular atrophy.

LABORATORY INVESTIGATIONS

- *Muscle enzymes*: Creatinine kinase, lactate dehydrogenase, and alanine aminotransferase
- *Autoantibodies*: Anti-Jo, anti-Mi 2, anti-SRP, anti-MDA5, anti-TIF -1, anti-SAE, and anti-NXP2
- *Electromyography*: Increased insertional activity, fibrillations, and positive sharp waves
- *Radiology*: Chest X-ray to rule out interstitial lung disease

DIFFERENTIAL DIAGNOSIS

- *Discoid lupus erythematosus*: Classical lesions on sun-exposed areas, absence of proximal muscle weakness, characteristic antinuclear antibody (ANA) profile, follicular plugging, and inflammatory infiltrate in the dermis
- Graft versus host disease
- *Lichen myxedematosus*: Deposition of mucin detectable on special stains
- *Lichen planus*: Absence of systemic involvement
- Multicentric reticulohistiocytosis
- Sarcoidosis
- Subacute cutaneous lupus erythematosus (SCLE)

COMPLICATIONS

Dermatomyositis may cause death because of muscle weakness or cardiopulmonary involvement. Patients with an associated malignancy may die of the malignancy. Calcinosis is more common in children.

TREATMENT

Therapy for dermatomyositis involves both general measures and specific measures to control the muscle disease and the skin disease. The muscle component is treated by administering corticosteroids (60 mg/day prednisolone), with or without immunosuppressive agents such as azathioprine (1.5–3 mg/kg/day in divided doses), methotrexate (7.5–15 mg/week), cyclosporine 5 mg/kg/day, and cyclophosphamide.

The skin disease is treated by avoiding sun exposure and by using sunscreens, topical corticosteroids, antimalarial agents (hydroxychloroquine and chloroquine), or mycophenolate mofetil. Sirolimus and leflunomide may also be of value in some patients.

Intravenous immunoglobulin (IVIg) not only benefits the muscle but also clears the skin lesions in the patients in whom it is used. Rituximab has been used for skin disease. Extracorporeal photochemotherapy and plasmapheresis may be useful in combination with other therapies. Methandienone, dapsone, and pentoxifylline are other options.

PROGNOSIS

Most patients with dermatomyositis survive, in which case they may develop residual weakness and disability. Children with severe dermatomyositis may develop contractures. The disease may spontaneously remit in as many as 20% of affected patients. About 5% of patients have a fulminant progressive course with eventual death.

SUGGESTED READING

1. Marvi U, Chung L, Fiorentino DF. Clinical presentation and evaluation of dermatomyositis. Indian J Dermatol. 2012:57(5): 375-81.

62 Dermatosis Papulosa Nigra

HISTORY

Dermatosis papulosa nigra (DPN) was first described by Castellani in 1925.

ETIOLOGY

The condition is probably genetically determined and considered a variant of seborrhoeic keratoses but has an earlier age of onset than seborrheic keratoses. A somatic activating mutation in FGFR3 has been found in lesions of DPN similar to seborrheic keratosis. Others view it as a variant of multiple fibroepithelial papillomata (acrochordons). The role of circulating growth factors and receptor interactions is under study.

EPIDEMIOLOGY

The incidence rises from the first decade to over 40% by the third and is rather higher in females than males.

CLINICAL FEATURES

Dermatosis papulosa nigra is a pigmented papular eruption of the face and neck caused by a nevoid developmental defect of the pilosebaceous follicles, with histology resembling seborrheic keratoses. The individual lesions are black or dark brown, flattened or cupuliform papules 1–5 mm in diameter seen over the malar regions and on the forehead. It occurs rarely on the lower parts of the face, chin, neck, chest, and back **(Fig. 1)**.

HISTOPATHOLOGY

There is a nevoid developmental defect of the pilosebaceous follicles, showing irregular acanthosis, papillomatosis, and hyperkeratosis. Pigment deposits are seen throughout the rete ridges and stratum basale.

DIFFERENTIAL DIAGNOSIS

- *Primarily multiple seborrheic keratoses*: Dermoscopic differences, larger lesions, and squamous eddies in histopathologic examination (HPE).
- *Acrochordons*: Usually skin colored, found in sites like the nape of the neck, axillae, and groin
- *Melanocytic nevi*: Presence of nevoid cells
- *Lentigines*: Flat lesions with mucosal involvement
- *Verrucae*: Koebnerization seen, koilocytes on biopsy

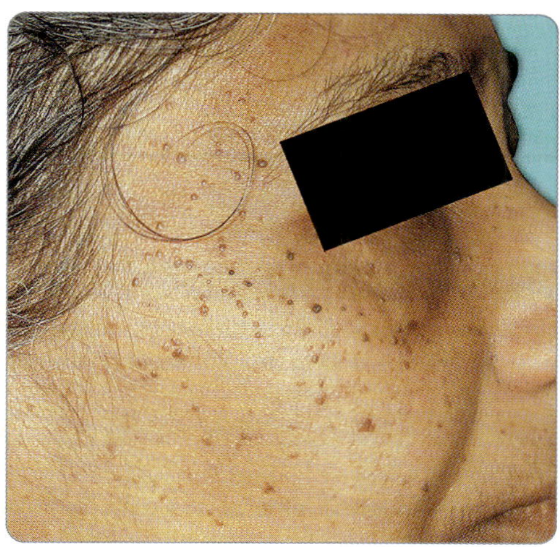

Fig. 1: Multiple hyperpigmented papules of dermatosis papulosa nigra (DPN) over the face.

- *Syringomas*: Angulated skin-colored papules, the proliferation of eccrine ducts with tadpole appearance
- Angiofibroma

TREATMENT

Snip excision with scissors, curettage, superficial liquid nitrogen application, and light electrodesiccation are the most common treatment modalities. DPNs are generally treated for cosmetic purposes. Complications of therapy include hyperpigmentation and hypopigmentation after cryotherapy.

SUGGESTED READING

1. Metin SA, Lee BW, Lambert WC, Parish LC. Dermatosis papulosa nigra: a clinically and histopathologically distinct entity. Clin Dermatol. 2017;35(5):491-6.

63 Dermoid Cyst

ETIOLOGY

Dermoid cysts result from sequestration of ectodermal tissue along embryonic fusion planes during development. Dermoid cysts are true hamartomas.

EPIDEMIOLOGY

Dermoid cysts are congenital defects and may be recognized at birth, these lesions often escape notice until they become enlarged, inflamed, or infected. Dermoid cysts are one of the most common pediatric skull tumors. This typically occurs in early childhood, but diagnosis may be delayed until as late as the sixth decade of life.

CLINICAL FEATURES

Dermoid cysts present as firm, noncompressible, nonpulsatile subcutaneous nodules that often reach a size of 1–4 cm in diameter. The lesions usually do not transilluminate. They are most commonly located around the eyes, particularly the lateral eyebrow but may also be found on the nose, scalp (often over the anterior fontanelle or the midline occiput), neck, sternum, sacrum, and scrotum. Dermoid cysts that are congenital and localized on the neck, head, or trunk are usually visible at birth. Hair protruding from a dermoid cyst punctum is pathognomic for dermoid cysts. Intracranial, intraspinal, or intra-abdominal dermoid cysts may be suspected after specific or nonspecific neurologic or gynecologic symptoms occur.

Occasionally, skin-related dermoid cysts are multiple and develop over periods as long as 20 years.

HISTOPATHOLOGY

Histologically, dermoid cysts are lined by keratinizing stratified squamous epithelium and contain mature adnexal structures. As a rule, these appendages are fully mature. Hair follicles containing hairs that project into the lumen of the cyst are often present. The dermis of dermoid cysts usually contains sebaceous glands, eccrine glands, and, in many patients, apocrine glands. Malignant degeneration in adulthood is extremely rare.

DIFFERENTIAL DIAGNOSIS

- *Metastatic carcinoma of the skin*: Histological evidence of abnormal cells
- *Pilar cyst*: Common in hear bearing area
- Trichilemmal cyst
- *Pilomatricoma*: Presence of shadow cells and lacks a cystic cavity

- *Steatocystoma multiplex*: Yellowish tinge to the appearance, extrusion of whitish material, not always at sites of embryological fusion
- Thyroglossal duct cyst
- Epidermoid cyst
- Lipoma

COMPLICATIONS

Dermoid cysts on the nose or midline scalp have a much higher likelihood of intracranial extension than those in periocular location. In addition to infectious complications, chemical meningitis or even hydrocephalus due to the release of keratinous and sebaceous material into the cerebrospinal fluid (CSF) can occur with intracranial dermoid cysts. Intralingual dermoid cysts can cause deglutition and speech problems. Malignant transformation is an unusual complication that may occur in patients with long-standing dermoid cysts.

TREATMENT

Surgical excision is the treatment of choice in any location, and preoperative imaging studies are required, particularly for lesions on the nose, midline scalp, or posterior axis, in order to exclude a connection to the central nervous system (CNS).

PROGNOSIS

If dermoid cysts are diagnosed early and treated with complete surgical excision, the prognosis is good, and no further complications are expected. In patients with carcinomatous transformation, the prognosis depends on the stage of the malignant disease and the success of therapy.

SUGGESTED READING

1. Shareef S, Ettefagh L. Dermoid Cyst. StatPearls. Treasure Island (FL): StatPearls Publishing; 2024.

64 Diabetic Dermopathy

➲ SYNONYMS

Diabetic shin spots, Binkley's spots.

➲ HISTORY

Atrophic skin lesions of the lower extremity, or shin spots, were first characterized and proposed as a cutaneous marker for diabetes in 1964. Shortly after, Binkley coined the term diabetic "dermopathy" to correlate the pathologic changes with those of retinopathy, nephropathy, and neuropathy.

➲ ETIOLOGY

The exact etiology is unknown. Antecedent traumatic injury in diabetics is the proposed etiology. Their presence does not correlate with blood glucose levels.

➲ EPIDEMIOLOGY

It is seen commonly in middle and elderly diabetic patients, more frequent in men than women. Isolated spots may be seen in normal individuals also.

➲ CLINICAL FEATURES

Lesions are predominantly situated on the shins, forearms, thighs, and over bony prominences. The initial lesion is an oval, dull-red papule 0.5–1 cm in diameter. It evolves slowly, producing a superficial scale, leaving an atrophic brownish scar. The color is due to hemosiderin in histiocytes near the vessels. The presence of four or more lesions has a high specificity for microvascular disease in skin and other tissues.

➲ DERMOSCOPY

Central white scar-like patch with peripheral brown pigmentation in a fishnet pattern.

➲ HISTOPATHOLOGY

There is a combination of vascular disease with periodic acid–Schiff (PAS)-positive thickening of the vessel wall and minor collagen changes. The presence of hemosiderin and melanin depositions in the epidermis of affected patients has also been reported.

COMPLICATIONS

A significant correlation exists between the presence of these lesions and other complications of diabetes, such as retinopathy, nephropathy, and neuropathy.

TREATMENT

No treatment is required.

PROGNOSIS

The lesions are persistent.

SUGGESTED READING

1. Pal R, Wal P, Pal Y, Wal A. Recent Insights on Diabetic Dermopathy. Open Dermatol J. 2019;13(1).

65 Diaper Dermatitis

➲ SYNONYMS

Napkin dermatitis, nappy rash, mechanical dermatoses.

➲ ETIOLOGY

Diaper dermatitis is an inflammatory reaction of the skin around the diaper area. Increased occlusive effects of a napkin, irritant effect of fecal enzymes (proteases and lipases), urinary pH, friction, hydration, temperature, chemical irritants (creams, oils, soaps, and antiseptics), microorganisms (*Candida albicans*), antibiotics, poor or misguided skin care, developmental anomalies of the urinary tract, and diarrhea (residual digestive enzymes) are predisposing factors. Even atopic dermatitis and seborrheic dermatitis can present as a diaper rash.

➲ EPIDEMIOLOGY

It is seen in infants and incontinent adult patients using diapers. It usually occurs between the 3rd and 12th weeks of life, and peaks between 9 and 12 months of age.

➲ PATHOPHYSIOLOGY

The most important predisposing factor for diaper dermatitis is the increased moisture which leads to increased friction and maceration. Also, an increase in pH around the diaper area from the breakdown of urinary urea can, in turn, increase fecal enzyme activity that can further damage the skin. This further results in colonization and infection from organisms such as *Staphylococci*, *Streptococci*, and *Candida*.

➲ CLINICAL FEATURES

Confluent glazed red erythematous skin is seen over the convexities of the buttocks, medial aspect of thighs, scrotum, and labia majora where the contact with the diaper is greatest. Deep folds of the groins and thighs are spared. Heals with postinflammatory hypopigmentation and wrinkling. Two variants are described. The edges of the napkin may lead to erythematous marks on the thighs and abdomen known as tidemark dermatitis or a more severe form of papuloerosive dermatitis known as Jacquet's dermatitis.

➲ DIFFERENTIAL DIAGNOSIS

- Allergic contact dermatitis
- Atopic dermatitis—involvement of other areas of the body

- Napkin psoriasis—the folds of the groins and thighs can also be involved, and biopsy shows specific features of psoriasis.
- Seborrheic dermatitis—lesions are more dry and scaly, other areas such as the scalp involved
- Candidal napkin dermatitis—the presence of fissures, pustules, and positive potassium hydroxide (KOH) mount
- Perianal streptococcal disease
- Acrodermatitis enteropathica—more of psoriasiform patches, perioral and other flexures involved, hair and nail changes seen, and low serum zinc levels
- Multiple carboxylase deficiency
- Langerhans cell histiocytosis—diffuse involvement, lesions refractory to treatment, systemic features, and Langerhans cell infiltrate on biopsy
- Congenital syphilis—the presence of bullae, other features, and positive venereal disease research laboratory (VDRL) test

COMPLICATIONS

Secondary infection with candidiasis and postinflammatory hypopigmentation.

TREATMENT

General Measures

Proper cleaning of the perianal area after passing feces, keeping the diaper area dry, avoidance of occlusive pants, use of a protective emollient ointment (white soft paraffin) or barrier creams (containing zinc oxide, titanium dioxide, and dimethicone), use of absorbent napkins, and talcum powders are best avoided.

Specific Treatment

It includes mild steroid cream such as hydrocortisone 1% for 1 week to 10 days and topical antifungal steroid combinations.

PROGNOSIS

Good prognosis if the underlying factor is removed.

SUGGESTED READING

1. Fölster-Holst R. Differential diagnoses of diaper dermatitis. Pediatr Dermatol. 2018;35(Suppl 1):s10-8.

66 Dilated Pore of Winer

➲ SYNONYMS

Winer's dilated pore.

➲ HISTORY

It was first described by Louis H Winer in 1954.

➲ ETIOLOGY

The exact etiopathogenesis is not known. Some have regarded it as a variant of infundibular cyst, while others consider it as a unique adnexal tumor of follicular differentiation.

➲ EPIDEMIOLOGY

It was common in males in the fourth to sixth decade.

➲ CLINICAL FEATURES

It presents as a solitary, asymptomatic, enlarged comedone without any perilesional inflammation or induration. Keratinaceous material can be expressed from the lesion at times. The head and the neck are the common sites affected **(Figs. 1 and 2)**.

➲ DERMOSCOPY

Dermoscopy shows central bluish-black central homogenous area of keratin plug with gray-white translucent halo around and a peripheral pigment network.

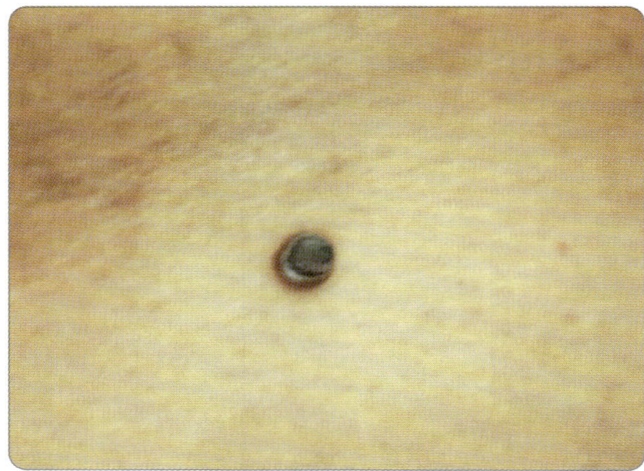

Fig. 1: Enlarged comedo-like lesion.

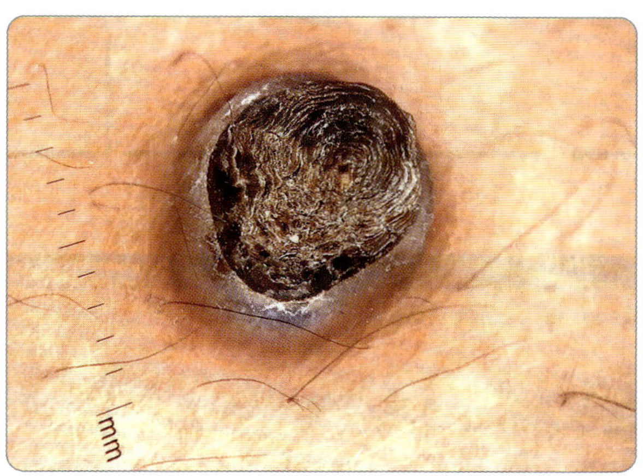

Fig. 2: Dermoscopy shows homogenous area of keratin plug with gray-white translucent halo.

HISTOPATHOLOGY

Markedly dilated follicular infundibulum extends into the dermis. The cavity is filled with lamellar keratin material lined by epithelium that is atrophic near the ostium and acanthotic at the deeper portion of the invagination. Radiating finger-like epithelial projections push into the surrounding dermis at regular intervals.

DIFFERENTIAL DIAGNOSIS

- Nevus comedonicus presents at birth or during childhood, with multiple keratin-filled openings.
- Pilar sheath acanthoma
- Comedo

TREATMENT

Excision can be performed for cosmetic purpose.

PROGNOSIS

The lesion is benign.

SUGGESTED READING

1. Tellechea O, Cardoso JC, Reis JP, Ramos L, Gameiro AR, Coutinho I, et al. Benign follicular tumors. An Bras Dermatol. 2015;90:780-98.

67 Discoid Lupus Erythematosus

SYNONYM

Cutaneous lupus erythematosus.

ETIOLOGY

The initiation of discoid lupus erythematosus (DLE) may result from somatic mutation or environmental factors such as trauma, stress, sun exposure, infection, drugs, pregnancy, and hormone replacement therapy. Positive associations with HLA-B7, -B8, -Cw7, -DR2, -DR3, and -DQw1 are reported.

EPIDEMIOLOGY

Discoid lupus erythematosus occurs commonly in young adults, and the prevalence is higher in women. 25% of patients with systemic lupus erythematosus (SLE) may develop typical discoid lesions at some point during their illness, and 1–5% of patients with discoid lupus may develop SLE.

CLINICAL FEATURES

Discoid lupus erythematosus is classified into generalized and localized lupus erythematosus.

Lesions begin as dull red macules or indurated plaques that develop an adherent scale and evolve with atrophy, scarring, and pigment changes. The hyperkeratosis characteristically extends into patulous follicles, producing spines on the undersurface of the scale. These spines are called carpet tacks or langue au chat (cat's tongue).

- *Localized discoid lupus erythematosus*: Discoid lesions are localized above the neck to the scalp, bridge of the nose, malar areas, lower lip, and ear. The concha of the ear and external canal are frequently involved. Few patients present with periorbital edema and erythema. Erythematous patches or plaques evolve into white, often depressed, scarring alopecia on the scalp. Perifollicular erythema and easily extractable anagen hair are the signs of active disease. About 24% of DLE patients may have mucosal involvement of the mouth, nose, eye, or vulva. On the lips, lesions may be gray or red and hyperkeratotic with erosions. Nails show subungual hyperkeratosis.
- *Generalized discoid lupus erythematosus*: Lesions are seen on the thorax, upper extremities, and neck. Diffuse scarring may involve the face and upper extremities. Elevated erythrocyte sedimentation rate (ESR), antinuclear antibody (ANA), anti(ss) DNA antibodies, or leukopenia are common with this form.

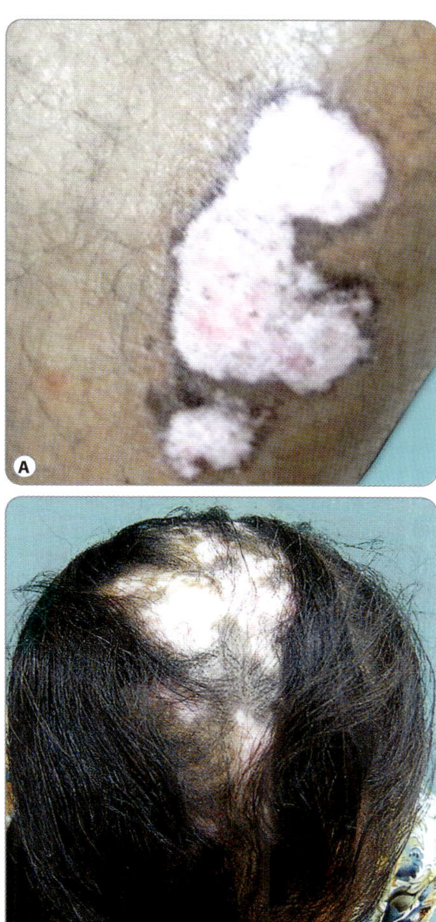

Figs. 1A and B: (A) Atrophic plaque with hyperpigmented border; and (B) Cicatricial alopecia due to discoid lupus erythematosus (DLE).

Other types include hypertrophic lupus, chilblain lupus, telangiectactic lupus, rosaceous type, and tumid lupus. Antinuclear antibodies are found in 5–60% of cases. The "homogenous" type of antinuclear factor is the most common ANA **(Figs. 1A and B)**.

DERMOSCOPY

- *Scalp DLE*: Follicular plugs (yellow dots), absence or reduced number of follicular ostia, fibrotic white dots, perifollicular scaling, perifollicular erythema, atrophy, thick arborizing vessels, dotted vessels, and hairpin vessels
- *Nonscalp DLE*: Follicular keratotic plugs, dilated follicles, white perifollicular halo, and linear vessels

HISTOPATHOLOGY

There is liquefaction degeneration of the basal cell layer of the epidermis, with hyalinization, edema, and fibrinoid changes, most marked immediately below the epidermis. A patchy dermal lymphocytic infiltrate with a few plasma cells and histiocytes is seen around the follicles. There is epidermal atrophy, thickening of the basement membrane, premature elastotic degeneration of collagen in light-exposed areas, and pigmentary incontinence.

Lupus band test can help to distinguish between DLE and SLE. It will be positive in both involved and uninvolved skin in SLE but positive only in involved skin in DLE.

DIFFERENTIAL DIAGNOSIS

- Seborrheic dermatitis—lacks the depigmentation and carpet tack-like scales, absence of follicular plugging, and can involve nonsun-exposed sites also.
- *Psoriasis*—profuse silvery white scales (Grattage test) and positive Auspitz sign
- *Superficial fungal infection*—demonstration of fungal hyphae
- *Rosacea*—absence of depigmented plaques and scaling
- *Lupus vulgaris*—granulomas on biopsy
- *Sarcoidosis*—naked granulomas on biopsy and raised angiotensin-converting enzyme (ACE) levels
- Drug eruptions
- Actinic keratosis
- Polymorphic light eruption (PMLE)

Histopathological differential diagnosis includes PMLE, lymphocytic lymphoma, Jessner's lymphocytic infiltrate, and lymphocytoma cutis.

COMPLICATIONS

Aggressive squamous cell carcinoma may develop in long-standing lesions of DLE.

TREATMENT

Topical steroids and intralesional corticosteroid injections are helpful in resistant lesions on the lips, mouth, and ears, along with sunscreens. Among other local measures, cryotherapy, surgical excision, painting small lesions with trichloracetic acid, and local laser therapy may be tried. Oral therapy includes prednisolone 0.5–1 mg/kg/day and hydroxychloroquine, initially at 200 mg twice daily, reducing to 200 mg/day once a response is achieved. Chloroquine sulfate is equally effective, usually at a dosage of 200 mg twice daily. Methylprednisolone 500–1,000 mg/day for 2 or 3 days can be given as intravenous pulse therapy.

PROGNOSIS

The untreated skin lesions resolve with scarring. Raynaud's phenomenon, scalp involvement, and chilblain-like lesions are slower to remit. Female patients may notice a premenstrual flare. Complete remission is seen in 50% of cases. The risk of developing overt SLE is 6.5%. The risk is higher with disseminated discoid lupus erythematosus (DDLE) (22%) than with DLE confined to the head and neck (1.2%). Females with DLE before the age of 40 years, with HLA-B8, have an increased risk of developing SLE.

➲ SUGGESTED READING

1. Vale ECSD, Garcia LC. Cutaneous lupus erythematosus: a review of etiopathogenic, clinical, diagnostic and therapeutic aspects. An Bras Dermatol. 2023;98(3):355-72.

68 Dowling–Degos Disease

➲ SYNONYMS

Dowling–Degos Kitamura disease, dark dot disease.

➲ HISTORY

Dowling–Degos disease was first described in 1938.

➲ ETIOLOGY

Dowling–Degos disease is caused by a loss-of-function mutation in keratin 5 gene (*KRT 5*).

Other genetic implications include mutations in *POFUT1*, *POGLUT1*, and *PSENEN*, which encode protein O-fucosyltransferase 1, protein O-glucosyltransferase 1, and presenilin enhancer protein 2 gene, respectively.

➲ PATHOPHYSIOLOGY

Dowling–Degos disease is a disorder of hyperpigmentation. The main pathophysiology involves the functioning of melanosomes. Due to haploinsufficiency of *KRT5*, there is an effect on the organization of cell adhesion, melanosome uptake into keratinocytes, organelle transport, and nuclear anchorage. The head domain of *KRT5* is thought to play a role in melanosome trafficking through its interaction with Hsc70. Also, the Notch signaling pathway plays an important role in skin homeostasis by regulating the proliferation and differentiation of melanocytes and keratinocytes and mediating their interactions with one another.

➲ CLINICAL FEATURES

Reticulate pigmentation of the skin in the flexural areas is associated with itching. Lentigo-like hyperpigmented macules and papules with hyperkeratosis will be seen in the intertriginous areas. The hyperpigmentation initially starts in the axilla and ground and gradually progresses to involve the other intertriginous regions. Comedone-like lesions on the neck and back, pitted perioral scars, and palmar pits can also be present **(Figs. 1A and B)**.

➲ DERMOSCOPY

Dermoscopy shows pigmented lesions—irregular, brown, star-shaped figures overlying a red background.

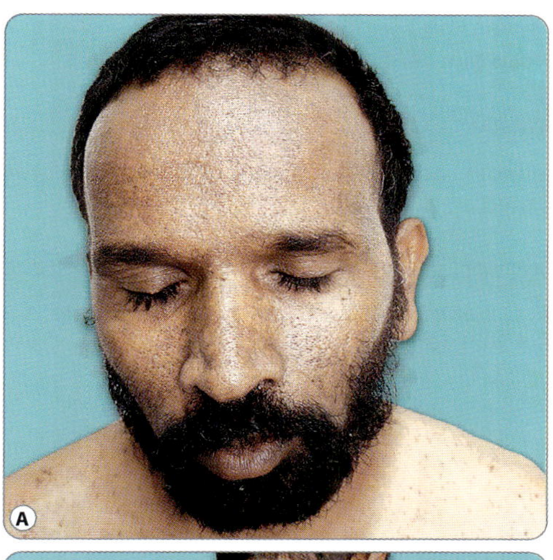

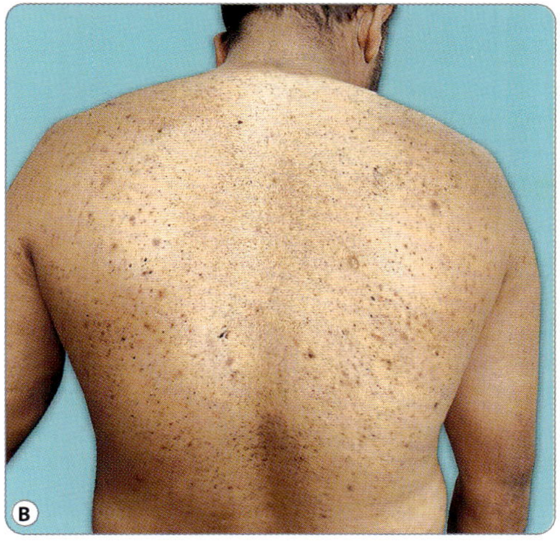

Figs. 1A and B: (A) Reticulate hyperpigmented macules and pitted scars on the face; and (B) Reticulate hyperpigmented macules with comedone-like lesions on back.

HISTOPATHOLOGY

- Increase in pigmentation of basal layer
- Downward elongation of rete ridges and thinning of suprapapillary epithelium
- Dermal melanophages and mild perivascular lymphohistiocytic infiltrates will be present.
- There will be haphazard distribution of irregularly placed melanosomes and keratinocytes.

DIFFERENTIAL DIAGNOSIS

- Reticulate pigmentation of Kitamura
- Neurofibromatosis type I

- Haber syndrome
- Acanthosis nigricans

TREATMENT

Topical tretinoin, adapalene, hydroquinone, and corticosteroids have been tried.

SUGGESTED READING

1. Stephan C, Kurban M, Abbas O. Dowling-Degos disease: A review. Int J Dermatol. 2021;60:944-50.

69 DRESS Syndrome (Drug Reaction with Eosinophilia and Systemic Symptoms)

➲ SYNONYMS

Drug-induced hypersensitivity syndrome (DIHS), drug-induced delayed multiorgan hypersensitivity syndrome (DIDMOHS), drug hypersensitivity syndrome (DHS), drug-induced pseudolymphoma.

➲ HISTORY

Initially, it was reported after taking hydantoin and drug-induced pseudolymphoma, and later, it was seen to occur with other anticonvulsants. However, as many drugs were later implicated in causing similar findings, the term drug reaction with eosinophilia and systemic symptoms (DRESS) was coined by Bocquest et al.

➲ PATHOGENESIS

Various hypotheses include:

- Genetic deficiency of detoxifying enzymes causes the accumulation of drug metabolites. Also, the activation of eosinophil and inflammatory cascade can be caused by interleukin 5 from T cells.
- Human leukocyte antigen (HLA) association
- Viral reactivation

➲ CLINICAL FEATURES

It presents with a varied spectrum of clinical features. The manifestations start after 2–8 weeks of the offending drug. The clinical features include fever, rash, lymphadenopathy, eosinophilia, and elevated liver function tests. The skin rashes can be urticarial, maculopapular eruption, or, sometimes, can be vesicular, pustular, and purpuric, target lesions cheilitis and even can develop erythrocytes. The systemic involvement will be in the form of hepatitis, pneumonitis, myocarditis, pericarditis, nephritis, and colitis. This could be the cause of major morbidity and mortality in this condition.

➲ MANAGEMENT

- Early recognition and withdrawal of the offending drug is the most important step in treating DRESS syndrome.
- Supportive and symptomatic treatment is based on the system involved.
- Systemic corticosteroids and other immunosuppressants like cyclosporine can be used.

➲ SUGGESTED READING

1. Calle AM, Aguirre N, Ardila JC, Cardona Villa R. DRESS syndrome: A literature review and treatment algorithm. World Allergy Organ J. 2023;16(3):100673.

70 Ecthyma

➲ SYNONYMS

Deep impetigo; in German, it is known as trench ulcer.

➲ HISTORY

Stokes described ecthyma.

➲ EPIDEMIOLOGY

Ecthyma is most common in children, especially those living in tropical countries. In industrialized countries, ecthyma may be seen in tourists returning from exotic vacations and in the homeless. It is also associated with poor hygiene, and it is more common in debilitated or immunosuppressed patients.

➲ ETIOLOGY

The causative organisms are group A streptococci or *Staphylococcus aureus*. The bacteria enter the skin through the areas of minor trauma. Thus, scabies, varicella, arthropod bites, and atopic dermatitis are common predisposing factors. Excoriation and manipulation by the patient also play a role.

➲ CLINICAL FEATURES

The initial lesion is similar to impetigo. Ecthyma begins as a vesicle or pustule on an erythematous base that deepens into a dermal ulceration with overlying gray-yellow crust, which is thicker and harder than the crust of impetigo. A shallow, punched-out ulceration is apparent when adherent crust is removed. The deep dermal ulcer has a raised and indurated surrounding margin. The shins are the most common site. Ecthyma lesions can remain fixed in size (sometimes resolving without treatment) or can progressively enlarge to 0.5–3 cm in diameter. It heals slowly and commonly produces a scar. Regional lymphadenopathy is common, even with solitary lesions.

➲ HISTOPATHOLOGY

Ecthyma lesions show dermal necrosis and inflammation. A deep and superficial granulomatous perivascular infiltrate occurs along with endothelial edema. In early lesions, *Streptococcus* can be cultured.

➲ DIFFERENTIAL DIAGNOSIS

- *Ecthyma gangrenosum*—demonstration of *Pseudomonas* on culture of the pus swab

- *Mycobacterium marinum* infection
- *Papulonecrotic tuberculids*—multiple small papules with central necrosis are seen.
- *Pyoderma gangrenosum*—ulcers with slough, violaceous border, and cigarette paper like atrophic scarring are seen.
- *Sporotrichosis*—linear distribution of ulcers and the presence of fungi
- *Leukocytoclastic vasculitis*—classical histopathological examination (HPE) findings
- Cutaneous diphtheria
- Erythema induratum

COMPLICATIONS

Complications include glomerulonephritis, bacteremia, cellulitis, and osteomyelitis.

TREATMENT

Topical mupirocin ointment is used for localized lesions. Wet compresses with disinfectant solutions should be used for debridement. The patients must refrain from manipulating the crust. Compression stockings are helpful in deep lesions.

Oral antibiotics, viz. antistaphylococcal agents (e.g., dicloxacillin, cephalexin, erythromycin, and clindamycin), have been used to cover possible secondary *S. aureus* infections.

ECTHYMA GANGRENOSUM

INTRODUCTION

Ecthyma gangrenosum is a cutaneous infection that most commonly occurs in immunocompromised individuals with fulminant bacteremia. It was first described in 1897 by Canadian pathologist Dr Lewellys Barker as a manifestation of *Pseudomonas aeruginosa*.

ETIOLOGY

Ecthyma gangrenosum is caused by *P. aeruginosa*. Other rare causes include *Pseudomonas cepacia*, and *Pseudomonas maltophilia*, *Serratia marcescens*, *Aeromonas hydrophila*, *Klebsiella pneumoniae*, *Escherichia coli*, *Vibrio vulnificus*, *Morganella morganii*, *Mucor*, *Aspergillus fumigatus*, *Fusarium*, *Scytalidium dimidiatum*, and *Candida albicans*.

EPIDEMIOLOGY

Infection can occur at any age; immunocompromised patients are at a greater risk.

CLINICAL FEATURES

Ecthyma gangrenosum can be classified into bacteremic and nonbacteremic forms. The bacteremic form is more common. The causative organism spreads hematogenously to the capillaries and

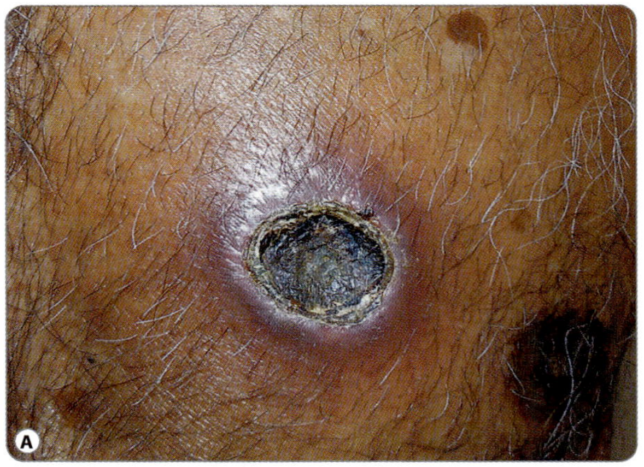

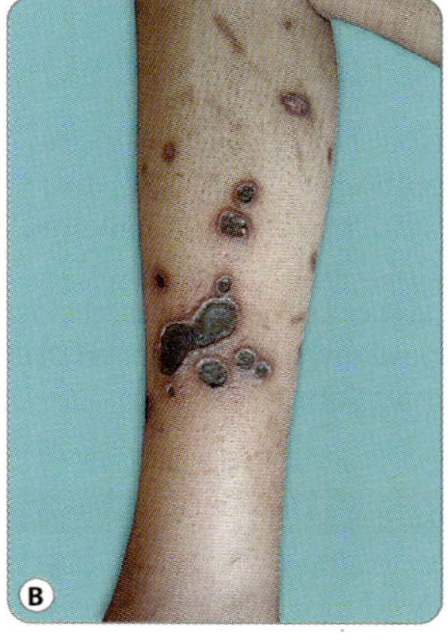

Figs. 1A and B: (A) Punched-out ulcer of ecthyma covered with eschar;
and (B) Ecthyma gangrenosum: Multiple ulcers with erythema in an immunocompromised child.

invades the media and adventitia of arteries and veins. Perivascular invasion ultimately leads to ischemic necrosis of the surrounding skin. In the nonbacteremic form, the lesions develop at the location of direct inoculation into the epidermis **(Figs. 1A and B)**.

Ecthyma gangrenosum is a cutaneous syndrome characterized by painless, minimally erythematous macules or thin papules or plaques that typically progress to bullous lesions, followed by hemorrhage and necrosis, often with retiform extensions from lesional margins. The anogenital area is a frequent site of involvement, but lesions can develop anywhere and at widespread cutaneous sites.

HISTOPATHOLOGY

Biopsies of ecthyma gangrenosum reveal minimal vascular neutrophilic infiltration despite necrotizing vessel injury, and special stains show extensive bacillary infiltration of the perivascular region, the adventitia, and the media of larger subcutaneous arterioles, with sparing of the lumen and intima.

DIFFERENTIAL DIAGNOSIS

- Necrotizing vasculitis
- Cryoglobulinemia—livedo reticularis-like picture and raised serum cryoglobulins
- *Herpes simplex* virus (HSV) infection in immunocompromised patients
- Pyoderma gangrenosum—absence of organism
- Trauma
- Nocardiosis—presence of nocardia species on Ziehl-Neelsen (ZN) stain
- Sporotrichosis

COMPLICATIONS

Complications include sepsis, hypoperfusion, multiorgan dysfunction, and death.

TREATMENT

One percent acetic acid compresses, potassium permanganate soaks, povidone, or silver sulfadiazine cream may be of value; in some cases, ceftazidime can also be used. Antipsuedomonal penicillin with aminoglycoside is preferred. In septicemia, systemic therapy with intravenous antibiotics is given. Ceftazidime, gentamicin, piperacillin, tobramycin, and amikacin may be used in appropriate combinations.

PROGNOSIS

Poor prognostic factors include multiple lesions, delay in instituting effective intravenous antipseudomonal therapy, and neutropenia. The mortality rate is nearly 100% if left untreated.

SUGGESTED READING

1. Hay R, Morris-Jones R. Bacterial infections. In: Griffiths C, Barker J, Bleiker T, Chalmers R, Cremer D (Eds). Rook's Textbook of Dermatology, 9th edition. United Kingdom: Wiley Blackwell Publishing House; 2016. pp. 26.1-26.85.

71 Ectodermal Dysplasias

➲ INTRODUCTION

Ectodermal dysplasias are genetic disorders resulting in structural or functional abnormalities in two or more of the major structures derived from the ectoderm. Organs affected include hair, teeth, nails, sweat glands, mucus glands, and sebaceous glands **(Figs. 1 to 4 and Table 1)**.

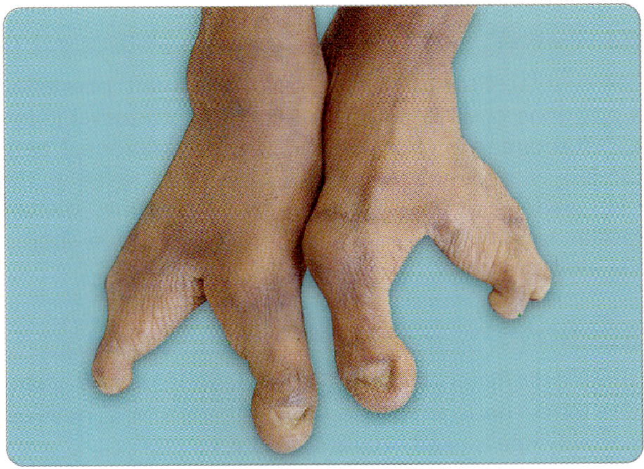

Fig. 1: Lobster claw anomaly in ectrodactyly–ectodermal dysplasia–cleft (EEC) syndrome.

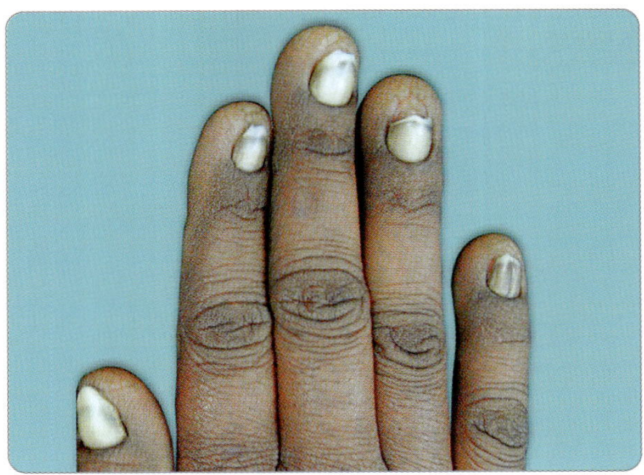

Fig. 2: Bulbous fingertips with thickened nails in hidrotic ectodermal dysplasia.

TABLE 1: Ectodermal dysplasia disorders.

Name	Inheritance	Protein product	Hair	Teeth	Sweating	Nails	Other
Hypohidrotic ED	XLR, AD, and AR	Ectodysplasin A	Sparse and thin	Abnormal and absent	Markedly decreased	Normal	Characteristic facies; neonates may have collodion membrane; and eczema is common
Hidrotic ED	AD	Connexin 30	Wiry, brittle, and pale	Normal	Normal	White during infancy, later thickened, distal separation	Palmoplantar keratoderma; conjunctivitis
AEC syndrome	AD	p63	Light, wiry, and coarse	Hypodontia	Normal	Hyperconvex, thickened, or absent; may be normal	Clefting of lip/palate (~80%), ankyloblepharon, neonatal erythroderma, and scalp dermatitis
EEC syndrome	AD	p63	Light, coarse, and dry	Hypodontia and premature loss	Usually normal	Transverse ridges and pitting	Clefting of lip/palate ectrodactyly and lacrimal duct abnormality; palm/sole hyperkeratosis
Rapp–Hodgkin syndrome	AD	p63	Light, wiry, and coarse	Hypodontia	Decreased	Ridging, pitting, and brittle	Clefting of lip/palate; scalp dermatitis less common; midfacial hypoplasia; and hypospadias in males

(AD: autosomal dominant; AEC: ankyloblepharon ectodermal dysplasia cleft lip/palate; AR: autosomal recessive; ED: ectodermal dysplasia; EEC: ectrodactyly–ectodermal dysplasia cleft; XLR: X-linked recessive)

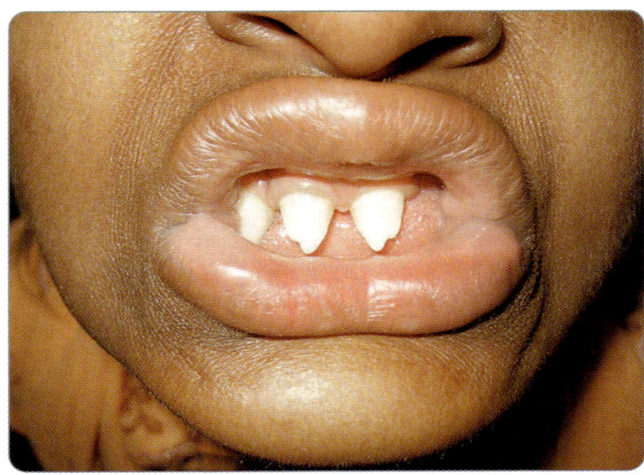

Fig. 3: Conical teeth.

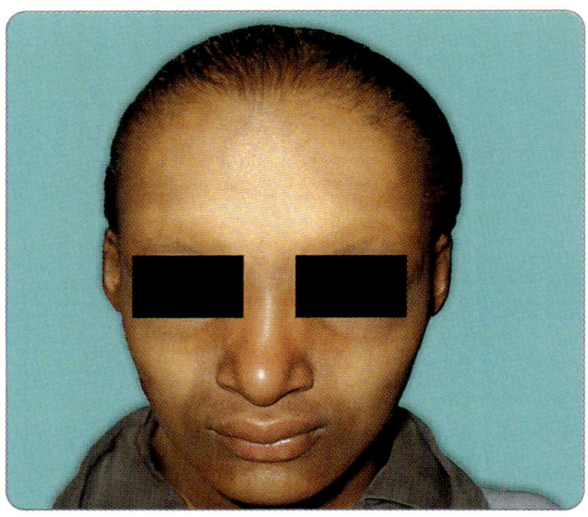

Fig. 4: Hypohidrotic ectodermal dysplasia (ED): Thinning of hair and senile appearance of face.

➲ SUGGESTED READING

1. Deshmukh S, Prashanth S. Ectodermal dysplasia: a genetic review. Int J of Clin Pediatr. 2012;5(3):197.

72 Eczema Herpeticum

SYNONYM

Kaposi's varicelliform eruption.

ETIOLOGY

Kaposi's varicelliform eruption (KVE) is caused by widespread infection with herpes simplex virus (HSV) type 1, HSV 2, coxsackie A16, and vaccinia (eczema vaccinatum). Atopic eczema is by far the most common predisposing condition. Other susceptible dermatoses include Darier's disease, pemphigus foliaceus, Hailey–Hailey disease, Grover's disease, ichthyosis vulgaris, congenital ichthyosiform erythroderma, allergic contact dermatitis, and irritant contact dermatitis. Topical and systemic immunosuppression has also been associated with eczema herpeticum, like topical tacrolimus or pimecrolimus.

EPIDEMIOLOGY

Cases are seen at all ages, most commonly in the second and third decades.

CLINICAL FEATURES

Eczema herpeticum is severe in patients with erythrodermic atopic eczema but frequently occurs in mild or quiescent cases. Recurrences of eczema herpeticum can occur. In severe cases, after an incubation period of about 10 days (range: 5–19 days), vesicles, which rapidly become pustular, erupt in massive crops. They may be localized or widespread. They may be hemorrhagic, and the face may become grossly edematous. New crops of vesicles may appear for 5–7 days. Fever commonly develops 2 or 3 days after the onset of the eruption, and constitutional symptoms may be severe. The regional lymph nodes are enlarged. The fever subsides after 4 or 5 days, and the pustules become crusted and slowly heal, leaving little permanent scarring. Rarely, they progress to potentially fatal systemic infection **(Fig. 1)**.

DIFFERENTIAL DIAGNOSIS

- Impetigo—not widespread to the whole body; *Staphylococcus aureus* is demonstrated in the pus.
- Contact dermatitis.
- Pemphigus vulgaris—acantholytic cells are seen, with positive direct immunofluorescence (DIF).
- Dermatitis herpetiformis—neutrophilic collection in dermal papillary tips; gluten sensitivity is seen.
- Bullous pemphigoid—subepidermal blister is seen with eosinophils, with positive DIF.

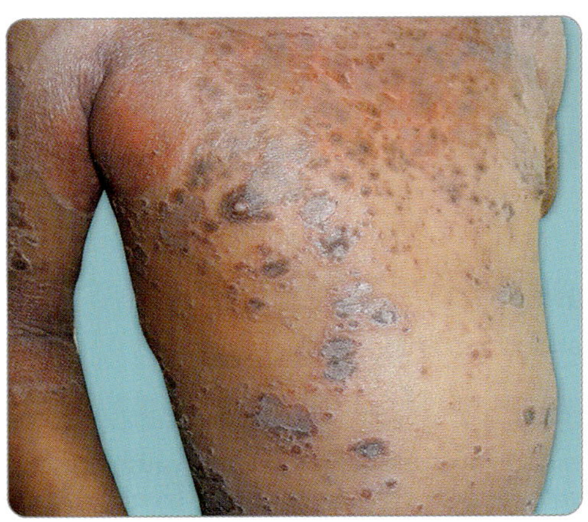

Fig. 1: Multiple crusted lesions in an atopic child.

COMPLICATIONS

Persistent ulcerative and verruciform lesions may occur.

TREATMENT

Awareness of the possibility of widespread herpetic infection should be encouraged in atopic eczema patients. Those with a history of eczema herpeticum should avoid close contact with relatives and friends with active herpes simplex. Severe cases should receive intravenous acyclovir as early as possible. Less ill patients respond well to oral acyclovir. Infection in pregnancy has been treated with acyclovir without adverse effect.

Bacterial infection and the underlying eczema or other dermatosis should be treated in the usual way with more cautious use of steroid therapy till viral infection heals.

SUGGESTED READING

1. Damour A, Garcia M, Seneschal J, Lévêque N, Bodet C. Eczema herpeticum: clinical and pathophysiological aspects. Clin Rev Allergy Immunol. 2020;59:1-18.

73 Ehlers–Danlos Syndrome

SYNONYM

Cutis hyperelastica.

HISTORY

The syndrome is named after two doctors, Edvard Ehlers of Denmark and Henri–Alexandre Danlos of France, who identified it at the turn of the 20th century.

ETIOLOGY

Ehlers–Danlos syndrome constitutes a group of inherited connective tissue disorders, caused by a defect in the synthesis of collagen (type I or III) **(Table 1)**.

Table 1: Types and clinical features of Ehlers–Danlos syndrome.

Type	*Gene*	*Clinical features*
I: Classical II: Classical	COL5A1 COL5A2/ COL1A1	AD. Affects type V and I collagen. Type 1 typically presents with severe skin involvement, and type 2 presents with mild-to-moderate skin involvement
III: Hypermobile	COL3A1 and TNXB	AD/AR. Hypermobility of varying degrees
IV: Vascular	COL3A1	AD. Type III collagen synthesis is affected. More serious form, because blood vessels and organs are more prone to tearing (rupture). Characteristic facial appearance (large eyes, small chin, thin nose and lips, and lobeless ears). More than 80% develop life-threatening complications by the age of 40 years
VI: Kyphoscoliosis	PLOD1	AR. Deficiency of an enzyme lysyl hydroxylase. Progressive curvature of the spine (scoliosis), fragile eyes, and severe muscle weakness
7A and B arthrochalasis	COL1A1 and COL1A2	It affects type I collagen, characterized by very loose joints and dislocations involving both hips
7C dermatospraxis		Extremely fragile and sagging skin

(AD: autosomal dominant; AR: autosomal recessive)

The common clinical features in the classical type include velvety-smooth skin, which may be stretchy, with abnormal wound healing and scar formation. Joints are loose, unstable, and prone to sprain, dislocation, subluxation (partial dislocation), and hyperextension (double-jointedness), with early onset of osteoarthritis. Low muscle tone and muscle weakness are seen. High and narrow palate, resulting in dental crowding, easy bruising, and valvular heart disease, especially mitral valve prolapse, are the other features.

DIFFERENTIAL DIAGNOSIS

- *Marfan's syndrome*—long extremities, Gorlin's sign positive, and ectopia lentis are seen
- *Osteogenesis imperfecta*—deformed bones and normally stretchable skin
- *Cutis laxa*—disease of elastic fibers
- Familial joint hypermobility
- *Pseudoxanthoma elasticum*—presence of characteristic skin lesions, angioid streaks in retina, and calcification of dermal vessels

MANAGEMENT

There is no cure for Ehlers–Danlos syndrome. The treatment is supportive. Close monitoring of the cardiovascular system, physical therapy, occupational therapy, and orthopedic instruments (e.g., wheelchairs and bracing) may be helpful. One should avoid activities that cause the joint to lock or overextend.

SUGGESTED READING

1. Malfait F, De Paepe A. The Ehlers–Danlos syndrome. Progress in heritable soft connective tissue diseases. Adv Exp Med Biol. 2014:129-43.

74 Epidermolysis Bullosa

➲ HISTORY

Koebner used the term epidermolysis bullosa (EB) hereditaria. Hallopeau distinguished EB simplex (nonscarring) and dystrophic (scarring).

➲ ETIOLOGY

Epidermolysis bullosa is an inherited connective tissue disease causing blisters in the skin and mucosal membranes, caused by a mutation in the keratin or collagen gene. Minor mechanical friction or trauma leads to the separation of the layers of the skin and formation of blisters.

➲ CLASSIFICATION (TABLE 1)

- *Epidermolysis bullosa simplex (EBS) (intraepidermal blisters):*
    - More common forms:
        - EBS of hands and feet (Weber–Cockayne) — Keratin 5, 14 autosomal dominant (AD)
        - EBS herpetiformis (Dowling–Meara) — Keratin 5, 14 AD
        - EBS Koebner — Keratin 5, 14 AD
    - Less common forms:

— EBS associated with neuromuscular disease	Plectin	Autosomal recessive (AR)
— EBS with mottled pigmentation		AD
— EBS superficialis	COL7A1	AD
— EBS Ogna		AD
— EBS with pyloric atresia		

- *Junctional epidermolysis bullosa (JEB):*
    - Autosomal recessive:
        - More common forms:
            - JEB gravis (Herlitz) — Laminin mutation
            - JEB mitis (non-Herlitz) — COL17A1
        - Less common forms:
            - JEB with pyloric atresia — α6β4 integrin
            - Inverse JEB
            - Progressive JEB
            - Cicatricial JEB

Junctional epidermolysis bullosa gravis (Herlitz): Blistering and erosions appear soon after birth and rapidly become generalized, and eroded areas heal slowly with atrophic scarring. Severe

Table 1: Common forms of epidermolysis bullosa simplex (EBS).

EBS of hands and feet (Weber–Cockayne): Most common type	*Koebner EBS: Subtype of generalized EBS*	*Dowling–Meara EBS/ EB herpetiformis: Tendency to occur in groups*
Heals without significant scarring or milia	60% heal with localized scarring, and 16% have milia	Heals with mild hyperpigmentation and localized atrophic scarring in 40% and milia in 20%
Mainly affects palms and soles	Occiput and back and legs are affected in infancy; hands and feet are affected in childhood; palms and soles are not preferentially involved	Spontaneous herpetiform, annular, or arcuate blistering on the trunk, limbs, and neck
Onset is in childhood	Blisters appear within first year or at birth	Infancy
Hot weather, friction, precipitate, and blister formation	Blistering is worse in warm weather, and in some people, it may improve with puberty	No exacerbation of lesions with exercise General condition improves with age
Hyperhidrosis of feet, calluses on balls of feet, and heel are very common	PPK with erosions	Confluent keratoderma, which appears in childhood and may lead to exion deformity of hands
The hair and nails are normal, with rarely nail dystrophy (localized and mild)	Nail dystrophy may be seen	Shedding of nails and formation of milia
Oral mucosal ulceration is rare	In AR cases, oral blistering with dental caries	Infancy with involvement of mucus membrane

(AR: autosomal recessive; EB: epidermolysis bullosa; PPK: palmoplantar keratoderma)

involvement of oral and pharyngeal mucosa leads to hoarseness and stridor, and nonhealing crusted erosions with exuberant granulation tissue are seen perioroficially.

- *Dystrophic epidermolysis bullosa (DEB)*: It is caused by the mutation in single gene *COL7A1*.
  - More common forms:
    - Severe generalized DEB (Hallopeau–Siemens) AR
    - Mild and nonmutilating generalized/ localized DEB AR
    - Classical DEB (Cockayne–Touraine; Pasini) AD
  - Less common forms:
    - Inverse DEB AR
    - Pretibial DEB
    - EB pruriginosa
    - Bart's syndrome
    - Transient bullous disease of childhood DEB

Bullae are present at birth, which heal with cigarette paper scars, mitten-like deformity of hands and feet, microstomia, loss of teeth, cicatricial alopecia, and renal and gastrointestinal tract (GIT) manifestations. Chronic lesions may undergo malignant transformation **(Figs. 1A to D)**.

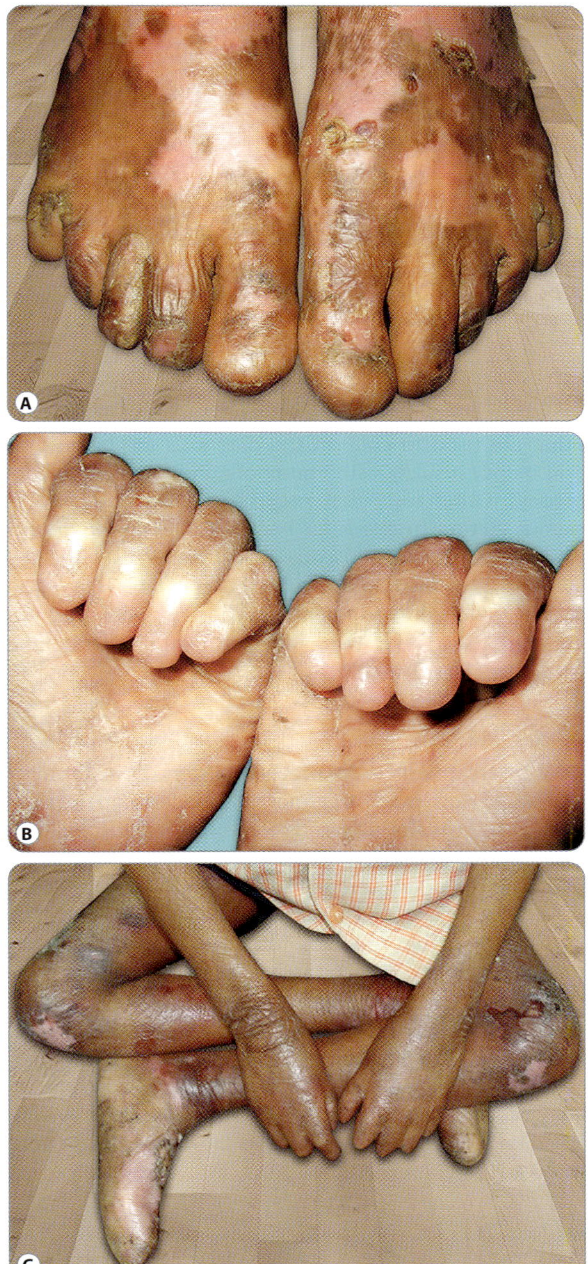

Figs. 1A to D: *Continued*

Continued

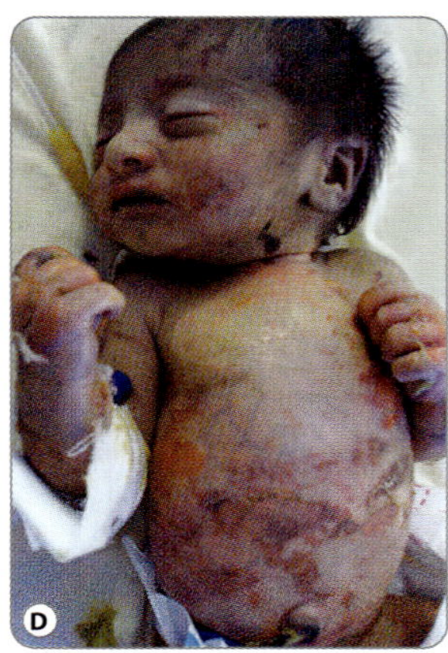

Figs. 1A to D: (A and B) Dystrophic epidermolysis bullosa (EB); (C) Dystrophic EB with mitten hands and feet with loss of nails; and (D) Bullae and peeling of the skin in a newborn.

INVESTIGATIONS

Tests that are used to confirm the diagnosis are genetic testing and skin biopsy (usually with immunofluorescent tests or electron microscopy). Other tests that may be done include blood test for anemia, culture to check for bacterial infection if wounds are healing poorly, upper endoscopy, or an upper GI series if there are swallowing or feeding difficulties, and growth curves should be carefully watched in an infant who has, or is believed to have, epidermolysis bullosa. If there are contractures, limb range of motion will be tested.

TREATMENT

The goal of treatment is to prevent blisters from forming and complications. How much treatment is needed depends on how severe the disease is. Recommendations often include avoiding skin damage (trauma) and hot environments. To prevent infection, the skin should be handled carefully, especially if any blistered areas become crusted or exposed (raw). Systemic therapies that are being tried include phenytoin, retinoids, tetracyclines, and antimalarials.

Research is taking place in the field of gene editing technology with the prospect of devising permanent, safe, tolerable, and feasible delivery of local and possibly systemic treatments for inherited diseases. If incorporated at an early stage, efficient gene therapies may prevent the development of symptoms, and at later stages, they may prevent disease progression involving the development of devastating chronic EB lesions and life-threatening cutaneous squamous cell carcinoma (SCC).

SUGGESTED READING

1. Bardhan A, Bruckner-Tuderman L, Chapple IL, Fine JD, Harper N, Has C, et al. Epidermolysis bullosa. Nat Rev Dis Primers. 2020;6(1):78.

75 Erysipelas

SYNONYMS

"Ignis sacer," "holy fire," "St. Anthony's fire."

ETIOLOGY

Most cases of erysipelas are due to *Streptococcus pyogenes* (also known as beta-hemolytic group A streptococci), although nongroup A streptococci can also be the causative agent.

EPIDEMIOLOGY

Erysipelas is the most common disease among the elderly, infants, and children. Risk factors include obesity, diabetes, trauma, lymphedema, leg ulcers, stasis eczema, intravenous (IV) drug abusers, and athlete's foot.

CLINICAL FEATURES

Patients typically develop symptoms including high fever, shivering, chills, fatigue, headaches, vomiting, and general illness within 48 hours of the initial infection. The erythematous lesion enlarges rapidly and has a sharply demarcated raised edge. It appears as a red, swollen, warm, hardened rash, similar in consistency to an orange peel. The leg is the most common site, followed by the face. More severe infections can result in vesicles, bullae, and petechiae, with possible skin necrosis. Lymph nodes may be swollen, and lymphedema may occur **(Table 1)**.

Table 1: Erysipelas and cellulitis.

Erysipelas	*Cellulitis*
Common in younger age group	Common in middle aged and elderly
Upper dermis and superficial lymphatics involved	Dermis and subcutaneous fat involved
More distinctive anatomical features, raised above the level of surrounding skin, and there is a clear line of demarcation between the involved and uninvolved skin	Ill-defined borders that merge with surrounding skin
Ear involved (Milan's sign)	Ear is spared
Acute onset of symptoms with systemic manifestations, including fever and chills	Indolent course

DIFFERENTIAL DIAGNOSIS

- Cellulitis—lacks well-defined border; it is spreading in nature
- Herpes zoster—presence of grouped vesicles on erythematous base in a dermatomal fashion
- Angioedema
- Contact dermatitis—history of (H/o) contact with allergen and more vesicular reaction with oozing and crusting
- Necrotizing fasciitis—fast spreading deeper infection and ulceration on the skin
- Insect bite

COMPLICATIONS

Without effective treatment, complications are common, which include fasciitis, myositis, thrombophlebitis, subcutaneous abscesses, and septicemia.

TREATMENT

Depending on the severity and culture sensitivity, oral or IV antibiotics using penicillin, clindamycin, or erythromycin are started. While systemic symptoms resolve in a day or two, the skin may take weeks to return to normal.

SUGGESTED READING

1. Gunderson CG, Martinello RA. A systematic review of bacteremias in cellulitis and erysipelas. J Infect. 2012;64(2):148-55.

76 Erythema Ab Igne

SYNONYMS

Ephelis ignealis, livedo reticularis et calore, head-induced circumscribed dermal melanosis, hot water bottle rash, fire stains, laptop thigh, toasted skin syndrome.

HISTORY

It was seen in the elderly who stood or sat close to open fires or electric heaters. The term is derived from Latin and means "redness from fire".

ETIOLOGY

It is caused by chronic exposure to moderate heat/recurrent infrared exposure short of causing thermal burn. People exposed to heat from sources such as heating pads, hot water bottles, laptops, hot stone massages, infrared lamps, and heated recliners developed this condition. It may be a valuable sign of hypothyroidism.

EPIDEMIOLOGY

This condition can occur at all ages including children.

CLINICAL FEATURES

A localized transient reticular erythema is initially blanchable, darkens, and becomes permanent eventually. Later, epidermal atrophy, scaling, and hyperpigmentation occur. Repeated exposure can lead to superficial epidermal atrophy or subepidermal blistering. Clinical variants include bullous, hyperkeratotic, and keloidal type. Long-standing lesions rarely develop malignant changes [squamous cell carcinoma (SCC), Merkel cell carcinoma, and cutaneous marginal zone lymphoma reported] **(Fig. 1)**.

DERMATOSCOPY

Erythema, polymorphous vessels (linear, dotted, glomeruloid, and comma shaped), red globules, telangiectasia, homogenous brown pigmentation, accentuated pigment network, dilated eccrine openings, and white structureless areas.

HISTOPATHOLOGY

In the early stages, epidermal atrophy, dermal pigmentation, and vasodilatation are evident. Basophilic degeneration of the connective tissue, focal hyperkeratosis, epithelial cellular atypia, and increased dermal elastin occur later.

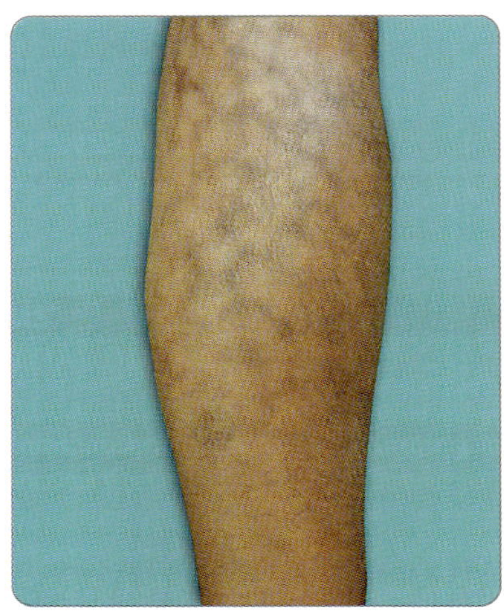

Fig. 1: Reticulate pigmentation over the arm of a patient who used to use heat pads for pain.

DIFFERENTIAL DIAGNOSIS

Livedo reticularis—more commonly found over dependent areas such as lower legs, vasculitis on histopathologic examination (HPE), ulcers, and healed atrophie blanche lesions seen.

TREATMENT

The heat source must be removed. Mild lesions may resolve spontaneously. Hypothyroidism should be excluded. 1064 QS Nd YAG laser with low fluence, ruby or alexandrite, systemic mesoglycan-based therapy, topical tretinoin, 5 fluorouracil, and steroids can be used for cosmetic improvement.

SUGGESTED READING

1. Harview CL, Krenitsky A. Erythema Ab Igne: A Clinical Review. Cutis. 2023;111(4):E33-8.

77 Erythema Elevatum Diutinum

➲ HISTORY

It was initially described by Hutchinson in 1888 and subsequently by Bury in 1889. The name erythema elevatum diutinum (EED) was first described by Radcliff–Crocker.

➲ ETIOLOGY

Erythema elevatum diutinum is a chronic leukocytoclastic vasculitis associated with a wide range of disease processes such as chronic bacterial infections, human immunodeficiency virus (HIV), human herpesvirus 6 (HHV 6), hepatitis B, syphilis, tuberculosis, malignancies, and connective tissue disorders.

➲ EPIDEMIOLOGY

It presents predominantly in males, in the fourth to sixth decade of life.

➲ CLINICAL FEATURES

It typically presents as multiple, persistent, symmetric, and erythematous or violaceous papules, nodules, and plaques on the extensor surface of the hands, elbows, wrists, knees, ankles, buttocks, face, ears, forearms, and genitals. Lesions may show temperature and diurnal variation (nocturnal aggravation). With time the lesions may become firmer and develop a yellowish-brown coloration, resembling xanthomata. These eventually heal with dyspigmentation. Constitutional symptoms including fever and arthralgia are seen commonly. EED is chronic and frequently relapsing. Extracutaneous involvement includes eyes (progressive keratolyis with pseudopterygium and peripheral ulcerative keratitis) and joints.

➲ HISTOPATHOLOGY

Early states show features of leukocytoclastic vasculitis, with thickening of blood vessel walls, mural and luminal neutrophilia, vascular occlusion, fibrinoid necrosis of blood vessel walls, endothelial swelling, leukocytoclasia, and dermal neutrophilia with lymphocytes. In later stages of fibrosis, macrophages containing lipids (lipophages) and histiocytes are seen.

➲ DIFFERENTIAL DIAGNOSIS

- Cutaneous small vessel vasculitis
- Sweet's syndrome
- Dermatitis herpetiformis (early stages)

➲ TREATMENT

Treatment is aimed at alleviating discomfort associated with the lesions, diminishing the damage to the skin, and eradicating underlying associated conditions. Dapsone and sulfone-based therapies are considered first-line treatment choices for EED.

➲ PROGNOSIS

Erythema elevatum diutinum may last from 5 to 35 years, with crops of new lesions developing every few weeks to months.

➲ SUGGESTED READING

1. Doktor V, Hadi A, Hadi A, Phelps R, Goodheart H. Erythema elevatum diutinum: a case report and review of literature. Int J Dermatol. 2019;58(4):408-15.

78 Erythema Infectiosum

➲ SYNONYMS

Fifth disease, slapped cheek syndrome, butterfly pox.

➲ HISTORY

The name "fifth disease" is not typically capitalized, since the name derives from its historical classification as the fifth of the classical childhood skin rashes or exanthemas. It was first described by Robert Willan in 1799 as "Rubeola, sine catarrh".

➲ ETIOLOGY

Erythema infectiosum is caused by Parvovirus B 19 belonging to the parvoviridae family.

➲ EPIDEMIOLOGY

The condition can affect all ages and tend to occur in epidemics, especially associated with school outbreaks in the late winter and early spring. It occurs by droplet infection by saliva, sputum or nasal discharge. The incubation period is 4–15 days.

➲ CLINICAL FEATURES

A prodrome of constitutional symptoms followed by bright red cheeks are a defining symptom of the infection in children (hence the name "slapped cheek disease"). Sparing of the bridge of the nose, periocular, and perioral area (circumoral pallor) seen. In addition to red cheeks, children often develop a red, lacy rash on the rest of the body, with the upper arms and legs being the most common locations. The rash typically lasts a couple of days and may itch. Teenagers and adults may present with self-limited arthritis.

➲ HISTOPATHOLOGY

The exanthema shows a perivascular mononuclear cell infiltrate with a focal interface dermatitis.

➲ DIFFERENTIAL DIAGNOSIS

- Rubella—maculopapular rash beginning behind the ears and spreading in a centrifugal fashion
- Drug reaction—widespread lesions, hepatic involvement, and lymphadenopathy
- Erysipelas of cheek
- Enteroviral infection
- Still's disease

- Infectious mononucleosis—generalized maculopapular rash and cervical lymphadenopathy present
- Lyme's disease—erythematous annular patch present mainly over shins
- Acute human immunodeficiency virus (HIV) seroconversion

COMPLICATIONS

It can cause aplastic crisis in immunocompromised individuals, sickle cell anemia, hereditary spherocytosis, G6PD deficiency, and thalassemia. In pregnant women, infection may lead to fetal hydrops, spontaneous abortion, self-limited anemia in the fetus, and stillbirth.

TREATMENT

Erythema infectiosum in itself is harmless and no treatment is required. Supportive treatment of fatigue, malaise, arthralgias, and pruritus is all that is usually required.

Intravenous immunoglobulin (IVIg) is administered in pregnancy and immunocompromised state.

PROGNOSIS

Parvovirus B19 infection in healthy individuals is self-limited. The rash of erythema infectiosum and the parvovirus arthropathy usually resolve in 1–2 weeks.

SUGGESTED READING

1. Leung AK, Lam JM, Barankin B, Leong KF, Hon KL. Erythema Infectiosum: A Narrative Review. Curr Pediatr Rev. 2024;20(4):462-71.

79 Erythema Multiforme

➲ HISTORY

It was first described by Ferdinand von Hebra in 1860. Bernard Thomas proposed the terms EM—major and minor.

➲ ETIOLOGY

Erythema multiforme (EM) is a skin condition of unknown cause, possibly mediated by deposition of immune complex [mostly immunoglobulin M (IgM)] in the superficial microvasculature of the skin and oral mucous membrane that usually follows an infection or drug exposure. The most common predisposing infection is herpes simplex, but bacterial infections (commonly *Mycoplasma*) and fungal diseases (histoplasmosis) are also implicated. Other causes include drug reactions, most commonly to sulfa drugs, phenytoin, barbiturates, penicillin, and allopurinol, or a host of internal ailments.

➲ EPIDEMIOLOGY

Erythema multiforme occurs in patients of all ages, but mostly in adolescents and young adults. There is a slight male preponderance (male-female sex ratio of approximately 3:2).

➲ CLINICAL FEATURES

Erythema multiforme minor represents a localized eruption of the skin with minimal or no mucosal involvement. The papules evolve into pathognomonic target lesions or iris lesions that appear within a 72-hour period and begin on the extremities. When the margins of the lesions are vesicular they are referred to as "Iris lesions of Bateman". Lesions remain in a fixed location for at least 7 days and then begin to heal. Mucosal lesions involve the lips, palate, and gingiva **(Figs. 1A and B)**.

➲ HISTOPATHOLOGY

Histopathology shows lymphocytic accumulation at the dermal-epidermal interface, with exocytosis into the epidermis, lymphocytes attached to scattered necrotic keratinocytes (satellite cell necrosis), spongiosis, vacuolar degeneration of basal cell layer, and focal junctional and subepidermal cleft formation, edema of the papillary dermis with ectasia of blood vessels and swollen endothelial cells. On direct immunofluorescence, degenerated keratinocytes appear as intradermal cytoid bodies showing homogenous IgM staining.

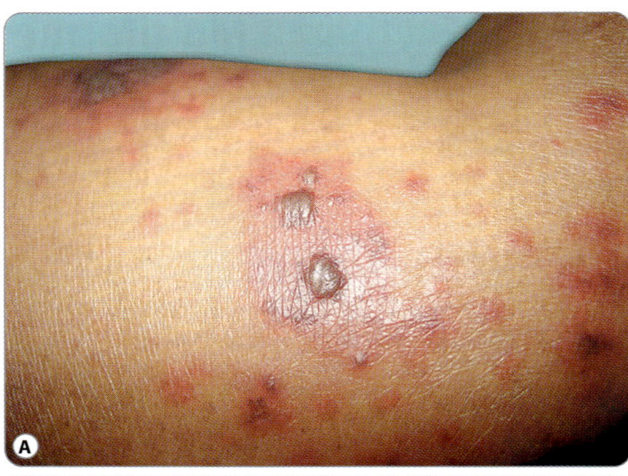

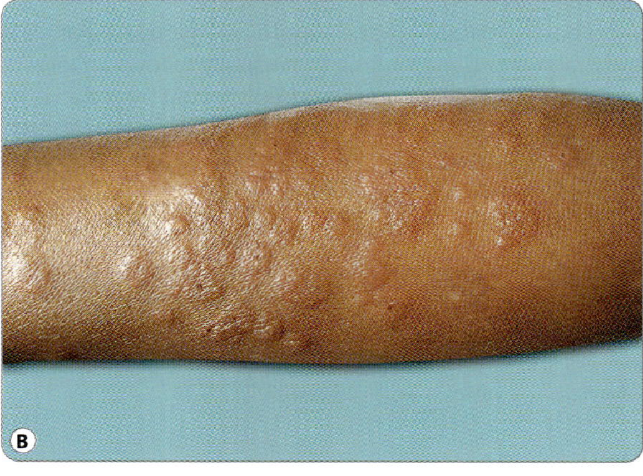

Figs. 1A and B: (A) Target lesions over the forearm; and (B) Erythema multiforme (EMF) with central hemorrhagic bulla.

DIFFERENTIAL DIAGNOSIS

- Urticaria—evanescent wheals seen
- Maculopapular drug eruption—absence of target lesions
- Sweet's syndrome—febrile episode is a must, neutrophilic infiltrated in the dermis
- Secondary syphilis
- Pityriasis rosea—absence of target lesions, classical herald patches seen
- Pemphigus vulgaris—acantholytic cells seen
- Serum sickness
- Granuloma annulare—skin-colored papules arranged in annular fashion, palisaded granuloma seen
- Viral exanthema
- Polymorphic light eruption

TREATMENT

Erythema multiforme is frequently self-limiting and requires no treatment. The appropriateness of glucocorticoid therapy can be uncertain because it is difficult to determine if the course will be self-limiting. Other drugs used include azathioprine, cyclosporine, thalidomide, levamisole, and dapsone. Herpes-associated EMF is treated with valacyclovir 500–1,000 mg/day, acyclovir 400 mg BD, or famciclovir 250 mg/day. Treatment should be given for 5–7 days.

PROGNOSIS

Erythema multiforme runs a mild course in most cases, and each individual attack subsides within 1–4 weeks. Recovery is complete, and there are usually no sequelae. Recurrences are common.

SUGGESTED READING

1. Trayes KP, Love G, Studdiford JS. Erythema multiforme: recognition and management. Am Fam Phys. 2019;100(2):82-8.

80 Erythema Nodosum

SYNONYM

Erythema contusiformis.

ETIOLOGY

Erythema nodosum (EN) is the most common clinicopathological variant of panniculitis triggered in response to a variety of internal infections, neoplasms, and other inflammatory multisystem diseases or may be drug induced. It is a delayed hypersensitivity reaction, causing immune complex deposition in septal venules of subcutaneous fat and granuloma formation.

EPIDEMIOLOGY

It is seen more commonly in females in the age group of 20–30 years.

CLINICAL FEATURES

The classical lesions are erythematous, warm, painful nodules, 1–5 cm in diameter, that are usually slightly elevated above the skin surface and occur bilaterally on the lower extremities, particularly on the anterior tibial surface. Spontaneous resolution occurs in 2–8 weeks.

CLASSIFICATION

- *Acute EN*: It is usually accompanied by fever, malaise, and joint pains mimicking arthritis. Arthralgia may persist up to 2 years after the resolution of skin lesions.
- *Chronic EN*: It presents as asymptomatic or minimally painful nodules and plaques on one leg and is usually not associated with constitutional symptoms.

Subacute nodular migratory panniculitis of Vilanova and EN migrans are other clinical variants.

ASLO titer, throat swab, chest X-ray, Mantoux test, and ESR should be done routinely in all patients.

HISTOPATHOLOGY

It is a prototype of septal panniculitis. There is widening of septa due to edema, lymphocytic infiltrate in early stages, and granulomatous infiltrate is seen as the lesions grow older. Meischer's radial granuloma is considered a histopathological hallmark. They are a collection of histiocytes around slit-like space or blood vessels forming granuloma at the junction of the fibrous septae and fat lobules.

DIFFERENTIAL DIAGNOSIS

- Insect bites
- Ecchymosis—flat lesions seen
- Weber Christian disease
- Fat necrosis due to pancreatitis
- Necrobiosis lipoidica—mostly seen in diabetics
- Subcutaneous granuloma annulare
- Lupus panniculitis—positive antinuclear antibody (ANA)

TREATMENT

It should be directed at the underlying disorder. Bed rest, aspirin, and nonsteroidal anti-inflammatory drugs (NSAIDs) may be helpful. Systemic corticosteroids are rarely indicated after ruling out underlying infection. Potassium iodide (400–900 mg daily) causes rapid pain resolution. Dapsone, colchicines, hydroxychloroquines (HCQs), and tumor necrosis factor (TNF)-alpha inhibitors can also be given for resistant, recalcitrant, or recurring cases.

SUGGESTED READING

1. Chowaniec M, Starba A, Wiland P. Erythema nodosum–review of the literature. Reumatologia/Rheumatology. 2016;54(2):79-82.

81 Erythrasma

➲ ETIOLOGY

Erythrasma is caused by gram-positive, nonspore forming, rod-shaped diphtheroid, *Corynebacterium minutissimum*.

➲ EPIDEMIOLOGY

Clinical infection may occur at any age but is more common among adults. Predisposing factors include diabetes mellitus, obesity, excessive sweating, and humid weather.

➲ CLINICAL FEATURES

Erythrasma presents with fine, brown scaling patches which are classically sharply demarcated. Lesions are typically found in intertriginous areas (axilla, groin, and inframammary), with the toe web spaces being most commonly involved. The patient is usually asymptomatic **(Fig. 1)**.

The diagnosis can be made based on the clinical picture alone. However, a simple side-room investigation with a Wood's lamp is additionally useful in diagnosing erythrasma. The ultraviolet light of a Wood's lamp causes the organism to fluoresce a coral red color (due to coproporphyrin III), differentiating it from fungal infections and other skin conditions. Gram stains show gram-positive rod-like organisms, filamentous and coccoid forms.

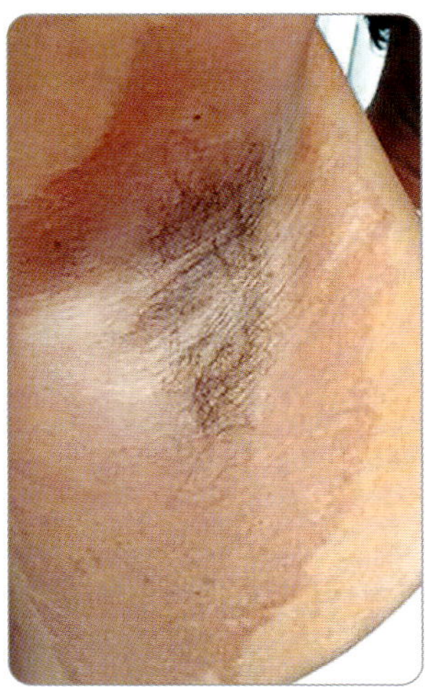

Fig. 1: Erythematous patch over the axilla with well-defined borders.

DIFFERENTIAL DIAGNOSIS

- Pityriasis versicolor—branny scales seen, banana and grapes appearance on potassium hydroxide (KOH) mount
- Tinea cruris—peripheral scaling and central clearing seen
- Intertrigo
- Seborrheic dermatitis—scaling seen
- Inverse psoriasis—negative Wood's lamp examination
- Candidiasis
- Pityriasis rosea—collarette scales seen, not limited to flexures

TREATMENT

Erythrasma responds well to most topically applied azole antifungal agents, such as clotrimazole 1% and miconazole 2%. Topical Fucidin and topical clindamycin are other alternatives. Oral erythromycin, 250 mg four times a day for 1 week, or tolnaftate solution applied twice a day for 2–3 weeks is equally effective.

PROGNOSIS

The disease may remain asymptomatic for years or may undergo periodic exacerbations. Relapses occasionally occur even after successful antibiotic treatment.

SUGGESTED READING

1. Forouzan P, Cohen PR. Erythrasma revisited: diagnosis, differential diagnoses, and comprehensive review of treatment. Cureus. 2020;12(9).

82 Erythroderma

➲ SYNONYMS

"Exfoliative dermatitis", "Dermatitis exfoliativa", "Red man syndrome".

➲ ETIOLOGY

The most common cause of erythroderma is exacerbation of an underlying skin disease, such as psoriasis, eczema, contact dermatitis, seborrheic dermatitis, lichen planus, pityriasis rubra pilaris, pemphigus group of disorders, lymphomas, leukemias, hereditary disorders, or a drug reaction. Antibiotics, antiepileptics, and nonsteroidal anti-inflammatory drugs (NSAIDs) have been commonly implicated.

➲ EPIDEMIOLOGY

Males are affected between two and three times more frequently than females and if hereditary disorders and atopic dermatitis are excluded, most patients are over 45 years of age.

➲ CLINICAL FEATURES

Patchy erythema, which rapidly generalizes, may be accompanied by fever, shivering, and malaise. The erythema extends rapidly and may be universal in 12–48 hours. Scales which may be large or fine and bran-like appear after 2–6 days, often first in flexures. Erythema and scaling involve >90% of the body surface area. Hypothermia may develop over a period of time. Skin is bright red, hot, dry, and palpably thickened. The general picture is modified according to the nature of any underlying disease and the patient's age and general physical condition **(Fig. 1)**.

➲ HISTOPATHOLOGY

It varies depending on the severity and duration of an inflammatory process. In the acute stage, spongiosis and parakeratosis are prominent, and a nonspecific inflammatory infiltrate permeates, to a variable depth, a grossly edematous dermis. In the chronic stage, acanthosis and elongation of the rete ridges become more prominent.

➲ COMPLICATIONS

Fluid and electrolyte imbalance, loss of barrier function of skin, hyperdynamic state, loss of temperature regulation, and dermatogenic enteropathy.

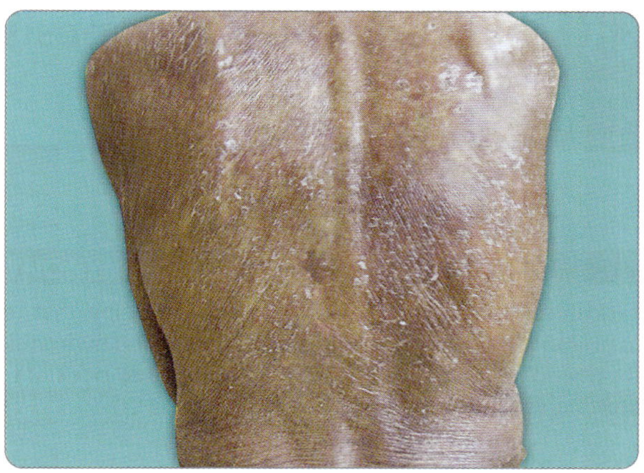

Fig. 1: Erythroderma.

➲ TREATMENT

Hospital admission with surveillance of protein, electrolyte imbalance, circulatory status, body temperature, and fluid balance. The cutaneous inflammation can be treated with soothing emollient creams or a mild topical steroid. Systemic steroids, though avoided may become necessary in severe persistent cases. Antibiotics are required to control secondary infection. The primary condition should be managed.

➲ PROGNOSIS

Erythroderma is a serious condition in itself, quite apart from hazards associated with the underlying disease, and is sometimes fatal despite skilled management. It is dangerous, particularly in elderly patients with more chances of systemic involvement and metabolic disturbances.

➲ SUGGESTED READING

1. Tan GF, Kong YL, Tan AS, Tey HL. Causes and features of erythroderma. Ann Acad Med Singap. 2014;43(8):391-4.

83 Exogenous Ochronosis

INTRODUCTION

A paradoxical localized cutaneous hyperpigmentation that results due to prolonged use of bleaching agents containing hydroquinone (HQ) or phenolic compounds. It is not inherited and does not have systemic manifestations.

HISTORY

Findlay reported the first case of exogenous ochronosis (EO) secondary to topical application of HQ in 1975.

ETIOLOGY

Use of products containing HQ, resorcinol, phenol, mercury, picric acid, and oral antimalarial agents.

PATHOGENESIS

Local competitive inhibition of homogentisic oxidase by topical HQ results in the accumulation of homogentisic acid and its metabolites in the papillary dermis causing their polymerization to form the characteristic brownish-yellow ochre pigment.

CLINICAL FEATURES

It appears as symmetric diffuse hyperpigmentation with sooty blue macules in a reticulate pattern over HQ-treated sun-exposed areas. The pigmentation can vary from gray-brown to blue-black with hyperchromic pinpoint caviar-like papules. Lesions may take up to 6 months to 3 years or even longer to develop.

The clinical classification of EO as suggested by Dogliotti and Leibowitz is as follows:

- *Stage I*: Erythema and mild hyperpigmentation
- *Stage II*: Progressive hyperpigmentation, pigmented colloid milium (caviar-like macules), and scanty atrophy
- *Stage III*: Papulonodular (sarcoid-like) lesions

DERMOSCOPY

The presence of amorphous blue-gray areas obliterating follicular openings to irregular gray-brown structures (globular, annular, or arciform) corresponds to the deposition of ochronotic pigment in the dermis.

HISTOPATHOLOGY

It shows pigment incontinence, solar elastosis, characteristic ochre pigment, and banana-shaped fibers in the papillary dermis. Colloid milium, granulomas, and eventual degeneration of collagen may also be seen.

Reflectance confocal microscopy shows hyporefractile oval to banana-shaped spaces in the dermis corresponding to the banana-shaped bodies on histology.

MANAGEMENT

- Improvement is gradual after the withdrawal of the offending agent
- Strict sun protection
- Topical agents such as retinoic acid and glycolic acid
- Procedures such as dermabrasion, glycolic acid peel, trichloroacetic acid peel, cryotherapy and CO_2 laser, Q-switched lasers like ruby, alexandrite, and Nd:YAG
- To prevent EO from developing, the use of HQ for pigmentation should always be under strict supervision of the dermatologist

SUGGESTED READING

1. Bhattar PA, Zawar VP, Godse KV, Patil SP, Nadkarni NJ, Gautam MM. Exogenous ochronosis. Indian J Dermatol. 2015;60(6):537-43.

84 Figurate Erythemas

INTRODUCTION

Figurate erythemas are characterized by lesions that are annular, arciform, or polycyclic in configuration.

The four "classic" figurate erythemas include:

1. Erythema annulare centrifugum
2. Erythema marginatum (rheumaticum)
3. Erythema (chronicum) migrans
4. Erythema gyratum repens

CLINICAL FEATURES

- *Erythema annulare centrifugum*: Slowly advancing lesions, asymmetrical elevated urticarial erythema with centrifugal spread with central fading. Commonly seen on the buttocks, thighs, and upper arms. Idiopathic or associated with infections/drugs/autoimmune disorders/malignancy. Histopathology shows perivascular mononuclear infiltrate referred as coat sleeve line arrangement. Treatment involves the identification and eradication of underlying causes.
- *Erythema gyratum repens (Gammel's disease)*: Regular waves of erythema spread over the body to produce a series of concentric figurate bands in a pattern resembling the grain of wood. Clearance of rash and relief of pruritus within 6 weeks subsequent to resolution of underlying illness. It may be associated with an internal tumor most commonly of the lung. Histology shows focal parakeratosis, neutrophilic exocytosis, and superficial perivascular lymphohistiocytic infiltration.
- *Erythema migrans (Afzelius' disease)*: Annular lesions arising at the location of a tick bite (Ixodes), having *Borrelia burgdorferi* as an indicator of Lyme disease. It has three stages of disease progression (early localized, early disseminated, and chronic disseminated). The organism has a predilection for skin, central nervous system (CNS), joints, heart, and eyes. It is treated with cephalosporin, tetracyclines, and macrolide antibiotics.
- *Erythema marginatum*: Specific to acute rheumatic fever, seen right before joint involvement. Annular lesions appear over the trunk, periumbilical area, and dorsum of the hands. Histology shows capillary dilatation and perivascular mild infiltrate.
- *Necrolytic migratory erythema*: Finding of glucagonoma, acral, and perioral location
- Annular erythema of infancy
- *Familial annular erythema*: Very rare, autosomal dominant

DIFFERENTIAL DIAGNOSIS

- Dermatophytosis—peripheral active border, central clearing, and positive potassium hydroxide (KOH) mount
- Annular urticaria—evanescent lesions
- Granuloma annulare—palisading granuloma with degenerated collagen and mucin
- Mycosis fungoides—the presence of Pautrier's microabscess, atypical lymphocytes, and epidermotropism
- Pseudolymphomas (especially erythema arciforme et palpable migrans)
- Bullous pemphigoid
- Pemphigus vulgaris
- Linear immunoglobulin A (IgA) disease—cluster of vesicles/bulla
- Erythema multiforme
- Sarcoidosis
- Still disease
- Annular psoriasis
- Erythrokeratoderma variabilis
- Chronic granulomatous disease
- Pityriasiform seborrheic dermatitis
- Neutrophilic dermatoses
- Vasculitides
- Leprosy-loss of sensation over the patch, granulomas in periappendageal, and perivascular location
- Leishmaniasis

SUGGESTED READING

1. Horii KA. Annular erythemas. In: Hoeger P, Kinsler V, Yan A, Harper J, Oranje A, Bodemer C, et al. (Eds). Harper's Textbook of Pediatric Dermatology. Wiley; 2019. pp. 764-70.

85 Fixed Drug Eruption

➲ ETIOLOGY

Although the exact mechanism is unknown, cell-mediated immune response initiates the lesions. CD8+ effector/memory T cells cause reactivation of lesions with reexposure to the offending drug. The drug acts as a hapten which binds to basal keratinocytes, leading to an inflammatory response. ICAM1 upregulation causes T-cell migration (CD4 and CD8), inflammatory cytokines, interferon-gamma, and tumor necrosis factor (TNF)-alpha release. As the inflammatory response dissipates, IL-15 ensures the survival of CD8 cells. Thus, when reexposure to the drug occurs, a more rapid response develops in the exact location of the prior lesions (recall phenomenon). If fixed drug eruption (FDE) fails to occur with drug challenge, it is called a refractory period, which may last weeks to months.

The common agents include antibiotics, antiepileptics, nonsteroidal anti-inflammatory agents, phenothiazines, over-the-counter medications, and nutritional supplements. Any route of medication can elicit FDE. Cases of FDE on the genitalia have been reported in patients whose sexual partner was taking the offending drug and was exposed to the drug through sexual contact.

➲ CLINICAL FEATURES

A specific mucocutaneous reaction pattern is characterized by erythematous patches following drug exposure, with new lesions occurring at the same site on repeated exposure to the same drug. The initial eruption is usually a solitary annular lesion located on the lips, genitalia, fingers, trunk, or gluteal area **(Fig. 1)**. Lesions may appear up to 2 weeks from the initial exposure to the drug and persist from days to weeks. They heal with postinflammatory hyperpigmentation. Subsequent reexposure to the medication results in a reactivation of the site, with inflammation occurring within 30 minutes to 16 hours. There may be pruritus, burning sensation, and pain in the lesions and rarely systemic symptoms.

Variants of FDE are generalized, bullous, urticarial, linear, pigmented, nonpigmented, inverse, wandering, eczematous, cellulitis like, erythema dyschromicum perstans–like, mucosal, and psoriasiform.

➲ HISTOPATHOLOGY

Histopathology shows dyskeratosis, spongiosis, necrotic keratinocytes, Civatte bodies, interface dermatitis with vacuolar change, lymphocytic infiltrate, dermal edema, and eosinophils. Pigmentary incontinence within the papillary dermis is a characteristic feature.

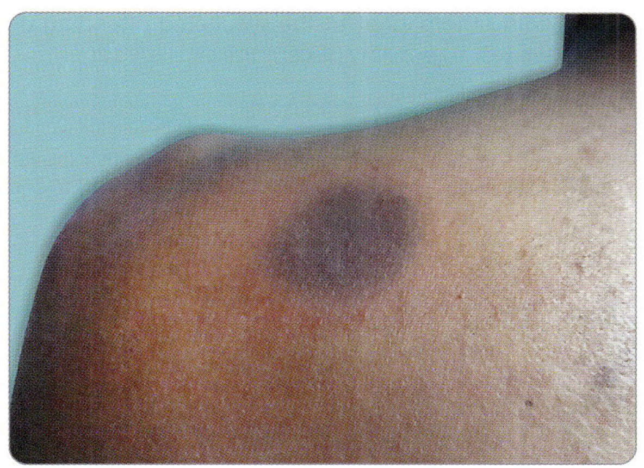

Fig. 1: Hyperpigmented annular patch with surrounding erythema.

Dermoscopy shows pigment dots and globules in various shades of brown and gray.

DIFFERENTIAL DIAGNOSIS

- Urticaria—no pigmentation
- Bullous pemphigoid—subepidermal bullae and positive direct immunofluorescence (DIF)
- Cellulitis
- Eczema—oozing and crusting seen
- Erythema annulare centrifugum
- Erythema multiforme
- Herpes simplex
- Insect bites
- Actinic lichen planus—hyperpigmented scaly halo around the lesion
- Discoid lupus erythematosus (DLE)
- Melasma—brownish macules and patches spread over the bridge of the nose, cheeks, and forehead
- Pemphigus vulgaris
- Pityriasis rosea
- Postinflammatory hyperpigmentation—lacks the erythematous ring
- Psoriasis—silvery white scales prominent and the scalp, nail changes seen
- Steven–Johnson syndrome—severe mucosal involvement

COMPLICATIONS

Hyperpigmentation may take many months to resolve. Incontinent pigment in the dermis responds poorly to topical bleaching agents such as hydroquinones.

TREATMENT

Lesions of FDE resolve spontaneously with avoidance of the inciting drug. Oral antihistamine and a topical corticosteroid are prescribed for symptomatic relief.

Rechallenging the patient to the suspected offending drug is the only known test to possibly discern the causative agent.

➲ SUGGESTED READING

1. Anderson HJ, Lee JB. A review of fixed drug eruption with a special focus on generalized bullous fixed drug eruption. Medicina. 2021;57(9):925.

86 Folliculitis

ETIOLOGY

The causative organisms of folliculitis are *Staphylococcus aureus* (most common), gram-negative organisms, pseudomonas (hot tub folliculitis), fungal (tinea barbae, pityrosporum folliculitis), and viral. Factors predisposing to folliculitis include occlusion, maceration, and hyperhydration of the skin. Also, shaving, plucking or waxing hair, use of topical corticosteroids, hot and humid weather, atopic dermatitis, and diabetes mellitus predispose an individual to folliculitis.

EPIDEMIOLOGY

Both sexes are equally affected and any age group may be involved.

CLINICAL FEATURES

Folliculitis is the superficial or deep infection of the hair follicle. It involves the face, chest, back, axillae, or buttocks. Palms and soles are spared. Lesions of superficial folliculitis are small, 1–4 mm pustules or crusted papules on an erythematous base. The lesions are frequently clustered and heal without scarring **(Fig. 1)**.

When infection is limited up to the infundibulum of the follicle, it is superficial folliculitis, and when it extends to the deeper aspect, it is deep folliculitis.

Clinical variants:

- Acute superficial folliculitis (Bockhart's folliculitis) is seen on scalp commonly due to *Staphylococcus aureus*.

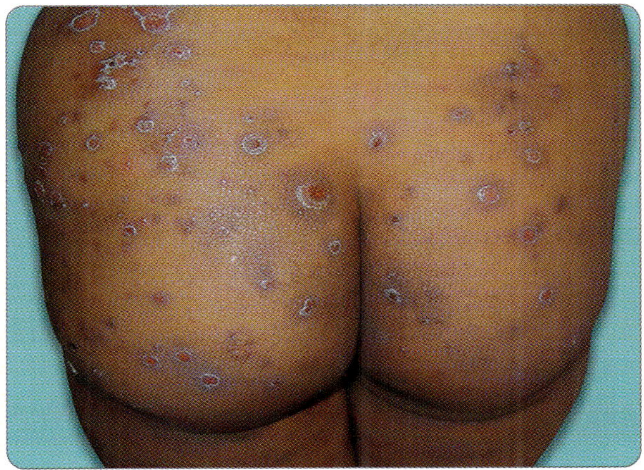

Fig. 1: Multiple crusted lesions over the gluteal area. Few pustules with erythema are also seen.

- Chronic folliculitis of the leg (dermatitis cruris pustulosa et atrophicans) is also a recalcitrant superficial form which causes atrophic scarring due to recurrent infection. It is associated with hypergammaglobulinemia and low complement levels.
- Gram-negative folliculitis is seen postacne, and hot tub folliculitis is due to *Pseudomonas aeruginosa*.
- Sycosis barbae (barber's itch) is a deep folliculitis, which presents as large, tender, erythematous papules, often with a central pustule. The lesions are painful. Lupoid sycosis is a deeper form associated with follicular destruction and atrophic scarring.

Perifolliculitis is the presence of inflammatory cells in perifollicular tissue, sometimes extending to the reticular dermis.

HISTOPATHOLOGY

On histopathology, neutrophils are present in the early stages, lymphocytes and macrophages in the late stages within the follicular ostium and upper regions of the follicle. The causative organism can be detected in the follicle.

DIFFERENTIAL DIAGNOSIS

- Acne vulgaris—presence of polymorphic lesions, comedones seen
- Rosacea—telangiectasias seen
- Chloracne
- Insect bite—papules with central punctum seen
- Milia—whitish papules seen
- Impetigo
- Papular urticaria—only on exposed areas, excoriated lesions seen
- Miliaria
- Superficial fungal infections—demonstration of fungal elements
- Keratosis pilaris—spiny papules with perifollicular erythema

COMPLICATIONS

Folliculitis may progress to form furuncles and abscesses.

TREATMENT

Antibacterial washes that contain chlorhexidine or triclosan should be used. Antibacterial ointments (bacitracin or mupirocin 2%) may also be used for 7–10 days. Widespread or recurrent staphylococcal folliculitis is treated with appropriate β-lactam antibiotics, macrolides, and lincosamides (e.g., clindamycin). Chronic *S. aureus* carriage can be treated with mupirocin 2% ointment applied twice daily to the nares, axillae/groin, and/or submammary area for 5 days or rifampicin 300 mg bd for 5 days.

SUGGESTED READING

1. Laureano AC, Schwartz RA, Cohen PJ. Facial bacterial infections: folliculitis. Clinics in dermatology. 2014;32(6):711-4.

87 Fordyce Disease

➲ SYNONYMS

Apocrine miliaria, Fox–Fordyce disease.

➲ HISTORY

Fordyce disease is named for George Henry Fox and John Addison Fordyce's report on the disease in 1902.

➲ ETIOLOGY

Hormonal factors are thought to have a role in its pathogenesis. Emotional and physical stimuli may also play a role in the disease course. The keratin plug in the follicular infundibulum obstructs the entrance of the apocrine duct. Depilatory laser hair removal has been found to damage the follicular infundibulum and cause keratin plugging.

➲ EPIDEMIOLOGY

It is observed primarily in women between the ages of 15 and 35 years and follows a prolonged course but usually remits after menopause and improves during pregnancy. Female-to-male ratio is 9:1.

➲ CLINICAL FEATURES

Fox–Fordyce disease is a chronic pruritic disorder of apocrine glands. It presents as dome-shaped, skin-colored, discrete perifollicular papules in the axillary, anogenital, and periareolar skin. A paucity of hair in affected areas is frequently observed. The condition is often intensely pruritic **(Fig. 1)**.

➲ HISTOLOGY

The blockage of the duct leads to apocrine sweat retention and subsequent rupture of the duct at the level of the epidermis. Epidermal spongiosis and vesiculation are seen. Associated findings include a perifollicular and periadnexal inflammatory infiltrate, consisting of lymphocytes with occasional histiocytes and eosinophils. Xanthomatous variant shows foamy macrophages. Stashower et al. proposed transverse histologic sectioning as the most effective way to demonstrate diagnostic features.

➲ DIFFERENTIAL DIAGNOSIS

- Acne
- Milia
- Miliaria

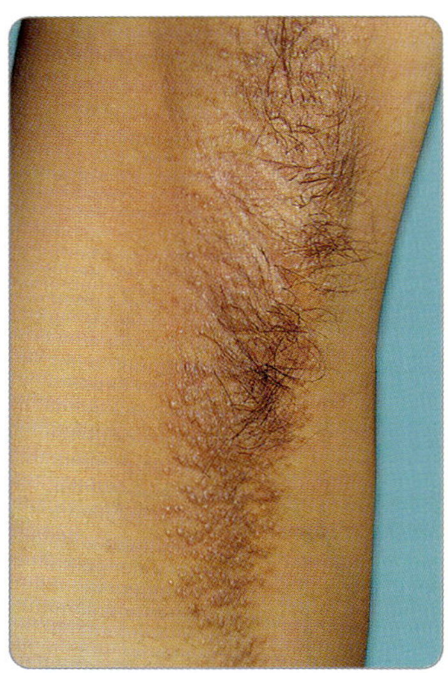

Fig. 1: Multiple skin-colored discrete papules over the axilla.

- Folliculitis
- Axillary perifollicular xanthomatosis (follicular variant of verruciform xanthomas)

➲ TREATMENT

Topical and intralesional corticosteroids are often the first line of therapy. Topical calcineurin and topical tretinoin 0.025%, pimecrolimus, and clindamycin have been shown to reduce pruritus. Oral isotretinoin and contraceptives are tried. Physical interventions that may be beneficial include phototherapy (hot quartz given once a week for 4–6 weeks), electrocautery, and excision of periareolar skin.

➲ SUGGESTED READING

1. Salloum A, Bouferraa Y, Bazzi N, Bou Zerdan M, Abi Chebl J, Chu T, et al. Pathophysiology, clinical findings, and management of Fox-Fordyce disease: A systematic review. J Cosmet Dermatol. 2022;21(2):482-500.

88 Fordyce Spots

➲ ETIOLOGY

These are ectopic sebaceous glands on lips, buccal, and genital mucosa. They lack an association with hair follicles with ducts opening directly onto the cutaneous surface.

➲ PATHOGENESIS

They are present at birth but become evident at puberty in response to gonadal and adrenal androgenic hormones. Enlargement of sebaceous glands renders them visible throughout the overlying epithelium.

➲ CLINICAL FEATURES

Asymptomatic, pinhead-sized, yellow, discrete isolated, or grouped papules. Occasionally, the papules are lobulated or form plaques. The lesions are usually bilateral and symmetrical. Sites include vermilion border of the lips and oral mucosa and, less commonly, on the penis, scrotum, and labia. On the penile shaft, papules become obvious on stretching the foreskin or during penile erection.

➲ HISTOPATHOLOGY

They show enlarged sebaceous glands, consisting of a group of mature sebaceous lobes surrounding small ducts that emerge at the epithelial surface and lack an association with a hair follicle.

➲ DERMOSCOPY

Small, whitish-yellow, structureless areas with a central opening representing the sebaceous gland, often clustered together, and with a lack of distinct pigment network, essentially showing enlarged sebaceous gland openings on a normal skin background.

➲ DIFFERENTIAL DIAGNOSIS

Milia, sebaceous hyperplasia, syringomas, molluscum contagiosum, lichen nitidus, closed comedones, cutaneous myxomas, and calcinosis cutis.

➲ TREATMENT

Treatment includes micro-punch surgery, electrodesiccation, cryotherapy, ablative laser, photodynamic therapy, topical bichloracetic acid, topical tretinoin, and oral isotretinoin.

➲ SUGGESTED READING

1. Leung AK, Barankin B. Fordyce Spots. Consultant. 2016;56:377-8.

89 Freckles

➲ SYNONYM

Ephelides.

➲ ETIOLOGY

Freckles are common in individuals with blond or red hair. They usually appear in the first 3 years of life. Since freckling can be seen in some families over generations, autosomal dominant inheritance is likely. Hyperpigmentation in ephelides is the result of increased sun-induced melanogenesis and transport of an increased number of fully melanized melanosomes from melanocytes to keratinocytes.

➲ CLINICAL FEATURES

They occur only on sun-exposed areas of the body, mainly on the face, the dorsal aspects of the arms, and the upper part of the chest and the back. They are well-demarcated, round, oval, or irregular in shape and 1–3 mm in diameter. They vary in color from light to dark brown **(Fig. 1)**. They decrease later in life. They are benign and show no propensity for malignant transformation. Ephelides are a marker of ultraviolet (UV)-induced damage and associated with the risk of melanoma.

Dermoscopy shows round brown globules, uniform pigmentation, and moth-eaten edges.

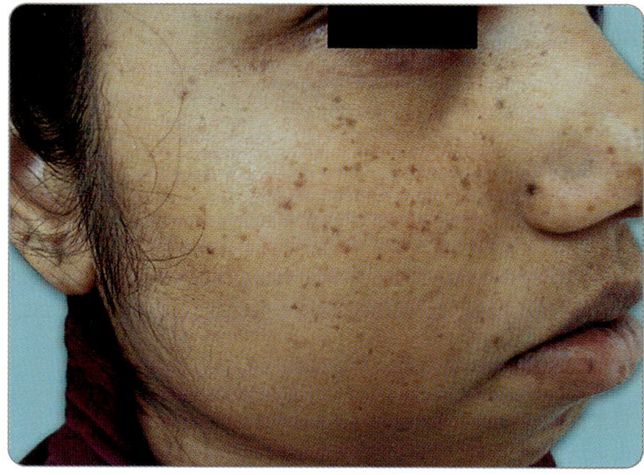

Fig. 1: Multiple well-demarcated hyperpigmented macules over the cheek, nose, and lips.

Table 1: Lentigines and freckles.

Lentigines	*Freckles*
No genetic predisposition	Common in fair skin and red hair individuals
No relation to sun exposure, seen all over the body	Exacerbated on sun exposure, seasonal; variation present, seen commonly in sun-exposed areas
Regular borders	Serrated borders
The number of melanocytes is increased	The number of melanocytes is normal
Elongation of rete ridges	No elongation of rete ridges
Associated with syndromes—LEOPARD, NAME, and LAMB	No such association
Mucosal lesions present	Mucosal lesions absent
Become darker in pregnancy	No relationship to pregnancy

HISTOPATHOLOGY

The keratinocytes show an increase in melanin content in the basal cell layer. Melanophages are seen in the papillary dermis. The number of melanocytes in ephelides does not differ significantly from normal. The melanocytes in ephelides are larger and have more branching of dendrites and higher dopa positivity.

DIFFERENTIAL DIAGNOSIS

- Lentigines—mucosal lesions are also seen
- Café-au-lait macules—larger lesions, can be in covered areas also
- Tinea versicolor—fine branny scaling seen
- Seborrheic keratosis
- Junctional nevi

Lentigines and freckles are described in **Table 1**.

TREATMENT

Sun exposure should be minimized and sunscreens should be used. The bleaching action of hydroquinone and topical retinoids may be beneficial. Pulsed lasers are used to remove pigmentation.

SUGGESTED READING

1. Kukla-Bartoszek M, Pośpiech E, Woźniak A, Boroń M, Karłowska-Pik J, Teisseyre P, et al. DNA-based predictive models for the presence of freckles. Forensic Sci Int Genet. 2019;42:252-9.

90 Furuncles

➲ SYNONYM

Boil.

➲ ETIOLOGY

Furuncles tend to occur in adolescents and young adults. *Staphylococcus aureus* (most common) and anaerobic bacteria are causative organisms. Predisposing factors include chronic bacterial carriage, diabetes mellitus, obesity, poor hygiene, and immunodeficiency states.

➲ CLINICAL FEATURES

It is defined as infection and inflammatory changes involving a hair follicle and surrounding tissue. Furuncles occur only in hair-bearing skin **(Fig. 1)**. The most common locations are the face, neck, axillae, buttocks, thighs, and perineum. Sites prone to friction or minor trauma, such as the area under a belt, are distinctly susceptible. Furuncles usually begin as a hard, tender, red nodule that enlarges and becomes painful and fluctuant; rupture results in decreased pain. Recurrent furunculosis seen in carriers of *S. aureus*.

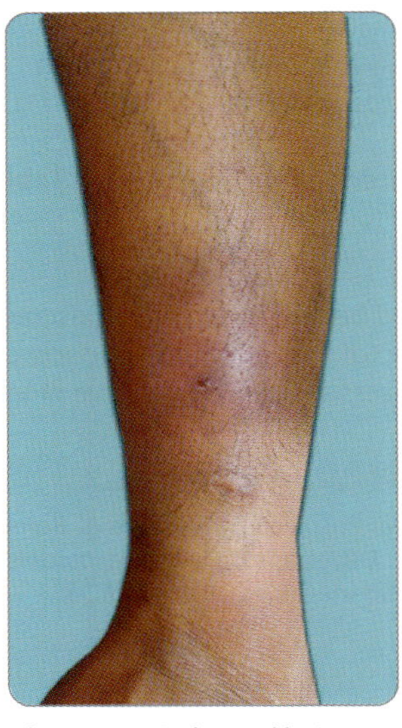

Fig. 1: Erythematous, indurated lesion over the leg.

HISTOPATHOLOGY

Furuncles are characterized by an acute, suppurative reaction involving the follicle with dense neutrophilic infiltrate below the infundibulum, as well as perifollicular necrosis with fibrinoid debris.

DIFFERENTIAL DIAGNOSIS

- Folliculitis—individuals pustules seen
- Pseudofolliculitis—ingrown hairs seen
- Foreign body reaction
- Acne—comedones, papules seen
- Hidradenitis suppurativa—polyporous comedones seen
- Epidermoid cyst—skin-colored swelling with central punctum seen

TREATMENT

Warm compresses may promote maturation, drainage, and resolution of symptoms. Fluctuant lesions require incision and drainage. Topical mupirocin or bacitracin is used for localized lesions. Systemic antibiotics are required for lesions on the nose, within the nares, or in the external auditory canal, large and recurrent lesions, lesions with surrounding cellulitis, and lesions not responding to local care.

PROGNOSIS

The lesions heal rapidly but with scarring.

SUGGESTED READING

1. Ioannides D, Lazaridou E. Furuncles and carbuncles. In: European Handbook of Dermatological Treatments. Cham: Springer International Publishing; 2023. pp. 339-44.

91 Gianotti–Crosti Syndrome

SYNONYMS

Infantile lichenoid dermatitis, papular acrodermatitis of childhood, papulovesicular acrolocated syndrome.

HISTORY

Ferdinando Gianotti and Agostino Crosti initially described Gianotti–Crosti syndrome (GCS) as an exanthem associated with a hepatitis B virus.

ETIOLOGY

Gianotti–Crosti syndrome is a cutaneous reaction pattern associated with viruses, bacteria, and vaccines. Common triggers include hepatitis B and Epstein–Barr virus (EBV). Other associated viruses are cytomegalovirus, *Enterovirus*, respiratory syncytial virus, rotavirus, adenovirus, echovirus, poxvirus, poliovirus, coxsackievirus, parvovirus, human immunodeficiency virus (HIV), hepatitis A, hepatitis C, and parainfluenza virus and bacteria like *Mycoplasma pneumonia*, *Borrelia burgdorferi*, *Bartonella henselae*, and group A β-hemolytic *Streptococcus*. The pathogenesis may be due to a viral antigenemia or circulating immune complexes (type IV hypersensitivity).

EPIDEMIOLOGY

Gianotti–Crosti syndrome is seen in infants and children between 6 months and 12 years, with a peak of 1–6 years of age. Incidence is more among atopic children.

CLINICAL FEATURES

Multiple coalescing, monomorphous, flat-topped or dome-shaped, red-brown papules and papulovesicles are distributed symmetrically on the cheeks, extensor surfaces of the extremities, and the buttocks **(Fig. 1)**. They can be pruritic and rarely hemorrhagic. They evolve over a few days and last for 2–8 weeks. Children with exclusive facial lesions may have EBV infection.

Diagnostic criteria are proposed for GCS wherein extensive truncal lesions and scaly lesions are negative findings. Hepatosplenomegaly and axillary or inguinal adenopathy are inconsistent findings.

HISTOPATHOLOGY

- Mild acanthosis and spongiosis with Langerhans cell-rich intradermal vesicle in vesicular variant
- Perivascular dense lymphocytic T-cell infiltrate and dendritic cells in papillary dermis

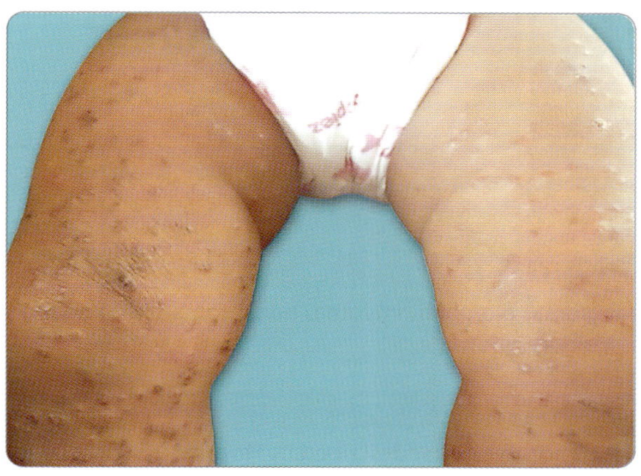

Fig. 1: Multiple papules bilaterally over both thighs.

DIFFERENTIAL DIAGNOSIS

- Papular urticaria
- Pityriasis rosea—herald patch is seen.
- Erythema multiforme—targetoid lesions are seen, followed by drugs/infection.
- Lichen planus—basal cell degeneration and lichenoid infiltrate are seen.
- Lichenoid drug eruption
- Molluscum contagiosum—umbilicated lesions are seen.
- Hand–foot–mouth disease—shallow ulcers with erythematous halo are seen on palms, soles, and mouth.
- Follicular eczema
- Erythema infectiosum

TREATMENT

Medium potency steroids may decrease the duration of lesions. In severe cases, systemic pulsed corticosteroids may be administered. Oral antihistamines or topical anti-itch lotions are used for symptomatic relief.

PROGNOSIS

Gianotti–Crosti syndrome is a self-limited and benign disease. The rash may last for 2–4 weeks.

SUGGESTED READING

1. Afonso A, Cachão J, Junior VL, Gouveia T. Gianotti-Crosti syndrome: a challenging exanthema. BMJ Case Rep. 2021;14(4):e240747.

92 Glomus Tumor

➲ SYNONYMS

Glomangioma, glomangiomyoma, nonchromaffin paraganglioma, Barre–Masson syndrome.

➲ HISTORY

Glomus tumors were first described by Hoyer in 1877, while the first complete clinical description was given by Masson in 1924.

➲ ETIOLOGY

Glomus tumor is a vascular hamartoma and arises from glomus bodies, which are specialized arteriovenous anastomoses found often in the fingers and palms and function as thermoregulatory receptors. Occurrence of familial cases with autosomal dominant inheritance and the association of multiple tumors with malformation of the same limb suggest the involvement of genetic factors. Glomulin gene mutation has been identified as the cause in multiple inherited glomangiomas.

➲ EPIDEMIOLOGY

The incidence increases from the age of 7 years onward, commonly seen around 30–50 years, among women.

➲ CLINICAL FEATURES

Glomus tumor is a pink or purple nodule varying in size from 1 to 20 mm, with paroxysmal pulsating pain precipitated by cold, pressure, or dependency. Triad of hypersensitivity to cold, heightened pinprick sensitivity, and paroxysmal pain. The most common site is the hands, particularly fingers, followed by other sites on the extremities, including the head, neck, and penis. Tumors beneath the nail are particularly painful, and the nail has a bluish-red flush. It may be associated with ridging and fissuring of the nail plate. Multiple glomus tumors are larger and usually dark blue in color and situated deep in the dermis.

Magnetic resonance imaging (MRI) is the investigation of choice. A pseudocapsule of surrounding reactionary tissue is seen on T2-weighted imaging.

➲ DERMOSCOPY

Digital glomus tumor shows linear and ramified vascular structures, longitudinal erythronychia, red subungual spot, and onycholysis; extradigital tumors can reveal homogenous white structure and peripheral telangiectasia.

➲ CLINICAL TEST FOR DIAGNOSIS

- Love's pin test (patient feels severe pain at the affected area and pain reduction when pressed elsewhere with pinhead)
- Hildreth's test (transient ischemia is induced along the arm using tourniquet, and the absence of pain is felt, which returns on removal of tourniquet)
- Cold sensitivity test

➲ HISTOPATHOLOGY

The tumor is lobulated, well-circumscribed, and situated in the dermis. The smaller painful lesions tend to be cellular. A glomus cell is cuboidal, with a well-marked cell membrane and a round central nucleus. The cells align themselves in rows around the single layer of endothelial cells of the vascular spaces surrounded by fibrous capsule. Numerous nonmyelinated nerve fibers course through the cellular masses.

➲ DIFFERENTIAL DIAGNOSIS

- *Leiomyoma*—painful tumor, skin-colored lesions, and whorled appearance of smooth muscles are observed.
- Eccrine spiradenoma
- *Cavernous hemangioma*—dilated veins are seen.
- *Schwannoma*—proliferation of nerve cells
- Blue nevus
- Melanoma
- *Angiolipoma*—absence of pulsating tumors

➲ COMPLICATIONS

There is a risk of malignant transformation and local recurrence following surgery. Sometimes, the nodule may erode the bone of the phalanx and cause pressure dystrophy of the overlying nail.

➲ TREATMENT

Treatment is surgical excision. Subungual lesions require nail avulsion. Treatment modalities used for multiple lesions include argon, carbon dioxide, or neodymium-doped yttrium aluminum garnet (Nd:YAG) laser therapy and sclerotherapy. Incomplete excision can cause recurrence.

➲ SUGGESTED READING

1. Lee WQ, Li Y, Yeo NE. Glomus tumour: an institutional experience of 31 cases. J Orthop Surg and Res. 2023;18(1):741.

93 Gonorrhea

➲ HISTORY

The word gonorrhea is derived from the Greek word meaning "flow of seed" (gonos—seed, rhea—flow), so named by Galen. The causative organism, *Neisseria gonorrhoeae*, was discovered by Albert Ludwig Neisser in 1879 from Poland.

➲ ETIOLOGY

Gonorrhea is caused by infection with *N. gonorrhoeae*, a gram-negative, aerobic, nonsporing, *coccus*-shaped *Bacterium* found in pairs. These are usually visualized intracellularly in the polymorphonuclear leukocytes. The disease is acquired through sexual contact, rarely via vertical transmission from mother to child during birth, accidental nonvenereal infection in adults, and children sharing beds or linen with infected parents.

➲ EPIDEMIOLOGY

Gonorrhea occurs commonly in women between the ages of 15 and 19 years and in men between the ages of 20 and 24 years.

➲ CLINICAL FEATURES

The average incubation period is 1–10 days; in most cases, it is <5 days. The most common manifestation in men is urethritis, characterized by cloudy or purulent discharge from the penile meatus **(Fig. 1)**. Mucosal inflammation in the anterior urethra

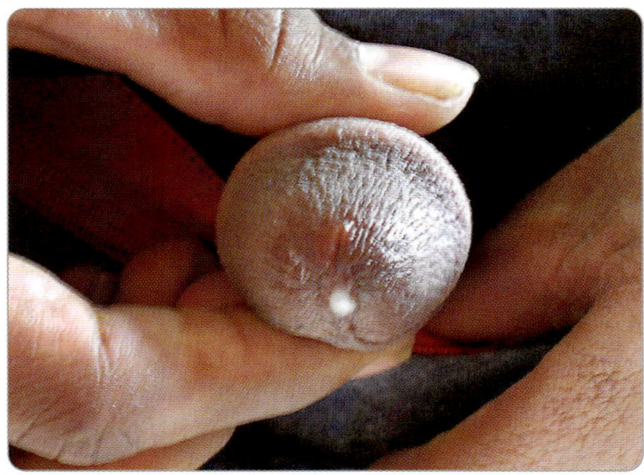

Fig. 1: Drop of pus at the urethral meatus in gonorrhea.

leads to painful urination and perimeatal redness and swelling. Proctitis is another manifestation, with symptoms including rectal mucopurulent discharge, pain on defecation, constipation, and tenesmus. In women, 50% of the cases are asymptomatic. Symptoms of urethritis include mucopurulent discharge, vaginal pruritus, and dysuria. Pelvic inflammatory disease (PID) occurs in 10–40% of uncomplicated infection and is characterized by fever, lower abdominal pain, back pain, vomiting, vaginal bleeding, dyspareunia, and adnexal or cervical motion tenderness on physical examination. Bartholinitis/Bartholin abscess can occur.

In newborns, ocular infections can occur during passage through the infected birth canal and are known as ophthalmia neonatorum. In children, pharyngeal or genital gonococcal infection may occur.

Disseminated gonococcal disease is associated with a classic triad of dermatitis, migratory polyarthritis, and tenosynovitis. It is also seen in complement deficiency states.

➲ ASSOCIATED SYNDROME

Fitz-Hugh–Curtis syndrome.

➲ DIAGNOSIS

Gram staining of the discharge, culture on Thayer–Martin media, Martin Lewis media, New York City (NYC) and GC-Lect media, hemoglobin (Hb)–yeast–liver (HYL) media, and Chacko–Nair media.

Centers for Disease Control and Prevention (CDC) criteria for diagnosis:

- Mucopurulent or purulent discharge
- Gram stain of urethral secretions demonstrating ≥5 white blood cells (WBCs) per oil immersion field; *Gonococcal* infection is established by documenting the presence of WBC-containing *gonococci*.
- Positive leukocyte esterase test on microscopic examination of first-void urine sediment demonstrating ≥10 WBC per high power field

Differential Diagnosis

- *Urinary tract infection*—absence of *diplococci*
- Chlamydia infection
- Pelvic inflammatory disease
- *Trichomoniasis*—presence of motile trichomoniasis vaginalis is seen.
- Herpes simplex virus
- *Bacterial vaginosis*—presence of clue cells
- *Mycoplasma* infection

➲ COMPLICATIONS

- *Women*: Infertility, disseminated disease, PID, tubo-ovarian mass, and pelvic abscess.
- *Men*: Littritis, fibrous stricture, periurethral abscess, chordee, acute prostatitis, gonococcal proctitis, epididymitis, penile lymphangitis, and penile edema (bull-headed clap).

➲ TREATMENT

Single dosage of any of the following drugs is effective: Cefixime 400 mg PO plus azithromycin 1 g, ceftriaxone 250 mg intramuscular (IM) plus azithromycin 1 g, ciprofloxacin 500 mg, ofloxacin 400 mg PO, and levofloxacin 250 mg PO.

Patients allergic to the above can be given spectinomycin, 2 g in a single IM dose.

In dual therapy for chlamydia, the following are added: Azithromycin, 1 g orally in a single dose, and doxycycline, 100 mg orally twice a day for 7 days.

In treatment failure cases, oral gemifloxacin 320 mg plus azithromycin 2 g single dose or IM gentamycin 240 mg plus azithromycin 2 g single dose.

➲ PROGNOSIS

Excellent if infection is treated early with appropriate antibiotics. Patient to be retested 3 months after treatment [culture or nucleic acid amplification test (NAAT)].

➲ SUGGESTED READING

1. Whelan J, Abbing-Karahagopian V, Serino L, Unemo M. Gonorrhoea: a systematic review of prevalence reporting globally. BMC Infect Dis. 2021;21(1):1152.

94 Gottron's Syndrome

➲ SYNONYM

Progressive symmetrical erythrokeratoderma.

➲ HISTORY

Progressive symmetrical erythrokeratoderma (PSEK) was first described by Darier in 1911.

➲ ETIOLOGY

Progressive symmetrical erythrokeratoderma is a rare cornification disorder, which has autosomal dominant inheritance. It occurs due to frameshift mutations in *Loricrin* gene.

➲ EPIDEMIOLOGY

Lesions appear in infancy, always before the age of 5 years. There is no sexual predilection.

➲ CLINICAL FEATURES

Skin is usually normal at birth. Large, geographic but symmetrical, fine, scaly plaques with an orange-red erythema appear in infancy. There is little pruritus. The shoulder girdle, cheeks, and buttocks are most often affected, with limited plaques on the ankles and wrists. Keratoderma may be present in about half the cases. Lesions can be triggered by temperature changes and mechanical irritation. The lesions regress after puberty **(Figs. 1A and B)**.

➲ ASSOCIATED SYNDROMES

Associated syndromes include Schneider's syndrome and Giroux–Barbeau syndrome.

➲ HISTOPATHOLOGY

The epidermis is acanthotic with preserved granular layer. The stratum corneum is hyperkeratotic with a basket-weave pattern and foci of parakeratosis. Perinuclear vacuolation of keratinocytes is present. Ultrastructurally, the granular cells contain swollen mitochondria, and corneocytes show lipid-like vacuoles. Labeling studies show increased epidermopoiesis with shortening of interphase.

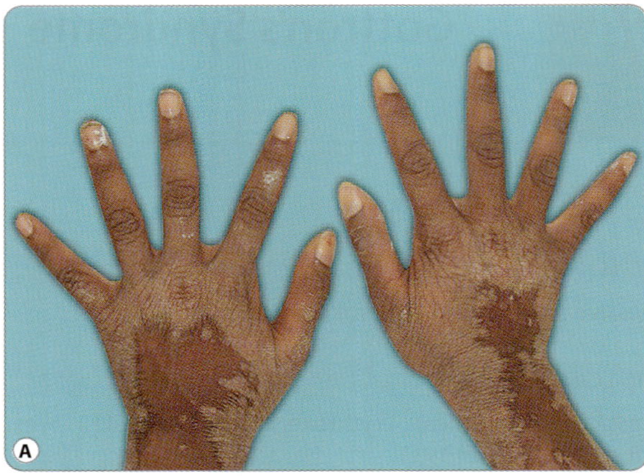

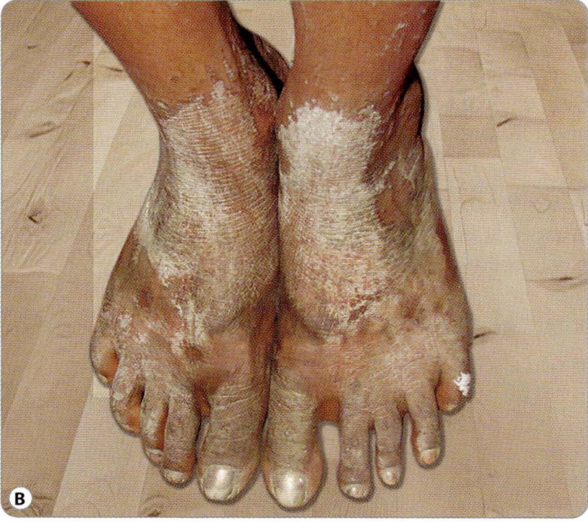

Figs. 1A and B: Bilaterally symmetric keratoderma over dorsum of (A) hands and (B) feet with well-demarcated borders.

➲ DIFFERENTIAL DIAGNOSIS

- Erythrokeratoderma variabilis (EKV)
- Localized pityriasis rubra pilaris
- Ichyosis linearis circumflexa (Netherton syndrome)
- Plaque psoriasis

➲ TREATMENT

Etretinate and acitretin are effective. Topical keratolytics like 2–3% salicylic acid, 10% urea, and psoralen and ultraviolet A (PUVA) treatment have also been tried.

➲ SUGGESTED READING

1. Boyden LM, Vincent NG, Zhou J, Hu R, Craiglow BG, Bayliss SJ, et al. Mutations in KDSR cause recessive progressive symmetric erythrokeratoderma. Am J Hum Genet. 2017;100(6):978-84.

95 Graft-versus-host Disease

➲ ETIOLOGY

Graft-versus-host disease (GVHD) is induced by donor immunocompetent T cells transferred into allogeneic hosts incapable of rejecting them. Acute GVHD develops in 25–40% of recipients of human leukocyte antigen (HLA)-identical sibling transplants. Chronic GVHD develops in 40% of patients. Major effector cells in the skin lesions of acute GVHD are CD8+ T cells that can release perforin upon recognition of allo major histocompatibility complex (MHC) class I molecules. In addition to perforin, FasL and natural killer (NK) cells also play a role in pathogenesis. High levels of tumor necrosis factor alpha (TNF-α) have been implicated in an increased incidence of GVHD.

➲ CLINICAL FEATURES

Graft-versus-host disease is classically divided into two forms: Acute, which occurs within 3 months post-transplantation, and chronic, which usually begins about 100 days post-transplantation. Risk factors for developing GVHD are an unrelated (but matched) donor, a related donor but with a mismatch at one or more HLA antigens, an unmodified (i.e., T-cell replete) graft, an older age of the donor or recipient, and a female donor with a male recipient.

Hyperacute GVHD, characterized by a generalized erythematous maculopapular eruption, high fever, hepatitis, and intestinal symptoms, has been reported to develop as early as the first week. Acute GVHD occurs commonly as a maculopapular (morbilliform) exanthem, folliculocentric, reflecting injury to hair follicle epithelium. The eruption favors the distal extremities, pinnae, sides of the neck, and upper back. In severe cases, the eruption progresses into a diffuse erythema, with bulla formation, a positive Nikolsky sign, and desquamation, resembling toxic epidermal necrolysis. Gastrointestinal and hepatic manifestations may precede, coincide or appear after the cutaneous eruption. Perifollicular papules, an erythematous palmoplantar rash, and a violaceous discoloration of the ears may be good indicators of the diagnosis of acute GVHD.

Acute GVHD has been graded clinically based on the involvement of the skin, liver, and gastrointestinal tract into five stages, 0–IV, with higher grades indicating a poorer prognosis. Grade 0 indicates no clinical evidence of disease. Grade I indicates rash involving <50% of body surface area and no gut or liver involvement; grade II indicates rash covering >50% of body surface area, bilirubin 2–3 mg/dL, diarrhea 10–15 mL/kg per day, or persistent nausea. Grade III or IV indicates generalized erythroderma, with a toxic epidermal necrolysis-like picture, bilirubin >3 mg/dL, or diarrhea >16 mL/kg per day. Chronic GVHD is classically divided into an early lichenoid form and a later sclerodermoid form. Lichenoid chronic GVHD is characterized by erythematous or violaceous lichenoid papules and plaques, usually affecting the dorsal aspects of the hands and feet, the forearms, and the trunk. Lacy white plaques and erosions of the oral mucosa may be seen; salivary gland dysfunction results in a Sjögren-like syndrome. Sclerodermoid chronic GVHD is characterized by plaques of dermal sclerosis, initially resembling morphea and/or lichen sclerosus and eventually by generalized scleroderma, often resulting in joint contractures. Poikilodermatous changes, multiple hemangiomas, nodular fibromas, subacute cutaneous lupus erythematosus (LE)-like eruptions, and scarring alopecia are the other features. Unlike systemic sclerosis, there is no Raynaud's phenomenon or acrosclerosis.

HISTOPATHOLOGY

Vacuolization of the basal cell layer, apoptotic keratinocytes adjacent to lymphocytes (satellite cell necrosis) in the suprabasal layer, exocytosis of mononuclear cells, and focal spongiosis are seen in acute GVHD. Hyperkeratosis, irregular hypergranulosis, mild acanthosis, basal layer vacuolar alteration, dyskeratotic epidermal cells (apoptotic keratinocytes), colloid bodies, and a dermal band-like lymphocytic infiltrate in direct apposition to the epidermis are seen in chronic lichenoid GVHD. Chronic sclerodermoid GVHD is characterized by epidermal atrophy and dermal fibrosis.

DIFFERENTIAL DIAGNOSIS

- *Acute GVHD*:
  - Drug eruptions (morbilliform, erythroderma, and toxic epidermal necrolysis)
  - Viral exanthems [including human herpesvirus (HHV)-6]
  - Eruption of lymphocyte recovery
- *Chronic GVHD*:
  - Lichenoid drug eruption
  - Pityriasis lichenoides chronica
  - Idiopathic lichen planus (LP)
  - Lichen sclerosus
  - Morphea
  - Scleroderma
  - Eosinophilic fasciitis

TREATMENT

Methotrexate or mycophenolate mofetil plus systemic tacrolimus or cyclosporine are used as prophylaxis for acute GVHD. The first line of treatment is systemic corticosteroids; additional immunosuppressive agents such as infliximab, mycophenolate mofetil, and daclizumab [anti-CD25, interleukin 2 receptor alpha (IL-2Rα)] can be used. For chronic GVHD, the standard first-line therapy is oral corticosteroids, either alone or in combination with cyclosporine or systemic tacrolimus. Other potential treatments include hydroxychloroquine, azathioprine and mycophenolate mofetil, etretinate, and acitretin. For cutaneous lesions, psoralen and ultraviolet A (PUVA), photopheresis, and synthetic retinoids can be employed.

➲ PROGNOSIS

Mortality is 30–50% in acute GVHD. After the onset of chronic GVHD, 25–40% of patients die within 2 years, often due to secondary infections.

➲ SUGGESTED READING

1. Gooptu M, Antin JH. GVHD prophylaxis 2020. Front Immunol. 2021;12:605726.

96 Gram-negative Folliculitis

HISTORY

Gram-negative folliculitis was first described by Fulton et al. in 1968.

ETIOLOGY

Gram-negative folliculitis is usually seen in patients who are receiving long-term systemic antibiotics. This antibiotic therapy disrupts the ecological balance by suppressing normal resident flora. The causative organisms are usually *Escherichia coli*, *Klebsiella* species, *Enterobacter* species, or *Proteus* species. This is more common in patients with acne or rosacea.

EPIDEMIOLOGY

It occurs more commonly in adult men with oily skin.

CLINICAL FEATURES

This condition is characterized by superficial papules and pustules extending from the infranasal area to the cheeks and chin. A patient with acne, who was initially responding to systemic antibiotics, later develops papules but no comedones. They are classified as follows:

- *Type 1 (80%)*: Superficial pustular lesions without comedones
- *Type II (20%)*: Deep, nodular, and cystic lesions

Diagnosis is by tissue Gram-stains and stains for fungi which may reveal pathogenic organisms. Culture and sensitivity studies should be performed and appropriate antibiotics given.

DIFFERENTIAL DIAGNOSIS

- Gram-positive folliculitis—gram stain shows gram-positive organisms
- Acne—presence of comedones
- Eosinophilic folliculitis—presence of eosinophils on gram-stain
- Acneiform eruptions—history of (h/o) topical or systemic drug intake, monomorphic lesions more on the back and face
- Rosacea—presence of telangiectasias
- Perioral dermatitis—lesions only around the mouth sparing the vermilion border

TREATMENT

Treatment includes topical application of antibiotics such as gentamycin, benzoyl peroxide, or systemic drugs such as quinolones (e.g., ciprofloxacin). In severe or recurrent cases, oral isotretinoin, 1 mg/kg/day for 16 weeks is prescribed.

➲ SUGGESTED READING

1. Kumar B, Sardana K, Gautam HK. Unique speciation and antibiotic susceptibility of acne complicated by gram-negative folliculitis.

97 Granuloma Annulare

HISTORY

Colcott Fox first described the "ringed eruption of the fingers" in 1895 and Radcliffe-Crocker gave the term granuloma annulare (GA) in 1902.

ETIOLOGY

There is no known specific etiological factor. Trauma, sunlight, insect bites, Bacillus Calmette–Guérin (BCG) vaccination, and viral infections including HIV, Epstein–Barr virus, hepatitis B virus, hepatitis C virus, and herpes zoster virus have been considered causative factors. Cases have been reported after gold therapy and treatment with allopurinol, diclofenac, quinidine, calcitonin, amlodipine, angiotensin-converting enzyme (ACE) inhibitors, daclizumab, and calcium channel blockers. Familial incidence is seen.

Theories in pathogenesis:
- Post-traumatic primary necrobiosis
- Immune complex-mediated vasculitis
- Cell-mediated delayed hypersensitivity
- Immunological dysregulation
- Enzyme-induced necrobiotic degeneration
- Elastic tissue injury with elastic fiber degeneration

EPIDEMIOLOGY

The incidence of GA is twice more common among women (2:1) than men. Generalized GA is seen in the elderly.

CLINICAL FEATURES

Lesions of GA are usually asymptomatic, there may be mild pruritus in the generalized form. Common sites involved are the dorsa of hands and feet. Closely set, skin-colored, firm, smooth papules 2–3 mm in size are arranged in a ring-like fashion to form annular lesions 1–5 cm in size **(Fig. 1)**. The mucous membranes, palms, and soles are usually spared. Koebner's phenomenon is seen. The lesions may resolve when a skin biopsy is taken. Lesions may improve in winter and worsen in summer.

The clinical variants include:
- Giant form
- The targetoid form resembles erythema multiforme.
- Perforating GA is seen commonly on dorsal hands and presents as papules with a central keratotic core. It occurs due to ischemic epidermal necrosis or transepithelial elimination.

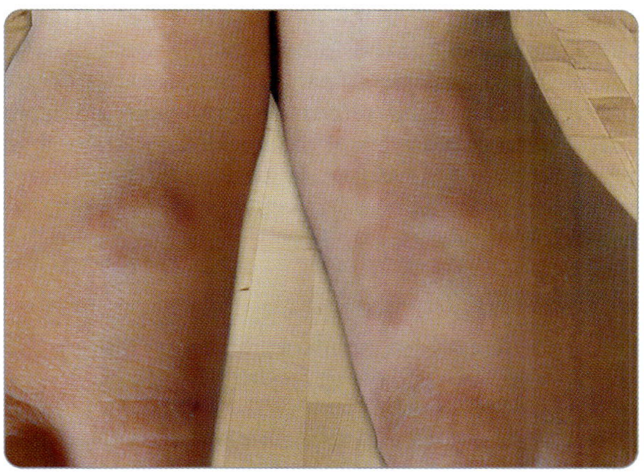

Fig. 1: Multiple papules in an annular arrangement over the feet in granuloma annulare.

- Generalized GA is seen after the fifth decade, with lesions ranging from 10 to 100. It has increased the prevalence of the HLA-Bw35 allele and diabetes mellitus.
- *Subcutaneous GA*: Lesions appear as subcutaneous nodules called "pseudorheumatoid nodule" seen commonly in children.
- Patch type or macular type/arcuate dermal erythema—seen on upper medial thighs and in bathing-trunk distribution. Lesions may closely simulate cutaneous T-cell lymphoma or morphea.
- Photodistributed
- Anetodermic
- Follicular pustular variant

ASSOCIATED CONDITIONS

Granuloma annulare has been reported in Mauriac's syndrome, necrobiosis lipoidica, type 1 diabetes mellitus, rheumatoid nodules, sarcoidosis, mycosis fungoides, malignant lymphomas, and carpal tunnel syndrome.

DERMOSCOPY

Whitish areas and yellow-orange structureless areas, unfocussed vessels (blurry vessels-dotted, linear irregular and branching) over pinkish-red background, whitish scaling, rosettes, and crystalline leaf venations.

BIOMARKERS

Acidophilin stains intracellular and extracellular histiocytes and helps to distinguish from necrobiosis lipoidica and sarcoidosis.

HISTOPATHOLOGY

The epidermis is normal except in the perforating type where it is broken. Multiple foci of incomplete collagen degeneration with mucin deposition are seen in the upper and mid dermis, surrounded by a palisading granuloma consisting of histiocytes, fibroblasts, and lymphocytes. Three histological patterns may occur viz necrobiotic palisading granuloma, an interstitial form, and granuloma of sarcoidal or tuberculoid type. In the interstitial pattern, there are no formed areas of necrobiosis, histiocytes and lymphocytes are present around blood vessels and between collagen bundles and collagen fibers are separated by mucin.

DIFFERENTIAL DIAGNOSIS

- Tuberculoid leprosy—presence of granulomas with lymphocytic cuff in perivascular and periappendageal location
- Lupus vulgaris—lesions with active expanding edge and healing at the other end, apple jelly nodules on diascopy
- Sarcoid granuloma—naked granulomas, raised ACE levels
- Gumma—the presence of collections of histiocytes, lymphocytes and plasma cells, venereal disease research laboratory (VDRL) positivity
- Tinea circinata—concentric scaly annular lesions with scaling
- Erythema annulare centrifugum
- Erythema elevatum diutinum
- Lichen planus

Papular GA can simulate arthropod bites, secondary syphilis, xanthomas, and non-X-histiocytoses such as eruptive histiocytomas.

COMPLICATIONS

The lesions may rarely leave atrophic scars on healing resembling mid-dermal elastolysis or anetoderma.

TREATMENT

Intralesional corticosteroids or steroids under occlusion are given. Other drugs tried in generalized GA are chlorpropamide, chloroquine, sulfones, systemic corticosteroids, potassium iodide, alkylating agents, etretinate, pentoxifylline, photochemotherapy, niacinamide, isotretinoin, dapsone, pentoxifylline, and cyclosporine. Surgical modalities such as cryosurgery, electrodessication, laser destruction, and radiation therapy may be effective.

PROGNOSIS

Individual lesions on an average remain for about 2 years but the duration could be as short as 3 months. On resolution, most lesions leave no telltale marks.

SUGGESTED READING

1. Joshi TP, Duvic M. Granuloma annulare: an updated review of epidemiology, pathogenesis, and treatment options. Am J Clin Dermatol. 2022:1-4.

98 Granuloma Faciale

➲ INTRODUCTION

The name granuloma faciale (GF) is a misnomer, as granulomas are never seen histologically. GF is a benign, inflammatory disease of unknown etiology. Suspected possible etiologies include actinic damage, trauma, allergies, and radiation therapy.

➲ HISTORY

It was first described by Wigley JE in 1945 as eosinophilic granuloma.

It is seen most commonly in the age group of 40–60 years.

➲ PATHOPHYSIOLOGY

A variant of leukocytoclastic vasculitis with a predominant eosinophilic infiltrate is confined to the skin or in the nasal cavity (extrafacial GF). It is mediated by interferon (IFN)-γ produced by CD4+ T-helper cells which express molecules such as intercellular adhesion molecule 1 (ICAM-1) on the surface of keratinocytes, promoting chemotaxis of lymphocytes. Basal keratinocytes do not express ICAM-1, restricting the migration of inflammatory cells into the epidermis and forming the characteristic grenz zone, which separates the inflammatory infiltrate from the epidermis and pilosebaceous appendages. Factors that may be responsible for the development of GF include hypersensitivity reactions, infections, trauma, actinic exposure, and radiation.

➲ CLINICAL FEATURES

Chronic, progressive, asymptomatic, isolated well-defined reddish-brown plaques or nodules with prominent follicular orifices and telangiectatic surface changes, or scaling is often present, but lesions never ulcerate. It may have itching, burning, or painful lesions. Lesions might darken upon sun exposure.

➲ DERMOSCOPY

Parallel, arborizing blood vessels, brown dots and globules, and dilated follicular openings.

➲ CLINICAL VARIANTS

- Extrafacial GF located on the scalp, back, shoulders, arms, breast, and trunk.
- *Intranasal lesions*: Eosinophilic angiocentric fibrosis (a mucosal variant of GF) that is found to occur in the nasal mucosa or upper airways in conjunction with skin lesions of GF. It leads to fibrotic stenosis of the affected site with localized extension

and damage. Epiphora and proptosis are complications in obstructive sinonasal eosinophilic angiocentric fibrosis.

➲ HISTOPATHOLOGY

- Dense, polymorphous inflammatory infiltrate is located in the papillary and mid-dermis below a narrow grenz zone.
- Infiltrate comprises neutrophils, lymphocytes, eosinophils, monocytes, and occasionally mast cells.
- Perivascular inflammation with nuclear dust and vessel wall damage. This chronic leukocytoclastic vasculitis which is localized and fibrotic is a vasculitic reaction pattern, extravasated RBCs, and hemosiderin deposition.
- Dilated follicular ostia and follicular plugs
- Chronic lesions may show fibrosis around venules.

Direct immunofluorescence (DIF) shows immunoglobulin G (IgG), fibrin, and rarely immunoglobulin M (IgM) deposition at the basement membrane zone and perivascular location.

➲ ASSOCIATED DISEASES

IgG4-related disease.

➲ DIFFERENTIAL DIAGNOSIS

Granulomatous rosacea, sarcoidosis, TB, cutaneous lupus erythematosus, and erythema elevatum diutinum.

➲ MANAGEMENT

Granuloma faciale may be recalcitrant, chronic with intermittent acute flares resistant to treatment requiring a multimodal approach:

- Calcineurin inhibitors (tacrolimus 0.1% ointment twice daily and pimecrolimus cream), topical dapsone gel also tried.
- Cryosurgery and pulsed-dye laser
- Systemic dapsone therapy at a dose of 100 mg daily
- Other treatment options include intralesional corticosteroid injections, intralesional 5 FU, dermabrasion, electrosurgery, surgical excision, and topical psoralen plus ultraviolet A (PUVA).

➲ SUGGESTED READING

1. Lindhaus C, Elsner P. Granuloma faciale treatment: a systematic review. Acta Derm Venereol. 2018;98(1):14-8.

99 Granuloma Venereum

➲ SYNONYMS

Granuloma venereum, lupoid form of groin ulceration, ulcerating granuloma of pudenda, granuloma genito-inguinale, granuloma venereum genito-inguinale, infective granuloma, ulcerating sclerosing granuloma, granuloma inguinale tropicum, Dravidian disease.

➲ HISTORY

McLeod first described donovanosis in 1882, and in 1905, Major Charles Donovan discovered the Donovan bodies. Maramell and Santora coined the term "Donovanosis".

➲ ETIOLOGY

It is caused by the bacillus *Calymmatobacterium granulomatis* (*Klebsiella granulomatis*)—intracellular gram-negative pleomorphic bacterium. It is pathogenic only for humans. The transmission is primarily through sexual contact, although it can be occasionally contracted via the fecal route or passage of the infant through an infected birth canal.

➲ EPIDEMIOLOGY

The disease is predominantly seen in the sexually mature age group of 20–40 years with a male-to-female ratio being 2.3:1.

➲ CLINICAL FEATURES

The incubation period of the disease varies from 8 days to 3 months. The primary lesion appears usually over the genital (90%) and inguinal (10%) regions as a painless papule or a nodule that breaks down to form an ulcer with a granulomatous base and beefy red margins and characteristically bleeds on touch. The early lesion may be a subcutaneous swelling that gradually softens and results in a small abscess (pseudobubo) with no lymphadenitis. The common sites affected are the prepuce, glans penis, and frenal folds in males and the vaginal introitus, labia majora, mons veneris, and fourchette in females.

Clinical types include ulcerogranulomatous/fleshy exuberant type which is the most common, necrotic type in which chronic plaque lesions undergo rapid necrosis leading to amputation of the organs, hypertrophic or verrucous type, and sclerotic type.

Almost 6% of patients may have extragenital lesions either by contiguous spread, autoinoculation, or dissemination through the hematogenous route. Commonly affected sites include the oral cavity, lips, gums, cheeks, palate, nose, chin, pharynx, larynx, thorax, bladder, pelvis, axillae, and feet.

Diagnosis is by demonstration of direct bilirubin (DB) by tissue smears, Wright stain, fine needle aspiration cytology (FNAC), and biopsy. Immunological tests such as complement fixation tests and polymerase chain reaction (PCR) can be done.

HISTOPATHOLOGY

Ulcerative lesions show acanthosis with elongated rete ridges, neutrophilic microabscesses, and plasma cells. Pseudoepitheliomatous hyperplasia of the marginal epithelium is seen. Nodular lesions show a massive inflammatory reaction in the dermis consisting of neutrophils and plasma cells with profuse granulation tissue. Large mononuclear cells with intracytoplasmic cysts containing characteristic Donovan bodies (Greenblatt cells) are seen in the granulation tissue. Hypertrophic lesions demonstrate an extensive granulomatous reaction and thick bundles of hyalinized collagen, and fibrous tissue is evident in a sclerotic lesion.

DIFFERENTIAL DIAGNOSIS

- Primary chancre—painless usually solitary ulcer with clean looking base, shotty nontender lymph nodes, and treponema on dark ground microscopy
- Herpes genitalis associated with HIV infection—irregular ulcers, hemorrhagic, positive Tzanck smear
- Cutaneous amoebiasis—ulcers and granulomatous lesions in perianal and perineal areas
- Tuberculosis—absence of Donovan bodies, granulomas on histopathological examination (HPE)
- Condylomata acuminata—koilocytes on biopsy
- Condylomata lata—venereal disease research laboratory (VDRL) positivity
- Gumma
- Lupus vulgaris
- Squamous cell epithelioma

COMPLICATIONS

Pseudoelephantiasis is more commonly seen in females (esthiomene). Stenosis of the urethral, vaginal, anal, and oral orifices due to fibrosis, and squamous cell epithelioma may develop in long-standing cases.

MANAGEMENT

National AIDS Control Organization Guidelines

Doxycycline 100 mg orally BD × 14 days or tetracycline hydrochloride 500 mg orally QID × 14 days or erythromycin stearate or base 500 mg QID × 14 days or trimethoprim-sulfamethoxazole DS orally BD × 14 days or until the lesions have completely healed. Pregnant women are treated with erythromycin 500 mg QID × 3 weeks.

This risk of acquiring HIV is 3–5 times more. In HIV-infected patients, there is high therapeutic failure rates to the first-line antibiotics and the mean time of healing and tissue destruction associated with ulcers is higher.

➲ PROGNOSIS

It is a chronic, indolent, and destructive condition with little or no tendency for spontaneous healing.

➲ SUGGESTED READING

1. Mangarov H, Broshtilova V, Batashki A, Velevska Y, Vatov P, Bezhanova S, et al. Donovanosis–A Case Report with a Review of Literature. Int J Clin Dermatol. 2023;6(1):10-3.

100 Granulomatous Cheilitis

➲ SYNONYMS

Orofacial granulomatosis, Miescher's cheilitis.

➲ HISTORY

The term granulomatous cheilitis was introduced in 1985 by Wiesenfeld.

➲ ETIOLOGY

Precise etiology is unknown. Genetic predisposition, sarcoidosis, ectopic Crohn's disease, a foreign body reaction to silica, contact antigens such as cobalt, gold, or mercury, and ultraviolet B (UVB) radiation are implicated.

➲ EPIDEMIOLOGY

The onset is in childhood or early adolescence without any sexual predilection.

➲ CLINICAL FEATURES

Granulomatous cheilitis begins as nontender swelling and enlargement of one lip usually upper or rarely both lips. The initial attack subsides within hours or days, but after recurrent attacks the swelling may persist and enlarge, eventually becoming permanent. The lip may become hard and fissured with reddish-brown discoloration **(Fig. 1)**. Rarely, the forehead, eyelids, or one side of the scalp may be involved. The regional lymph nodes are enlarged (usually minimally in 50% of patients).

➲ ASSOCIATED SYNDROMES

Melkersson–Rosenthal syndrome (a triad of recurrent lip edema, facial paralysis, and scrotal tongue).

➲ HISTOPATHOLOGY

Histology reveals a perivascular and interstitial infiltrate of lymphocytes, plasma cells, and histiocytes with focal noncaseating epithelioid granulomas.

➲ DIFFERENTIAL DIAGNOSIS

- Angioedema—recurrent attacks of swelling of lips with or without wheals
- Ascher's syndrome
- Lymphoma

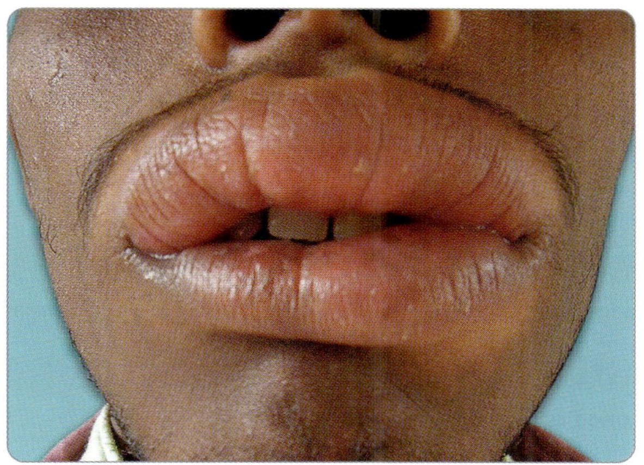

Fig. 1: Enlargement of the lips in granulomatous cheilitis.

- Crohn's disease
- Leprosy
- Rhinosporidiosis—associated with fleshy masses in the nasal cavity, presence of sporangia on tissue biopsy
- Sarcoidosis—naked granulomas seen
- Tuberculosis

TREATMENT

Intralesional corticosteroids 10 mg/mL, reduction cheiloplasty is helpful. Clofazimine in a dose of 100 mg twice daily for 10 days, then twice weekly for 4 months has been tried. Other drugs used are metronidazole, erythromycin, ketotifen, azathioprine, mycophenolate mofetil, dapsone, sulfapyridine, hydroxychloroquine, thalidomide, fumaric acid esters, and tumor necrosis factor inhibitors.

When lesions are fixed and nonevolving cheiloplasty reduction done.

PROGNOSIS

The swelling is typically chronic but may regress very slowly after some years.

SUGGESTED READING

1. Pathania YS. Current treatment modalities in granulomatous cheilitis. Int J Dermatol. 2022;61(6):755-9.

101 Grover's Disease

➲ SYNONYMS

Transient acantholytic dermatosis, papular acantholytic dermatosis.

➲ HISTORY

The condition was described by Grover in 1970.

➲ ETIOLOGY

The precise etiology is unknown. Heat, sweating, fever, and malignancy are predisposing factors. It is seen more frequently in patients with atopic dermatitis, asteatotic dermatitis, and allergic contact dermatitis. Rare associations with lymphoma and also the use of BRAF inhibitors and cytotoxic chemotherapeutic drugs are reported.

➲ EPIDEMIOLOGY

Middle-aged men with solar damage are affected three times more often than women.

➲ CLINICAL FEATURES

Pruritus is the most common symptom which usually does not corelate to the degree of cutaneous involvement. Erythematous to red-brown keratotic papules with crusting that remain discrete are seen on the anterior part of the chest, upper back, and the lower part of the rib cage. Palms, soles, and scalp are almost always spared. Oral lesions that resemble aphthae may be seen. Occasionally, lesions may be acneiform, vesicular, pustular, bullous, or blaschkoid.

➲ DERMOSCOPY

The presence of several polygonal, star-like, or roundish-oval-shaped yellowish or brownish areas of various sizes surrounded by a thin whitish halo regardless of the histopathological subtype of the disease, corresponding to focal acantholysis with different degrees of dyskeratosis or keratinocytes dismaturation.

➲ HISTOPATHOLOGY

Focal acantholysis and dyskeratosis are seen. The presence of spongiosis and acantholysis in the same specimen should raise the possibility of transient acantholytic dermatosis. Five distinct histologic patterns have been described: (1) Simulating Hailey–Hailey disease; (2) simulating Darier disease; (3) mainly spongiotic dermatitis; (4) simulating pemphigus vulgaris; and (5) simulating pemphigus foliaceus.

Immunofluorescence studies are negative.

DIFFERENTIAL DIAGNOSIS

- Dermatitis herpetiformis—neutrophilic abscess in dermal papillae
- Folliculitis—papules and pustules with follicular orientation
- Galli–Galli disease
- Herpes simplex—multiple grouped vesicles associated with pain, burning sensation, and multinucleated giant cells on Tzanck smear
- Herpes zoster—dermatomal distribution of vesicles
- Insect bites—fewer lesions, associated with punctum
- Milia
- Miliaria—widespread lesions associated with itching
- Pityriasis rosea
- Scabies—classical nocturnal itching, circle of Hebra involved, pathognomonic burrows seen
- Syphilis
- Prurigo simplex
- Darier's disease—corps ronds and grains seen
- Hailey–Hailey disease—dilapidated brick wall appearance on histopathological examination (HPE)
- Pemphigus foliaceus—acantholytic cells seen, subcorneal blister present

COMPLICATIONS

Lesions resolve with postinflammatory pigmentary alteration or with no residual change.

TREATMENT

Counseling to keep cool and wearing suitable clothes to prevent sweat rash. Potent topical corticosteroids, menthol, or pramoxine-containing lotions may be effective in diminishing inflammation and in controlling itching. Vitamin A 50,000 U 3 times a day for 2 weeks then daily for up to 12 weeks, isotretinoin 40 mg/day for 2–12 weeks can be given.

Triamcinolone (16 mg daily tapered to 2–4 mg daily) is reported to be more effective than prednisone, UVB exposure, psoralen plus ultraviolet A light (PUVA), UVA-1, ALA-PDL, grenz radiation, methotrexate, acitretin, calcipotriol, and cryotherapy and have all been reported to be effective in severely resistant cases. If the patient is on BRAF inhibitors, the addition of MEK inhibitors seems to protect. Dupilumab and etanercept have been recently tried.

PROGNOSIS

It is a self-limited disorder that resolves over weeks to months. Some cases may be chronic and persistent.

SUGGESTED READING

1. Aldana PC, Khachemoune A. Grover disease: review of subtypes with a focus on management options. Int J Dermatol. 2020;59(5):543-50.

102 Hairy Tongue

➲ SYNONYM

Lingua villosa.

➲ ETIOLOGY

Hairy tongue is a result of defective desquamation of the filiform papillae due to a variety of precipitating factors such as poor oral hygiene, broad-spectrum antibiotics, therapeutic radiation of the head and the neck, tobacco use, coffee and tea drinking, mouth breathing, chronic use of bismuth-containing antacids, and lack of dietary roughage.

➲ EPIDEMIOLOGY

Hairy tongue is reported more often in males, and the incidence increases with age.

➲ CLINICAL FEATURES

Hairy tongue is characterized by the hypertrophy and elongation of filiform papillae to >15 mm, i.e., in the anterior two-thirds of the tongue **(Fig. 1)**. It is usually asymptomatic, but patients may complain of a tickling or gagging sensation and halitosis. Papillae often retain pigments from food, beverages, and candies, resulting in the varying colors associated with the condition (e.g., black, brown, white, green, and pink). The tongue has a thick coating in the middle, with a greater accentuation toward the back. In extreme cases, a blast of compressed air results in the papillae "waving in the breeze."

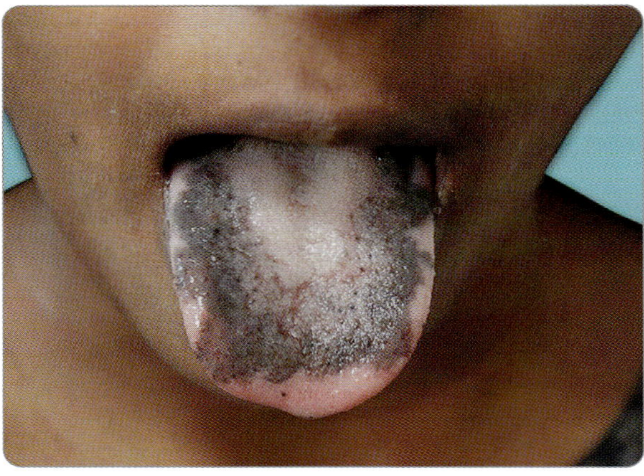

Fig. 1: Hairy tongue in a 16-year-old girl.

A culture of the tongue's dorsal surface should be performed if superimposed oral candidiasis or other specific oral infection is suspected. Cytologic smears stained with Gram-stain or periodic acid-Schiff stain, potassium hydroxide preparations may reveal candidal organisms.

DERMOSCOPY

Dermoscopy reveals brownish hair-like elongation of filiform papillae with whitish lingual papillae.

HISTOPATHOLOGY

Histopathology shows elongated filiform papillae, with mild hyperkeratosis and occasional inflammatory cells. Accumulated debris intermingled among the papillae and candidal pseudohyphae may be seen.

DIFFERENTIAL DIAGNOSIS

- Oral candidiasis
- Oral hairy leukoplakia—lesions mainly over lateral borders of the tongue, not easily scrapable, caused by Epstein–Barr virus (EBV)
- Lichen planus—more erosions seen, reticulate lacy network present over buccal mucosa
- Pseudo black tongue (darkly stained tongue in the absence of elongated filiform papillae)
- Acanthosis nigricans

COMPLICATIONS

Candidal overgrowth, altered taste sensation.

TREATMENT

Treatment consists of identification and stoppage of the offending agents as well as brushing the tongue with a toothbrush to remove elongated filiform papillae and retard the growth of additional ones. 1–2% hydrogen peroxide or 40% aqueous solution of urea, topical triamcinolone acetonide, gentian violet, salicylic acid, podophyllin, and tretinoin gel can be used. Surgical removal of the papillae by using electrodesiccation, carbon dioxide laser, or even scissors is the treatment of last resort. If *Candida albicans* is present, topical antifungal medications can be used.

PROGNOSIS

The prognosis is excellent.

SUGGESTED READING

1. Schlager E, St. Claire C, Ashack K, Khachemoune A. Black hairy tongue: predisposing factors, diagnosis, and treatment. Am J Clin Dermatol. 2017;18:563-9.

103 Hand, Foot, and Mouth Disease

➲ HISTORY

Hand, foot, and mouth disease (HFMD) was first described in Canada in 1957 by Robinson. Alsop coined the term hand, foot, and mouth disease in 1959.

➲ ETIOLOGY

Hand, foot, and mouth disease is most frequently caused by coxsackie virus A16 and less commonly by other coxsackie viruses (A5, A7, A9, A10, B1, B3, and B5) and enterovirus A17. Transmission is mainly via fecal-oral contact and less commonly by respiratory droplets. During epidemics, transmission can occur from mother to fetus.

➲ EPIDEMIOLOGY

Children from 2 to 10 years old are commonly affected.

➲ CLINICAL FEATURES

The incubation period ranges from 2 to 5 days with viral shedding lasting for up to 5 weeks. Infection begins with fever and sore mouth. 90% of cases have small vesicles, which rapidly ulcerate with ragged borders surrounded by a red areola on the buccal mucosa, tongue, soft palate, and gingiva. Hands and feet have asymptomatic red papules that quickly become vesicles surrounded by a red halo. They are often oval (football-shaped), linear, triangular, or crescentic and run parallel to the skin lines on the ventral aspect of fingers and toes **(Figs. 1 to 3)**. The lesions crust and heal in 7–10 days. In children who wear diapers, vesicles, and erythematous, edematous papules occur on the buttocks.

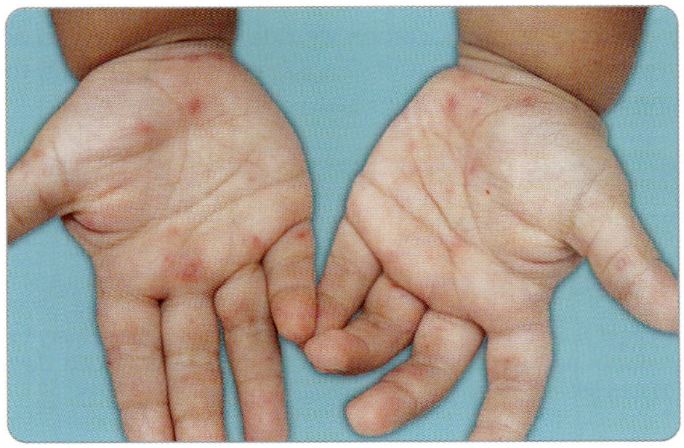

Fig. 1: Multiple vesicles over the palms, few vesicles are oval.

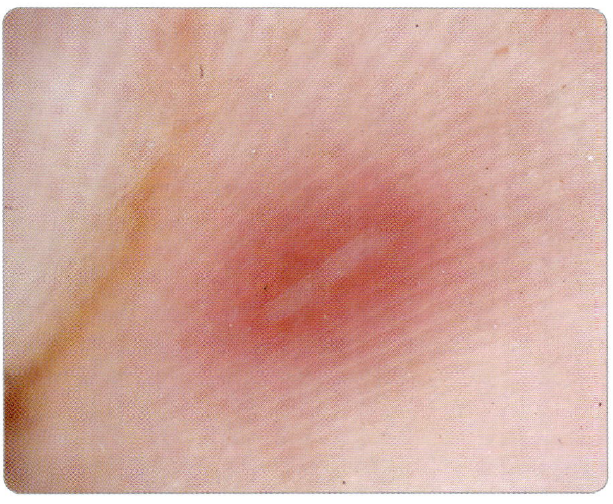

Fig. 2: Dermoscopy—note oblong vesicle on erythematous base on the palm.

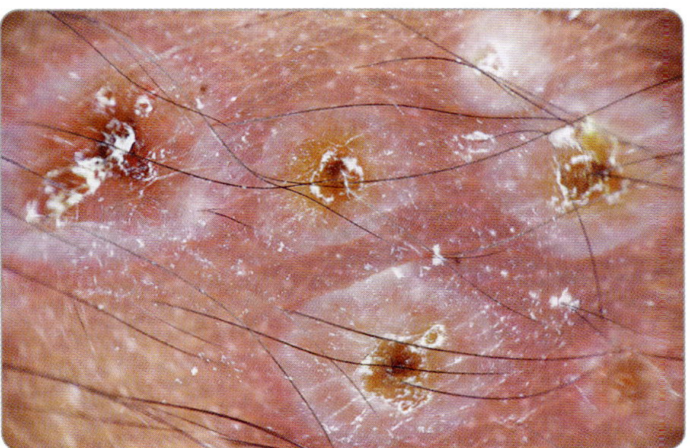

Fig. 3: Dermoscopy—white halo, perifollicular crusting, and peripheral erythema.

The diagnosis is confirmed by the isolation of the virus from the vesicles, the detection of antigens from the vesicles, or antibodies in the serum by enzyme-linked immunosorbent assay (ELISA) tests. The viral nucleic acid may be detected by reverse transcriptase polymerase chain reaction (PCR). The virus grows well on human epithelial cells and monkey kidney cell cultures.

➲ DERMOSCOPY

Central bluish-gray globules, black/gray dots, white halo, crusting, and peripheral erythema.

➲ HISTOPATHOLOGY

An intraepidermal blister is formed by vacuolar and reticular degeneration of keratinocytes. Inclusion bodies and multinucleated giant cells are absent **(Fig. 4)**.

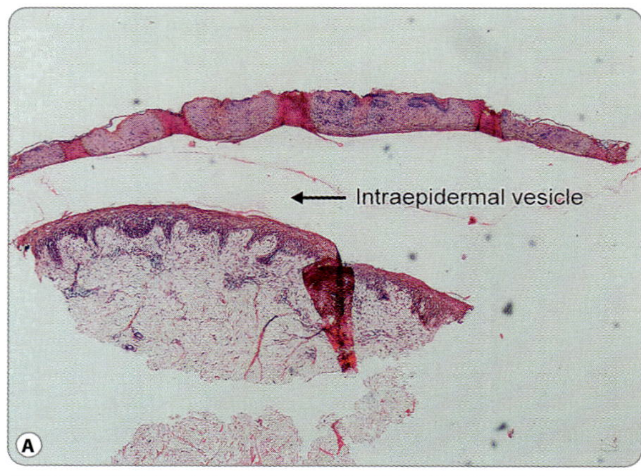

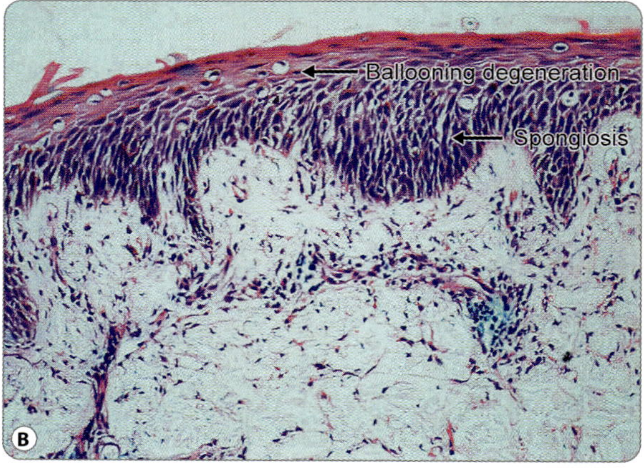

Figs. 4A and B: Histopathology.

DIFFERENTIAL DIAGNOSIS

- Herpangina—only oral cavity involved
- Erythema multiforme—target lesions seen with history of (h/o) preceding drug intake or infections
- Varicella—crops of vesicles with pleomorphic appearance seen all over the body
- Aphthous ulcer—can be seen in any age group
- Herpetic gingivostomatitis—palms and soles also involved
- Behçet's disease—pathergy test positive, ocular symptoms present
- Pemphigus vulgaris—acantholytic cells seen
- Allergic contact dermatitis

COMPLICATIONS

Complications are very rare. Eczema coxsackium, aseptic meningitis, infection caused by enterovirus 71 is associated with encephalitis, flaccid paralysis, pulmonary edema, and hemorrhage. Spontaneous abortions may occur if infections occur in the first trimester.

➲ TREATMENT

Supportive therapy, with the use of topical anesthetics for oral mucosa. Indications of hospitalization are inability to maintain hydration and complications.

➲ PROGNOSIS

The infection is usually mild and seldom lasts more than a week.

➲ SUGGESTED READING

1. Saguil A, Kane SF, Lauters R, Mercado MG. Hand-foot-and-mouth disease: rapid evidence review. Am Fam Phys. 2019;100(7):408-14.

104 Hemangiomas

HISTORY

Mulliken et al. categorized vascular anomalies into two families: A family of self-involuting tumors, and another family of malformations that are essentially permanent.

ETIOLOGY

Hemangiomas are benign hamartomatous proliferations of vascular endothelial cells. Vascular anomalies are vascular malformations.

EPIDEMIOLOGY

Female patients outnumber male patients with hemangiomas by a ratio of 3:1.

CLINICAL FEATURES

Hemangiomas are typically absent at birth and characteristically have rapid growth (proliferative phase) in infancy from 8 to 18 months with spontaneous involution later in life. 80% of lesions are present on the head and neck area. 50% of the lesions will involute by the age of 5 years, and 75% will involute by 7 years. During this phase, mast cell numbers decrease to normal and there is a decrease in endothelial and mast cell activity. These vascular spaces become lined with endothelial cells without muscular support. The lesions typically blanch with pressure, unlike the lesions seen with port-wine stains. They are also referred to as strawberry hemangiomas.

Vascular malformations such as lymphangiomas and arterio-venous malformations are present at birth and are characterized by very slow growth with persistence into adult life **(Figs. 1A and B)**.

ASSOCIATED SYNDROME

- PHACES syndrome—*P*osterior fossa abnormalities, *H*emangiomas, *A*rterial lesions, *C*ardiac abnormalities, *E*ye abnormalities, and *S*ternal clefting
- LUMBAR association—*L*ower body hemangioma and other cutaneous defects; *U*rogenital anomalies, ulceration; *M*yelopathy; *B*ony deformity; *A*norectal malformations; arterial anomalies; and *R*enal anomalies
- SACRAL association—*S*pinal dysraphism, *A*nogenital anomalies, *C*utaneous anomalies, *R*enal and urologic anomalies, associated with *A*ngioma of *L*umbosacral localization
- PELVIS association—*P*erineal IH, *E*xternal genital malformations, *L*ipomyelomeningocele, *V*esicorenal abnormalities, *I*mperforate anus, and *S*kin tag

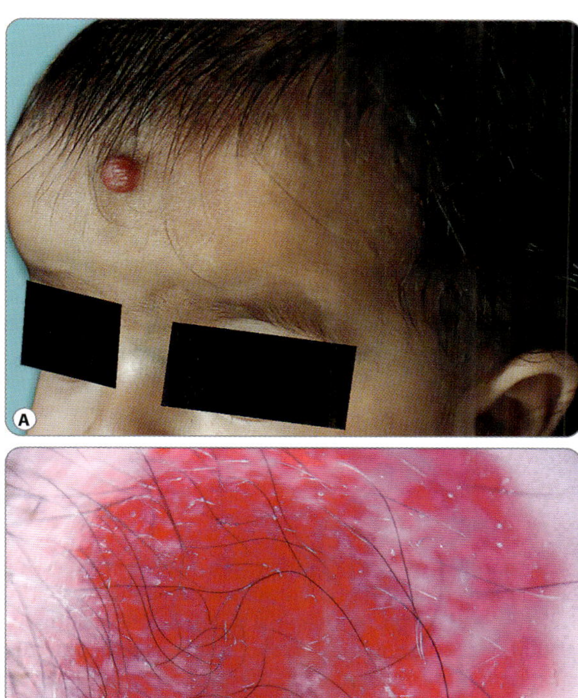

Figs. 1A and B: (A) Infantile hemangioma on the forehead; and (B) Dermoscopy of infantile hemangioma. Red-white background, clustered red lacunae; polymorphous vascular structures.

➲ DERMOSCOPY

Red/red-blue/red-white background, clustered red lacunae; polymorphous vascular structures: red globular and helical vessels; and clustered serpentine vessels.

➲ HISTOPATHOLOGY

Pathological findings include the proliferation of a single layer of endothelial cells and pericytes. Endothelial cells of the basement membrane characteristically have large amounts of endoplasmic reticulum.

➲ DIFFERENTIAL DIAGNOSIS

- Capillary malformation—proliferation of capillaries seen instead of dilated vascular channels
- Cherry hemangioma—much smaller lesions
- Angiosarcoma
- Teratoma
- Arteriovenous malformations—not compressible, bruit can be heard

- Neonatal rhabdomyosarcoma
- Cobb syndrome
- Dabska tumor
- Lipomas—skin-colored swellings which are mobile, adipocytes on biopsy
- Oral lymphangiomas
- Pyogenic granuloma—lesions are smaller, noncompressible, bleeds on touch

COMPLICATIONS

Ulceration, bleeding, secondary infection of ulcers, erosion of bone, Kasabach–Merritt syndrome—consumption coagulopathy and thrombocytopenia, disseminated intravascular coagulation; high-output congestive heart failure; nasopharyngeal hemangiomas can be associated with respiratory obstruction; amblyopia due to periorbital hemangiomas.

TREATMENT

Risk stratification: Classified as high risk if evidence of the following: Life-threatening complications (compromising vital organ function of the airway, liver, or gastrointestinal tract), functional impairment (e.g., periorbital hemangiomas) or ulceration, associated structural anomalies, risk of permanent disfigurement, very large (≥5 cm) or rapid growing hemangioma.

Treatment for low-risk and uncomplicated hemangioma—active nonintervention (serial observation), topical beta blockers (topical propranolol, topical timolol, and topical carteolol), high-potency topical corticosteroids, and intralesional corticosteroids.

Treatment of High-risk/complicated hemangiomas—oral propranolol at 1 mg/kg/day in two divided doses, increasing to 2 mg/kg/day given in two divided doses after 1 week, and then up to 3 mg/kg/day divided twice daily, dependent on hemangioma severity and response. Atenolol (a selective beta-1 blocker) and nadolol (a nonselective beta blocker) may be as effective as propranolol. Systemic corticosteroids are used (where beta blockers are contraindicated). Other options include: Topical imiquimod, topical becaplermin (0.01% gel), vincristine, recombinant interferon-α (2a and 2b), embolization, radiotherapy, cryotherapy, compression bandage, pulsed dye laser, and surgical excision.

SUGGESTED READING

1. George A, Mani V, Noufal A. Update on the classification of hemangioma. J Oral Maxillofac Pathol. 2014;18(Suppl 1):S117-20.

105 Henoch–Schönlein Purpura

➲ SYNONYMS

Anaphylactoid purpura, purpura rheumatica.

➲ HISTORY

The disease is named after Eduard Heinrich Henoch (1820–1910), a German pediatrician, and his teacher Johann Lukas Schönlein (1793–1864), who described it in the 1860s.

➲ ETIOLOGY

Henoch–Schönlein purpura (HSP) frequently presents 1–2 weeks following an upper respiratory tract infection.

➲ EPIDEMIOLOGY

Henoch–Schönlein purpura is the most common form of vasculitis in children. The peak age of onset for the disease is 4–7 years. HSP can also occur in adults.

➲ CLINICAL FEATURES

The initial presentation of HSP is often characterized by an acute onset of purpura, arthralgias, and colicky abdominal pain. Cutaneous lesions have a symmetric distribution and begin as macular erythema or urticarial papules. They subsequently progress to inflammatory purpuric macules and papules that can range in size from pinpoint to several millimeters. Urticaria, vesicles, bullae, and foci of necrosis can also be seen. There is a predilection for the lower extremities and buttocks **(Fig. 1A)**, but lesions can also occur on the trunk, upper extremities, and face. Individual lesions regress within 10–14 days, with resolution of skin involvement over a period of several weeks to months, although recurrences are observed in 5–10% of patients.

In up to 75% of patients with HSP, there is gastrointestinal and/or musculoskeletal involvement. Common manifestations include abdominal pain, vomiting, and gastrointestinal bleeding (occasionally complicated by intussusception) in association with arthritis of the ankles and knees and edema of the lower extremities. Fever occurs in approximately 20% of adults and 40% of children. Renal involvement is also common, but it is usually mild (microscopic hematuria and minimal proteinuria) and self-limited. While only 2% of patients will develop long-term renal impairment, the risk is 10-fold greater in those presenting with nephritic or nephrotic syndrome.

➲ DERMOSCOPY

Early/evolving lesions show a dull red background, red globules, and red dots. Findings in established lesions are red to red-purple background, yellow and white structureless areas, red globules, and red dots **(Fig. 1B)**.

➲ HISTOPATHOLOGY

Histologically, leukocytoclastic vasculitis involving the capillaries and postcapillary venules of the upper and mid dermis is observed. By direct immunofluorescence, immunoglobulin A (IgA) deposits in a vascular pattern are seen in up to one-third of cases.

➲ DIFFERENTIAL DIAGNOSIS

- Arthropod bites—absence of palpable purpura, no systemic involvement
- Morbilliform drug eruptions with hemorrhage independent sites

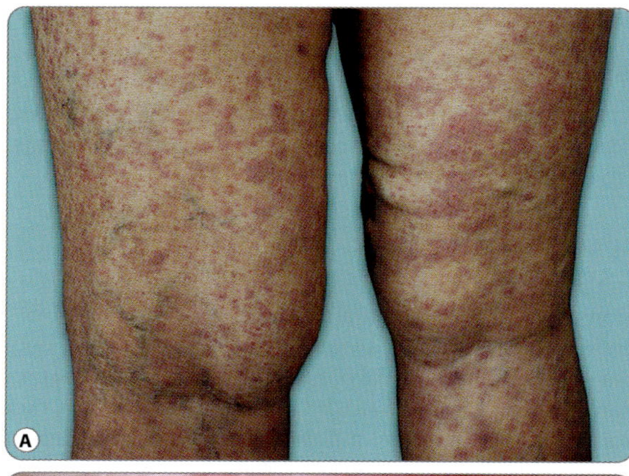

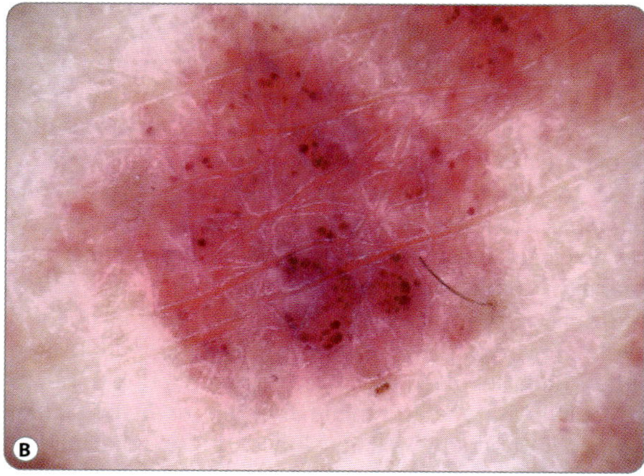

Figs. 1A and B: (A) Purpura over the legs; and (B) Dermoscopy—red background with white structureless areas, red dots, and globules.

- Erythema multiforme—target lesions seen, palms and soles involved
- Urticarial vasculitis—petechiae seen, pigmentation remains on healing
- Erythema elevatum diutinum
- Pityriasis lichenoides et varioliformis acuta—trunk also involved, papules with surmounted vesicles
- Polyarteritis nodosa—medium vessel vasculitis present, glomerulonephritis conspicuously absent
- Meningococcemia—retiform purpura present, patient is usually toxic
- Thrombocytopenic purpura—decreased platelet count, history of (h/o) bleeding manifestation

TREATMENT

Because the cutaneous and musculoskeletal symptoms of HSP are generally self-limited, resolving over the course of weeks to months, treatment is mainly supportive. Systemic corticosteroids are effective in treating arthritis and abdominal pain associated with HSP and reducing the duration of skin lesions but do not prevent recurrences of purpura. Management of HSP also depends in large part on the severity of the associated renal involvement. Corticosteroids and/or cytotoxic medications (especially cyclophosphamide or azathioprine) are often used to treat severe renal disease. Corticosteroid-sparing drugs such as colchicine, dapsone, azathioprine, methotrexate, cyclophosphamide, intravenous gamma globulin, antimalarials, rituximab, mycophenolate mofetil, and plasmapheresis can be used.

SUGGESTED READING

1. Hetland LE, Susrud KS, Lindahl KH, Bygum A. Henoch-Schönlein purpura: a literature review. Acta Derm Venereol. 2017;97(10):1160-6.

106 Herpes Simplex

HISTORY

The word "herpes" was first defined by Greek scholars as "to creep or crawl" in reference to the spreading nature of the skin lesions.

ETIOLOGY

Herpes simplex viruses are ubiquitous, host-adapted pathogens that cause a wide variety of disease states. Two types exist: Herpes simplex virus type 1 (HSV-1) and type 2 (HSV-2). HSV-1 is traditionally associated with orofacial disease, while HSV-2 is traditionally associated with genital disease.

EPIDEMIOLOGY

Herpes simplex virus type 1 infections transmitted via saliva are common in children, although primary herpes gingivostomatitis can be observed at any age. HSV-2 infections are clustered perinatally (from a maternal episode at delivery) and primarily once sexual activity begins.

CLINICAL FEATURES

The clinical course of herpes simplex infection depends on the age and immune status of the host, the anatomic site of involvement, and the antigenic virus type. Primary HSV-1 and HSV-2 infections are accompanied by systemic signs, longer duration of symptoms, and a higher rate of complications. Recurrent episodes are milder and shorter. Both HSV-1 and HSV-2 can cause similar genital and orofacial primary infections after contact with infectious secretions containing either HSV-1 (usually oral secretions) or HSV-2 (usually genital secretions).

In primary infections, symptoms typically occur within 3–7 days after exposure. A prodrome of tender lymphadenopathy, malaise, anorexia, and fever, as well as localized pain, tenderness, and burning, often occurs before the onset of mucocutaneous lesions. Initially, painful, sometimes umbilicated, vesicles on an erythematous base appear, followed by progression to pustules and/or ulcerations. Multiple grouped and scattered vesicles typically develop. Crusting of lesions and resolution of symptoms occur within 2–6 weeks.

Primary orolabial herpes infections usually present as gingivostomatitis in children or as pharyngitis and a mononucleosis-like syndrome in young adults. In general, the mouth and lips are the most common sites of involvement. Significant edema, pain, and ulceration of the oropharyngeal membranes can lead to dysphagia and drooling. Recurrent lesions appear most often on the vermilion border of the lip **(Fig. 1A)**.

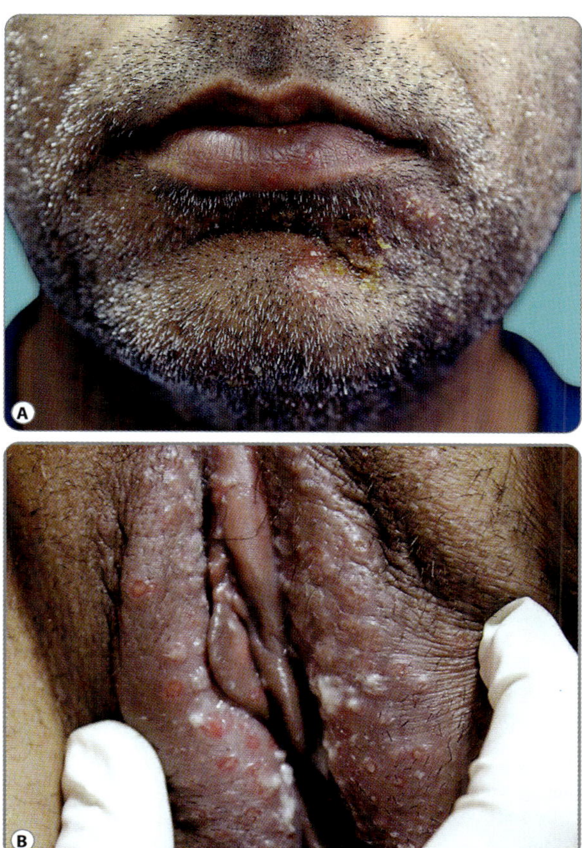

Figs. 1A and B: (A) Multiple grouped vesicles near the angle of the mouth; and (B) Multiple small superficial erosions over the labia majora and minora.

Primary genital herpes infection produces a severe clinical picture and presents as an excruciatingly painful, erosive balanitis, vulvitis, or vaginitis **(Fig. 1B)**. In women, lesions can also involve the cervix, buttocks, and perineum and are associated with inguinal adenopathy and dysuria. Genital lesions in men typically occur on the glans penis or penile shaft. Recurrent genital infections can be subclinical or limited in severity. Usually, a limited number of vesicles will reappear on the genitalia or buttocks with resolution within 1 week.

HISTOPATHOLOGY

Ballooning of the cytoplasm of keratinocytes, nuclear degeneration, and margination of chromatin to form intranuclear inclusion bodies are seen. Multinucleated giant cells form by fusion of the infected keratinocytes. Intraepidermal vesicles appear as a fluid containing large quantities of virus. A variably dense inflammatory response of lymphocytes, neutrophils, and eosinophils infiltrates the dermis.

Table 1: Treatment of herpes simplex.

Disease context	*Drug and dosage*
Herpes simplex infections:	
Orolabial herpes (first episode)	• Acyclovir: 200 mg 5×/day or 400 mg PO TDS × 7–10 days • Famciclovir: 250 mg PO TDS or 500 mg BD × 7–10 days • Valacyclovir: 1 g PO BD × 7–10 days
Orolabial herpes (recurrence)	• Acyclovir: 400 mg PO TDS × 5 days • Famciclovir: 750 mg BD or 1.5 g OD × 1 day • Valacyclovir: 2 g BD × 1 day
Genital herpes (first episode)	• Acyclovir: 200 mg PO 5×/day × 10 days or 400 mg PO TDS × 10 days • Famciclovir: 250 mg PO TDS × 10 days • Valacyclovir: 1 g PO BD × 10 days
Genital herpes (recurrence)	• Acyclovir: 800 mg BD × 5 days or 800 mg TDS × 2 days • Famciclovir: 1 g BD × 1 day or 125 mg PO BD × 5 days or 500 mg orally once followed by 250 mg BD × 2 days • Valacyclovir: 500 mg BD × 3 days or 1 gm OD × 5 days
Chronic suppression (≥6 episodes/year) should be discontinued after 12 months to reassess symptom episode frequency	• Acyclovir: 400 mg BD • Famciclovir: 250 mg BD • Valacyclovir: 500 mg OD for <10 outbreaks/year or 1 g PO OD for 10 or more outbreaks/year

(BD: twice daily; OD: once daily; PO: orally; TDS: three times daily)

COMPLICATIONS

Pharyngitis, headache, meningism, encephalitis, dissemination of infection, eczema herpeticum, monoarticular arthritis, radiculo-neuropathy, sacral radiculopathy (Elsberg syndrome), urinary retention, constipation in females, and in men, impotence, recurrent infection are known complications.

TREATMENT

As per the Centers for Disease Control and Prevention (CDC) 2021, the treatment of herpes simplex is mentioned in **Table 1**.

PROGNOSIS

Recurrences are common, especially in the first 2 years after infection.

SUGGESTED READING

1. Halford WP, Gebhardt BM, Carr DJ. Mechanisms of herpes simplex virus type 1 reactivation. J Virol. 1996;70(8):5051-60.

107 Herpes Zoster

➲ SYNONYMS

Shingles, zona.

➲ HISTORY

Herpes means creeping. Kundratiz (1922) and Bruusgarrd (1932) demonstrated the association between varicella and herpes zoster lesions. Weller et al. identified in vitro the same virus in both diseases.

➲ ETIOLOGY

Zoster is the result of the reactivation of latent varicella zoster virus in the sensory nerve ganglion cells. Lesions are precipitated by pressure or trauma to nerve roots, by neoplastic deposits, radiotherapy, surgery, or other trivial trauma.

➲ EPIDEMIOLOGY

The incidence increases with age.

➲ CLINICAL FEATURES

Herpes zoster often begins with a prodrome of intense pain associated with pruritus, tingling, tenderness, or hyperesthesia followed by eruption of grouped vesicles on an erythematous base **(Fig. 1)**. It occurs within a sensory dermatome usually on the trunk supplied by T3 to L2; face supplied by trigeminal nerve, particularly the ophthalmic division; neck, scalp or an extremity, typically

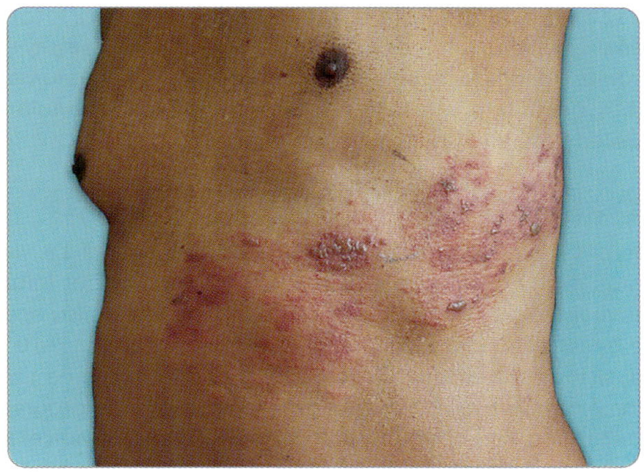

Fig. 1: Grouped vesicles on an erythematous base in herpes zoster distributed along the sixth and seventh thoracic dermatome.

involving a single dermatome unilaterally. Rarely, pain is not followed by cutaneous eruption and is known as "zoster sine herpete". Herpes zoster oticus, also known as Ramsay Hunt syndrome, is a triad of ipsilateral facial palsy, otalgia, and vesicles near the ear and auditory canal. The presence of vesicles on the tip of the nose indicates the involvement of the nasociliary nerve called Hutchinson's sign.

In immunocompromised hosts, herpes zoster may be quite severe and can have unusual clinical presentations, e.g., persistent, crusted, verrucous, hyperkeratotic, ecthymatous lesions, involving multiple dermatomes sometimes bilaterally, with postherpetic hyperhidrosis. Disseminated cutaneous disease (defined as >20 vesicles outside the area of primary or adjacent dermatomes) and/or visceral involvement occurs in approximately 10% of immunocompromised patients.

Tzanck smear shows characteristic multinucleated epithelial giant cells by light microscopy but cannot be differentiated from those due to herpes simplex virus (HSV) infection. Additional laboratory tests include viral culture, serology, and polymerase chain reaction (PCR).

DIFFERENTIAL DIAGNOSIS

- Zosteriform herpes simplex (vesicles are smaller and recurrent)
- Localized contact dermatitis—absence of neuralgia
- Bacterial skin infections (e.g., bullous impetigo and cellulitis)—negative Tzanck smear, no dermatomal distribution
- Insect bites—papules with central punctum are classical.
- Burns
- Papular urticaria—spread discretely over exposed areas
- Erythema multiforme—target lesions seen
- Drug eruptions

COMPLICATIONS

Complications include zoster-associated pain (within 4 weeks), postherpetic neuralgia [major risk factors for postherpetic neuralgia (PHN) are: Age >60 years, severe or incapacitating pain with acute herpes zoster, more severe rash with acute herpes zoster], secondary bacterial infection, scarring, ophthalmic zoster, Ramsay–Hunt syndrome, meningoencephalitis, motor paralysis, pneumonitis, hepatitis, granuloma annulare/scar sarcoidosis/fungal granuloma at the healed sites, and Guillain–Barré syndrome.

TREATMENT

For herpes zoster, early treatment with antiviral agents, i.e., within 72 hours of the onset of the first vesicle, is optimal, but initiation of antiviral therapy after 72 hours but within 7 days also appears to be beneficial. Aciclovir 800 mg five times a day for 7–10 days or valaciclovir 1 g or famciclovir 250 mg or 500 mg three times a day for 7 days is useful. Such treatment prevents the progression of the eruption, reduces the systemic complications of varicella and zoster, lessens zoster pain, and can reduce the risk of development of postherpetic neuralgia.

Intravenous acyclovir 500 mg/m^2 or 10 mg/kg 8th hourly in one-hour infusions for 7 days and vidarabine 12-hour infusion of 10 mg/kg for 7 days is indicated for the treatment of zoster in immunocompromised patients as well as those with serious complications. Administration of systemic steroids in immunocompetent adults >50 years of age reduces the incidence of postherpetic neuralgia.

Foscarnet 40 mg/kg intravenously (IV) 8th hourly for 10 days is effective in acyclovir-resistant cases.

Multiple treatments are available for postherpetic neuralgia which include 5% lidocaine patches, topical capsaicin (0.025–0.075%), capsaicin (8%) patch-FDA approved, narcotics, nerve blocks, biofeedback, analgesics, EMLA cream, tricyclic antidepressants (amitriptyline, nortriptyline, and desipramine), gabapentin 300–3,600 mg, and pregabalin 75–600 mg. Other modalities include antiseizure medications (valproic acid, carbamazepine, oxcarbazepine, and lamotrigine), serotonin-norepinephrine reuptake inhibitors (duloxetine and venlafaxine), botulinum toxin injections, oral or transdermal opioid analgesics, intrathecal glucocorticoid injections, neuromodulation and nerve stimulation (transcutaneous electrical nerve stimulation, pulsed radiofrequency, and spinal cord stimulation), cognitive and behavioral therapies, shave removal, surgical excision, curettage, cryotherapy, imiquimod 5%, intralesional steroids, sclerotherapy. Sympathetic blocks with 0.25% bupivacaine and rhizotomy are performed for severe postherpetic neuralgia.

➲ PREVENTION

Vaccination is indicated to reduce the risk of developing herpes zoster and postherpetic neuralgia in those at increased risk for disease (immunocompetent individuals ≥50 years of age—indiction stronger for ≥60 years old, immunocompromised patients ≥19 years of age at increased risk of herpes zoster). Types of vaccine include nonlive recombinant glycoprotein E vaccine [designated recombinant zoster vaccine (RZV)] and a live attenuated vaccine [designated zoster vaccine live (ZVL)].

➲ SUGGESTED READING

1. Patil A, Goldust M, Wollina U. Herpes zoster: a review of clinical manifestations and management. Viruses. 2022;14(2):192.

108 Hidradenitis Suppurativa

SYNONYMS

Acne inversa, Verneuil's disease, pyoderma fistulans significa, apocrinitis, apocrine acne.

HISTORY

Velpeau first described the condition in 1839.

EPIDEMIOLOGY

The incidence is four times more in women and begins after puberty.

ETIOLOGY

Hidradenitis suppurativa is not a true infectious process, and bacterial infection is only secondary. Genetic factors, HLA-A1 and HLA-B8, are associated with severe disease. The role of hormonal influences is controversial, with improvement during pregnancy and premenstrual and postnatal flare-ups. Smoking and lithium therapy are known to exacerbate the disease.

Rupture of the follicular infundibulum distended by keratin occurs and results in the extrusion of follicular bacteria, apocrine sweat, sebaceous matter, and keratinous material into the adjacent dermis. This leads to the development of a foreign body inflammatory reaction. Secondary bacterial infection with *Staphylococcus aureus*, *Streptococcus pyogenes*, and various gram-negative organisms may occur.

CLINICAL FEATURES

Initial lesions are "blind boils" or erythematous tender nodules of 0.5–1.5 cm, which grow in size, and if untreated, break through the overlying skin yielding purulent or seropurulent discharge forming chronic draining sinuses. Double-ended comedones are also present. Healing occurs with fibrosis and band-like scars, causing ropelike elevation of the skin. Common sites are the apocrine gland-bearing areas such as axillae, areola of the nipple, groin, perineum, perianal, and periumbilical region. Rarely submammary folds, scalp, zygomatic and malar areas of the face, nape of the neck, external auditory meatus, and shoulders may be involved **(Figs. 1A to C)**.

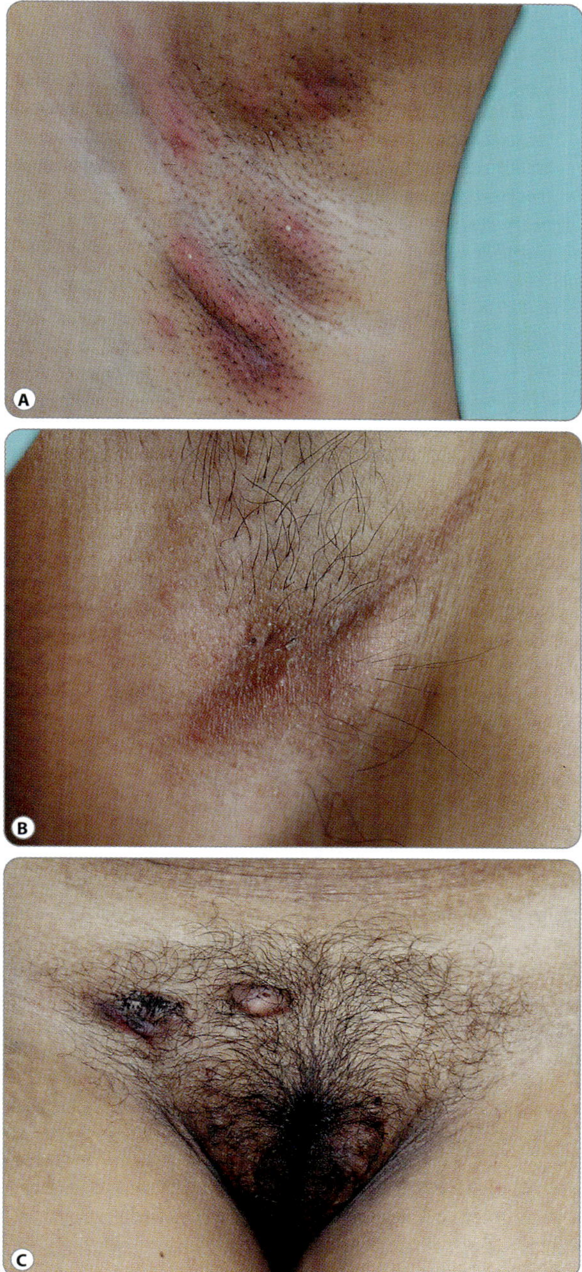

Figs. 1A to C: (A) Erythematous papules and pustules over the axilla in hidradenitis suppurativa; (B) Erythematous papules and sinus over the axilla in hidradenitis suppurativa; and (C) Scarring with sinus over the genital region in hidradenitis suppurativa.

SEVERITY SCORING

- Hurley's staging of hidradenitis suppurativa:
  - *I*: Isolated abscess without scarring
  - *II*: Recurrent abscesses, with sinus tract formation and cicatrization
  - *III*: Diffuse involvement, with multiple interconnected sinus tracts and abscesses
- Sartorius staging is based on the anatomical region involved, the number and type of lesions, the longest distance between two relevant lesions and if lesions are clearly separated by normal skin in each region.
- *Modified sartorius staging*—treatment response taken into account
- HS physician's global assessment (PGA) system
- HiSCR (Hidradenitis Suppurativa Clinical Response) score
- HIdradenitis SuppuraTiva cORe outcomes set International Collaboration (HISTORIC) has identified six core domains to measure

ASSOCIATED CONDITIONS

- *Follicular occlusion triad of pillsbury*: Acne conglobata, hidradenitis suppurativa, and dissecting cellulitis of the scalp. The tetrad consists of pilonidal cysts.
- *HIV-associated follicular syndrome*: Pityriasis rubra pilaris, acne conglobata, hidradenitis suppurativa, and lichen spinulosus
- Other associated conditions are pityriasis rubra pilaris, acanthosis nigricans, steatocystoma multiplex, Dowling–Degos disease, Crohn's disease, pyoderma gangrenosum, and acromegaly.

HISTOPATHOLOGY

There is hyperkeratosis of the infundibulum that results in comedo-like horny impaction. There is a heavy mixed inflammatory cell infiltrate in the lower half of the dermis, usually with extension into the subcutis. Abscesses are present in active cases, and they may connect to the skin surface via a sinus tract. Granulation tissue with inflammatory cells and occasional foreign body giant cells may be seen.

DIFFERENTIAL DIAGNOSIS

- Crohn's disease—granulomas seen on biopsy, no involvement of sweat glands, intestinal lesions seen on endoscopy
- Actinomycosis—multiple sinuses discharging granules (colonies of organisms)
- Catscratch disease
- Cutaneous blastomycosis—sites are usually extremities, demonstration of the fungi
- Granuloma inguinale—presence of genital lesions, Donovan bodies on Giemsa stained crush smear
- Lymphogranuloma venereum—presence of bubo
- *Nocardia* infection
- Noduloulcerative syphilis

- Furunculosis—absence of polyporous comedones, responds to treatment
- Mycetoma—discharging sinuses with grains seen
- Tuberculosis—tubercular granuloma on histopathologic examination (HPE)

COMPLICATIONS

Extensive scarring may restrict mobility, lymphedema of the associated limb, spondyloarthropathy, interstitial keratitis, anemia, secondary systemic amyloidosis, and squamous cell carcinoma.

TREATMENT

General measures include weight reduction, avoidance of tight-fitting clothing, topical antiseptic washes, such as chlorhexidine 4%, benzoyl peroxide, bleach baths or zinc pyrithione, to cleanse the skin, smoking cessation, eradication of *S. aureus* carriage status, screen for CVS risk factors, depression and anxiety. Axillary hair may be clipped but avoid shaving or depilating. Nonsteroidal anti-inflammatory drugs (NSAIDs) may be used to relieve pain. Wound care in hidradenitis suppurativa (HS) aims to manage odor, pain, and exudate (which is sometimes profuse), and minimize bacterial colonization and secondary infection.

Hurley stage I or mild disease can be treated with topical clindamycin gel (1%) or resorcinol (15%), intralesional triamcinolone may also be given. Oral antibiotics such as doxycycline/minocycline (100 mg OD/BD), or tetracycline (500 mg twice daily) and antiandrogenic therapies that may improve the disease including combined oral contraceptives, spironolactone, and finasteride may be tried.

Inflammatory lesions with skin tunnels or scarring (Hurley Stage II or III, moderate-to-severe disease): The initial approach often consists of oral antibiotic therapy, usually tetracyclines or a combination of clindamycin 300 mg BD and rifampin 300 mg BD for 10 weeks. Antiandrogens (for female patients) or metformin are commonly added as adjunctive therapies. Adalimumab is approved by the US Food and Drug Administration (FDA), the recommended dosing schedule for adults with HS is an initial 160 mg subcutaneous dose (given at one time or split into two 80 mg doses given over two consecutive days), then 80 mg on day 15, and then 40 mg once weekly starting on day 29. Acitretin (25–50 mg) is the primary oral retinoid utilized for HS. In 2023, the European Commission approved secukinumab for adults with active, moderate to severe HS, and an inadequate response to conventional systemic HS therapy, with suggested dosing for secukinumab as 300 mg at weeks 0, 1, 2, 3, and 4 followed by once monthly maintenance dosing. Other biologics tried are infliximab, ustekinumab, anakinra, and bimekizumab.

For patients with refractory, severe (Hurley stage III) disease, wide excision can be beneficial in conjunction with medical therapy. In addition, multiple procedures may be employed as a second line such as excision, carbon dioxide laser evaporation, drainage of abscesses, deroofing of sinus tracts, sinus tract excision, or STEEP surgery. Patients with severe suppurative disease unresponsive to the oral combination of clindamycin and rifampin may require rescue therapy with intravenous antibiotics such as intravenous ertapenem. Systemic glucocorticoids are an additional option for treating highly symptomatic, acute flares.

Other therapies that have been tried are neodymium-doped yttrium aluminum garnet (Nd:YAG) laser therapy, apremilast, zinc supplementation, acitretin, isotretinoin, alitretinoin, fumarates, vitamin D3 supplementation, ionizing radiation, photodynamic therapy, botulinum toxin injections, cryoinsufflation, golimumab, risankizumab, Janus kinase inhibitors, and the glucagon-like peptide-1 agonist liraglutide, and combination therapy with rifampin, moxifloxacin, and metronidazole.

PROGNOSIS

The disease is chronic with frequent recurrences.

SUGGESTED READING

1. Sabat R, Jemec GB, Matusiak Ł, Kimball AB, Prens E, Wolk K. Hidradenitis suppurativa. Nat Rev Dis Primers. 2020;6(1):18.

109 Hirsutism

SYNONYMS

Hirsutes, hirsuties, pilosis.

INTRODUCTION

Hirsutism is a clinical diagnosis defined by the presence of excess terminal hair growth (dark, coarse hairs) in androgen-dependent areas (e.g., upper lip, chin, midsternum, upper and lower abdomen, upper arms, upper and lower back, and inner thigh/buttocks) in which women typically have little or no hair.

ETIOLOGY

Hirsutism is a marker of increased androgen levels in females from increased production of androgens (i.e., testosterone) either by the adrenals or due to an ovarian disease:

- Ovarian causes—polycystic ovarian syndrome (PCOS), ovarian tumors (Sertoli–Leydig cell, granulosa-theca cell, and hilus cell)
- Adrenal causes—Cushing's syndrome, androgen-producing tumors, congenital adrenal hyperplasia (CAH) (most commonly due to 21-hydroxylase deficiency)
- Hyperandrogenic-insulin-resistant acanthosis nigricans syndrome (HAIRAN)
- Hyperprolactinemia—by increasing adrenal dehydroepiandrosterone sulfate (DHEA-S)
- Drugs [androgens, glucocorticosteroids, progestins, estrogen antagonists (clomiphene and tamoxifen), minoxidil, cyclosporine, danazol, diazoxide, phenytoin, D-penicillamine, and interferon]
- Acromegaly
- Cushing's syndrome

20% of the patients may have idiopathic hirsutism (IH) with normal androgen levels and ovarian function.

EPIDEMIOLOGY

It affects around 5–10% of women.

CLINICAL FEATURES

Hirsute women usually present with increased growth of terminal hair at the sides of the face, upper lip, chin, upper back, shoulders, sternum, and upper abdomen **(Fig. 1)**. Most also have an underlying endocrine disorder that should be identified. Important clues to the severity of androgen excess and the presence of an underlying disorder can be obtained by history, physical examination, and appropriate laboratory testing. Signs of virilization, including frontal

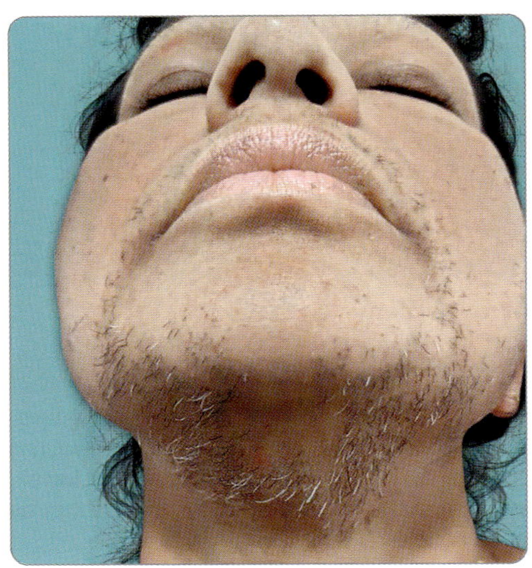

Fig. 1: Terminal hair over the face.

balding, clitoromegaly, increased muscle mass, or deepening of the voice, are seen when the serum testosterone concentration is more severely elevated like in cases of tumors. PCOS is the underlying disorder in approximately 75–80% of women who present with hirsutism.

Diagnostic Criteria for Polycystic Ovary Syndrome

Diagnostic criteria for polycystic ovary syndrome are mentioned in **Table 1**.

- *Biochemical hyperandrogenism*: Elevated total or free testosterone, or calculated free androgen index. Dehydroepiandrosterone sulfate and androstenedione can be considered.
- Clinical Hyperandrogenism—hirsutism, acne
- Polycystic ovaries (USG)—12 or more follicles 2–9 mm in size or an ovarian volume > 10 cm^3 for either ovary
- Oligoamenorrhea (cycles >35 days apart or <8 menses a year)

➲ PHYSICAL EXAMINATION

Modified Ferriman–Gallwey score: Nine androgen-sensitive sites are graded from 0 to 4. A Ferriman–Gallwey score >8 is considered abnormal. Scores between 8 and 15 are usually considered to be mild hirsutism, 16 to 25 moderate, and scores >25 severe hirsutism **(Fig. 2)**.

- Additional signs of androgen excess—acne, keratosis pilaris, or seborrhea
- Body mass index (BMI)—may be increased in PCOS
- Abdominal and pelvic exam—for tumoral mass

Table 1: Diagnostic criteria for polycystic ovary syndrome.

NIH consensus criteria 1990 (all required)	*Revised Rotterdam criteria 2003 (require exclusion of other conditions that mimic PCOS) (two out of three required)*	*AES definition 2008 (all required)*
Menstrual irregularity due to oligo- or anovulation	Oligo- or anovulation	Clinical and/or biochemical signs of hyperandrogenism
Clinical and/or biochemical signs of hyper-androgenism	Clinical and/or biochemical signs of hyperandrogenism	Ovarian dysfunction—oligo/anovulation and/or polycystic ovaries on ultrasound
Exclusion of other disorders: NCCAH and androgen-secreting tumors	Polycystic ovaries (by ultrasound)	Exclusion of other androgen excess or ovulatory disorders

(AES: Androgen Excess Society; NCCAH: nonclassic congenital adrenal hyperplasia; NIH: National Institutes of Health; PCOS: polycystic ovary syndrome)

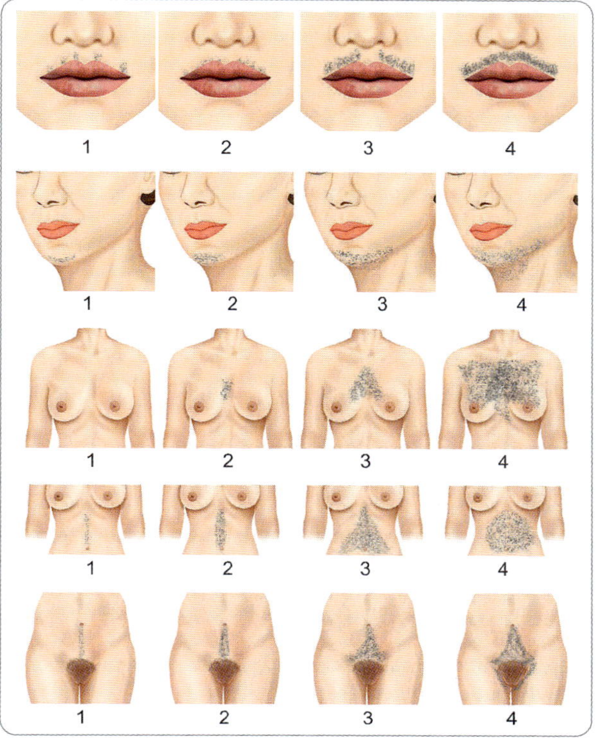

Fig. 2: *Continued*

Continued

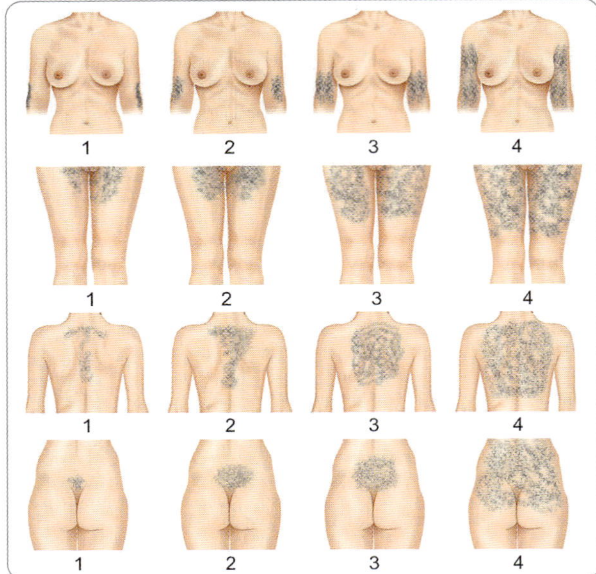

Fig. 2: Modified Ferriman–Gallwey scoring.

INVESTIGATIONS

- Serum total testosterone
- Human chorionic gonadotropin (hCG)
- Prolactin
- Luteinizing hormone (LH)
- Follicle-stimulating hormone (FSH)
- Thyroid-stimulating hormone (TSH))
- Early morning 17-hydroxyprogesterone (around 8 AM)
- Serum DHEAS—to identify an adrenal source of excess androgens. Mild elevations may not affect the treatment.
- Sex hormone-binding globulin levels
- Twenty-four-hour urine-free cortisol
- Pelvic ultrasonography—to detect PCOS and other ovarian tumors
- Adrenal CT—if the woman has a markedly elevated serum testosterone or serum DHEAS concentration

DIFFERENTIAL DIAGNOSIS

There are conditions that are characterized by generalized or excess hair growth but do *not* represent hirsutism:

- *Vellus (lanugo) hair*: Soft, androgen-independent unpigmented hair that covers the entire body of a fetus or newborn. It may also be seen in women with disorders such as anorexia nervosa.
- *Hypertrichosis*: The excessive growth of androgen-independent hair that is vellus, prominent in nonsexual areas. It is most commonly familial or caused by systemic disorders (hypothyroidism, anorexia nervosa, malnutrition, porphyria, and dermatomyositis) or oral medications (acetazolamide,

phenytoin, latanoprost, streptomycin, psoralen, minoxidil, cyclosporine, and diazoxide).

TREATMENT

Nonpharmacologic Treatment

- Reasonable expectations should be discussed.
- Diet and exercise should be advised to all women with PCOS.
- For overweight females recommend lifestyle interventions with a goal of weight loss; weight loss results in improved insulin sensitivity, a decrease in serum androgens, and, in some cases, a return of ovulatory cycles.

Pharmacologic Treatment

Drugs are indicated for treatment when hyperandrogenism is confirmed.

- Oral contraceptives (OCP) are the first-line treatment for hirsutism. It is preferable to use an OC containing a progestin with low androgenic activity (e.g., norethindrone acetate, ethynodiol diacetate, desogestrel, gestodene, and norgestimate). Side effects include breast tenderness, irregular vaginal bleeding, mood changes, and mild fluid retention.
- Spironolactone (androgen blocker and competes with DHT for binding to the androgen receptor). The starting dose is 50 mg twice daily and may be increased to a total daily dose of 200 mg. It takes at least 6 months to have any beneficial effect. Side effects include hyperkalemia, gastrointestinal discomfort, and irregular menstrual bleeding.
- Flutamide (nonsteroidal androgen receptor antagonist) is used primarily in the management of prostate cancer, but it has been used off-label for managing hirsutism in doses of 500 mg daily.
- Cyproterone acetate (strong progestogenic and antiandrogen properties)—available in combination with ethinyl estradiol (2 mg CPA and 35 µg EE/tablet).
- Finasteride (5-alpha reductase inhibitor)—for treatment of IH
- Glucocorticoid—to treat hirsutism associated with CAH
- GnRH agonists—This therapy is parenteral and reserved for women with severe hirsutism who do not respond to the OC and antiandrogens.
- Eflornithine hydrochloride cream (13.9%) a potent, irreversible inhibitor of the enzyme ornithine decarboxylase. The cream is applied to the face twice a day.
- Insulin-lowering agents are not an effective therapy for hirsutism.

Direct or Mechanical Methods of Hair Removal

- Electrolysis is recommended for hair that is naturally white or blonde.
- Photoepilation therapies (laser and intense pulsed non-coherent light sources) can be used to reduce hair via selective photothermolysis.

SUGGESTED READING

1. Matheson E, Bain J. Hirsutism in women. Am Fam Phys. 2019;100(3):168-75.

110 Histoplasmosis

➲ SYNONYMS

Cave disease, Darling's disease, Ohio valley disease, Reticulo-endotheliosis, Spelunker's Lung, Caver's disease.

➲ HISTORY

Histoplasma was discovered in 1905 by Darling.

➲ ETIOLOGY

Histoplasma capsulatum var. *capsulatum* causes American histoplasmosis, and *Histoplasma capsulatum* var. *duboisii* causes African histoplasmosis.

➲ EPIDEMIOLOGY

It can affect individuals of any age.

➲ CLINICAL FEATURES

Histoplasmosis is a systemic infection that can affect multiple organs and tissues; nevertheless, in majority of cases, the most affected are the lungs and the tissues of the reticuloendothelial system such as the spleen, liver, bone marrow, and the lymph nodes. There are two types of histoplasmosis: The primary pulmonary type and the progressive secondary type.

Primary cutaneous histoplasmosis is very rare and has been reported in cases of accidental inoculation in the laboratory. The most common type is mucocutaneous which spreads from disseminated chronic forms in which ulcers and nodules with erythema and exudates are observed in different parts of the skin and mucosae, most frequently in the oral mucosa.

➲ DERMOSCOPY

Scaling and peripheral arborizing telangiectasias.

➲ HISTOPATHOLOGY

In smears or impressions stained with Wright or Giemsa stains, intracellular yeasts of 3–4 μ in size can be seen. The nucleus stains red-violet and the cytoplasm becomes a very faint, almost colorless blue that looks like a capsule. Microscopically, an abundance of tuberculated macroconidia is observed. They are 8–14 μ in diameter, round or oval, and they emerge from short conidiophores at right angles. Also, microconidia can be observed which are 2–4 μ in diameter, spherical or oval, have smooth walls, and emerge from short, narrow conidiophores arranged at right angles with respect to the hypha.

DIFFERENTIAL DIAGNOSIS

- Blastomycosis
- Coccidioidomycosis
- Sarcoidosis
- Tuberculosis

TREATMENT

In mild-to-moderate primary pulmonary infection, it is not always necessary to administer antimycotic drugs as remission is spontaneous. In moderate and chronic forms, itraconazole and fluconazole are useful in dosages of 200–400 mg/day until the remission of symptoms. In patients with severe pulmonary histoplasmosis with respiratory insufficiency or in disseminated cases, intravenous amphotericin B is required. The initial dosage is 0.1 mg/kg, increased by 0.1 mg/kg with each dose until 0.8 or 1 mg/kg, with a maximum of 50 mg per regimen is achieved.

SUGGESTED READING

1. Kauffman CA. Histoplasmosis: a clinical and laboratory update. Clin Microbiol Rev. 2007;20(1):115-32.

Hyperhidrosis

➲ EPIDEMIOLOGY

Persons of all ages can be affected by hyperhidrosis. Localized hyperhidrosis, unlike generalized hyperhidrosis, usually begins in childhood or adolescence.

➲ CLINICAL FEATURES

Hyperhidrosis is excessive sweating from the skin. The most widely used classification system divides it into primary and secondary types. Primary hyperhidrosis, the most common type, is characterized by excessive sweating localized to the palms, soles, and/or axillae **(Figs. 1A and B)**. It is stimulated by intense emotion

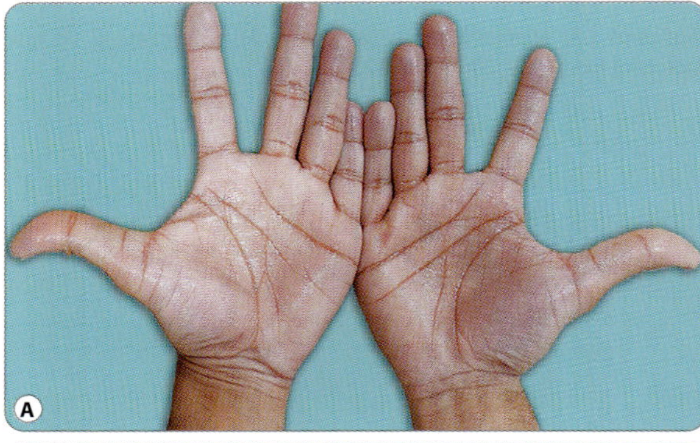

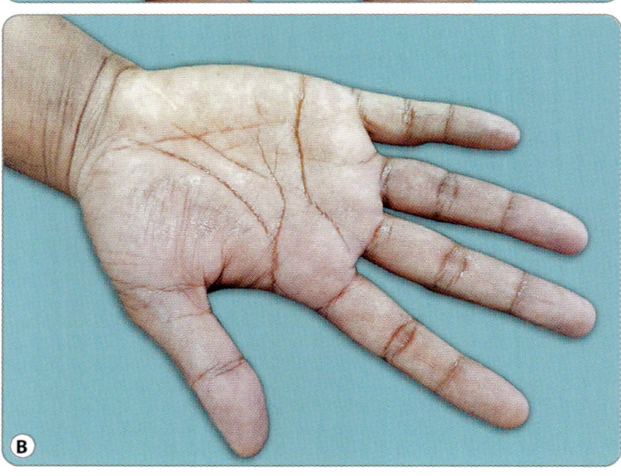

Figs. 1A and B: Hyperhidrosis over palms.

or stress, and in general, patients only have excessive sweating during waking hours. Primary hyperhidrosis is thought to arise from increased neural impulses from the cerebral cortex to the eccrine gland (hence the term "cortical" hyperhidrosis). The glands themselves are normal in structure. Secondary hyperhidrosis may be localized or generalized and is associated with medical conditions such as genetic syndromes, malignancy, or infection.

Criteria for the Diagnosis of Primary Hyperhidrosis

- Focal, visible excess sweating
- Present for at least 6 months
- No apparent secondary causes
- At least two of the following:
  - Bilateral and symmetric
  - Impairs activities of daily life
  - At least one episode per week
  - Age of onset <25 years
  - Positive family history
  - Stops during sleep

Secondary Hyperhidrosis

Causes of generalized hyperhidrosis are:

- *Thermal hyperhidrosis*: Sweating follows any rise in body temperature, whether this is caused by exercise, environmental heat, or an illness, e.g., acute infections and some chronic illnesses (Hodgkin's disease).
- Emotional stimuli, hypoglycemia, opiate withdrawal, and shock cause sweating by a direct or reflex stimulation of the sympathetic system at hypothalamic or higher centers.
- Lesions of the central nervous system (e.g., a cerebral tumor or cerebrovascular accident)
- Phaeochromocytoma, the carcinoid syndrome, diabetes mellitus, thyrotoxicosis, Cushing's syndrome, and the hot flushes of menopausal women.
- *Drugs*: Propranolol, physostigmine, pilocarpine, tricyclic anti-depressants, and serotonin reuptake inhibitors

Causes of localized hyperhidrosis are:

- Gustatory stimuli (associated with Frey syndrome, encephalitis, syringomyelia, diabetic neuropathies, herpes zoster parotitis, and parotid abscess)
- Eccrine nevus
- Eccrine angiomatous hamartoma and Blue rubber-bleb nevus
- Glomus tumor
- Peripheral neuropathy, organomegaly, endocrinopathy, monoclonal plasma-proliferative disorder, and skin changes (POEMS) syndrome
- Burning feet syndrome
- Pachydermoperiostosis
- Pretibial myxedema

The treatment of hyperhidrosis is described in **Table 1**.

Table 1: Treatment of hyperhidrosis.

	Therapy	Frequency	Side effects	Duration	Comments
First-line	• Topicals • 20% aluminum chloride hexahydrate 6.25% aluminum tetrachloride Zirconium salts Aldehydes	Use nightly for 3–5 nights, then every few days as needed	Burning irritant contact dermatitis	Days	Blocks sweat ducts Aldehydes not recommended due to sensitization
	• Glycopyrronium 2.4% (premoistened cloth)	Once daily	Local skin irritation Anticholinergic symptoms		
Second-line	Iontophoresis	2–3 times a week	Discomfort during procedure	Days	Blocks sweat ducts
	Botulinum toxin A	Every 4–6 months	Discomfort during injection weakness of underlying muscles	Months	Prevents release of acetylcholine
	Microwave thermolysis	Administered in two 20- to 30-minute treatment sessions separated by 3 months	• Altered skin sensation • Discomfort • Local reactions		Microwave energy can be utilized to destroy eccrine glands in axillae
	Oral therapy	As needed		Hours	
	Oxybutynin	1.25–5 mg bid	Dry mouth and urinary retention most common; also confusion and decreased mental status		Anticholinergic
	Glycopyrrolate	1–2 mg bid			Anticholinergic
	Clonidine	0.1–0.3 mg bid	Hypotension, rebound hypertension		α_2-adrenergic agonist
	Clonazepam	0.25–0.5 mg bid	Sedation		Anxiolytic
Third-line	Local excision	Once	Scarring	Permanent	Last resort
	Sympathectomy		Compensatory hyperhidrosis Horner's syndrome	Usually permanent	

Emerging therapies: Topical botulinum toxin, ultrasound, use of iontophoresis or phonophoresis to facilitate delivery of botulinum toxin A (Btx A) percutaneously for palmar hyperhidrosis (HH) and laser therapy.

➲ SUGGESTED READING

1. McConaghy JR, Fosselman D. Hyperhidrosis: management options. Am Fam Phys. 2018;97(11):729-34.

112 Hypertrichosis

➲ ETIOLOGY

There are two distinct types of hypertrichosis: Generalized hypertrichosis and localized hypertrichosis. Hypertrichosis can be either congenital or acquired later in life.

Generalized hypertrichosis and localized hypertrichosis are discussed in **Table 1**.

➲ CLINICAL FEATURES

Hypertrichosis describes the growth of an excessive amount of hair on any area of the body **(Figs. 1 and 2)**. Generalized hypertrichosis

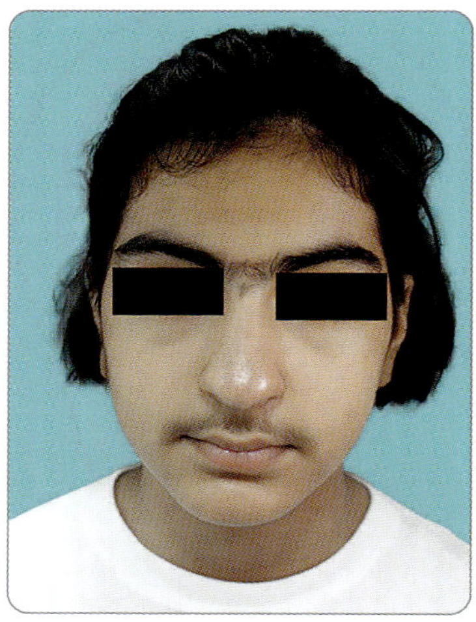

Fig. 1: Hypertrichosis over lips.

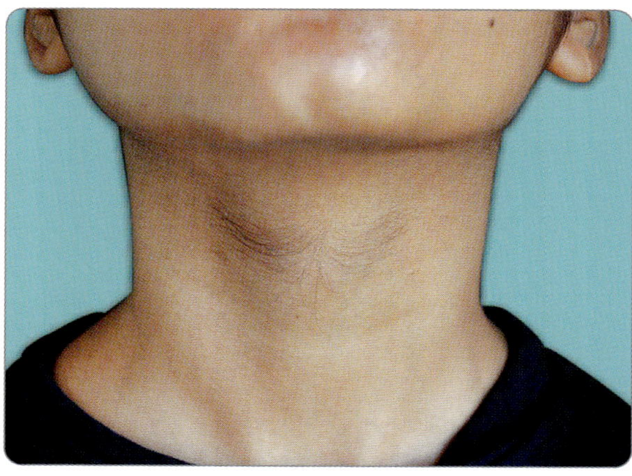

Fig. 2: Anterior cervical hypertrichosis.

Table 1: Generalized hypertrichosis and localized hypertrichosis.

Congenital generalized hypertrichosis	*Acquired generalized hypertrichosis*	*Congenital localized hypertrichosis*	*Acquired localized hypertrichosis*
Congenital hypertrichosis lanuginosa	CNS (e.g., traumatic brain injuries)	Hypertrichosis cubiti	After repeated trauma, friction, irritation, or inflammation
Universal hypertrichosis	POEMS syndrome	Hypertrichosis of the auricle	Vaccination sites
Ambras syndrome	Internal malignancies, most often carcinoma of the lung, colon, or breast	Trichomegaly of the eyelashes	Varicella scars as well as sites of wart removal and laser epilation
X-linked hypertrichosis	Juvenile dermatomyositis and hypothyroidism	Hypertrichosis of the eyebrows	Post-PUVA therapy
Gingival fibromatosis with hypertrichosis	Advanced HIV infection	Anterior cervical hypertrichosis	Potent topical corticosteroids or tacrolimus, repeated irritation from anthralin, and creams containing mercury or iodine.
Mucopolysaccharidoses	Malnutrition (including anorexia nervosa)	Posterior cervical hypertrichosis	
Fetal hydantoin syndrome	Drugs: Cyclosporine, minoxidil, and phenytoin	Porphyria cutanea tarda, CEP	

(CEP: congenital erythropoietic porphyria; CNS: central nervous system; HIV: human immunodeficiency virus; POEMS: Polyneuropathy, Organomegaly, Endocrinopathy, Monoclonal plasma cell disorder, and Skin changes; PUVA: psoralen plus ultraviolet A) is the presence of lanugo hair, excess vellus hair, or terminal hair on much of the cutaneous surface, including an acquired transformation of terminal hair into lanugo hair. Drug-induced hypertrichosis is characterized by slow growth of terminal hair of medium thickness. The findings are most evident on the forehead, temples, and flexor aspects of the extremities and trunk. Drug-related hypertrichosis is usually reversible and differs in distribution from drug-induced hirsutism.

➲ TREATMENT

Treatment of hypertrichosis may include shaving, depilatories, bleaching, plucking, waxing, laser, and electrolysis. Electrolysis may require more than one treatment session. Shaving, contrary to popular belief, does not increase the amount of hair that regrows. Chemical depilatories (calcium or potassium thioglycolate) and bleaching agents are available over-the-counter and frequently prove effective but may irritate the skin of some users. LASERs [long pulsed 1,064 nm Nd:Yag laser, Alexandrite laser, intense pulsed light (IPL), and diode laser are the most efficacious] may be helpful in selected cases, especially dark hair in fair-skinned patients. A newer topical cream for the treatment of hypertrichosis is eflornithine hydrochloride 13.9%, an irreversible inhibitor of ornithine decarboxylase that slows (but does not remove hair) hair growth.

➲ SUGGESTED READING

1. Saleh D, Yarrarapu SN, Cook C. Hypertrichosis. StatPearls. Treasure Island (FL): StatPearls Publishing; 2025.

113 Ichthyosis

➲ HISTORY

The word is derived from Greek "*ichthys*", meaning fish.

The first historic reference to ichthyosis as "Ekakushtha" appears in an Indian text in 250 BC. Willan introduced the term "ichthyosis". The first account of a harlequin fetus was in 1750. Wells and Kerr defined groups of ichthyoses with autosomal recessive, sex-linked, and autosomal dominant inheritance patterns.

➲ ETIOLOGY

Ichthyoses are disorders of cornification with abnormal differentiation and desquamation of the epidermis.

➲ EPIDEMIOLOGY

It starts at birth or develops later in life.

Diagnosis, onset, defect, clinical features, and histopathology of ichthyosis are described in **Table 1**.

➲ TREATMENT

The mainstay of symptomatic management is the continual use of lubricants and emollients. Patients are advised nonsoap cleansers (soap may exacerbate dryness). Ceramide-containing lipid creams, therapeutic emollients such as ammonium lactate 12%, preparations containing urea and keratolytics, such as α-hydroxy, lactic acid, propylene glycol, and salicylic acid are beneficial. Topical retinoids (trifarotene which was granted Orphan Drug Designation by FDA for the treatment of congenital ichthyoses) may be valuable but can cause skin irritation. Systemic treatment with acitretin or isotretinoin, and the use of moisturizing cleansers and humidifiers may be helpful.

Table 1: Diagnosis, onset, defect, clinical features, and histopathology of ichthyosis (Figs. 1A to D).

Diagnosis	*Onset*	*Defect*	*Clinical features*	*Histopathology*
Congenital ichthyoses				
Ichthyosis vulgaris	Infancy childhood	Absence of filaggrin	• Fine or centrally tacked down scale with superficial fissuring • Relative flexural sparing, worse on lower extremities **(Fig. 1A)** • Hyperlinear palms and soles	Hyperkeratosis, reduced or absent granular layer
Epidermolytic hyperkeratosis/bullous congenital ichthyosiform erythroderma	Birth	Keratin 1, 10 In Vorner type-keratin 9	Verrucous firm hyperkeratotic spines, linearly arranged in flexural creases, blisters, erythroderma, palmoplantar keratoderma	Hyperkeratosis, vacuolar degeneration of epidermal granular layer, and large irregular keratohyalin granules
X -linked recessive ichthyosis	Birth	Steroid sulfatase	• Fine to large scales, comma-shaped corneal opacities on the posterior capsule • Cryptorchidism	Hyperkeratosis and hypergranulosis
Nonbullous ichthyosiform erythroderma	Birth	Transglutaminase 1	Frequently collodion membrane at birth; fine, white scale in generalized distribution; variable erythroderma and palm/sole involvement	Compact hyperkeratosis, parakeratosis, normal or prominent granular layer

Continued

Continued

Diagnosis	***Onset***	***Defect***	***Clinical features***	***Histopathology***
Lamellar ichthyosis	Birth	Loricrin and involucrin	Frequently collodion membrane at birth; fine to large or plate-like scale in generalized distribution; variable color of scale; palmoplantar involvement; variable degree of erythroderma **(Fig. 1B)**	Compact orthohyperkeratosis with variable focal parakeratosis
Harlequin ichthyosis	Birth	ATP-binding cassette A-12	• Markedly thickened skin with geometric deep fissures • Restricted respiration, neonatal sepsis, and death. Survivors develop CIE	Massively thickened orthohyperkeratotic stratum corneum with acanthosis and decreased granular layer
Ichthyosiform syndromes				
Netherton syndrome	Birth	LEKTI-serine protease inhibitor	Ichthyosis linearis circumflexa, trichorrhexis invaginata, atopy, aminoaciduria, failure to thrive	Nonspecific
Sjögren–Larsson syndrome	Birth	Fatty aldehyde dehydrogenase	Generalized fine scale to coarse hyperkeratosis, spastic diplegia, mental retardation, retinal glistening white dots, and seizures	Nonspecific
Refsum disease	Adult	Phytanoyl COA hydroxylase	Progressive neurologic dysfunction, cardiac, renal skeletal abnormalities, and retinitis pigmentosa	Lipid-containing vacuoles in basal keratinocytes
Keratosis icthyosis and deafness syndrome	Birth	Connexins 26,30	Progressive corneal opacification, generalized hyperkeratosis, discrete erythematous plaques, and neurosensory deafness	Nonspecific

Continued

Continued

Diagnosis	*Onset*	*Defect*	*Clinical features*	*Histopathology*
CHILD syndrome	Birth	3β hydroxysteroid dehydrogenase	Congenital hemidysplasia, ichthyosiform erythroderma, and limb defects	Nonspecific
• Acquired ichthyosis • Drugs (e.g., nicotinic acid, hypocholesterolemic agents, and maprotiline) • Chronic hepatic disease, renal failure, and thyroid and parathyroid disease • Malabsorption states • Sarcoidosis, leprosy • Acquired immune deficiency syndrome (AIDS) • Lymphoma and other malignancies				

(ATP: adenosine triphosphate; COA: coarctation of the aorta; CHILD: congenital hemidysplasia with ichthyosiform erythroderma and limb defects)

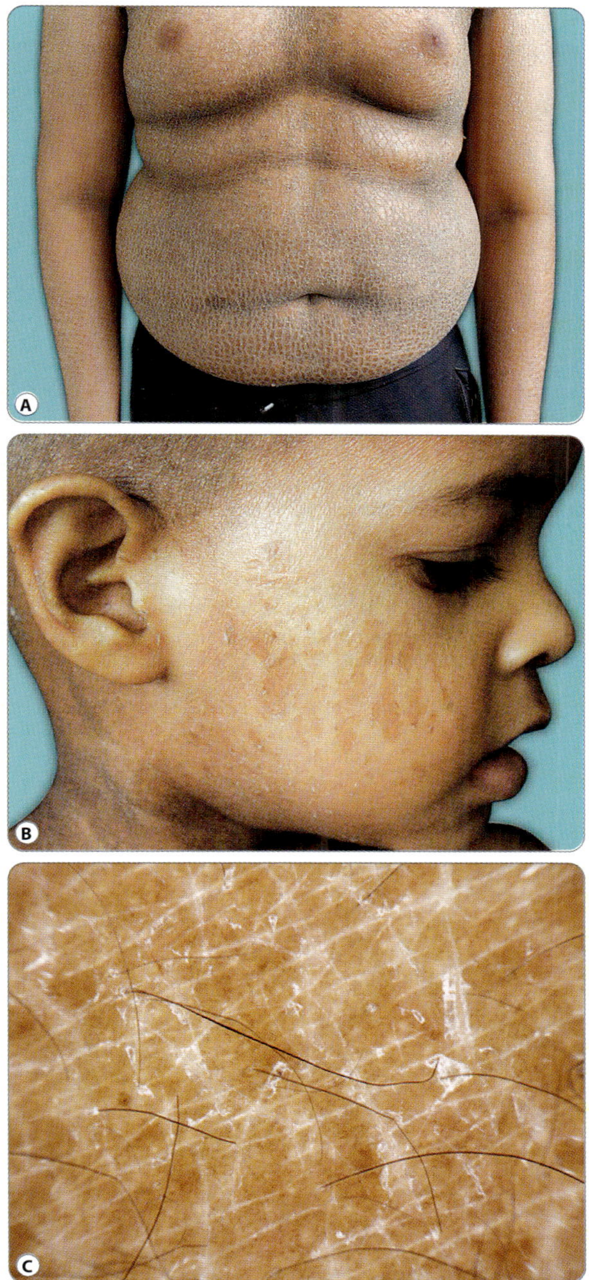

Figs. 1A to D: *Continued*

Continued

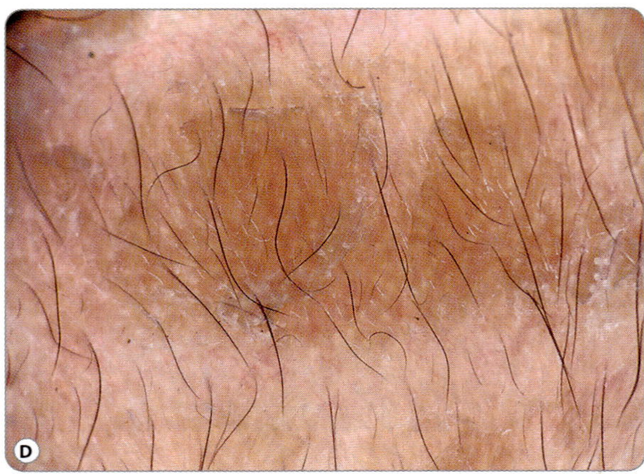

Figs. 1A to D: (A) Ichthyosis vulgaris; (B) X-linked ichthyosis; (C) Large plate-like scales in lamellar ichthyosis; and (D) Large plate-like scales in lamellar ichthyosis.

SUGGESTED READING

1. Oji V, Traupe H. Ichthyosis: clinical manifestations and practical treatment options. Am J Clin Dermatol. 2009;10:351-64.

114 Idiopathic Guttate Hypomelanosis

➲ SYNONYM

Disseminate lenticular leukoderma.

➲ ETIOLOGY

The cause of IGH is unknown, but normal aging or photoaging probably plays a role. Age-related somatic mutation of melanocytes may explain the etiology. A familial tendency has been noted.

➲ EPIDEMIOLOGY

Incidence increases with age. It is seen in up to 80% of patients over the age of 70 years. IGH occurs in all races and skin types but is more striking in darkly pigmented skin. An apparent female predominance is probably the result of the heightened perception of a cosmetic problem.

➲ CLINICAL FEATURES

The typical IGH lesion is a circumscribed, sharply defined, asymptomatic porcelain white macule that usually begins over lower limbs. The lesions are usually 0.5–6 mm in diameter and are often delineated by the skin furrows. Occasionally lesions are up to 2.5 cm **(Fig. 1A)**. Once present, they do not change in size and do not coalesce. Their surface is smooth but not atrophic. No spontaneous repigmentation has been observed. Vellus hairs within the lesions usually retain their pigment. In most patients, there are multiple lesions on the photoexposed regions such as extensor forearms and shins. Rarely the face, neck, and shoulders can be affected.

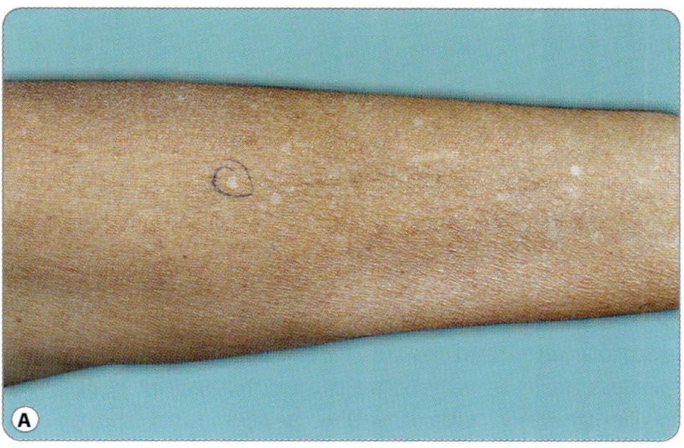

Figs. 1A to D: *Continued*

Continued

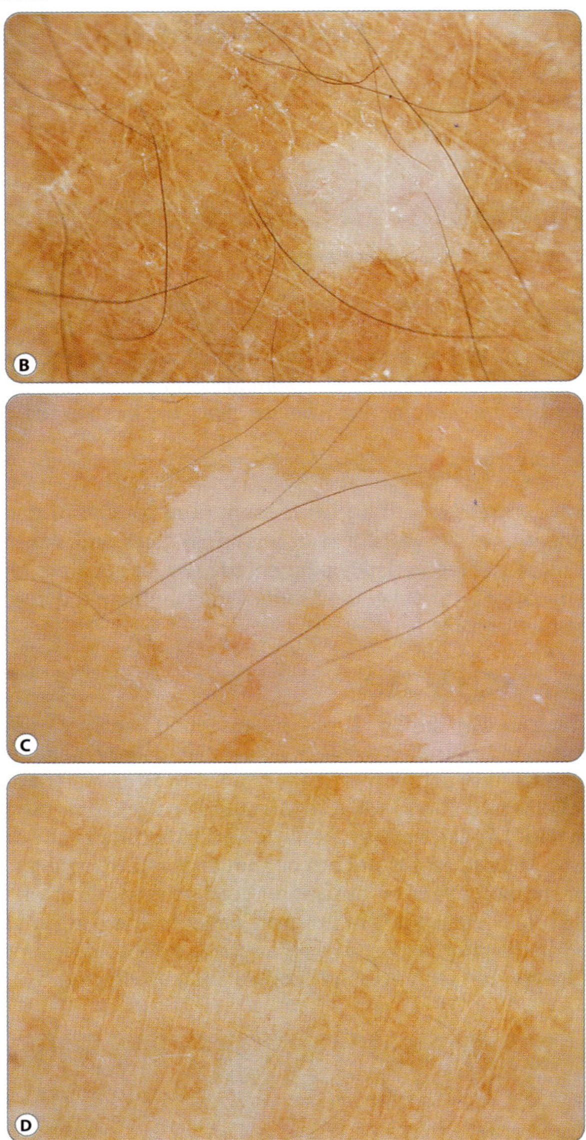

Figs. 1A to D: (A) Multiple porcelain white hypopigmented macules over upper limbs; (B) Dermoscopy showing ameboid pattern; (C) Dermoscopy showing patelloid pattern; and (D) Dermoscopy showing nebuloid pattern.

➲ DERMOSCOPY

The dermoscopic features of IGH are characterized by white structureless areas in which the pigment network is absent. They extend peripherally with irregular borders and shapes. Various patterns have been described which are as follows:

- *Amoeboid pattern*: White structureless area with a pseudopod-like periphery resembling an amoeba

- *Feathery pattern*: White structureless area with feather-like linear extensions and irregular margins
- *Petaloid pattern*: White structureless areas resemble the petals of a flower.
- *Nebuloid pattern*: White structureless areas have indistinct borders like a cloud. Other descriptions include "cloudy sky-like" and "cloudy" patterns **(Figs. 1B to D)**.

HISTOPATHOLOGY

The most consistent histological features of IGH are a flattening of the dermoepidermal junction, moderate to marked reduction or focal absence of melanin granules in the basal and suprabasal layers, and a basket-weave hyperkeratosis. There is a moderate to relatively marked reduction in the number of dihydroxyphenylalanine (DOPA)-positive epidermal melanocytes (10–50% compared with normal skin), but these cells are never totally absent. At the ultrastructural level, some of these melanocytes have normal melanogenic activity, while others lack mature melanosomes. The keratinocytes show a marked variation in melanin content, which may be absent or markedly decreased.

DIFFERENTIAL DIAGNOSIS

- Guttate vitiligo—hair overlying lesions may be affected
- Achromic verruca plana—the presence of koilocytes on biopsy, koebnerization seen
- Pityriasis lichenoides chronica—scaling is seen, lesions are larger, widespread
- Disseminated hypopigmented keratoses that follow psoralen plus ultraviolet A (PUVA) therapy
- Atrophie blanche—porcelain white atrophic lesions with angulated margins seen, history of (h/o) preceding ulcers present

TREATMENT

Patients should be reassured that lesions of IGH are benign and no treatment necessary. As sunlight is most likely a precipitating factor, the use of sunscreens and physical barriers should be strongly recommended. Cryotherapy, topical steroids/retinoids/calcineurin inhibitors, superficial dermabrasion, topical 88% phenol, fractional carbon dioxide lasers, nonablative fractional photothermolysis via fractional 1,550-nm ytterbium/erbium fiber laser, microneedling with microinfusion of 5-fluorouracil, skin grafting, and excimer light treatment are the various treatments tried. The risk of leukoderma induced by cryotherapy or postinflammatory hyperpigmentation should be considered.

SUGGESTED READING

1. Juntongjin P, Laosakul K. Idiopathic guttate hypomelanosis: a review of its etiology, pathogenesis, findings, and treatments. Am J Clin Dermatol. 2016;17:403-11.

115 Impetigo

➲ SYNONYMS

School sores, impetigo contagiosa of Tilbury Fox.

➲ HISTORY

The word impetigo is derived from Latin word "impetere" meaning "assail".

➲ ETIOLOGY

The primary pathogens in nonbullous and bullous impetigo are *Staphylococcus aureus* and less commonly, group A β-hemolytic *Streptococcus* (*Streptococcus pyogenes*). Methicillin-resistant *Staphylococcus aureus* (MRSA) which is hospital or community acquired is the most common cause.

➲ EPIDEMIOLOGY

It primarily affects children.

Nonbullous impetigo and bullous impetigo are described in **Table 1**.

Table 1: Nonbullous impetigo and bullous impetigo.

	Nonbullous impetigo	*Bullous impetigo*
Clinical features	• The initial lesion is a very thin-walled vesicle on an erythematous base. The vesicle ruptures so rapidly that it is seldom seen as such • The exuding serum dries to form yellowish-brown crusts (**Figs. 1A and B**). Gradual, irregular, peripheral extension occurs without central healing, and multiple lesions, which are usually present, may coalesce. The crusts eventually dry and separate to leave erythema, which fades without scarring. The face, especially around the nose and mouth, and the limbs are the sites most commonly affected. In severe cases, there may be regional adenitis with fever and other constitutional symptoms	In bullous impetigo, the bullae are less rapidly ruptured and become much larger; a diameter of 1–2 cm is common and persist for 2 or 3 days. The contents are at first clear, later cloudy. After rupture thin, flat, brownish crusts are formed. Central healing and peripheral extension may give rise to circinate lesions. Although the face is often affected, the lesions may occur anywhere regional adenitis is rare

Continued

Continued

	Nonbullous impetigo	*Bullous impetigo*
Histopathology	Within the epidermis, neutrophilic vesiculopustules are present. Spongiosis frequently underlies the pustule. The upper dermis contains an intense infiltrate of neutrophils and lymphocytes. Gram-positive cocci are present in the lesions	Cleavage of the uppermost epidermis, typically within the granular layer, is seen. Secondary acantholysis may be observed, mimicking pemphigus foliaceus. Usually, few inflammatory cells and no bacteria are present within the blister cavity. The upper dermis may contain neutrophils
Differential diagnosis	• Varicella • Insect bites • Eczema • Candidiasis • Herpes simplex infection	• Bullous insect bites • Thermal burns • Herpes simplex infection

➲ COMPLICATIONS

Cellulitis, lymphangitis, and bacteremia resulting in osteomyelitis, septic arthritis, septicemia, staphylococcal scalded skin syndrome, poststreptococcal acute glomerulonephritis, scarlet fever, urticaria, and erythema multiforme are the known complications **(Figs. 1A and B)**.

➲ TREATMENT

Removal of crusts and maintenance of good hygiene are general measures. First-line topical therapy includes fusidic acid, mupirocin 2% ointment, and retapamulin 1%. Ozenoxacin, a topical quinolone, was approved by the US Food and Drug Administration (FDA) in 2017 for the treatment of impetigo. Oral antibiotics such as flucloxacillin, erythromycin 500 mg QID, dicloxacillin 250 mg QID, and cephalexin 250 mg QID may be prescribed in the following indications: Widespread infection, lymphadenopathy, or nephritogenic *Streptococcus*.

For MRSA, trimethoprim-sulfamethoxazole DS, clindamycin, or doxycycline can be given. For *S. aureus* carriers, mupirocin ointment 2% BID is applied to their nares.

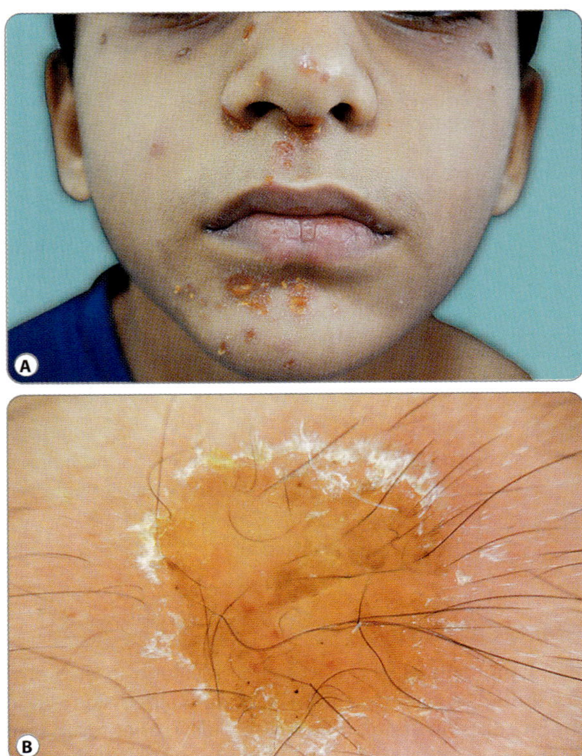

Figs. 1A and B: (A) Pustules and crusted erosions of impetigo contagiosa; and (B) Dermoscopy of impetigo contagiosa.

SUGGESTED READING

1. Hartman-Adams H, Banvard C, Juckett G. Impetigo: diagnosis and treatment. Am Fam Phys. 2014;90(4):229-35.

116 Incontinentia Pigmenti

➲ SYNONYMS

Bloch–Sulzberger syndrome, Bloch–Siemens syndrome.

➲ HISTORY

Incontinentia pigmenti (IP) was described by Garrod et al. in 1906. However, it was Bloch who first used the term "incontinentia pigmenti" for this condition, and Sulzberger who provided a more detailed account of Bloch's patient.

➲ ETIOLOGY

Incontinentia pigmenti is an X-linked dominant multisystem disease caused by mutations in the *NEMO* gene (NF-κB essential modulator) on chromosome Xq28, the protein product of which confers protection against apoptosis induced by the tumor necrosis factor family of cytokines.

➲ EPIDEMIOLOGY

Incontinentia pigmenti occurs during infancy or early childhood. It is reported primarily in females and is lethal for hemizygous affected males.

➲ CLINICAL FEATURES

The skin changes often present between the first weeks and the first 2 months of birth. Four distinct clinical stages are recognized:

- *Stage 1*: Inflammatory macules, papules, vesicles, and pustules (from birth or shortly thereafter), most prominently on lower extremities **(Fig. 1A)**
- *Stage 2*: Hyperkeratotic and verrucous lesions (between 2 and 8 weeks of age)
- *Stage 3*: Gray-brown pigmentation (several months of age into adulthood), linear or whorled, most often on the trunk
- *Stage 4*: Atrophic, hypopigmented, and depigmented bands or streaks that are hairless and anhidrotic and fail to tan on sun exposure (from infancy through adulthood) **(Fig. 1B)**.

The various clinical stages of IP can overlap, occur in utero, or occasionally be skipped entirely. Associated cutaneous findings include patchy scarring alopecia, woolly hair nevi, nail dystrophy, and anhidrosis in atrophic streaks. Extracutaneous features include dental abnormalities such as partial anodontia and conical or peg-shaped teeth; the central nervous system (CNS) abnormalities, including seizures, delayed psychomotor development, mental retardation, and spastic hemiplegia; and ocular disease, characterized by retinal vascular abnormalities and blindness.

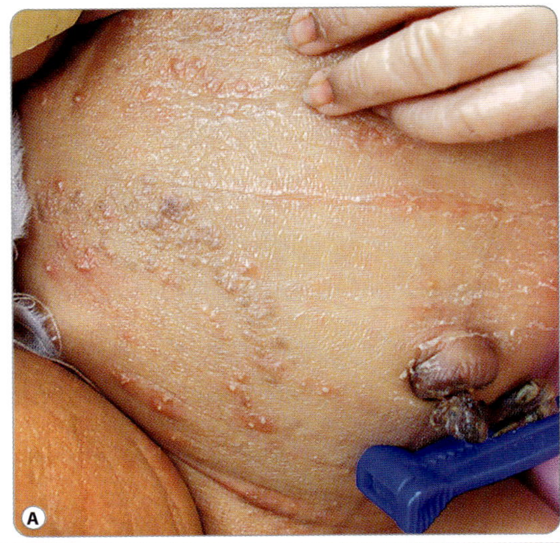

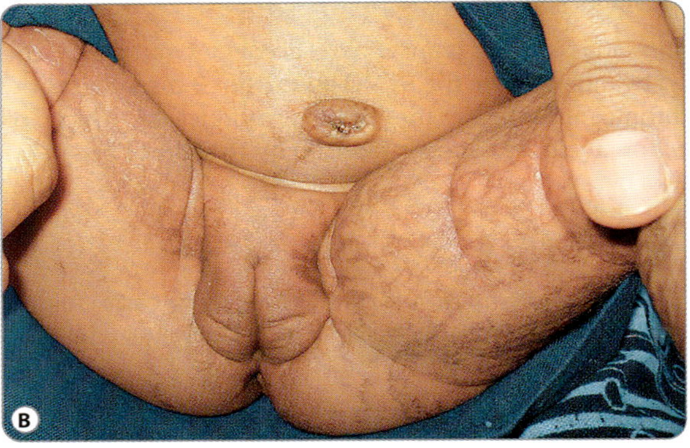

Figs. 1A and B: (A) Vesicles in a whorled arranged in stage I; and (B) Linear hyperpigmentation bilaterally on thighs.

HISTOPATHOLOGY

The bullae are situated beneath the horny layer or within a spongiotic epidermis. The dermis shows nonspecific inflammatory changes with a cellular infiltrate, including numerous eosinophils. The lichenoid papules show hyperkeratosis, acanthosis, and edema of the basal layer. Macrophages laden with melanin are present in the upper dermis. In the warty lesions, the hyperkeratosis is further increased, and within the irregularly acanthotic epidermis are hyaline bodies representing individual cell keratinization. The epidermal changes at this stage may suggest pseudoepitheliomatous hyperplasia. The pigmented patches show diminution or absence of pigment in the basal cells and large quantities of melanin in melanophages in the upper dermis. In all three stages, melanophages are present.

DIFFERENTIAL DIAGNOSIS

- *Infantile pemphigoid*—subepidermal blister is seen with eosinophils.

- *Herpes simplex infection*—grouped vesicles associated with burning sensation, pain; positive Tzanck smear
- Mastocytosis—Darier's sign is positive, and dermal mast cell infiltrate is seen.
- *Langerhans' cell histiocytosis*—histiocyte infiltration in dermis, absence of different stages
- *Epidermolysis bullosa*—larger bullae, scarring, and milia are seen; hair and nail involvement are present.

TREATMENT

Individuals affected with IP and families should be offered genetic consultation for consideration of mutation testing. Usually, no treatment is necessary other than the control of secondary infection and regular follow-up. Cross-referral and follow-up by other specialties like neurology, ophthalmology, and dental are essential.

PROGNOSIS

Those with neurological features tend to do less well than those with more minor manifestations of the syndrome. The pigmentary changes typically fade during childhood years.

SUGGESTED READING

1. Minić S, Trpinac D, Obradović M. Incontinentia pigmenti diagnostic criteria update. Clin Genet. 2014;85(6):536-42.

117 Kaposi's Sarcoma

➲ HISTORY

Kaposi's sarcoma (KS) was described initially in 1872 by a Hungarian dermatologist, Moritz Kaposi.

➲ ETIOLOGY

Kaposi's sarcoma is a spindle cell tumor thought to be derived from endothelial cell lineage. Human herpesvirus 8 (HHV-8) and human immunodeficiency virus (HIV) are implicated in etiology. Cigarette smoking may be protective for KS risk in HHV-8 seropositive patients infected with HIV.

➲ EPIDEMIOLOGY

Before the acquired immunodeficiency syndrome (AIDS) epidemic, KS was seen mainly in elderly men. African KS is fairly common in young adult males living near the equator.

➲ CLINICAL FEATURES

There are four types of KS:

1. *The classic type* affects elderly men of Mediterranean and Middle European descent and in men in Sub-Saharan Africa.
2. *HIV-associated* KS mainly affects men who have sex with men.
3. *Endemic or African KS* arises in some parts of Africa in children and young adults.
4. *Iatrogenic* KS is due to drug treatment causing immune suppression.

The tumors most often appear as bluish-red or purple bumps on the skin. They are reddish-purple, because they are rich in blood vessels. The lesions may first appear on the feet or ankles, thighs, arms, hands, face, or any other part of the body **(Figs. 1A and B)**.

➲ DERMOSCOPY

Common dermoscopic features of KS are bluish-red-purple pigmentation, white lines, white clods, and surface scale. Some areas show "rainbow pattern" where various colors of the rainbow spectrum are juxtaposed next to each other.

➲ HISTOPATHOLOGY

The typical histology of KS includes spindle-shaped cells, with vascular channels lined by abnormal endothelial cells (slit-like spaces and promontory sign). Extravasated erythrocytes, hemosiderin, and fibrosis can often be seen.

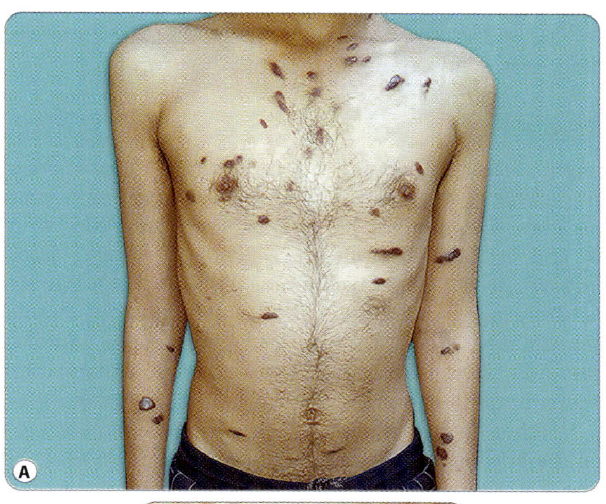

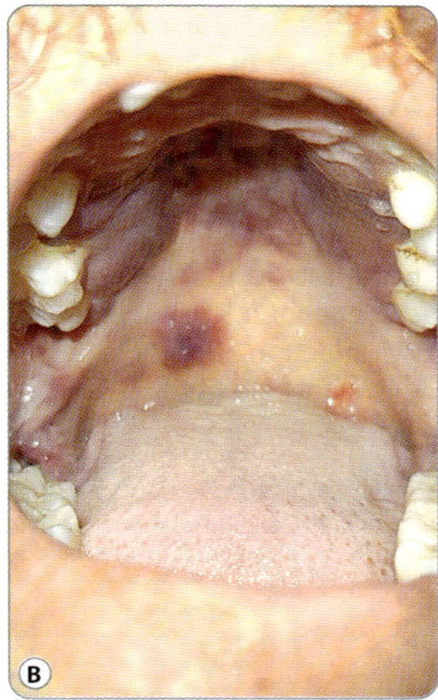

Figs. 1A and B: (A) Vascular lesions of Kaposi sarcoma over the trunk and limbs; and (B) Vascular lesions of Kaposi sarcoma over oral mucosa.

➲ DIFFERENTIAL DIAGNOSIS

- Acquired immunodeficiency syndrome-related angiomatosis
- *Hemangiomas*—dilated vascular channels with normal endothelial cells are present.
- *Pyogenic granulomas*—smaller lesions and bleeds on trauma
- Nevi
- *Melanomas*—atypical melanocytes in sheets and nests
- *Cutaneous lymphomas*—atypical lymphocytes are seen.
- Stasis dermatitis
- Postinflammatory hyperpigmentation
- *Prurigo nodularis*—no proliferation of vessels and vertically oriented collagen
- Angiosarcomas

➲ COMPLICATIONS

Bleeding, obstruction, or perforation of an organ.

➲ TREATMENT

Treatment decisions depend on the extent and location of the lesions, as well as the person's symptoms and degree of immunosuppression. Antiretroviral therapy against the AIDS virus can shrink the lesions. Chemotherapy with pegylated liposomal doxorubicin, paclitaxel, pomalidomide, oral etoposide, vinblastine, or vincristine (alone or in combination with bleomycin), vinorelbine, or gemcitabine. Radiation therapy, cryotherapy, intralesional interferon 2 alpha/vinblastine/bleomycin/vincristine/doxorubicin, electrochemotherapy, and excision can be used for lesions in certain areas. If other treatment approaches are contraindicated, then topical therapy with alitretinoin, imiquimod, timolol, silver nitrate, nicotine patches, and rapamycin may be used. Investigational approaches are HIV protease inhibitors, mechanistic (previously called mammalian) target of rapamycin (mTOR) inhibitors, molecularly targeted antiangiogenic agents (e.g., pazopanib), and immune checkpoint inhibitor immunotherapy.

➲ PROGNOSIS

Treatment and remission of KS do not improve survival in AIDS patients. The appearance of KS is a poor prognostic sign for individuals with HIV infection. Prognosis also depends on the immune status and HIV viral load of the patient.

➲ SUGGESTED READING

1. Schneider JW, Dittmer DP. Diagnosis and treatment of Kaposi sarcoma. Am J Clin Dermatol. 2017;18(4):529-39.

118 Kawasaki Disease

SYNONYMS

Mucocutaneous lymph node syndrome, infantile polyarteritis, Kawasaki syndrome.

HISTORY

Kawasaki disease was first described in 1967 by Dr Tomisaku Kawasaki, who reported 50 cases of a distinctive illness in children seen at the Tokyo Red Cross Medical Center in Japan.

ETIOLOGY

The cause has not been determined. It may be an autoimmune disorder causing medium vessel vasculitis of the mucus membranes, lymph nodes, walls of the blood vessels, and the heart. Microorganisms and toxins have been suspected, but none has been identified to date. Kawasaki disease is not felt to be a contagious illness. Genetic factors and the immune system seem to play roles in the disease, which is characterized by immune activation.

EPIDEMIOLOGY

It is commonly seen in children <5 years.

CLINICAL FEATURE

Kawasaki disease has telltale symptoms and signs that appear in phases. The first phase, which can last for up to 2 weeks, usually involves a persistent fever >104°F (39°C) and lasts for at least 5 days. Other symptoms that typically develop include severe redness in the eyes, a rash on the stomach, chest, and genitals, red, dry, cracked lips, swollen tongue with a white coating and big red bumps (strawberry tongue), sore throat, swollen palms and soles with a purple-red color, and lymphadenopathy. During the second phase, which usually begins within 2 weeks of fever, the skin on the hands and feet may begin to peel in large pieces. The child also may experience joint pain, diarrhea, vomiting, or abdominal pain.

DIFFERENTIAL DIAGNOSIS

- Scarlet fever
- *Steven–Johnson syndrome*—severe mucosal lesions, bullae, and erosions are seen over the body.
- Drug rash
- *Henoch–Schönlein purpura*—palpable purpura on buttocks and extremities, IgA on direct immunofluorescence (DIF), and abdominal and renal involvement

- Measles
- Toxic shock syndrome
- Infectious mononucleosis

COMPLICATIONS

Echocardiographic studies have shown that 20–25% of untreated children develop cardiovascular sequelae, including coronary artery (CA) aneurysms, depressed myocardial contractility and heart failure, myocardial infarction, arrhythmias, and peripheral arterial occlusion.

TREATMENT

Intravenous immunoglobulin (IVIg) (2 g/kg administered as a single infusion over 8–12 hours) and aspirin (30–100 mg/kg daily divided into four doses) have constituted the mainstay of therapy, which has to be given within the first 10 days of illness. In patients who do not defervesce within 48 hours, a second dose of IVIg 2 g/kg over 8–12 hours should be considered. Corticosteroids, cyclosporin, and ulinastatin (urinary trypsin inhibitor) have been used in patients with disease refractory to IVIg.

PROGNOSIS

With prompt treatment, the prognosis is good. The rate of mortality is <1%.

SUGGESTED READING

1. Newburger JW, Takahashi M, Burns JC. Kawasaki disease. J Am Coll Cardiol. 2016;67(14):1738-49.

119

Keloid

➲ HISTORY

Keloids were described by Egyptian surgeons around 1700 BC. Baron Jean-Louis Alibert in 1806 coined the term keloid, meaning "crab claw." The Olmec of Mexico in pre-Columbian times used keloid scarification as a means of decoration.

➲ ETIOLOGY

Changes in the cellular signals that control growth and proliferation may be related to the process of keloid formation, viz. transforming growth factor beta (TGF-β), tissue inhibitor of metalloproteinase (TIMP), matrix metalloproteinase (MMP), vascular endothelial growth factor (VEGF), and platelet-derived growth factor (PDGF). They may arise spontaneously, result from direct trauma, and follow inflammatory conditions like acne vulgaris or chickenpox scars. In some cases, the tendency to form keloids seems to run in families.

➲ EPIDEMIOLOGY

Keloids are equally common among women and men. People with darker skin are more likely to develop keloids. It is more common in adolescents and young adults.

➲ CLINICAL FEATURES

Keloid is a reactive lesion that represents exuberant scar formation that extends beyond the site of the original injury. Common sites are the head and neck area, ears (dumbbell keloids), upper chest, and arms. Keloids are raised and look shiny and dome-shaped, ranging in color from pink to red. Some become quite large and unsightly. Aside from causing potential cosmetic problems, these exuberant scars tend to be itchy, tender, or even painful **(Figs. 1A to C)**.

➲ ASSOCIATED SYNDROMES

Associated syndromes include Turner syndrome, Rubinstein–Taybi, Goeminne syndrome, conjunctivocorneal dystrophy, and multiple endocrine syndrome type 2B.

➲ DERMOSCOPY

The presence of different vascular structures in a background of a white scarring patch is the most characteristic dermoscopic finding in keloidal scarring. In contrast, hypertrophic scar shows erythematous or white patches with scanty or absent vascularization.

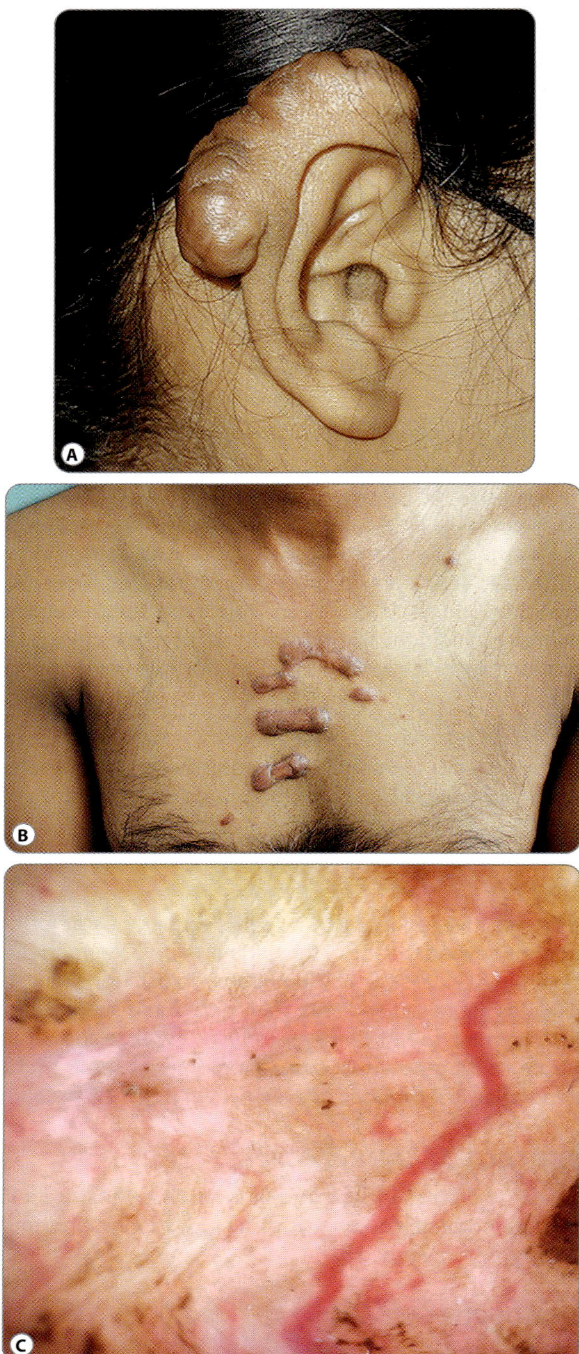

Figs. 1A to C: (A) Keloid due to ear piercing; (B) Keloid over the sternum; and (C) Dermoscopy of keloid.

HISTOPATHOLOGY

The epidermis is normal; collagen bundles in the dermis are thicker and more abundant, yielding acellular, node-like structures in the deep dermal region. The most consistent histologically distinguishing feature of keloids is the presence of random organization of type I and type III collagen. In addition to collagen, proteoglycans are deposited in excess amounts in keloid scars. A tongue-like advancing edge is seen underneath the normal-appearing epidermis and papillary dermis.

DIFFERENTIAL DIAGNOSIS

- *Hypertrophic scar*—fibrous tissue limits to the original defect, does not progress, is nonitchy, does not arise spontaneously, and is not familial/racial. Histopathological examination (HPE)—organized parallel pattern of type III collagen
- Dermatofibrosarcoma protuberans
- *Sarcoidosis*—naked granulomas; angiotensin-converting enzyme (ACE) levels are raised, and collagen is normal.
- *Squamous cell carcinoma*—horn pearls are seen.
- Fibromatosis
- *Lobomycosis*—demonstration of the fungus
- Keloidal scleroderma

COMPLICATION

Complications include pain, secondary infection, and ulceration.

TREATMENT

Treatment options include intralesional corticosteroids—triamcinolone acetonide 10–40 mg/mL with or without hyaluronidase, bleomycin, intralesional and topical (with tattooing) 5-fluorouracil, topical imiquimod, topical mitomycin C occlusive dressings, compression therapy (with elastic wrap bandages, custom pressure earmold, earring, and magnets), radiation therapy, cryosurgery (spray, contact, and intralesional), pulse dye laser, ablative laser, laser-assisted drug delivery (LADD), platelet-rich plasma (PRP) postexcision, excision, or silicone gel sheets.

PROGNOSIS

The rate of recurrence varies from 10 to 40%.

SUGGESTED READING

1. Tsai CH, Ogawa R. Keloid research: current status and future directions. Scars Burn Heal. 2019;5:2059513119868659.

120 Keratoacanthoma

➲ SYNONYMS

Molluscum sebaceum, Self-healing squamous-cell carcinoma (SCC), and Keratocarcinoma.

➲ HISTORY

Keratoacanthoma was originally described by Sir Jonathan Hutchinson in the 1880s, and the name was given by Freudenthal of Wroclaw.

➲ ETIOLOGY

Both sunlight and chemical carcinogens have been implicated as pathologic factors. Trauma, human papilloma virus, genetic factors, and immunocompromised status have also been implicated.

➲ EPIDEMIOLOGY

Keratoacanthoma has been reported in all age groups, but the incidence increases with age. M:F ratio is 2:1.

➲ CLINICAL FEATURES

Lesions typically are solitary and begin as firm, round, skin-colored, or reddish papules that rapidly progress to dome-shaped nodules with a smooth, shiny surface and a central crateriform ulcer or keratin plug that may project like a horn **(Fig. 1)**. They may heal spontaneously over 4–6 months. Most keratoacanthomas occur on sun-exposed areas. The face, neck, and dorsum of the upper extremities are common sites. Truncal lesions are rare.

Various types include giant, mucosal, pseudorecidive, occupational, keratoacanthoma centrifugum marginatum, multiple keratoacanthomas (Ferguson–Smith type), generalized eruptive keratoacanthoma of Grzybowski, subungual keratoacanthoma, agglomerated form, multiple familial keratoacanthoma of Witten and Zak, and distal digital keratoacanthoma.

➲ DERMOSCOPY

Dermoscopy shows white background, central keratin plug (amorphous, yellow-white to light brown), white circles around follicular openings, and vascular loops that are hairpin-like or made of linear irregular vessels.

➲ HISTOPATHOLOGY

Keratoacanthomas are composed of singularly well-differentiated squamous epithelium that show only a mild degree of

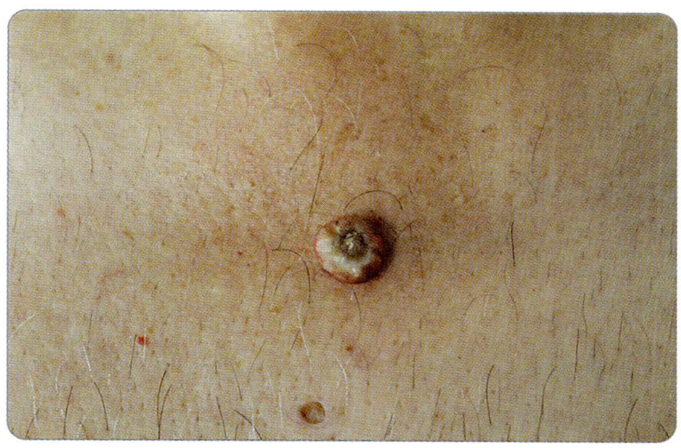

Fig. 1: Solitary keratoacanthoma: Dome-shaped nodule with central keratin plug projecting like a horn surrounding central depigmented atrophic skin.

pleomorphism and are likely to form masses of keratin that constitute the central core of keratoacanthoma. A fully developed lesion shows epidermal extension on the sides of the keratin-filled crater like a lip or buttress. There are many horn pearls. The base is regular and well demarcated, with a sharp outline between the tumor and the stroma. The stroma has a mixed inflammatory infiltrate, including neutrophils and eosinophils, with neutrophils forming epidermal microabscesses.

➲ DIFFERENTIAL DIAGNOSIS

- *Actinic keratosis*—only on sun-exposed areas and smaller lesions
- *Cutaneous horn*—massive hyperkeratosis with underlying changes
- *Basal cell carcinoma*—ulcer with rolled out edges and islands of basaloid cells
- *Molluscum contagiosum*—smaller umbilicated lesions and koebnerization are seen.
- Muir–Torre syndrome
- *Prurigo nodularis*—intensely itchy, mainly on the extremities
- *Sporotrichosis*—demonstration of the fungi
- *Squamous cell carcinoma*—horn pearls in biopsy
- Verrucous carcinoma
- Verruca vulgaris

➲ COMPLICATIONS

Subungual keratoacanthoma may cause pressure erosion in the terminal phalanx.

➲ TREATMENT

Treatment is primarily surgical. Reserve medical treatment for exceptional cases where surgical intervention is either not feasible or desirable. Intralesional methotrexate (MTX), 5-fluorouracil, bleomycin, interferon alpha-2a and alpha-2b, and steroids have been used with success. Electrodesiccation and curettage, laser therapy, radiation, cryotherapy, photodynamic therapy, topical

5-fluorouracil, and imiquimod have been used successfully. Systemic agents are an additional option for multiple and large keratoacanthomas—systemic retinoids, MTX plus prednisone, cyclophosphamide, and intravenous fluorouracil.

➲ PROGNOSIS

Keratoacanthoma is believed to have a good prognosis. 6% of keratoacanthomas present as squamous cell carcinoma if left untreated.

➲ SUGGESTED READING

1. Kwiek B, Schwartz RA. Keratoacanthoma (KA): an update and review. J Am Acad Dermatol. 2016;74(6):1220-33.

121 Keratolysis Exfoliativa

➲ SYNONYMS

Exfoliative keratolysis, focal palmoplantar keratoderma, dyshidrosis lamellosa sicca, lamellar dyshidrosis, recurrent focal palmar peeling.

➲ ETIOLOGY

The exact cause of keratolysis exfoliativa (KE) remains unclear. However, several factors have been proposed to contribute to its development. These factors include excessive sweating, occlusive footwear, hot and humid environments, prolonged water exposure, bacterial or fungal infections, and exposure to irritants. Recent histopathologic and molecular studies have linked KE to premature corneodesmosomal disruption.

➲ EPIDEMIOLOGY

Keratolysis exfoliativa can affect individuals of all ages and genders, but it is more commonly observed in young adults in the summer season. Occupations that involve frequent handwashing or prolonged glove use may increase the risk of developing this condition. It is more prevalent in tropical and subtropical regions due to the climatic conditions favoring increased sweating.

➲ CLINICAL FEATURES

The clinical presentation of KE primarily involves the palms and soles. The condition typically begins as an erythematous ring bordering the imminent lesions followed by small, discrete, superficial air-filled blisters that later coalesce and rupture, leaving behind irregularly shaped collarette scales. The condition is essentially asymptomatic but may be associated with mild itching or burning sensations. Lesions are usually symmetrical and may affect multiple fingers or toes **(Figs. 1A and B)**.

➲ DERMOSCOPY

Dermoscopy shows superficial erosions, air bubbles beneath the stratum corneum, collarette scales, and focal areas of erythema. The dermoscopic examination aids in differentiating KE from other dermatological conditions with similar clinical features **(Fig. 1C)**.

➲ HISTOPATHOLOGY

Histopathological examination of KE reveals intracorneal splitting and focal separation of the stratum corneum. The epidermis appears normal in other aspects.

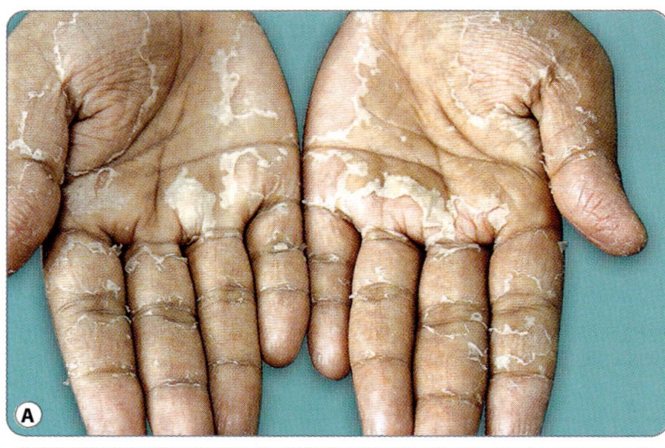

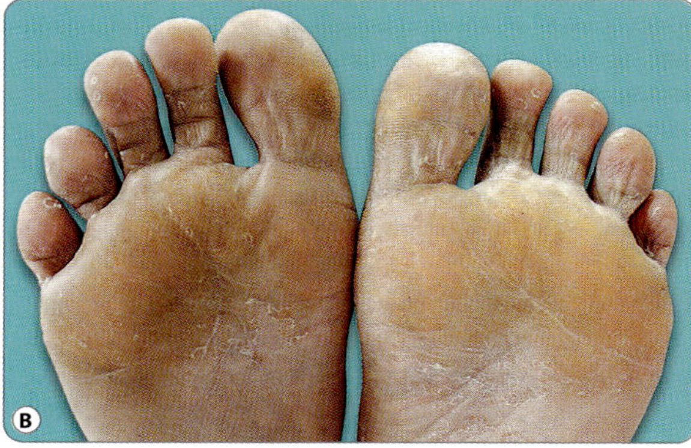

Figs. 1A to C: (A) Palms showing focal peeling and collarette scales; (B) Soles showing focal peeling and collarette scales; and (C) Dermoscopy showing collarette scales.

DIFFERENTIAL DIAGNOSIS

- *Dyshidrotic eczema*: It is characterized by vesicles on the palms and soles but lacks collarette scales.
- *Tinea manuum/pedis*: It is a fungal infection that typically shows scaling and erythema with positive fungal cultures.
- Contact dermatitis
- Acral skin peeling
- Localized epidermolysis bullosa simplex

- Palmoplantar psoriasis
- Keratolytic winter erythema
- Circumscribed palmar hypokeratosis

TREATMENT

The treatment of KE aims to reduce excessive sweating, control bacterial or fungal infections if present, protect from irritants, and enhance skin barrier function. Treatment options include the use of antiperspirants or aluminum chloride solutions to reduce sweating, topical keratolytic agents, such as salicylic acid, urea, or lactic acid, topical corticosteroids, acitretin, and photochemotherapy.

SUGGESTED READING

1. Hausauer AK, Cohen DE. Keratolysis exfoliativa. Dermatol Online J. 2015;21(12).

122 Keratosis Pilaris

➲ ETIOLOGY

Keratosis pilaris (KP) is a genetic autosomal dominant disorder of keratinization of hair follicles. It is more common in people who have very dry skin or atopic dermatitis. The condition is generally worse in winter and often clears in summer. The individual follicular bumps are caused by a hair that is unable to reach the surface and becomes trapped beneath the keratin debris. Often, patients develop mild erythema around the hair follicles, which is indicative of the inflammatory condition.

➲ EPIDEMIOLOGY

Keratosis pilaris affects nearly 50–80% of all adolescents and approximately 40% of adults. Symptoms particularly intensify during puberty.

➲ CLINICAL FEATURES

Keratosis pilaris is a common benign condition that manifests as 10–100 small, rough, folliculocentric keratotic papules, often described as chicken bumps, chicken skin, or goose bumps, in characteristic areas of the body, particularly the posterolateral upper arms, anterior thighs, buttocks, and facial cheeks. The single most characteristic area in KP is the upper-outer arms **(Fig. 1)**.

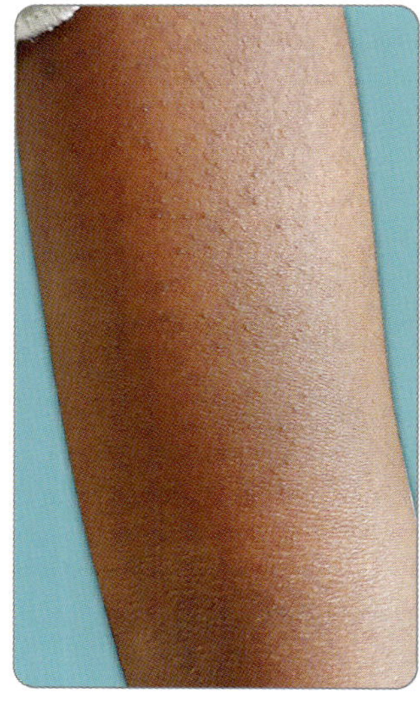

Fig. 1: Multiple skin-colored papules of keratosis pilaris over the arm.

Palpation may reveal a fine, sandpaper-like texture to the area. Perifollicular erythema is often present, indicating inflammation. Individual follicles show long strand of keratin glinting when examined inside light called the "antenna sign."

The variants include:

- KP rubra (red, inflamed bumps on the arms and legs)
- KP alba (rough, bumpy skin with no irritation)
- KP rubra faceii (reddish rash on the cheeks)
- *KP atrophicans*: Keratotic follicular papules with nonpurulent inflammation and atrophic end stages that are characterized by irreversible hair loss and atrophic depressions. This entity includes KP atrophicans faciei, keratosis follicularis spinulosa decalvans, and atrophoderma vermiculatum.

ASSOCIATED CONDITIONS

Associated conditions include ichthyosis, atopic dermatitis, Noonan/cardiofacial syndrome, renal insufficiency, prolidase deficiency, Down syndrome, monilethrix, pachyonychia congenita, and ectodermal dysplasia.

DERMOSCOPY

Dermoscopic features of KP include the presence of hairs that are frequently coiled, semicircular, or looped, or embedded in the stratum corneum and perifollicular erythema. Hairs may emerge in groups of two or three.

HISTOPATHOLOGY

A triad of hyperkeratosis, hypergranulosis, and follicular plugging is seen on histopathology. The upper dermis may have some mild superficial perivascular lymphocytic inflammatory changes.

DIFFERENTIAL DIAGNOSIS

- *Acne vulgaris*—facial lesions are also present, but not present on thighs
- *Atopic dermatitis*—other features of atopy
- Eruptive vellus hair cysts
- *Folliculitis*—pustules are prominent.
- Keratosis follicularis
- *Kyrle disease*—can be found at any site; elimination of keratin and underlying liver/renal disease
- *Lichen nitidus*—hypopigmented papules in groups over extremities, claw-clutching ball appearance on histopathological examination (HPE)
- Lichen spinulosus
- Milia
- *Perforating folliculitis*—elimination of keratin from hair follicle
- *Pityriasis rubra pilaris*—widespread lesions with islands of sparing and keratotic sandal are seen.
- Trichostasis spinulosa
- *Ulerythema ophryogenes*—lesions are mainly over the face and neck; atrophic lesions are seen.
- Xerosis

➲ TREATMENT

Moisturizing lotions soothe the skin and help it look better; skin creams that contain urea, lactic acid, glycolic acid, salicylic acid, retinoids, or vitamin D are used. Steroid creams reduce redness. Minor surgical procedures, such as gentle acne extractions, microdermabrasion, and chemical peels, may be useful in resistant KP. Systemic retinoids, laser therapy, or other ablative procedures may be tried in severe and resistant cases.

➲ PROGNOSIS

Keratosis pilaris becomes more exaggerated at puberty; it frequently improves with age.

➲ SUGGESTED READING

1. Maghfour J, Ly S, Haidari W, Taylor SL, Feldman SR. Treatment of keratosis pilaris and its variants: a systematic review. J Dermatolog Treat. 2022;33(3):1231-42.

123 Koilonychia

SYNONYMS

Thin spoon-shaped nails, Koilos = hollow.

ETIOLOGY

Koilonychias may be inherited as an autosomal dominant trait, or it may be associated with other syndromes. It is seen commonly with anemia (Plummer–Vinson syndrome), hyperthyroidism, cachexia, cheilosis, glossitis, chemotherapy, malnutrition, and as an occupational nail disorder in automotive workers, coil winders, glass workers, hairdressers, organic chemists, rickshaw pullers (especially the toenails), and slaughterhouse workers. Temporary koilonychias are normal in early childhood, especially of the great toenail.

The changes may be due to anoxia of the distal nail matrix.

CLINICAL FEATURES

Koilonychia is dystrophy of the fingernails in which they are thinned and concave with raised edges. In a sense, it is the opposite of clubbing. Koilonychia affects fingers more frequently than toes. The thumb, index, and middle fingernails are commonly involved. The affected nails may be thickened, thinned, softened, or normal **(Fig. 1)**.

ASSOCIATED CONDITIONS

Koilonychia is associated with trichothiodystrophy, palmoplantar keratoderma, progeria, pangeria, incontinentia pigmenti, psoriasis, alopecia areata, focal dermal hypoplasia, LEOPARD syndrome, monilethrix, nail–patella syndrome, Cronkhite–Canada syndrome, Nezelof syndrome, Oliver–Mcfarlane syndrome, lichen planus, lichen striatus, Darier's disease, acanthosis nigricans, and Raynaud's phenomenon.

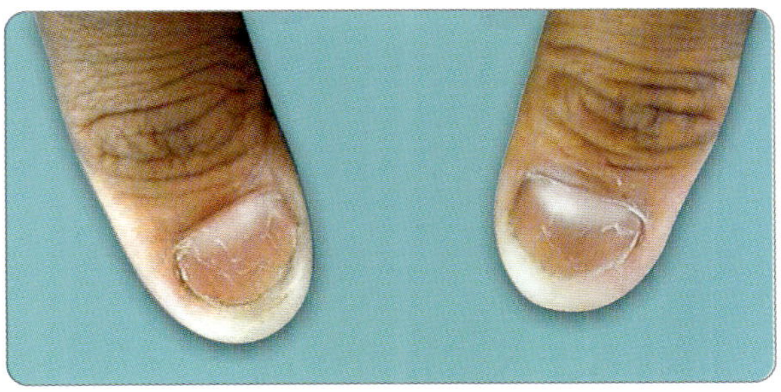

Fig. 1: Flat spoon-shaped nails in koilonychia.

The serrated koilonychia syndrome combines spooning of the nails with transverse grooves.

➲ TREATMENT

Koilonychia is treated by buffing the surface of the nail plate and applying acrylic gel. Preformed prosthetic plastic nails may be employed for short periods.

➲ SUGGESTED READING

1. Walker J, Baran R, Vélez N, Jellinek N. Koilonychia: an update on pathophysiology, differential diagnosis and clinical relevance. J Eur Acad Dermatol Venereol. 2016;30(11):1985-91.

124 Leishmaniasis

SYNONYMS

Old World Cutaneous Leishmaniasis (*Synonyms: Oriental Sore, Biskra Button, Delhi Boil, and Baghdad Boil*).

ETIOLOGY

Leishmaniasis is a protozoal infection caused by the genus *Leishmania*, transmitted by the bite of the sandfly.

CLINICAL FEATURES

The vector of Indian kala-azar is *Phlebotomus argentipes*; those for cutaneous leishmaniasis are *Phlebotomus papatasi* and *Phlebotomus sergenti*.

- *Cutaneous leishmaniasis of Leishmania major*: The initial lesion is a nodule, which gradually enlarges to form a crust and ulcer with raised red margins. Healing occurs in 2–6 months with scarring.
- *Cutaneous leishmaniasis of Leishmania tropica*: The lesion presents as an itchy brown papule or nodule and forms an infiltrated plaque 1–2 cm in diameter over a period of about 6 months; it ulcerates at the center, forming a crust. It heals with a typical depressed cribriform scar. Leishmaniasis recidivans is a chronic, relapsing form of *L. tropica* infection affecting usually the face and presenting with much scarring.
- *Cutaneous leishmaniasis of Leishmania aethiopica*: Cutaneous lesions resemble those due to *L. tropica*.

INVESTIGATIONS

Diagnostic methods include visualization of the characteristic amastigote in smears or tissue (histopathology), parasite isolation by in vitro culture, and molecular detection of parasite DNA.

Slit skin smears can be used to identify parasites and confirm diagnosis. Serological tests include direct agglutination test, enzyme-linked immunosorbent assay (ELISA), and the rK39 rapid diagnostic ELISA. Histopathology shows upper dermal mixed chronic infiltrate of lymphocytes, macrophages, plasma cells, and sometimes necrotizing granulomas. *Leishmania donovani* bodies in macrophages or extracellularly can confirm the diagnosis.

Other tests which can be employed are DNA amplification methods [polymerase chain reaction (PCR), nested PCR, quantitative PCR (qPCR), loop-mediated isothermal amplification (LAMP)], serum interleukin-10 (IL-10), and adenosine deaminase (ADA) levels.

Disseminated Cutaneous Leishmaniasis

Disseminated cutaneous leishmaniasis starts as a single nonulcerating nodular lesion on the face. The lesions disseminate over the whole body, affecting the face, limbs, and buttocks mainly. Mucous membranes are usually spared.

Differential Diagnosis

- *Pyodermas*—gram-positive organisms
- Tropical ulcers
- *Buruli ulcers*—demonstration of mycobacteria on Ziehl–Neelsen (ZN) stain
- Syphilis
- Yaws
- Tuberculosis (cutaneous)
- Nocardiosis
- Sporotrichosis
- Basal cell and squamous cell epitheliomas

Visceral Leishmaniasis (*Synonym: Kala-Azar*) and Post-kala-azar Dermal Leishmaniasis (*Synonym: Dermal Leishmanoid*)

Visceral leishmaniasis is caused by viscerotropic leishmania of the *L. donovani* complex.

- *Visceral Leishmaniasis*: A majority of infections are inapparent and subclinical. If untreated, it ends fatally due to massive parasite load.
- The incubation period for visceral leishmaniasis varies from 1 to 3 months. Symptoms include high-grade fever, fatigue, cough, diarrhea, and epistaxis. There is massive splenomegaly, a smaller hepatomegaly, and generalized lymphadenopathy.
- *Post Kala-azar Dermal Leishmaniasis (PKDL)*: PKDL is a late cutaneous manifestation.
- *African PKDL:* It starts toward the end of treatment, with an incubation period ranging from 0 to 9 months. A papular rash develops in convalescence, appearing on the face and limbs, and heals spontaneously over a period of a few months. The Montenegro reaction is positive, and the histology of the papules is tuberculoid.
- *Indian PKDL:* It appears 2 years or more following recovery from visceral leishmaniasis. The lesions include hypopigmented macules, nodular lesions, verrucous, papillomatous, hypertrophic, and xanthomatous lesions.

Differential Diagnosis

Differential diagnosis includes leprosy, pityriasis versicolor, pityriasis rosea, phrynoderma, scars, nevi, pityriasis alba, nutritional dyschromias, onchocerciasis, postherpes zoster hypopigmentation, nevus anemicus, syphilis, onchocerciasis, mycosis fungoides, leukemia cutis, secondary deposits of internal malignancies, nodular lesions of neurofibromatosis, and sarcoidosis.

MANAGEMENT

- Local treatments are recommended for uncomplicated/simple cutaneous leishmaniasis [infection with species not likely to be associated with mucosal leishmaniasis (ML), no mucosal involvement, single lesion or a few lesions, small lesion size (<1 cm), and immunocompetent host], while systemic treatment is recommended for complex cutaneous leishmaniasis [infection with species associated with ML, >4 lesions of significant size (>1 cm), individual lesions ≥5 cm, subcutaneous nodules, regional adenopathy >1 cm size, size or location of lesions for which local treatment is not feasible, lesions on the face, fingers, toes, or genitalia, immunosuppressed host, and clinical failure of local therapy after 2–3 months post-treatment].
- *Local treatment for simple leishmaniasis*: Eschars should be debrided, and secondary wound infection should be managed prior to the administration of local therapy to maximize treatment effect. Modalities used are cryosurgery, thermotherapy [a radiofrequency instrument, ThermoMed, has received the Food and Drug Administration (FDA) approval for this purpose], intralesional injection of sodium stibogluconate or meglumine antimoniate, topical paromomycin, topical WR279,396 (15% paromomycin and 0.5% gentamicin), and photodynamic therapy (PDT).
- Complex cutaneous leishmaniasis warrants systemic therapy like oral fluconazole (200–400 mg OD for 6 weeks), oral ketoconazole (600 mg OD for 28 days), oral miltefosine (2.5 mg/kg/day for 28 days), sodium stibogluconate/meglumine antimoniate [20 mg/kg/day intravenous/intramuscular (IV/IM) for 10–20 days], amphotericin B deoxycholate, liposomal amphotericin B, and pentamidine isethionate.

SUGGESTED READING

1. Torres-Guerrero E, Quintanilla-Cedillo MR, Ruiz-Esmenjaud J, Arenas R. Leishmaniasis: a review. F1000Res. 2017;6:750.

125 Lentigo

SYNONYMS

Lentigine, beauty spot, liver spots, or age spots; derived from Latin word for lens, "lentil."

ETIOLOGY

Lentigo is caused by chronic sun exposure. Heredity does seem to play a role, as fair-skinned individuals may develop them more easily. Although age is sometimes blamed for lentigo, older individuals have more cumulative sun exposure and therefore are more likely to have lentigo.

EPIDEMIOLOGY

Lentigo is most frequently seen in adults >30 years, and it occurs most commonly on the sun-exposed skin, the face, the back of the hands, the arms, the chest, and the lower legs.

CLINICAL FEATURES

- *Lentigo simplex* is the most common form, which may be acquired or congenital. The lesions are sharply circumscribed, pigmented, light brown or dark brown macules, <5 mm, occurring as isolated lesions on the skin, nails, and mucous membranes. Unique varieties of lentigo simplex on genitalia have been called genital lentiginosis.
- *Nevus spilus*: The tan macular background pigmentation ranges from <1 to >10 cm in diameter, primarily on the torso and extremities.
- *Agminated lentigines* are a circumscribed group of small, pigmented macules arranged often in a segmental pattern, each macule consisting of a lentiginous epidermal proliferation of melanocytes.
- *Solar lentigo* directly correlates with increasing age and sun exposure.
- *PUVA lentigines*: Phototoxic doses of photochemotherapy lead to the development of lentigines 6–8 months later.
- *Ink spot lentigo*: It is also known as reticulated lentigo, fewer in number, dark brown to black, irregular ink spot-like macule.
- *Tanning bed lentigo*: It follows indoor tanning.
- *Generalized lentigines*—also known as lentigines profusa or multiple lentigines. They are found on an exposed or covered site from childhood.

- *Patterned lentigines*—inherited tendency to lentigines on the face, lips, buttocks, palms, and soles
- *Centrofacial neurodysraphic lentiginosis*: It is associated with intellectual disability.

➲ ASSOCIATED SYNDROMES

Associated syndromes include LEOPARD (lentigines, ECG conduction defects, ocular hypertelorism, pulmonary stenosis, abnormal genitalia, growth retardation, and deafness) syndrome, NAME (nevi, atrial myxoma, myxoid neurofibroma, and ephelides), LAMB (lentigines, atrial and mucocutaneous myxomas, and blue nevi) syndrome, Peutz–Jeghers syndrome, FACES syndrome, Tay's syndrome, Sotos syndrome, Laugier–Hunziker, Moynahan, Xeroderma pigmentosum, Ruvalcaba–Myhre–Smith, Bannayan–Zonana syndrome, and Cowden disease **(Fig. 1)**.

➲ DERMOSCOPY

Dermoscopy shows faint pigmented fingerprint structures or a structureless pattern. Frequently, a delicate, light brown pseudo-network with well-defined borders and a "moth-eaten" edge is recognizable.

➲ HISTOPATHOLOGY

Lentigo simplex consists of intraepidermal melanocytic hyperplasia in the basal layer of elongated epidermal rete ridges, without nest formation.

➲ DIFFERENTIAL DIAGNOSIS

- *Actinic keratosis*—crusted lesions
- *Ephelides (freckles)*—only photoexposed areas are seen; mucosa is spared, and seasonal variation is seen.
- Seborrheic keratosis

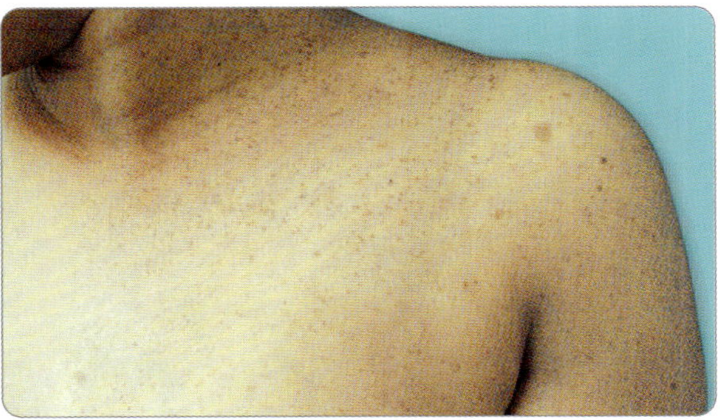

Fig. 1: Unilateral lentiginosis.

➲ COMPLICATIONS

There are no known complications from lentigo simplex. Complications arise from the associated syndromes. Atypical varieties of lentigo simplex (in any anatomic site) may be potential precursors or masqueraders of melanoma.

➲ TREATMENT

Photoprotection is important. Topical retinoids, cysteamine, hydroquinone, alpha hydroxyl acids, azelaic acids, chemical peels, cryotherapy, pigment lasers, intense pulse light, or simple surgical excision are the treatment options. Combination therapy gives the best results.

➲ PROGNOSIS

The long-term course and malignant potential of agminated lentigines are unknown.

126 Leukocytoclastic Vasculitis

SYNONYMS

Cutaneous small-vessel vasculitis (CSVV), hypersensitivity angitis, cutaneous necrotizing venulitis.

ETIOLOGY

Leukocytoclastic vasculitis is the most common form of vasculitis. About 50% are idiopathic, 15–20% due to infection, 15–20% related to inflammatory diseases (such as collagen vascular disorders), 10–15% due to medications and other drugs, and <5% are associated with malignancy. Circulating immune complexes are identified in a majority of patients.

CLINICAL FEATURE

Patients present 7–10 days after exposure to an inciting agent with a single crop of lesions consisting of palpable purpura, erythematous papules, vesicles, or urticarial lesions **(Fig. 1)**. Occasionally, pustules and erythema multiforme-like lesions are seen. Palpable purpura is the hallmark cutaneous sign. Lesions favor dependent areas, as well as areas affected by trauma (pathergy) or under tight-fitting clothing. It persists for 1–4 weeks and heals with postinflammatory hyperpigmentation that may persist for months.

Constitutional and/or musculoskeletal symptoms, such as fever, weight loss, arthralgias, and myalgias, may accompany flares

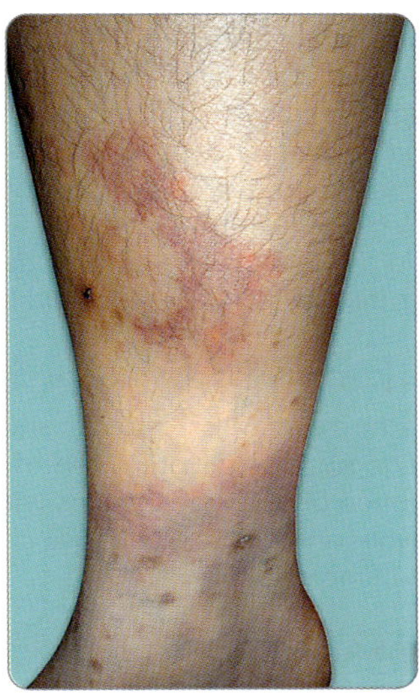

Fig. 1: Purpura and ulcers over the leg in leukocytoclastic vasculitis.

of CSVV. Gastrointestinal, genitourinary, or neurologic symptoms should raise the suspicion of systemic vasculitis.

DERMOSCOPY

Red globules and blotches in a mottled distribution on a milky-red background without scales.

HISTOPATHOLOGY

Biopsy of lesion within 18–24 hours duration shows infiltration of the vessel wall by neutrophils, deposition of fibrinoid [periodic acid–Schiff (PAS) positive] material in and around vessels, segmental inflammation in angiocentric pattern, swelling of endothelium, dermal infiltrate of neutrophils with fragmented nuclei (leukocytoclasia and nuclear dust), extravasations of RBCs. Resolving lesions may only show perivascular lymphocytic infiltrate.

Direct immunofluorescence shows immunoglobulin G (IgG) deposition. Sometimes immunoglobulin M (IgM) and immunoglobulin A (IgA) can be deposited.

Diagnosis of CSSV is a process of exclusion.

DIFFERENTIAL DIAGNOSIS

- Infective endocarditis—presence of Osler's nodes and Janeway lesions
- Wegener's granulomatosis—upper respiratory tract and kidneys involved classically
- Insect bites
- Septic vasculitis
- Benign pigmented purpura—absence of palpable purpura and negative histopathology examination (HPE) findings

TREATMENT

In the active stage of the disease, the basic instructions include avoiding stress, bed rest, elevation of the foot end, compression hosiery, and keeping extremities warm.

Lesions resolve with control of the infection, withdrawal of the causative drug, or removal of a tumor. Antihistamines and nonsteroidal anti-inflammatory drugs (NSAIDs) reduce symptoms such as pruritus and joint pain. Dapsone (50–200 mg/day in divided doses), colchicine (0.6–1.8 mg/day in divided doses), low-dose corticosteroid (<10 mg on alternate days), azathioprine, cyclophosphamide, methotrexate, or cyclosporine can be given.

PROGNOSIS

It depends upon the severity of systemic involvement, but in general, it is quite good. Approximately 90% of patients will have spontaneous resolution of cutaneous lesions within several weeks or a few months, while another 10% will have chronic or recurrent disease at intervals of months to years.

SUGGESTED READING

1. Fraticelli P, Benfaremo D, Gabrielli A. Diagnosis and management of leukocytoclastic vasculitis. Intern Emerg Med. 2021;16(4):831-41.

127 Leukonychia

➲ SYNONYMS

White nails, Greek words *leuko* ("white") and *onyx* ("nail").

➲ ETIOLOGY

True leukonychia is the result of defective keratinization of a distal matrix with the persistence of parakeratotic cells in the ventral nail plate. Apparent leukonychia is due to changes in subungual tissue, especially nail bed or from underlying onycholysis or subungual hyperkeratosis.

Pseudoleukonychia—nail plate/bed alterations of external origin as in onychomycosis and following application of fresh coats of enamel on top of old, worn enamel.

It is not due to any deficiency.

➲ CLINICAL FEATURES

- Leukonychia is a very common nail dyschromia. It is more common on fingernails than toe nails. True leukonychia is divided into total leukonychia and subtotal leukonychia.
- Total leukonychia may be due to hypoalbuminemia, familial, or drug-induced (sulfonamides).
- Subtotal leukonychia may be punctuated which is the most common type viz. alopecia areata, trauma; striate—due to a manicure (gift spots), transverse—arsenic and thallium poisoning, or longitudinal-parakeratotic focus in the matrix, seen in Darier's disease or a small tumor.
- Congenital leukonychia totalis—autosomal dominant/familial, it is a rare developmental anomaly where the nail plate is milky/porcelain white.

➲ ASSOCIATED CONDITIONS

Pili torti, multiple sebaceous cysts, renal calculi, palmoplantar keratoderma with deafness, LEOPARD syndrome, keratosis pilaris, congenital hypoparathyroidism.

Apparent leukonychia includes Terry's nail, half and half nail, Muehrcke's nail (lines run across the entire nail bed and occur in more than one nail), pallor of anemia, and macrolunula of leprosy.

➲ TREATMENT

No treatment besides attending to the cause of the problem.

➲ SUGGESTED READING

1. Iorizzo M, Starace M, Pasch MC. Leukonychia: What Can White Nails Tell Us? Am J Clin Dermatol. 2022;23(2):177-93.

128 Leukoplakia

➲ ETIOLOGY

Tobacco use, trauma, and mechanical irritation through dental stumps/ill-fitting dentures are the predisposing factors.

➲ EPIDEMIOLOGY

It is common in adults (50–70 years), with a 2:1 male predominance.

➲ CLINICAL FEATURES

Leukoplakia is a white patch/plaque on the mucosa that cannot be rubbed off and that is not recognized as a specific disease entity, thus more of a diagnosis of exclusion. Clinically it is divided into two subtypes:

1. *Homogenous leukoplakia*: White, flat, uniform lesion that may have a shallow crack and a smooth wrinkled or corrugated surface that is consistent throughout.
2. *Nonhomogenous leukoplakia/speckled/verrucous*: White and red lesions that may be irregular and flat, nodular (speckled), ulcerative, or verrucous. This has 4–5 times the malignancy risk compared to homogenous types **(Fig. 1)**.

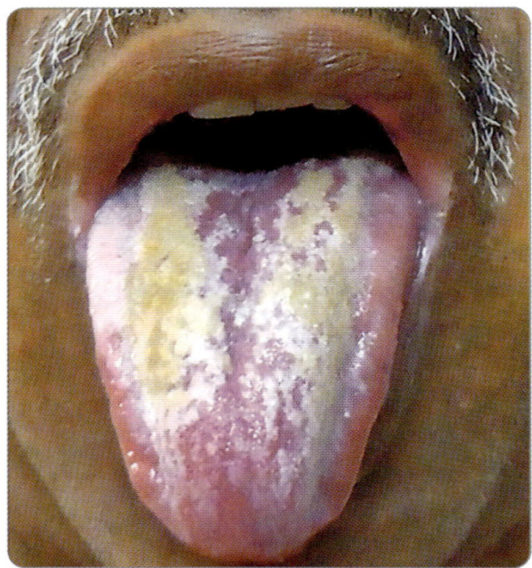

Fig. 1: White-coated tongue in leukoplakia.

DERMOSCOPY

White structureless areas of irregular shapes and translucency, whitish-pink veil at the periphery, whitish-pink clods, and thick lines.

HISTOPATHOLOGY

About 80% of the lesions usually demonstrate benign features with simple hyperkeratosis. Rest show epithelial dysplasia, in situ carcinoma, and invasive squamous cell carcinoma (SCC) picture.

DIFFERENTIAL DIAGNOSIS

- Candidiasis—easily removable white pseudomembrane which contains budding yeast cells
- Lichen planus—white patches classically in a reticulate pattern and not scrapeable
- Leukoderma
- Oral hairy leukoplakia—patches more on the lateral borders of the tongue, caused by Epstein–Barr virus (EBV)
- Habitual cheek biting

COMPLICATION

Squamous cell carcinoma.

TREATMENT

If there is no dysplasia or mild dysplasia, then regular clinical follow-up and cessation of potentially carcinogenic habits.

In moderate-to-severe dysplastic lesions, complete removal (surgical excision, CO_2 laser, and cryotherapy) and continued monitoring are advised.

PROGNOSIS

The rate of malignant transformation is 5–20%, 1 in 30 years. DNA aneuploidy is the most promising prognostic indicator.

SUGGESTED READING

1. Parlatescu I, Gheorghe C, Coculescu E, Tovaru S. Oral leukoplakia - an update. Maedica (Bucur). 2014;9(1):88-93.

129 Lichen Nitidus

➲ SYNONYM

Pinkus disease.

➲ HISTORY

In 1901, Pinkus described a peculiar papular eruption and termed it "lichen nitidus".

➲ ETIOLOGY

The etiology of lichen nitidus (LN) is unknown. It has been associated with and considered a variant of lichen planus as the early lesions of both conditions have clinical and histopathological similarities. Some unknown antigenic stimulus activates a cell-mediated immune response resulting in a collection of lymphocytes and other inflammatory cells. There is activation of Th2 type of immune response, which may explain the granulomatous response seen in LN.

➲ EPIDEMIOLOGY

Lichen nitidus is more prevalent among children or young adults, and a female predominance is described in the generalized or confluent type of eruption.

➲ CLINICAL FEATURES

It is characterized by numerous tiny, discrete, skin-colored, uniform, pinhead-sized, flat shiny papules distributed in groups over the flexor aspects of the upper extremities as well as the genitalia, chest, abdomen, and dorsal aspects of the hands **(Fig. 1)**. Pruritus can occur. The papules may exhibit a variety of pink, yellow, red–blue or brown hues. In darkly pigmented individuals, the papules tend to be hypopigmented, but sometimes they are hyperpigmented. They exhibit the Koebner phenomenon, especially in generalized form. Nail involvement is observed in up to 10% of patients (primarily adults) and changes include pitting, ridging, splitting, and linear striations.

Linear, spinous, keratodermic, vesicular, follicular, perforating, hemorrhagic, mucosal, and actinic are rare morphological variants. Lesions may be confined to the palms and soles, with a varied presentation such as bilateral hyperkeratotic, fissured eczema, pompholyx-like or purpuric.

➲ DERMOSCOPY

Smooth, white, well-circumscribed 1–2 mm circular areas are seen with a brown shadow reflected.

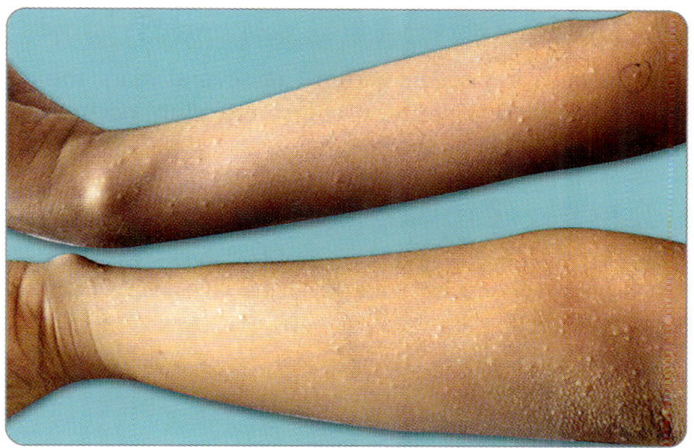

Fig. 1: Multiple discrete, skin-colored papules of lichen nitidus.

ASSOCIATED CONDITIONS

Lichen planus (25–30%), Crohn's disease, atopic dermatitis, juvenile chronic arthritis, trisomy 21, and congenital megacolon.

HISTOPATHOLOGY

It is very distinctive and characterized by a well-circumscribed infiltrate composed of lymphocytes, epithelioid cells, and occasional Langhans giant cells typically "clutched" by the surrounding hyperplastic rete ridges in a "ball and claw" configuration. In most lesions, the infiltrate is confined to the width of two to three dermal papillae. There is hydropic degeneration of the basal layer.

DIFFERENTIAL DIAGNOSIS

- Lichen planus—only focal basal cell degeneration and infiltrate seen
- Lichen striatus—linear erythematous papules along Blashko lines
- Guttate lichen sclerosus
- Lichen spinulosus
- Lichen scrofulosorum
- Verruca plana
- Papular sarcoidosis
- Id reaction
- Lichen amyloidosis
- Keratosis pilaris
- Guttate psoriasis
- Lichenoid secondary syphilis
- Frictional lichenoid dermatitis (elbows and knees)
- Papular eczema (especially in skin types V and VI)

TREATMENT

When significant pruritus is present, topical corticosteroids and oral antihistamines may be helpful. Topical calcineurin inhibitors are also effective in children. Generalized LN can be treated with either narrowband ultraviolet B (UVB) or photochemotherapy [psoralen plus ultraviolet A (PUVA)], steroids, retinoids, and cyclosporine.

➲ PROGNOSIS

Spontaneous clearing occurs within 1 or several years; the disease runs a chronic and persistent course. Healing occurs without scarring or pigmentary changes.

➲ SUGGESTED READING

1. Payette MJ, Weston G, Humphrey S, Yu J, Holland KE. Lichen planus and other lichenoid dermatoses: Kids are not just little people. Clin Dermatol. 2015;33(6):631-43.

130 Lichen Planus

HISTORY

It was described by Erasmus Wilson.

ETIOLOGY

Cell-mediated immunity plays a major role. The following sequence of events results:

- Specific antigen recognition
- Cytotoxic lymphocytic activation
- Keratinocyte apoptosis

EPIDEMIOLOGY

There is no racial and sexual predilection. It commonly affects patients in the age group of 30–60 years.

CLINICAL FEATURES

It presents as a purple, polygonal, pruritic, plane-topped, papulosquamous disorder. Wickham striae over the surface is visible after applying mineral oil. Lesions are symmetrically distributed over the flexural areas of wrists, arms, and legs. Koebner's phenomenon is seen **(Fig. 1A)**.

Clinical variants:

- Based on the configuration of the lesion—annular and linear
- *Based on the morphology of lesions*:
    - Hypertrophic lichen planus (LP)—verrucosus is the most pruritic form of lichen planus. "Fountain sign" is seen during the intralesional injection **(Fig. 1C)**.
    - Atrophic LP—is rare and may resemble lichen sclerosus.
    - Erosive and ulcerative LP—presents with chronic painful bullae and ulcerations over the feet **(Fig. 1D)**.
    - In vesiculobullous LP—vesicles and bullae develop over the lesions. It should be differentiated from lichen planus pemphigoides.
    - Follicular LP (lichen planopilaris, LP follicularis, peripilaris, and acuminatus)—may occur alone or in association with other forms. It is associated with cicatricial alopecia. Its variants are:
        - Pseudopelade form of Brocq
        - LP follicularis tumidus with oval pseudotumoral plaques of mastoid area
        - Postmenopausal frontal fibrosing alopecia
        - Lichen planoporitis with the lichenoid reaction centered over the acrosyringium and eccrine ducts entering the epidermis.
    - Lichen planus pigmentosus presents with dark brown macules in sun-exposed and flexural folds.

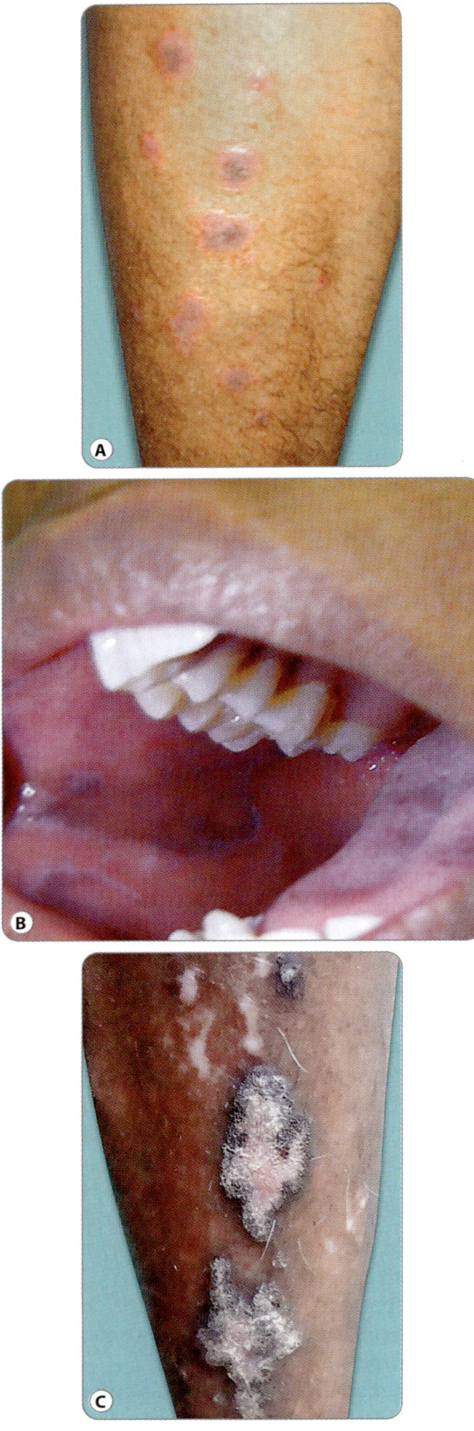

Figs. 1A to D: *Continued*

Continued

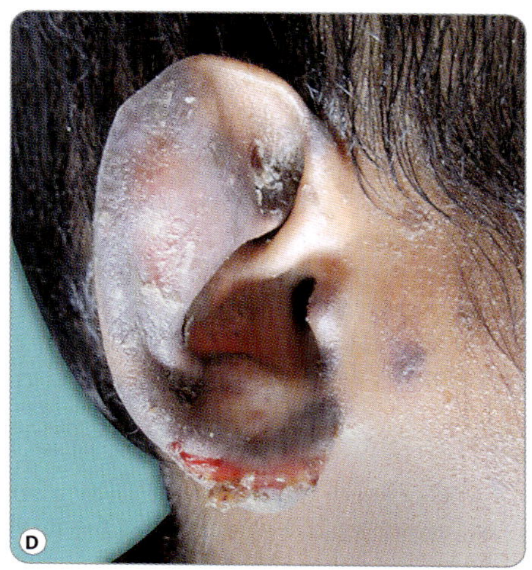

Figs. 1A to D: (A) Papules of lichen planus over shin with violaceous hue; (B) White lacy network in mucosal lichen planus; (C) Hypertrophic lichen planus; and (D) Erosive lichen planus.

- In actinic LP—pruritus is minimal, and annular lesions are seen commonly over the face.
- Perforating variant, guttate LP, and exfoliative and exanthematous form.

- *Based on the site of involvement*:
  - LP of scalp
  - Mucosal LP—only oral manifestation is seen in 20–30%. Reticular, plaque-like atrophic, papular, erosive, ulcerative, bullous, and gingival are various forms of oral LP **(Fig. 1B)**.
  - LP of nails—thinning, longitudinal ridging, onychoschizia, twenty-nail dystrophy, pterygium, and pup tent sign
  - Inverse LP—lesions occurring in flexural areas such as axillae, groin, and inframammary areas
  - Palmoplantar LP—yellowish compact keratotic papules/papulonodular lesions

Special forms of LP include drug-induced, LP-lupus erythematous overlap syndrome, LP pemphigoid, keratosis lichenoides chronic (Nekam's disease) lichenoid reaction, and the lichenoid reaction of graft-versus-host disease (GVHD).

➲ DERMOSCOPY

Polymorphic pearly white structures corresponding to Wickham's striae (rounded, arboriform "fern leaf" projections, reticular, and annular), vascular structures (red dots and radial capillaries), and brown or blue-gray globules. In addition, perifollicular scaling can be seen in lichen planopilaris.

➲ ASSOCIATED SYNDROMES

Graham-Little–Piccardi–Lassueur syndrome (lichen planus spinulosus, cicatricial alopecia of scalp, nonscarring alopecia of axillary, and pubic areas), vulvovaginal syndrome, Grinspan syndrome (hypertension and diabetes with lichen planus), and frontal fibrosing alopecia.

HISTOPATHOLOGY

On histopathology, there is hyperkeratosis, focal wedge-shaped areas of hypergranulosis, and elongation of rete ridges that resemble sawtooth patterns. Civatte bodies (apoptotic bodies or colloid bodies) are seen in the dermis. Separation of the epidermis in small clefts (Max–Joseph cleft formation) is occasionally seen. Basal epidermal keratinocyte damage and band-like lichenoid interface lymphocytic reaction are the two main features.

DIFFERENTIAL DIAGNOSIS

- Psoriasis—well defined plaques with silvery white scaling, mainly on extensors, scalp, and nail involvement seen
- Lichen simplex chronicus—signs of lichenification evident
- Lichen nitidus—hypopigmented papules in groups present, koebnerization seen, and claw clutching ball appearance on biopsy
- Granuloma annulare—skin-colored lesions, not very pruritic, palisading granulomas on biopsy
- Lichenoid drug eruptions—mainly over extensors, larger psoriasiform lesions seen, Wickham's striae absent, oral lesions rare, parakeratosis, and eosinophils seen in histopathologic examination (HPE)
- Lichen amyloidosis—hyperpigmented papules seen mainly on shins, homogenous eosinophilic masses seen at dermal papillae, positive apple green birefringence on Congo red staining and polarized microscopy
- Pityriasis lichenoides—scaly hypopigmented patches on the trunk
- Secondary syphilis—lymphoplasmacytic infiltrate seen, venereal disease research laboratory (VDRL) positive
- GVHD

COMPLICATIONS

The 0.5–5% of oral LP patients may develop squamous cell carcinoma.

TREATMENT

- *Cutaneous LP*: Topical corticosteroids fluocinonide 0.05% cream, clobetasol propionate cream, with occlusion can be given. Intralesional triamcinolone acetonide, systemic steroids, acitretin 30 mg/day, phototherapy, and cyclosporine.
- *Mucosal LP*: Good oral hygiene, topical steroids, systemic steroids, retinoids, oral griseofulvin, dapsone, and thalidomide.

SUGGESTED READING

1. Boch K, Langan EA, Kridin K, Zillikens D, Ludwig RJ, Bieber K. Lichen Planus. Front Med (Lausanne). 2021;8:737813.

131 Lichen Sclerosus

➲ SYNONYMS

Lichen sclerosus et atrophicus (LSEA), balanitis xerotica obliterans (men), kraurosis vulvae (women), lichen albus, white spot disease.

➲ HISTORY

The initial description of the disease was given by Hallopeau in 1889. Histological features were described by Darier in 1892.

➲ ETIOLOGY

The exact etiology is unknown, strong association with autoimmune disorders is seen. It may be familial (HLA-DQ7) or due to hormonal influence. The ratio of genital to extragenital lesions is 5:1.

➲ EPIDEMIOLOGY

It is 6–10 times more prevalent in women than in men. There are two peaks of onset, childhood and after menopause or fourth and fifth decades in men.

➲ CLINICAL FEATURES

Genital

The disease runs a relapsing and remitting course. Polygonal papules and porcelain white plaques with atrophic fragile skin, fissures, telangiectasia, purpura, erythema, erosions, and varying degrees of sclerosis are present in the anogenital area. Involvement of the vulva and anus in the figure of 8 patterns may be observed. Mucosal involvement at the edge of the mucocutaneous junction may lead to initial narrowing also referred to as a keyhole or hourglass appearance. Women experience intractable pruritus and dyspareunia. In men, lesions are usually seen on the glans and prepuce and are asymptomatic. Sometimes there may be phimosis, paraphimosis, painful erections, and decreased penile sensitivity. The end stage may manifest with balanitis xerotica obliterans.

Extragenital

Extragenital lichen sclerosus occurs on the thigh, neck, and trunk. Erythema may be the only initial sign. Lesions begin as white papules which later form plaques with follicular plugs on the surface (dells). Eventually, these dells disappear to leave behind smooth porcelain white skin. Telangiectasia may be seen **(Fig. 1A)**.

Koebner's phenomenon has been described in this condition.

ASSOCIATED CONDITIONS

Autoimmune thyroid disease, alopecia areata, pernicious anemia, morphea, and vitiligo.

DERMOSCOPY

- *Early lesion (<2 years)*: White, yellowish, or pale brown follicular plugs, homogeneous structureless white to pinkish white background, linear or dotted vessels, blue-gray peppered dots and globules.
- *Late lesion (>2 years)*: Poorly defined bright white or red structureless areas, white shiny streaks, linear curved or branching vessels, scattered blue-gray dots, and pigment network in sclerotic lesions.

HISTOPATHOLOGY

Compact orthokeratosis, follicular plugging, a thinned epidermis, hydropic degeneration of basal cells, homogenization of collagen in the upper dermis, and a lichenoid infiltrate at the dermoepidermal junction (DEJ) are seen **(Figs. 1B and C)**.

DIFFERENTIAL DIAGNOSIS

For extragenital manifestations:

- Guttate morphea—absence of follicular plugging, no lichenoid infiltrate, and thickened collagen in almost the entire dermis
- Atrophic lichen planus (LP)—lack follicular plugging, band-like lymphocytic infiltrate seen in the dermis
- Anetoderma—atrophic wrinkled skin seen over lesions
- Atrophoderma of Pasini and Pierini—cliff-like borders made out
- Idiopathic guttate hypomelanosis—angulated macules seen, no atrophy
- Psoriasis
- Bowen's disease
- Discoid lupus erythematosus (DLE)—mainly in sun-exposed areas

  For genital lesions refer to the section on balanitis xerotica.

COMPLICATIONS

Premalignant changes and squamous cell carcinoma.

TREATMENT

Ultrapotent topical corticosteroids, e.g., clobetasol propionate 0.05%, emollients, tacrolimus, tretinoin, calcipotriol, systemic retinoids, oral stanozolol, antimalarials, cryotherapy, and PUVA and UVA-1 phototherapy are given.

PROGNOSIS

It is a chronic condition with periodic waxing and waning. 4–5% of the cases may have a risk of developing squamous cell carcinoma.

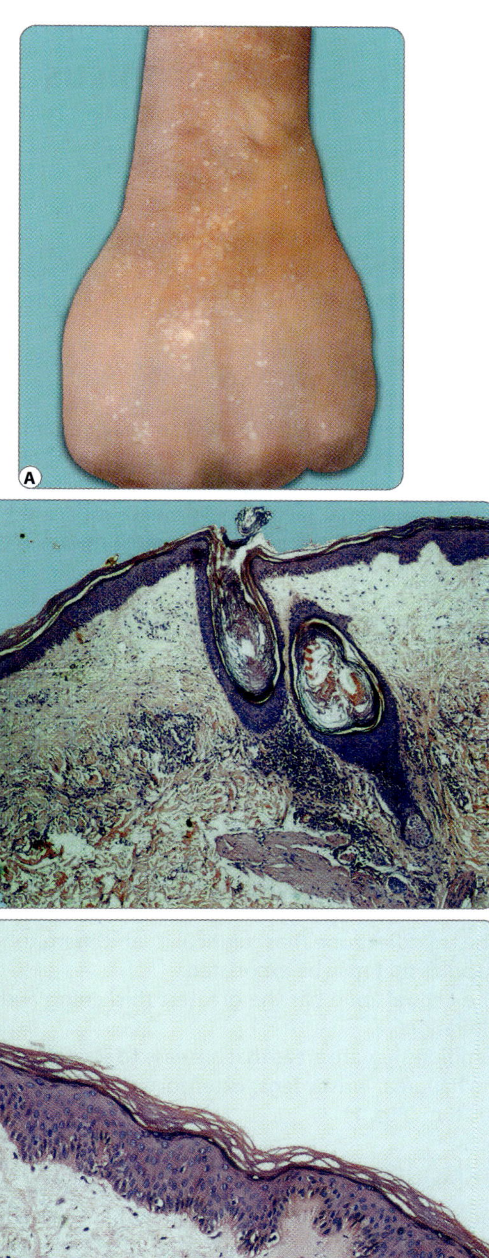

Figs. 1A to C: (A) White hypopigmented macules of lichen sclerosis. Koebnerization is also seen; (B) Thinning of rete with follicular plugging; and (C) Hydropic degeneration of basal cells.

➲ SUGGESTED READING

1. De Luca DA, Papara C, Vorobyev A, Staiger H, Bieber K, Thaçi D, et al. Lichen sclerosus: The 2023 update. Front Med (Lausanne). 2023;10:1106318.

132 Lichen Simplex Chronicus

SYNONYMS

Circumscribed neurodermatitis, lichen vidal, habit tic.

ETIOLOGY

The exact etiology is not known. It has been postulated that neurotransmitters that affect mood such as dopamine, serotonin, or opioid peptides modulate the perception of itch via the descending spinal pathway. Environmental factors such as heat, sweat, and emotional factors have been implicated. Atopics are more prone. Constant itching and scratching are responsible for lichenification.

EPIDEMIOLOGY

The condition affects adults between 30 and 50 years. Women are affected more than men.

CLINICAL FEATURES

Present with intensely pruritic, hyperpigmented, lichenified, and circumscribed plaques that may be surrounded by lichenoid papules. Each plaque may have three zones.

1. A 2–3 cm wide peripheral zone that is barely thickened may have isolated papules.
2. The middle zone has lenticular and hemispheric prurigo papules that may be excoriated.
3. The central zone has the greatest thickening and pigmentary alteration.

Common sites are areas that are easy to scratch such as occipital and nuchal area, wrists, legs, extensor aspects of arms, perineum, and scrotum **(Fig. 1)**.

DERMOSCOPY

Scalp lesion—erythema and scaling associated with shaft breakage, at the level of the scalp, into two or three shafts, hence appearing as short hair emerging from the single follicular unit—"broom fibers".

HISTOPATHOLOGY

On histopathology, there is hyperplasia of all epidermal layers. Hyperkeratosis, acanthosis, lengthening of rete ridges, and vertically arranged collagen bundles in the thickened papillary dermis are present. The chronic inflammatory infiltrate is in the dermis. The silver impregnation technique shows the proliferation of Schwann cells.

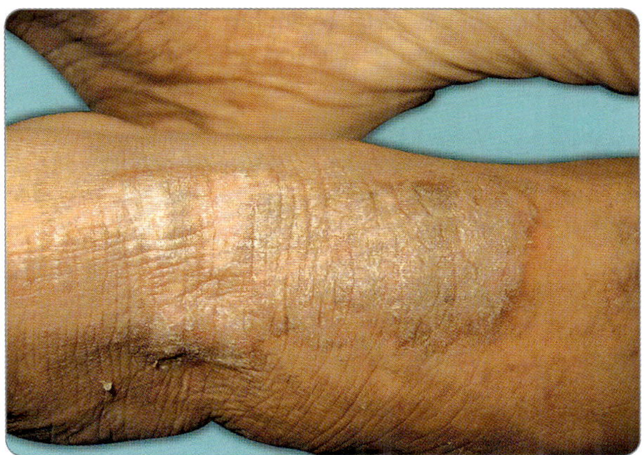

Fig. 1: Lichenified skin over the ankle joint showing increased skin markings, thickening, and hyperpigmentation.

DIFFERENTIAL DIAGNOSIS

- Atopic eczema—mainly involves extensors in infants and flexures in children, remissions and exacerbations seen, personal or family history of (h/o) atopy present
- Psoriasis—well-circumscribed plaques with silvery white scales, positive grattage test, and Auspitz sign
- Hypertrophic lichen planus—lichenoid band-like infiltrate and basal cell degeneration seen
- Contact dermatitis—flexures mainly involved, spongiosis seen mainly in histopathologic examination (HPE)
- Parapsoriasis
- Acanthosis nigricans—velvety hyperpigmented plaques seen, usually nonitchy
- Amyloidosis—patches with rippled appearance present, no lichenification
- Acne keloidalis nuchae
- Alopecia mucinosa
- Extramammary paget disease
- Phytophotodermatitis
- Pretibial myxedema—nonpitting edema present, mucin deposition demonstrated
- Stasis dermatitis—varicosities seen, hyperpigmentation, oozing, venous ulcers, atrophie blanche lesions evident

COMPLICATIONS

Sleep is disturbed. Violent scratching may cause excoriation, secondary infection, and depigmentation. Solid tumor-like plaques and giant lichenification of Pautrier may occur if the subcutaneous tissues are lax as in the genitocrural region.

TREATMENT

The main aim is to interrupt the itch-scratch cycle. Potent topical corticosteroids, menthol, pramoxine, emollients, intralesional triamcinolone acetonide, sedative antihistamines, capsaicin, calcipotriene, tacrolimus, cryotherapy, and UVB therapy help to break the cycle.

➲ PROGNOSIS

The disease has a chronic course and exacerbation may occur in response to emotional stress.

➲ SUGGESTED READING

1. Ju T, Vander Does A, Mohsin N, Yosipovitch G. Lichen Simplex Chronicus Itch: An Update. Acta Derm Venereol. 2022;102:adv00796.

133 Lichen Spinulosus

➲ SYNONYM

Keratosis spinulosa

➲ HISTORY

This condition was first recorded in the literature by Crocker in 1883. He named it "lichen pilaris seu spinulosus".

➲ ETIOLOGY

The exact etiology is not known. Atopy, infections, and hereditary factors play a role. Additional associations include seborrheic dermatitis, drug reaction, Hodgkin's disease, Crohn's disease, syphilis, and human immunodeficiency virus (HIV).

➲ EPIDEMIOLOGY

It is seen in children and adolescents.

➲ CLINICAL FEATURES

The disease presents with an asymptomatic lesion which measures about 2–6 cm in diameter and is composed of minute flesh-colored follicular horny papules, each with a central spinous process. The papules are grouped and are distributed symmetrically on the trunk, limbs and buttocks. The classic lesion of lichen spinulosus is a keratotic plug located within the dilated follicular orifice **(Fig. 1)**.

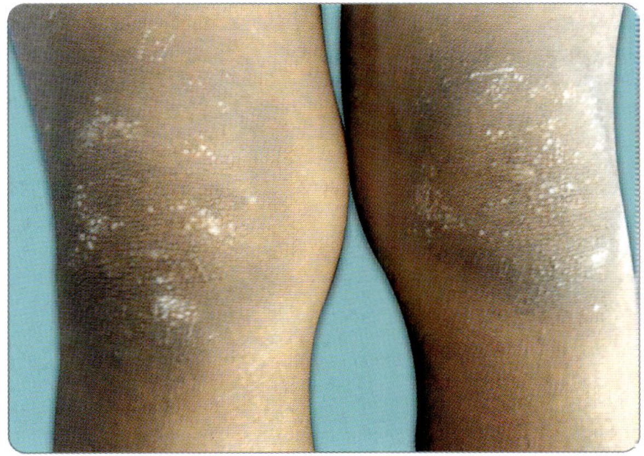

Fig. 1: Grouped hyperkeratotic papules in lichen spinulosa showing koebnerization.

DERMOSCOPY

Perifollicular scaling, normal interfollicular area, keratotic plug, and perifollicular white areas may be seen.

HISTOPATHOLOGY

Histopathological features are nonspecific and resemble keratosis pilaris. The hair follicle is dilated with a keratin plug. Mild perifollicular infiltration is present.

DIFFERENTIAL DIAGNOSIS

- Keratosis circumscripta
- Follicular ichthyosis—absence of keratotic plug
- Pityriais rubra pilaris—widespread lesions, a checkerboard pattern of hyperkeratosis seen
- Disseminate and recurrent infundibular folliculitis
- Frictional lichenoid dermatitis of children
- Hypovitaminosis A
- Phrynoderma—spiny papules mainly over elbows. Knees; other signs of deficiency such as bitot's spots in the eye may be seen
- Keratosis pilaris—mainly over posterolateral aspect of arms, and thighs; antenna sign positive, perifollicular erythema noted
- Lichen nitidus—hypopigmented grouped smooth papules seen, classical histopathologic examination (HPE) picture of ball in claw appearance
- Pityrosporum folliculitis—diffuse erythematous papules/ pustules seen over seborrheic areas
- Trichostasis spinulosa—dilated pore with retention of hair seen

TREATMENT

Keratolytic agents and emollients such as 12% lactic acid, 20–40% urea, and 6% salicylic acid are used. CO_2 laser helps in resistant cases.

SUGGESTED READING

1. Chu Antony C, Teixeira F. Acquired disorders of epidermal keratinization. In: Griffiths C, Barker J, Bleiker T, Chalmers R, Cremer D (Eds). Rook's Textbook of Dermatology, 9th edition. Wiley Blackwell Publishing House; 2016.

134 Lichen Striatus

➲ SYNONYMS

Linear lichenoid dermatosis, Blaschko linear acquired inflammatory skin eruption (BLAISE).

➲ HISTORY

In 1898, Balzer and Mercier first described a peculiar linear papular eruption that they termed "lichenoid trophoneurosis". Later, Senear and Caro proposed the name "lichen striatus".

➲ ETIOLOGY

The distribution of lichen striatus along Blaschko's lines points to somatic mosaicism. Environmental agents, particularly viruses, have been implicated. It may represent a manifestation of an atopic diathesis.

➲ EPIDEMIOLOGY

It is seen primarily in children between the ages of 4 months and 15 years; the median age of onset is 2–3 years, and the female:male ratio has varied from 1.6:1 to 2:1.

➲ CLINICAL FEATURES

The eruption consists of an asymptomatic, continuous, or interrupted band composed of discrete or clustered pink, skin-colored, or tan papules that are flat-topped, smooth, or scaly, and range in diameter from 2 to 4 mm. Typically, there is a single, unilateral streak on an extremity along Blaschko's lines affecting the limbs. Occasionally, a bilateral distribution or multiple parallel bands may be seen. Nail changes may include longitudinal ridging, splitting, onycholysis, nail loss, hyperkeratosis of the nail bed, thinning or thickening of the nail plate, nail pitting, onychodystrophy, punctuate and striate leukonychia, and overcurvature of the nail plate **(Fig. 1)**.

➲ DERMOSCOPY

Brown to gray granular pigmentation, dotted vessels, and white scales.

➲ HISTOPATHOLOGY

Histopathology depends on the age of the lesion. The earliest change is spongiosis. Generally, there is a lichenoid tissue reaction with varying degrees of involvement of the hair follicles and sweat glands and ducts; the lichenoid inflammation that is occasionally

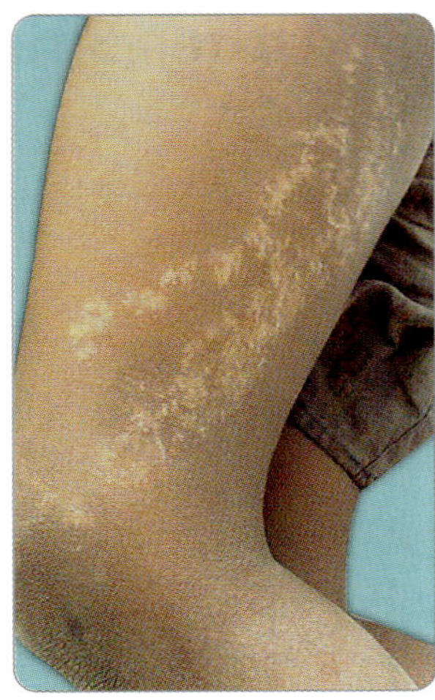

Fig. 1: Linear band of papules with hypopigmentation in lichen striatus.

present around hair follicles is indistinguishable from that seen in lichen planopilaris. Sweat gland and hair follicle involvement is a helpful diagnostic feature.

The epidermis shows intercellular and intracellular edema, exocytosis, parakeratosis, dyskeratosis, and focal or diffuse lysis of the basal layer in areas where the lichenoid infiltrate invades the epidermis.

DIFFERENTIAL DIAGNOSIS

- Linear lichen planus—classical lichenoid reaction pattern on histopathologic examination (HPE)
- Linear porokeratosis—lesions with raised furrowed hyperkeratotic rim, cornoid lamella on biopsy
- Linear psoriasis—psoriasiform reaction pattern on biopsy
- Inflammatory linear verrucous epidermal nevus—more hyperpigmented papules with warty surface, nevus cells on biopsy
- Linear Darier disease—corps ronds and grains in HPE
- Lichen nitidus
- Warts—koilocytes seen in HPE

COMPLICATIONS

Postinflammatory hypopigmentation, particularly in those with more darkly pigmented skin.

TREATMENT

No treatment is required. Topical corticosteroids under occlusion and calcineurin inhibitors have been used to hasten spontaneous resolution.

➲ PROGNOSIS

Most lesions resolve spontaneously. It does not usually recur; some relapses may occur either in the same site or in the same lateral side of the body.

➲ SUGGESTED READING

1. Payette MJ, Weston G, Humphrey S, Yu J, Holland KE. Lichen planus and other lichenoid dermatoses: Kids are not just little people. Clin Dermatol. 2015;33(6):631-43.

135 Linear IgA Disease

➲ SYNONYMS

Chronic bullous disease of childhood, juvenile dermatitis herpetiformis, juvenile pemphigoid, linear dermatitis herpetiformis, linear IgA bullous dermatosis.

➲ HISTORY

In 1970, Jordon et al. proposed the name "benign chronic bullous dermatosis of childhood".

➲ ETIOLOGY

- Autoimmune, associated with haplotype HLA-B8, -CW7, and -DR3.
- Autoantibodies are IgA1 and monomeric against BPAG2. In bullous pemphigoid, the pathogenic IgG antibodies bind the NC16 domain of BP antigen 2 (BPAG2; BP180), whereas the epitopes that have stimulated an IgA response in linear IgA disease (LAD) are more toward the carboxy terminus, i.e., toward the collagenous domain of the same molecule.

➲ CLINICAL FEATURES

Chronic Bullous Disease of Childhood

The mean age of onset is under 5 years. It is usually acute and the initial attacks are more severe than subsequent recurrences. Symptoms vary from absent or mild pruritus to severe burning. The face, perineum, perioral area, eyelids, ears, and scalp may be affected. The eruption may spread to the trunk, thighs, limbs, hands, and feet.

The lesions comprise urticated plaques and papules; annular or polycyclic lesions often have blistering around the edge, the string of pearls, or cluster of jewels sign. Mucosal involvement is common (oral mucosal ulcers and erosions, nasal stuffiness and bleeding, and conjunctivitis) **(Fig. 1)**.

Adult Linear IgA Disease

The lesions comprise urticated plaques, papules, vesicles, and blisters. The trunk is almost always involved, and the limbs, face, scalp, hands, and feet are also affected. The characteristic annular lesions with blistering around the edge are less common than in children. Mucosal involvement is similar to those in children.

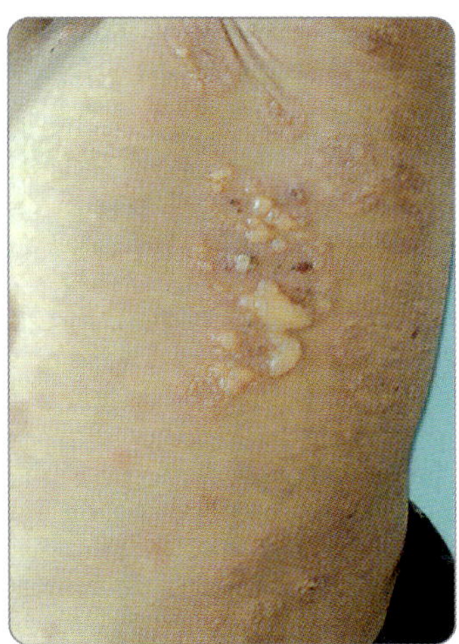

Fig. 1: Vesicles and bulla arranged in an annular pattern in linear IgA dermatosis.

Drug-induced Linear IgA Bullous Dermatosis

Vancomycin is the most frequently implicated drug. Others include penicillins, cephalosporins, angiotensin-converting enzyme (ACE) inhibitors, and non-steroidal anti-inflammatory drugs (NSAIDs).

HISTOPATHOLOGY

The subepidermal vesicles contain numerous eosinophils suggestive of bullous pemphigoid. In some blisters, neutrophils predominate, and dermal capillary microabscesses are seen, suggesting dermatitis herpetiformis. Others show subepidermal blisters with nonspecific features.

Direct immunofluorescence shows linear deposition of IgA along the basement membrane zone. Indirect immunofluorescence for IgA basement membrane zone antibodies is more often positive in children (about 80%) than adults.

DIFFERENTIAL DIAGNOSIS

- *Children—Bullous impetigo—demonstration of organisms*:
  - Genetic epidermolysis bullosa—scarring, hair and nail dystrophies, and negative direct immunofluorescence (DIF)
  - Papular urticaria—discrete lesions, no blister on histopathologic examination (HPE), and negative DIF
  - Childhood bullous pemphigoid—subepidermal blister with linear IgG and C3 deposits at basement membrane on DIF
- *Adults—atypical erythema multiforme*:
  - Dermatitis herpetiformis—smaller discrete vesicles that excoriate fast, papillary tip neutrophilic abscess, and granular IgA deposits at dermal papillae on DIF

- Bullous pemphigoid—linear IgG and C3 deposits in DIF
- Prurigo nodularis—negative DIF, absent bullae/vesicles

TREATMENT

- Topical steroids are used in mild disease.
- Low-dose corticosteroids 0.2–0.5 mg/kg/day, equivalent to prednisolone
- Dapsone 0.5 mg/kg, in young children, and 25–50 mg/day in an adult, may be slowly increased to a dose of 1 mg/kg or a little more in a child and 100–150 mg in an adult.
- Sulfamethoxypyridazine (0.5–1.5 mg/day)
- Other drugs include azathioprine, cyclophosphamide, tetracycline, mycophenolate mofetil, colchicine, etanercept, systemic retinoids, dicloxacillin, oxacillin, nicotinamide, methotrexate, cyclosporine, erythromycin, and intravenous immunoglobulin (IVIg).
- Monoclonal antibodies such as omalizumab can also be used.
- Rituximab is used in severe and recalcitrant cases.

SUGGESTED READING

1. Shin L, Gardner JT, Dao H. Updates in the diagnosis and management of linear IgA disease: a systematic review. Medicina. 2021;57(8):818.

136 Lipodystrophy

➲ INTRODUCTION

The term lipoatrophy is used when describing the loss of fat from one area (usually the face). This condition is also characterized by a lack of circulating leptin which may lead to osteosclerosis.

Lipodystrophy may be divided into the following types:

- *Congenital lipodystrophies*:
  - Congenital generalized lipodystrophy (Berardinelli–Seip syndrome)
  - Familial partial lipodystrophy
- *Acquired lipodystrophy*:
  - Acquired partial lipodystrophy (Barraquer–Simons syndrome)
  - Acquired generalized lipodystrophy
  - Centrifugal abdominal lipodystrophy (Lipodystrophia centrifugalis abdominalis infantilis)
  - Lipoatrophia annularis (Ferreira–Marques lipoatrophia)
  - Localized lipodystrophy
  - Human immunodeficiency virus (HIV)-associated lipodystrophy

LOCALIZED LIPOATROPHY

➲ INTRODUCTION

Localized atrophy may be seen following injection of medications viz. insulin, corticosteroids, antibiotics, heparin, growth hormone, and glatiramer; following panniculitis and morphea; or as primary idiopathic lipoatrophy.

➲ CLINICAL FEATURES

Lesions may vary from only a small dimple to an extensive, disfiguring area with much local loss of fat or firm fatty induration.

➲ HISTOPATHOLOGY

There is a loss of fat tissue, and inflammatory changes are conspicuously absent. In lipohypertrophy, there may be a replacement of mid-dermal collagen by hypertrophic fat cells.

➲ TREATMENT

Prevention is by constant alteration of the site of injection or by the use of more purified insulins.

LOCALIZED "IDIOPATHIC" LIPOATROPHY

This group of disorders predominantly affects the thighs, ankles, or abdomen.

CLINICAL FEATURES

- *Lipoatrophia semicircularis*: These patients show lesions on the anterolateral aspects of the thighs, characterized by a band-like circular depression, 2–4 cm in width.
- *Centrifugal lipodystrophy*: Lipodystrophia centrifugalis abdominalis infantilis affects the subcutaneous fat, usually of the abdomen and upper groin **(Fig. 1)**.

HISTOPATHOLOGY

Two histological subsets exist: Involutional and inflammatory. The adipocytes are small and embedded in hyaline connective tissue with many capillaries.

TREATMENT

Treatment is disappointing, although after the disease activity has ceased there seems to be regrowth of fat in 75% of cases.

The mainstay of treatment includes cosmetic surgery and management of complications.

CONGENITAL GENERALIZED LIPODYSTROPHY

SYNONYMS

Lipoatrophic diabetes, Berardinelli–Seip syndrome.

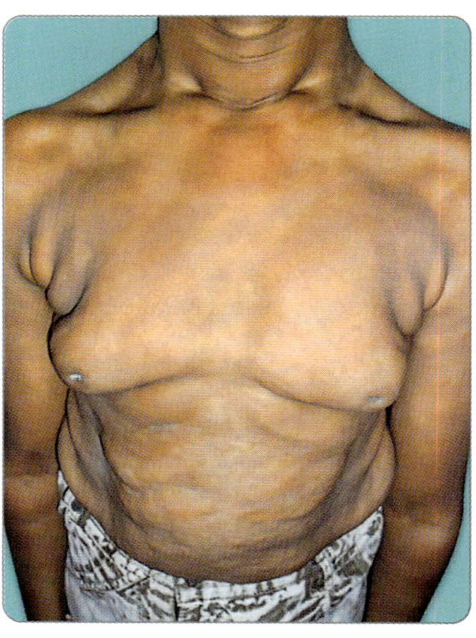

Fig. 1: Lipodystrophy.

➲ ETIOLOGY

Congenital generalized lipodystrophy type I (CGL1) was mapped to chromosome 9q34 and CGL2 to chromosome 11q13. CGL1 is caused by mutations in the *AGPAT2* gene.

➲ CLINICAL FEATURES

There is complete loss of subcutaneous and other fat, present at birth or before the age of 2 years.

➲ DIFFERENTIAL DIAGNOSIS

Donohue syndrome (leprechaunism).

ACQUIRED GENERALIZED LIPODYSTROPHY

➲ ETIOLOGY

- Type 1, acquired generalized lipodystrophy (AGL) with panniculitis (25%) **(Fig. 1)**
- Type 2, AGL with autoimmune disease (25%)
- Type 3 idiopathic (50%)

PARTIAL LIPOATROPHY

➲ SYNONYMS

Partial lipodystrophy, Barraquer–Simons disease, progressive lipodystrophy.

➲ ETIOLOGY

This rare lipoatrophy occurs as an incidental part of a widespread mesodermal atrophy. The condition is sometimes familial. It may follow an acute specific fever such as measles.

➲ CLINICAL FEATURES

The disease is characterized by the relatively slow, symmetrical disappearance of the facial fat, producing a cadaverous appearance and complete loss of the subcutaneous fat in the upper half of the body.

➲ HISTOPATHOLOGY

There is usually complete loss of adipose tissue over the affected areas.

➲ TREATMENT

New plastic surgical techniques, including free radial forearm adipofascial flaps, can markedly improve the facial appearance.

PARTIAL FACE-SPARING LIPODYSTROPHY

SYNONYM

Kobberling–Dunnigan syndrome.

ETIOLOGY

- Familial partial lipodystrophy type 1 (FPLD1)—no known molecular genetic basis
- FPLD2—results from heterozygous mutations in the *LMNA* gene encoding nuclear lamin A/C usually of an autosomal dominant pattern
- FPLD3—many different heterozygous mutations in the *PPARG* gene encoding peroxisome proliferator-activated receptor-γ (PPARγ)

CLINICAL FEATURES

It is characterized by a widespread but partial absence of subcutaneous fat usually sparing the face and neck but has a normal facial appearance.

TREATMENT

Management involves genetic counseling, attention to metabolic consequences, and exclusion of associated syndromes.

HUMAN IMMUNODEFICIENCY VIRUS-ASSOCIATED LIPODYSTROPHY SYNDROME

ETIOLOGY

The mechanisms of human immunodeficiency virus (HIV) lipodystrophy are complex. Lipoatrophy is associated with impaired adipocyte differentiation, increased apoptosis, insulin resistance, lipolysis, altered adipocyte cytokine expression, and mitochondrial toxicity.

CLINICAL FEATURES

Three patterns are described: Lipoatrophy, lipohypertrophy, and mixed.

They show marked loss of fat in the face, extremities and central subcutaneous fat accumulation. Omental fat accumulation produces a protuberant abdomen and an increased waist-to-hip circumference ratio **(Fig. 1)**.

HISTOPATHOLOGY

There is a diminution in the volume of subcutaneous fat. Foci of lymphoid infiltrates and lipogranulomas are seen. Scattered apoptotic adipocytes may also be present. Ultrastructurally, buffalo hump lipohypertrophy shows adipocytes intermediate between those in brown and white fat.

DIFFERENTIAL DIAGNOSIS

Human immunodeficiency virus-wasting syndrome.

MANAGEMENT

Choosing the right combination of newer highly active antiretroviral therapy (HAART) drugs and avoiding stavudine and zidovudine reduce the risk of developing lipoatrophy. The addition of a thiazolidinedione (pioglitazone) may be beneficial in lipoatrophy. Cessation of smoking, diet, and exercise help to achieve an appropriate body mass index (BMI). A statin or fibrate if triglyceride and cholesterol levels are high should be introduced. Metformin should be introduced for an overweight patient and pioglitazone for a lipoatrophic one. In severe cases, who do not respond to conservative treatment, tesamorelin can be considered. This is a growth hormone-releasing hormone (GHRH) analog that can be used to treat excess abdominal fat. Surgical interventions include autologous fat injection, flaps, and injection of fillers such as polylactic acid. Liposuction is helpful for buffalo humps. Simple lipectomy treats gynecomastia and lipomas.

SUGGESTED READING

1. Araújo-Vilar D, Santini F. Diagnosis and treatment of lipodystrophy: a step-by-step approach. J Endocrinol Invest. 2019;42:61-73.

137 Lipoma

➲ ETIOLOGY

It has been demonstrated that loss of negative-feedback control regulatory enzymes (by citrate or phosphofructokinase) may be an early feature in the development of lipoma.

➲ EPIDEMIOLOGY

Lipomas are more common in females after the age of 40 years.

➲ CLINICAL FEATURES

Lipomas are benign tumors composed of mature fat cells. They are found in the subcutaneous tissue and less commonly in internal organs. Lipomas are often lobulated, with a characteristic soft, putty-like consistency **(Fig. 1)**. The overlying skin is normal and moves freely over the tumor and feels cooler than the surrounding skin. The "slip sign", i.e., slipping of the edge of the lesion when pressure is applied with the finger, is positive. The common sites are the neck, shoulders, upper arms, back, and thighs. There are rarely any subjective symptoms, but pain from pressure on the nerves is sometimes experienced.

Another rare event is infiltration of adjacent tissues, particularly muscle. In these patients, there is a high recurrence rate after surgical intervention because of its diffuse infiltration. Thus,

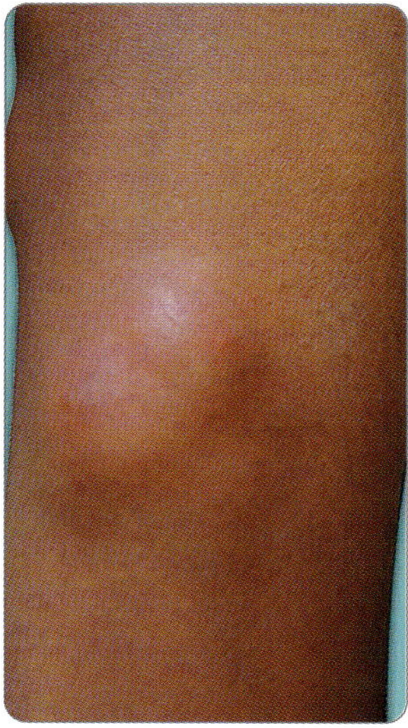

Fig. 1: Lipoma over the forearm.

complete surgical excision is often impossible. Variants include angiolipoleiomyoma, angiolipoma, chondroid lipomas, corpus callosum lipoma, intradermal spindle cell lipoma, neural fibrolipoma, pleomorphic lipomas, and superficial subcutaneous lipoma.

ASSOCIATED CONDITIONS

Gardner's syndrome, Proteus syndrome, Cowden's disease, Bannayan's syndrome, lipomatosis, adiposis dolorosa, and benign symmetric lipomatosis (Madelung disease).

HISTOPATHOLOGY

Fat cells in groups slightly larger than the normal lobule are typically enclosed within a capsule of connective tissue, but the capsule may be deficient and the tumor then appears locally invasive. Relatively large blood vessels are seen traversing the connective tissue septa. Xanthomatous and mucinous changes appear in many lipomas.

DERMOSCOPY

Under dermoscopy, a lipoma generally has nonspecific features, but a few characteristics might help in recognizing it:

- *Yellowish homogeneous background*: This reflects the fat content within the lipoma. The yellowish color is due to the fatty tissue being closer to the skin's surface.
- *Vascular patterns*: Lipomas may exhibit mild vascularity, showing *linear or arborizing vessels* due to the increased vascular supply around the benign tumor. These vessels tend to be finer and more scattered than those seen in malignant lesions **(Fig. 1)**.

DIFFERENTIAL DIAGNOSIS

- Neurofibroma—painful tumor, moves only along the nerve course
- Angiolipomas—proliferation of vessels seen along with mature adipocytes
- Lipofascial herniae in the natal or perianal region
- Epidermoid cyst

COMPLICATIONS

Fat necrosis may cause enlargement, pain, and tenderness. A large lipoma on the exposed skin of the lower legs is susceptible to nodular perniosis.

TREATMENT

This usually depends on the patient's desire for the lipoma to be surgically removed. Options range from steroid injection to surgical excision including liposuction. Other options such as laser-assisted lipolysis, radiofrequency ablation, cryotherapy, and ultrasound-assisted liposuction are also available.

SUGGESTED READING

1. Charifa A, Azmat CE, Badri T. Lipoma Pathology. 2022 Dec 5. In: StatPearls [Internet]. Treasure Island (FL): StatPearls Publishing; 2025.

138 Lupus Vulgaris

➲ SYNONYM

Tuberculosis cutis luposa.

➲ ETIOLOGY

Lupus vulgaris is a chronic progressive postprimary form of cutaneous tuberculosis occurring in a person with a moderate or high degree of immunity. It can also appear at sites of inoculation and in scrofuloderma scars as well.

➲ CLINICAL FEATURES

The acral areas, such as the nose, cheeks, rim of the ear, extensor surfaces of the limbs, lateral surfaces of buttocks, and breasts are favored. Usually, the lesions are solitary and very slow growing. The initial lesion is a soft erythematous nodule of 3–4 mm size which is slightly elevated above the surface. A few surrounding nodules may appear and later coalesce to form a soft plaque; the initial nodule may also enlarge and form a plaque. Healing occurs with atrophic scarring. Apple jelly nodules are seen in the dermis, floating like a piece of sago in tapioca pudding. On diascopy, findings become prominent; another clinical diagnostic technique is the use of a thin, blunt, or rounded probe. If the lesion is present on the nose, there may be central atrophy and shrinkage (the so-called "parrot beak" appearance). When gentle pressure is applied to the center of the lesion, the probe penetrates the skin; when it is withdrawn, often a drop of blood appears (match stick test). This is due to central epidermal atrophy. The other disorders with lupoid nodules such as sarcoidosis, lupus erythematosus, rosacea, and pseudolymphomas have an intact epidermis and are not easily penetrated.

The different types include:

- Lupus spot—the initial lesion which is a very small nodule.
- Lupus vulgaris planus—lupus spot slowly grows and becomes a patch.
- Plaque form—Nodules coalesce to form plaque
- Lupus vulgaris verrucosus—warty lesions appear due to pseudoepitheliomatous hyperplasia
- Lupus vulgaris tumidus (hypertrophicus)—large nodules and plaques
- Lupus vulgaris ulcerosus—necrosis of older parts of the lesions occur resulting in mutilation
- Lupus vulgaris vegetans—multiple papillomas develop at the edge of erosion
- Lupus vulgaris mutilans—ears and nose can be destroyed.
- Mucus lupus vulgaris—the most common site is nasal mucosa.

Often, the vestibule is affected. Oral lesions can occur. Lacrimal gland involvement can occur.

A positive tuberculin test will be seen.

➲ HISTOPATHOLOGY

Classical caseating tubercular granulomas composed of lymphocytes, plasma cells, epithelioid cells, and giant cells are seen. The epidermis may be flattened or atrophied. Acid-fast bacilli (AFB) are usually not found. The reticular dermis shows dense fibrosis.

➲ DERMOSCOPY

- Yellow-orange areas ("apple-jelly" nodules)
- Telangiectasias (*linear or arborizing vessels*)
- White structureless areas (*indicative of fibrosis*)
- Fine white scales (*in ulcerative areas*)
- Brownish pigmentation (*postinflammatory changes*)
- Erosions or ulcerations

➲ DIFFERENTIAL DIAGNOSIS

- Sarcoidosis—naked granulomas seen
- Leprosy—lymphocyte and macrophage granulomas mainly around neurovascular bundles, AFB can be seen
- Leishmaniasis—presence of LD bodies in a tissue sample
- Tertiary syphilis
- Lymphocytoma—collections of atypical lymphocytes in the dermis
- Discoid lupus erythematosus—mainly on sun-exposed areas, follicular plugging and dermal infiltrate seen
- Blastomycosis—demonstration of fungi, pseudoepitheliomatous hyperplasia seen
- Chronic vegetating pyodermas.

➲ COMPLICATIONS

Ulceration, crusting, and scarring with the destruction of underlying tissues and cartilage are seen (ulcerative and mutilating forms). Destruction and deformity occur less commonly in lesions on the trunk than on the face. Ectropion and distortion of the mouth are also possible in mutilating form. Development of squamous cell carcinoma known as lupus carcinoma can occur.

➲ TREATMENT

Category 1 ATT-2 $(HRZE)_{3+}$ $4(HR)_3$. Antitubercular treatment with 8 weeks of intensive therapy with rifampicin, isoniazid, pyrazinamide, and ethambutol. Continuation phase of 4 months with isoniazid and rifampicin. Surgical excision is done for single lesion cases.

Shortened regimens and newer drugs such as *rifapentine* and *bedaquiline* are being investigated for resistant or complicated cases.

Adjunctive treatments such as *photodynamic therapy, corticosteroids*, and *surgical interventions* are considered in specific cases.

For *drug-resistant lupus vulgaris*, more aggressive, second-line drugs may be needed.

➲ SUGGESTED READING

1. Couppoussamy KI, Shanmugam S, Devanda R, Murugan R. Lupus vulgaris: a narrative review. Int J Dermatol. 2024;63(4):431-7.

139 Lyme Disease

SYNONYMS

Erythema migrans, Lyme arthritis, Lyme borreliosis.

HISTORY

The disease is named after the town of Lyme, Connecticut, USA, where a number of cases were identified in 1975.

ETIOLOGY

Lyme disease is caused by a spirochete, *Borrelia burgdorferi sensu lato,* which is transmitted by Ixodidae ticks.

CLINICAL FEATURES

The only skin finding that is diagnostic is erythema migrans. 50% of patients recall a tick bite at the site of the lesion. The incubation period is about 3–32 days after the bite. Gradually expanding annular erythema appears around the papule of the tick bite. Classically, the innermost portion remains dark red and becomes indurated (thicker and firmer); the outer edge remains red; and the portion in between clears, giving the appearance of a bull's eye. It can grow up to 15 cm or more. Secondary annular lesions may appear ranging from 2 to 100. It gradually fades over months. Malaise, fever, fatigue, headache, stiff neck, myalgia, and lymphadenopathy can occur in the early stages. The chronic stage is acrodermatitis chronic atrophicans. Chronic arthritis of the knees, cardiac involvement, and neurologic involvement can occur.

In the late persistent infection, the cutaneous feature is acrodermatitis chronica atrophicans (ACA). ACA begins as a reddish-blue patch of discolored skin, often on the back of the hands or feet. The lesion slowly atrophies over several weeks or months, with the skin becoming first thin and wrinkled and then, if untreated, completely dry and hairless.

Two blood tests used to diagnose Lyme disease are a screening test [Lyme enzyme-linked immunosorbent assay (ELISA)] and, if that test is positive, a more specific Western blot assay. Cerebrospinal fluid (CSF) analysis and electrocardiogram (ECG) are needed to rule out nervous and cardiac involvement.

HISTOPATHOLOGY

There is superficial and deep perivascular and interstitial mixed cell infiltrate containing lymphocytes, plasma cells, and eosinophils. Warthin starry staining may show spirochetes in the upper dermis.

DIFFERENTIAL DIAGNOSIS

- Granuloma annulare
- Insect bite
- Erythema annulare
- Erythema marginatum

COMPLICATIONS

After treatment, some patients may still have muscle or joint aches and nervous system symptoms. This is called post-Lyme disease syndrome (PLDS).

TREATMENT

Oral antibiotics including doxycycline 100 mg BD, amoxicillin 500 mg TID, or erythromycin are useful in early stages. Treatment is given for at least 2 weeks. *Combination antibiotic therapy* is used to treat persistent or hard-to-treat cases of Lyme disease.

SUGGESTED READING

1. Steere AC, Strle F, Wormser GP, Hu LT, Branda JA, Hovius JW, et al. Lyme borreliosis. Nat Rev Dis Primers. 2016;2(1):1-9.

140

Lymphangioma Circumscriptum

SYNONYM

Superficial lymphatic malformation.

HISTORY

It was described by Fox and Fox in 1879.

ETIOLOGY

Lymphangioma circumscriptum results due to congenital malformation of superficial lymphatics.

EPIDEMIOLOGY

About 50% of lesions are present at birth and most of the rest manifest by the age of 5 years.

CLINICAL FEATURES

The characteristic lesion is groups of deep-seated vesicle-like papules resembling frog spawn. These vesicles represent superficial saccular dilations from the underlying lymphatic vessels that occupy the papilla and push upward against the overlying epidermis. The color varies from red to blue–black due to the presence of blood. Common sites are the abdomen, axillae, genitals, and mouth, particularly the tongue. Magnetic resonance imaging (MRI), lymphangiography, and ultrasound have to be performed to evaluate the lymphatic channels **(Fig. 1)**.

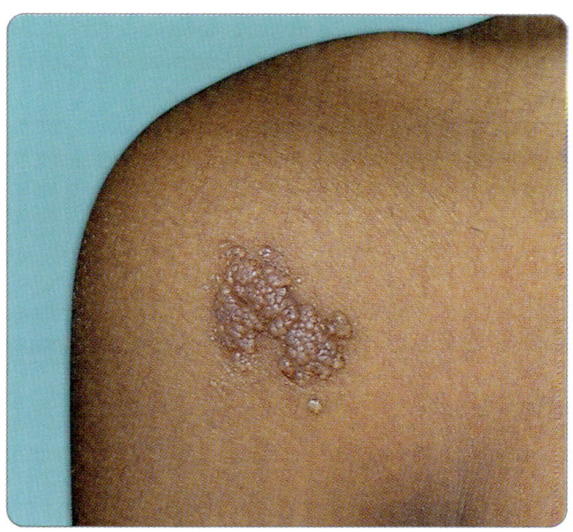

Fig. 1: Grouped papules resembling frog spawn in lymphangioma circumscriptum.

HISTOPATHOLOGY

The epidermis may be hyperkeratotic, with cystic places lined by endothelial cells in the papillary dermis which often contain lymph and RBCs.

DERMOSCOPY

The hallmark dermoscopic feature of lymphangioma circumscriptum is the presence of *multiple translucent or skin-colored vesicles*, often clustered in a group. These vesicles can have a *"frog spawn" appearance*, resembling clusters of small, fluid-filled sacs. Other features are *polychromatic vesicles, dark or reddish-brown areas* within the vesicles which represent dilated lymphatic channels.

Unlike melanocytic lesions, lymphangioma circumscriptum does not display a *pigment network* under dermoscopy, which helps differentiate it from pigmented lesions such as melanomas or pigmented nevi.

DIFFERENTIAL DIAGNOSIS

- Molluscum contagiosum—central umbilication will be seen
- Warts
- Herpes simplex—grouped lesions, symptomatic
- Herpes zoster
- Lymphangiectasia
- Metastatic carcinoma of the skin

COMPLICATIONS

Infection, hemorrhage, and malignant transformation.

TREATMENT

Excision and grafting, fulguration and coagulation, CO_2 laser vaporization, pulsed dye laser, and sclerotherapy result in the resolution of the lesion.

- *Surgical excision*: Definitive but may lead to scarring and recurrence if deep components are not removed
- *Laser therapy (CO_2, PDL, and Nd)*: Effective for superficial and deeper lesions with good cosmetic results
- *Sclerotherapy*: Good for larger or deeper lesions, often used in combination with other treatments
- *Radiofrequency ablation*: Minimally invasive with fewer recurrences
- *Cryotherapy and electrosurgery*: Useful for small or superficial lesions
- *Topical therapy*: Experimental and used for small lesions, especially in patients not suitable for invasive procedures

PROGNOSIS

Recurrences after treatment are common due to its deep component.

SUGGESTED READING

1. Patel GA, Schwartz RA. Cutaneous lymphangioma circumscriptum: frog spawn on the skin. Int J Dermatol. 2009;48(12):1290-5.

141 Lymphogranuloma Venereum

⊃ SYNONYMS

Climatic bubo, tropical bubo, lymphopathia venereum, lymphogranuloma inguinale, Durand–Nicolas–Favre disease, poradenitis inguinale.

⊃ HISTORY

Nélaton in 1890 and L' Hardy in 1894 pointed out the venereal nature of the disease. Durand, Nicolas, and Favre established its clinicopathologic entity in 1913. In 1930, the causative organism was identified.

⊃ ETIOLOGY

Lymphogranuloma venereum (LGV) is a sexually transmitted disease caused by *Chlamydia trachomatis serovars* L1, L2 (most common), and L3.

⊃ CLINICAL FEATURES

- *Primary stage:* The incubation period is 7–12 days. Primary lesion may be an asymptomatic transient papule, pustule, herpetiform ulcer, or nodular ulceration. The most common type is herpetiform, a superficial, painless, and evanescent lesion that leaves no scar.
- *Secondary stage (Inguinal syndrome):* This stage begins within 2–6 weeks of the primary stage. It is characterized by enlarged and tender regional lymphadenopathy or bubo. In one-third of the patients, enlargement of inguinal lymph nodes above and femoral lymph nodes below the Poupart's ligament occurs, resulting in the characteristic "groove sign of Greenblat." Inguinal bubo is unilateral in two-thirds of cases. Impending rupture is characterized by livid color (blue balls) of overlying skin. Perilymphangitis leads to the formation of adhesion with the surrounding pelvic organ, resulting in frozen pelvis.
- *Tertiary stage (Genitoanorectal syndrome):* It is seen in 25% of the untreated patients. Genital syndrome includes penile and scrotal elephantiasis, esthiomene, ramrod penis, and saxophone penis. Anorectal syndrome includes lymphorrhoids/perianal condyloma and hyperplastic and ulcerative changes in anorectal mucosa.

Papillary follicular conjunctivitis, episcleritis, and keratitis are the ocular manifestations.

Cutaneous manifestations include generalized exanthemata, widespread papules, pustules, nodules, scarlatiniform eruptions, urticaria, erythema multiforme, erythema nodosum, and erythema annulare centrifugum.

DIAGNOSIS

Chlamydial species can be isolated from bubo, rectum, and cervix using HeLa 229, baby hamster kidney cells, and McCoy cells. Elementary bodies and reticulate bodies are visualized in tissue scrapings by staining with Giemsa, Warthin–Starry, and Grocott's methenamine silver. Antigen detection is done by enzyme immunoassays, rapid assay, sure cell *Chlamydia* test, and clear view *Chlamydia* test. Antibody detection is done by complement fixation test, microimmunofluorescence test, single L-type chlamydial fluorescence test, radioisotope precipitation test, immunoperoxidase test, polymerase chain reaction (PCR), and restriction fragment length polymorphism (RFLP).

HISTOPATHOLOGY

The major diagnostic feature in lymph nodes is the presence of vacuolated macrophages with intravacuolar organisms.

DIFFERENTIAL DIAGNOSIS

- Genital herpes
- Primary syphilis
- Chancroid
- Tuberculosis
- Filariasis
- Granuloma inguinale
- Inflammatory bowel disease
- Actinomycosis
- Cat scratch disease
- Schistosomiasis

TREATMENT

The lesions heal with doxycycline, 100 mg BD for 3 weeks, or erythromycin/tetracycline 500 mg 4 times a day for 3 weeks. Azithromycin 1 g orally once weekly for 3 weeks is also an effective alternative regimen. In children and pregnancy, erythromycin stearate is prescribed.

Chronic manifestations of LGV, such as genital elephantiasis, vulval growths, esthiomene or rectal strictures, and stenosis, which do not respond to oral antibiotics, require surgical intervention and plastic reconstruction.

MANAGEMENT OF SEXUAL PARTNERS OF LYMPHOGRANULOMA VENEREUM

All exposed partners of LGV probable or confirmed patients in the last 60 days should receive testing and empiric treatment with a chlamydial regimen (doxycycline 100 mg PO BID for 7 days or 1 g azithromycin stat).

PROGNOSIS

Patients are followed up clinically until signs and symptoms resolve. This may occur within 3–6 weeks. However, routine morphological test of cure is usually not done.

➲ SUGGESTED READING

1. Rawla P, Thandra KC, Limaiem F. (2023). Lymphogranuloma Venereum. Treasure Island (FL): StatPearls Publishing. [online] Available from https://www.ncbi.nlm.nih.gov/books/NBK537362 [Last accessed January, 2025].

142 Lymphocytoma Cutis

SYNONYMS

Cutaneous lymphoid hyperplasia, Spiegler–Fendt sarcoid.

HISTORY

Cutaneous lymphoid hyperplasia (CLH) was first reported by Spiegler in 1894.

ETIOLOGY

Cutaneous lymphoid hyperplasia reflects an exaggerated local immunologic reaction to a stimulus, often unrecognized. Inciting agents include arthropod bites, reaction to tattoo dye, jewelry (especially gold), arthropod bites, medications, folliculitis, trauma, infections (*Borrelia burgdorferi*, herpes simplex, and herpes zoster), vaccinations, and acupuncture.

EPIDEMIOLOGY

Male to female ratio is approximately 2:1. It is a disease seen commonly after the fourth decade.

CLINICAL FEATURES

Cutaneous lymphoid hyperplasia is seen most often in adults over the face and neck. It presents as soft, doughy, or firm nodules (lumps). These range from skin-colored to red-brown or red-purple in color and occasionally have a scale or crust on the surface. Single nodules or a small number of lesions appear 72% of the time, and more numerous lesions are uncommon.

DERMOSCOPY

On dermoscopy, white reticular lines on pinkish background and some fine linear vessels crossing white reticular lines, perifollicular vessels, and white dots are seen in pseudolymphoma folliculitis.

HISTOPATHOLOGY

Normal epidermis separated by a grenz zone from the dermis is seen. Dense mixed infiltrate of lymphocytes, eosinophils, plasma cells, and histiocytes forming follicular arrangement is present in the upper dermis. The majority of lymphocytes are B cells.

DIFFERENTIAL DIAGNOSIS

- Jessner lymphocytic infiltrate
- Cutaneous lupus erythematosus

- Plaque form of polymorphous light eruption
- Syphilis
- Cutaneous T- and B-cell lymphomas (the follicles have only lymphocytic infiltrate, which is bottom heavy).

TREATMENT

Cutaneous lymphoid hyperplasia is a self-limiting condition. The first step is to remove any potential cause or offending agent. Topical or injected corticosteroids, topical immunomodulators such as tacrolimus, local radiation therapy, hydroxychloroquine sulfate, cryotherapy, photodynamic therapy with delta aminolaevulinic acid (ALA), surgical excision, and radiotherapy are available options.

PROGNOSIS

Benign course; a small proportion progresses to B-cell lymphoma.

SUGGESTED READING

1. Oliveira EV, Badiale GB, Moraes MM. Lymphocytoma cutis – case report. An Bras Dermatol. 2013;88(6 Suppl 1):128-31.

143 Melanoma

➲ HISTORY

The French physician René Laennec was the first to describe melanoma as a disease entity.

➲ ETIOLOGY

In light-skinned races, the risk factors include high exposure to sunlight in childhood, multiple sunburns later in life, multiple nevi, dysplastic nevi, large nevi, family history of melanoma, and immune deficiency. CDKN2A/p16 on chromosome 9 and CDK4 on chromosome 12 gene mutations are noted in familial melanomas.

➲ EPIDEMIOLOGY

Melanoma is slightly more common in men than in women (1.2:1). The average age of diagnosis is in the fifth decade.

➲ CLINICAL FEATURES

Melanoma is the malignant neoplasm of the melanocytes. Melanoma is relatively rare and makes up 10% of all skin cancer cases. It can start in an existing mole or develop in normal-looking skin. "ABCD" rule indicates malignant transformation of preexisting mole.

- *Asymmetry*: The shape of one half does not match the other.
- *Border:* The edges are ragged, blurred, or irregular.
- *Color*: The color is uneven and may include shades of black, brown, and tan.
- *Diameter*: There is a change in size, usually an increase of >6 mm.
- Evolving over time and elevated above skin surface
- Firm to touch

  E and F are for nodular melanomas.

There are four types of cutaneous melanoma:

1. *Superficial spreading melanoma (70–75%)*: It presents as a slightly raised lesion with an irregular border and variable, unevenly distributed pigmentation with shades of red, blue, brown, purple, and black. There is a long phase of horizontal growth prior to vertical growth and metastasis.
2. *Lentigo maligna melanoma (5–10%)*: It is a flat pigmented lesion, which gradually enlarges, light tan to dark brown or black with irregular notched borders. It is usually located on the face, neck, or arms of the elderly.
3. *Acral lentiginous melanoma (7–10%)*: Early lesion is flat, with irregular margins and pigmentation; the lesion rapidly becomes raised and nodular. The soles, the palms of the hands, the nailbeds, and the oral mucosa are usual locations. Early vertical growth and rapid metastasis are the characteristic features **(Fig. 1)**.

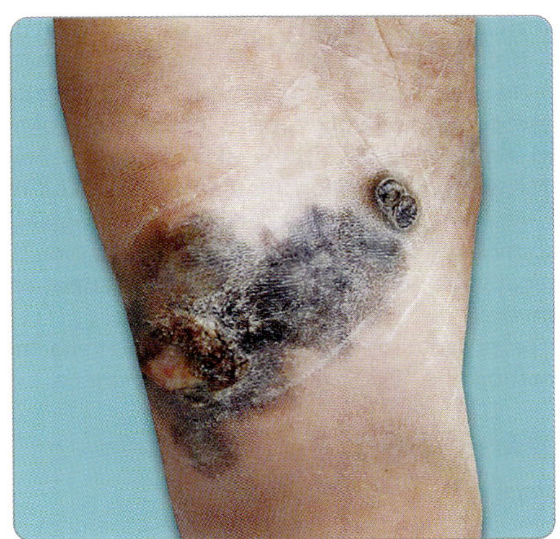

Fig. 1: Malignant melanoma.

4. *Nodular melanoma (15–20%)*: Raised, nodular lesion and sometimes ulcerated. Borders are irregular and color variegated. Occasionally, the tumor has no apparent pigmentation (amelanotic malignant melanoma). It does not seem to have a horizontal growth phase, and it usually grows vertically quickly with metastasis.

Lesions which greatly deviate from the common characteristics are labeled as an "Ugly Duckling," and the "Little Red Riding Hood" sign suggests that individuals with fair skin and light-colored hair might have difficult-to-diagnose amelanotic melanomas.

DERMOSCOPY

The Consensus Net Meeting on Dermoscopy in 2000 proposed a two-step algorithm for dermoscopic diagnosis of pigmented skin lesions.

Marghoob and Braun subsequently put forward a revised two-step algorithm, including polarized dermoscopy and blood vessel morphology. In this pattern analysis, the ABCD rule, the Menzies method, and the seven-point checklist are employed to diagnose melanoma.

- *Seven-point checklist* is based on seven melanoma-specific criteria and is classified into major or minor.
  - Major criteria (each given a score of 2): Atypical pigment network, blue-whitish veils, and atypical vascular patterns
  - Minor criteria (each given a score of 1): Irregular dots/globules, irregular streaks, irregular blotches, and regression structures
  - A score of 3 or more should be considered suspicious.
- *Lentigo maligna melanoma* shows asymmetric pigmented follicular openings, dark rhomboidal structures, slate gray globules, and slate gray dots.
- *Nodular melanoma* shows blue-black color within the lesion, ulceration, homogenous disorganized patterns, homogenous blue-pigmented structureless areas, multiple (>3) colors, a

combination of polymorphous vessels, and milky red globules/areas.

- *Acral melanoma*: Parallel ridge pattern (PRP) is the most specific dermoscopic finding. PRP consists of band-like pigmentation located on the ridges of the skin markings. The BRAAFF checklist was proposed for the diagnosis of acral melanoma, which includes four positive features, i.e., irregular blotches, PRP, asymmetry of structures, and asymmetry of colors, and two negative features, i.e., parallel furrow pattern and fibrillar pattern.

Other proposed diagnostic dermoscopic criteria include the Menzies method, the ABCD rule, and the CASH criteria.

HISTOPATHOLOGY

- *Clark staging*:
  - Level I: All tumor cells are above the basement membrane (in situ).
  - Level II: Tumor extends to the papillary dermis.
  - Level III: Tumor extends to interface between papillary and reticular dermis.
  - Level IV: Tumor extends between bundles of collagen of reticular dermis.
  - Level V: Tumor invasion of subcutaneous tissue (87% metastases)
- *Breslow staging*:
  - Thin: <0.75 mm depth of invasion
  - Intermediate: 0.76–3.99 mm depth of invasion
  - Thick: >4 mm depth of invasion

DIFFERENTIAL DIAGNOSIS

- *Dysplastic nevus*—absence of atypical melanocytes
- *Keratoacanthoma*—crateriform lesion
- *Pigmented basal cell carcinoma (BCC)*—basaloid cells in nests with peritumoral lacuna
- *Pyogenic granuloma*—reddish papules that bleed on touch
- Blue nevus
- *Lentigo*—focally increased melanocytes only in the epidermis
- *Seborrheic keratosis*—flat papules with wart surface and no atypical cells
- *Cherry angioma*—multiple reddish papules

COMPLICATIONS

Melanomas may spread by the lymph system or the bloodstream. The liver, lung, bone, and brain are the common sites of metastases.

TREATMENT

Wide surgical excision with regional lymph node removal is the treatment of choice. Adjuvant therapies are interferon alpha (2a or 2b), pegylated interferon, granulocyte-macrophage colony-stimulating factor, ipilimumab, dacarbazine, and interleukin 2.

Agents that can be considered in the treatment of advanced-stage (stage 4) melanoma include temozolomide, cisplatin, vinblastine, carmustine, tamoxifen, pembrolizumab, trametinib, vemurafenib, dabrafenib, and nivolumab.

➲ PROGNOSIS

With early diagnosis, the 5-year survival rate approaches 95%.

➲ SUGGESTED READINGS

1. Heistein JB, Acharya U, Mukkamalla SKR. (2023). Malignant Melanoma. Treasure Island (FL): StatPearls Publishing. [online] Available from https://www.ncbi.nlm.nih.gov/books/NBK470409/ [Last accessed January, 2025].
2. Kato J, Horimoto K, Sato S, Minowa T, Uhara H. Dermoscopy of Melanoma and Non-melanoma Skin Cancers. Front Med. 2019;6:180.

144 Melasma

SYNONYMS

Mask of pregnancy, chloasma.

ETIOLOGY

The exact etiology is not known. Contributing factors are hormonal therapy, pregnancy, and sun exposure.

EPIDEMIOLOGY

Melasma is more common in women (90% of cases), and the incidence increases after puberty.

CLINICAL FEATURES

Classification:

- *Based on distribution*: Centrofacial pattern (63%), malar (21%), **(Fig. 1)** and mandibular (16%)
- *Based on Wood's lamp examination*: Epidermal, dermal, and mixed patterns
- *Histopathological*: Epidermal and dermal

Melasma is symmetric, acquired hypermelanosis characterized by irregular, light-to-dark brown confluent or speckled macules with sharply demarcated or moth-eaten irregular margins, seen over sun-exposed areas.

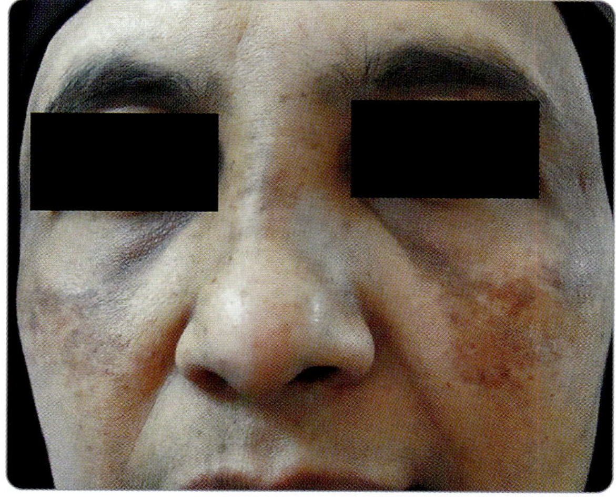

Fig. 1: Macular hyperpigmentation over the malar area and nose in melasma.

The Melasma Area and Severity Index (MASI) is a common outcome measure used to assess melasma patients.

HISTOPATHOLOGY

Hyperpigmented basal layer of the epidermis with slightly increased number of melanocytes. Some pigment is present within the papillary dermis as well (free pigment, scattered melanophages).

DERMOSCOPY

Dermoscopic features of the melasma reveal diffuse light-to-dark brown pseudoreticular network, multiple brown dots, granules, globules, and arcuate and annular structures, with sparing of the perifollicular region and around the sweat gland openings, increased vascularity, and telangiectasias.

DIFFERENTIAL DIAGNOSIS

- *Pigmented cosmetic dermatitis*—diffuse pigmentation
- Postinflammatory hyperpigmentation
- *Acanthosis nigricans of the face*—velvety pigmentation in patches
- Pigment demarcation lines
- *Poikiloderma*—presence of mottled pigmentation, atrophy, and telangiectasia
- *Lichen planus pigmentosus*—slaty gray diffuse pigmentation
- *Addison's disease*—hyperpigmentation of the palmar creases, mucosa, and knuckles
- Ashy dermatosis
- Solar melanosis

TREATMENT

Avoidance of sunlight, discontinuation of provocative factors, and the use of opaque sunscreens are the primary measures. Topical hydroquinone 1%, 2%, or 4%; azelaic acid; Kligman's formula (5% hydroquinone, 0.1% tretinoin, and 0.1% dexamethasone in hydrophilic ointment); chemical peels with trichloroacetic acid (TCA) or glycolic acid; and erbium-doped yttrium aluminum garnet (Er:YAG) laser are indicated.

Tablet tranexamic acid 250 mg twice daily has shown promising results in melasma.

PROGNOSIS

Epidermal melasma responds well to treatment. Recurrences are common.

SUGGESTED READINGS

1. Yalamanchili R, Shastry V, Betkerur J. Clinico-epidemiological Study and Quality of Life Assessment in Melasma. Indian J Dermatol. 2015;60(5):519.
2. Sarkar R, Arora P, Garg VK, Sonthalia S, Gokhale N. Melasma update. Indian Dermatol Online J. 2014;5(4):426-35.

145 Melanocytic Nevi

SYNONYM

Moles

CLINICAL FEATURES

Congenital melanocytic nevi are present at birth and are of large size. Tardive nevi are not present at birth but appear in the first 2 years of life. They are larger than acquired nevi and may have hypertrichosis. Neurocutaneous melanocytosis is associated with epilepsy, mental retardation, raised intracranial pressure, spinal dysraphism, meningocele, and clubfoot. Nevi are present commonly over the head, neck, and trunk of males, **(Fig. 1)** whereas in females; it occurs commonly over the upper and lower limbs.

Acquired type is classified into junctional, compound, and intradermal varieties. Junctional nevus appears as a flat pigmented macule 3 mm–1 cm in size with well-preserved surface markings. Compound nevi appear as slightly raised circular plaques with a darker center and lighter periphery. Occasionally, coarse hair may project from the surface. Intradermal nevi are dome-shaped, skin-colored, smooth papules.

ASSOCIATED SYNDROMES

Associated syndromes include carney complex [NAME (nevi, atrial myxoma, myxoid neurofibromas, ephelides) and LAMB (lentigines,

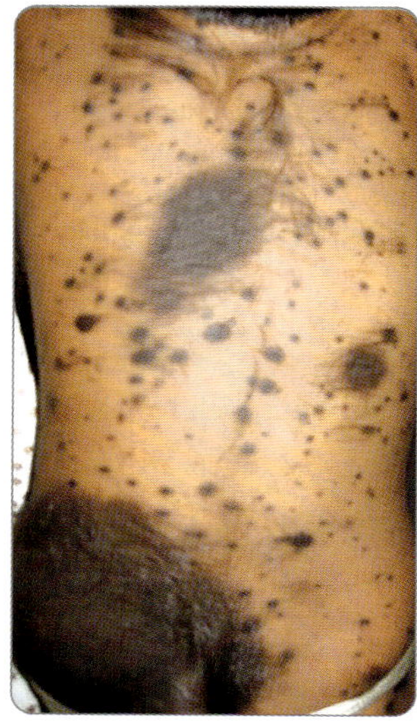

Fig. 1: Giant congenital melanocytic nevi with hypertrichosis.

atrial myxoma, mucocutaneous myxomas, blue nevi) syndromes], epidermal nevus syndrome, neurocutaneous melanosis, and premature aging syndromes.

DERMOSCOPY

General dermoscopic patterns seen in congenital melanocytic nevi are:

- Globular pattern with central dark globules
- Peripheral reticular pattern with central homogenous area

HISTOPATHOLOGY

Nevus cells are present in the reticular dermis and extend into the collagen bundles in a single row (Indian file appearance), sheets, or combinations. In congenital nevus, the nevus cells are found deeper in the dermis, along with neurovascular bundles, with both surrounding hair follicles, sebaceous glands, and subcutaneous fat.

DIFFERENTIAL DIAGNOSIS

- *Lentigines*—mucosa is also involved.
- *Actinic keratosis*—crusted papules over sun-exposed areas
- *Freckles*—flat macules and lighter in color
- *Basal cell carcinoma*—basaloid cells
- *Melanoma*—dysplastic melanocytes

COMPLICATIONS

The rate of malignant transformation in congenital variety is about 2–40%.

TREATMENT

Careful follow-up to identify any malignant transformation is essential. Serial excision, curettage, CO_2 laser ablation, excision and grafting, and Q-switched ruby laser can be tried.

SUGGESTED READING

1. Macneal P, Patel BC. (2023). Congenital Melanocytic Nevi. Treasure Island (FL): StatPearls Publishing. [online] Available from https://www.ncbi.nlm.nih.gov/books/NBK563168/ [Last accessed January, 2025].

146 Milia

➲ ETIOLOGY

Some milia (singular—milium) arise in undeveloped sebaceous glands, while some arise in the proximal part of divided sweat ducts after ductal damage, which is usually secondary to subepidermal blistering disorders. Destruction of skin appendages by radiotherapy may result in a ring of milium-like lesions at the margin of the area treated.

➲ EPIDEMIOLOGY

Milia are quite common at all ages from infancy onward.

➲ CLINICAL FEATURES

Milium is a small subepidermal keratin cyst. Milia are classified as primary milia, which arise spontaneously on the face in predisposed individuals and are also linked with specific inherited genetic skin disorders like orofacial digital syndrome and congenital hereditary trichodysplasia, and secondary milia, **(Fig. 1)** which occur either in diseases associated with subepidermal bullae, such as bullous pemphigoid, dystrophic epidermolysis bullosa, and porphyria cutanea tarda, or after dermabrasion and other trauma.

These present as multiple, superficially located, white, globoid, firm lesions, 1–2 mm in diameter. They are usually noticed only on the face and occur in the areas of vellus hair follicles, particularly on the cheeks and eyelids. In the oral cavity, they may be found on

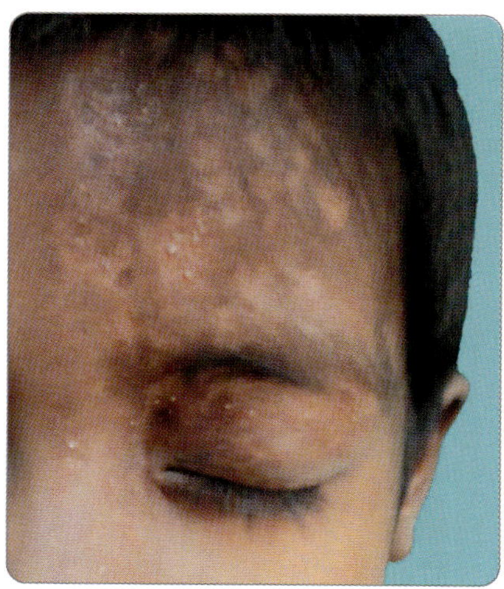

Fig. 1: Milia over scar of herpes zoster.

the palate (Epstein pearls and Bohn nodules). Secondary mil a are scattered randomly according to the affected area.

Milia en plaque is a plaque-like inflammatory variant of milia commonly located on the ear.

HISTOPATHOLOGY

Milia are lined by a stratified epithelium, a few cell layers thick, and contain concentric lamellae of keratin.

DIFFERENTIAL DIAGNOSIS

- *Syringomas*—translucent, angulated papules, and watery discharge on puncturing the lesions
- Trichoepitheliomas
- *Molluscum contagiosum*—umbilication is seen, and molluscum bodies are present in Giemsa stain of the crush smear.

TREATMENT

Incision of the epidermis over the milium with a cutting-edge needle or sharp-pointed scalpel and squeezing out the contents is usually effective. Tangential pressure applied with a comedone extractor or curette can also be used to squeeze out the contents. Radiofrequency ablation and topical retinoids are also effective. Milia en plaque may improve with tetracycline (minocycline) antibiotic.

SUGGESTED READING

1. Gallardo Avila PP, Mendez MD. (2023). Milia. Treasure Island (FL): StatPearls Publishing; 2023. [online] Available from https://www.ncbi.nlm.nih.gov/books/NBK560481/ [Last accessed January, 2025].

147 Miliaria

➲ SYNONYMS

Sudamina (miliaria crystallina), prickly heat (miliaria rubra), mammillaria (miliaria profunda).

➲ ETIOLOGY

Miliaria occurs due to the obstruction of sweat glands. Depending on the level of obstruction, various types of miliaria are shown in **Table 1**.

➲ EPIDEMIOLOGY

The incidence of miliaria is the greatest during the first few weeks of life, largely the result of the relative immaturity of the eccrine sweat duct apparatus, which favors poral occlusion and sweat retention.

➲ CLINICAL FEATURES

- Miliaria crystallina is often seen in febrile illnesses associated with profuse sweating. They are clear, thin-walled vesicles, 1–2 mm in diameter, without an inflammatory areola, **(Fig. 1)**

Table 1: Correlation between type of miliaria and level of obstruction.

Type of miliaria	*Level of obstruction*
Miliaria crystallina	Stratum corneum
Miliaria rubra	Stratum granulosum and below
Miliaria profunda	Dermoepidermal junction

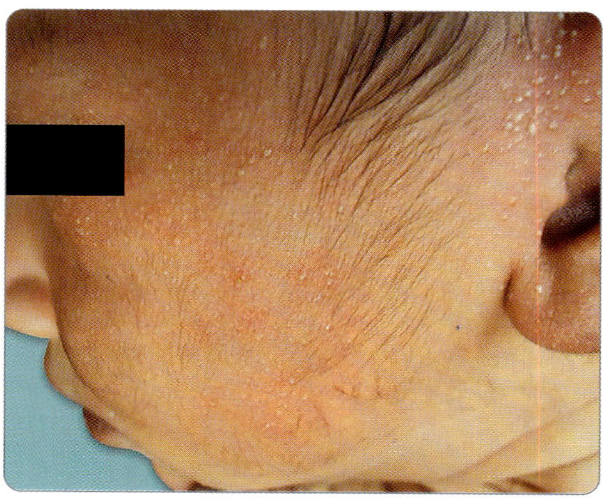

Fig. 1: Miliaria.

and usually symptomless, which develop in crops and mainly on the trunk. The vesicles soon rupture and are followed by superficial, branny desquamation.

- Miliaria rubra are minute, discrete, nonfollicular erythematous papules developing in areas of friction with clothing, in flexures, and after occlusive therapy with polythene. Characteristically, the lesions produce intense discomfort in the form of an unbearable pricking sensation. Some of the eruptions of miliaria rubra become pustular, resulting in miliaria pustulosa.
- The eruption of miliaria profunda consists of pale or flesh-colored, 1–3 mm-sized papules that resemble gooseflesh.

HISTOPATHOLOGY

Miliaria crystallina is histologically typified by an intracorneal or subcorneal vesicle that is in direct communication with the underlying sweat duct. In miliaria rubra, spongiotic vesicles that are in continuity with a sweat duct are found in the stratum malpighii. A chronic inflammatory infiltrate is seen around and within the vesicles and in the subjacent dermis. In miliaria profunda, sweat retention vesicles form within the superficial dermis.

DERMOSCOPY

Dermoscopy findings include large white globules with surrounding darker halos, giving the appearance of "white bull's eye".

DIFFERENTIAL DIAGNOSIS

- *Insect bite reaction*—fewer lesions and papules with classical central punctum are seen.
- *Viral exanthema*—diffuse, blanchable, erythematous maculo-papular rash is seen.
- *Folliculitis*—follicular-oriented papules/pustules with hair emerging from the center.
- *Drug eruptions*—preceding history of drug intake and may be associated with fever, icterus, and hepatomegaly
- *Candidiasis*—frank pustules and the demonstration of budding yeast cells
- *Milia*—fewer in number and nonerythematous

COMPLICATIONS

The most important complications of miliaria are secondary infection and the disturbance of heat regulation. Periporitis staphylogenes refers to multiple staphylococcal abscesses superimposed on miliaria rubra in young infants.

TREATMENT

The most effective prevention or treatment for miliaria is the avoidance of further sweating. Avoidance of excessive exposure to heat, humidity, and exercise and avoiding the use of tight or occlusive clothing are frequently curative. A cool bath often helps in alleviating pruritus. Oral ascorbic acid 500 mg twice daily was found to diminish the severity of miliaria. Calamine lotion is as effective as anything for the relief of discomfort.

➲ SUGGESTED READINGS

1. Guerra KC, Toncar A, Krishnamurthy K. Miliaria. (2024). In: StatPearls. Treasure Island (FL): StatPearls Publishing. [online] Available from https://www.ncbi.nlm.nih.gov/books/NBK537176/ [Last accessed January, 2025].
2. Shilpashree P, Gupta D, Sharma H, Noorian E. Clinical Study Of Miliaria. Int J Acad Med Pharm. 2022;4(5):319-22.

148 Molluscum Contagiosum

SYNONYMS

Water wart, molluscum sebaceum, epithelioma contagiosum, Bateman's disease.

HISTORY

Bateman differentiated it from molluscum fibrosum in 1814. In 1841, Henderson and Paterson independently described intracytoplasmic inclusion bodies (Henderson–Paterson bodies). In 1905, Juliusberg established the viral etiology of molluscum contagiosum (MC).

ETIOLOGY

Molluscum contagiosum is a common viral infection of the skin caused by molluscum contagiosum virus (MCV), a DNA virus belonging to the Poxviridae family and the genera of Molluscipoxvirus. There are four subtypes: MCV 1–4. MCV-1 infection is common in children and MCV-2 in adults and immunocompromised individuals. MCV enters the basal keratinocyte and increases the rate of cell division to twice that of normal skin, probably by the inhibition of the normal keratinocyte apoptotic differentiation program by specific MCV-encoded proteins. This cellular proliferation produces lobulated epidermal growth.

EPIDEMIOLOGY

Molluscum contagiosum commonly occurs in children, sexually active adults, and immunocompromised individuals. It is rare under the age of 1 year, perhaps due to maternally transmitted immunity and a long incubation period.

CLINICAL FEATURES

Transmission of infection in children is by skin-to-skin contact and sometimes by fomites. In adults, transmission is through sexual contact, but it may occur via nonsexual contact also.

The incubation period of MC varies from 2 weeks to 6 months. Common sites in children are the face, neck, sides of the trunk, axillae, lower abdomen, and thighs. They can also occur over the eyelids, scalp, lips, and even tongue and buccal mucosa. Sexually acquired lesions are confined to the pubic area and genitals. The characteristic lesions are discrete, dome-shaped, shiny, pearly white umbilicated papules varying in size from 1 to 10 mm. They may be skin-colored or pink. The lesions may be single or multiple and are asymptomatic **(Figs. 1 and 2)**.

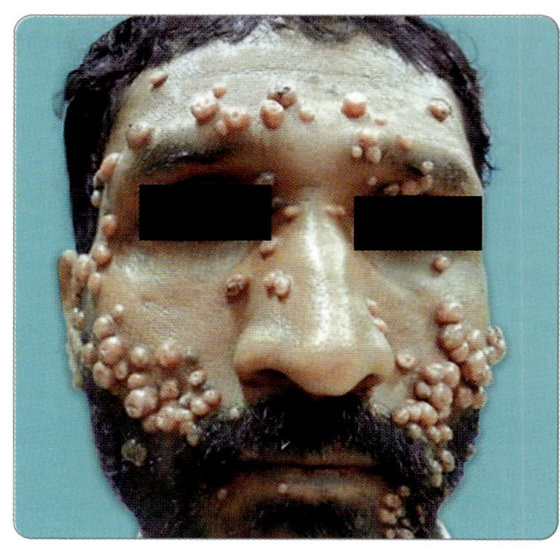

Fig. 1: Extensive molluscum contagiosum over the face in an immunocompromised patient.

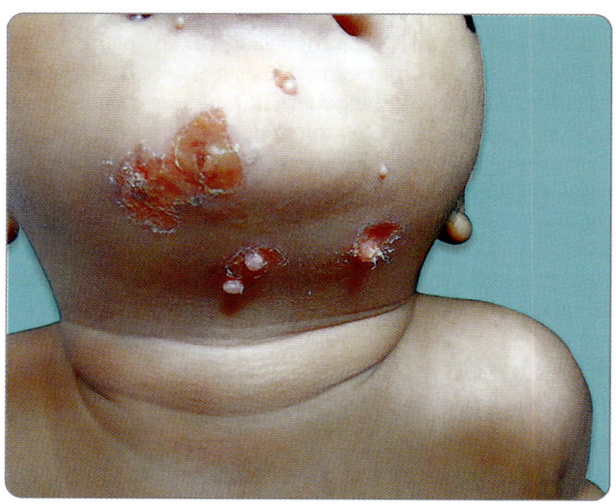

Fig. 2: Secondary infection in molluscum contagiosum lesions.

Most lesions resolve spontaneously over a period of 6–9 months; rarely do they persist for several years. Resolution may follow inflammation, suppuration, and crusting. In immunocompromised patients, the lesions are extensive, larger, and persistent.

➲ PATHOLOGY

Histopathological examination or direct examination of the expressed material, stained or unstained, reveals large, intracytoplasmic, eosinophilic, smooth, ovoid, and homogenous inclusion bodies (molluscum bodies or Henderson–Paterson bodies) in epidermal keratinocytes **(Figs. 3A and B)**.

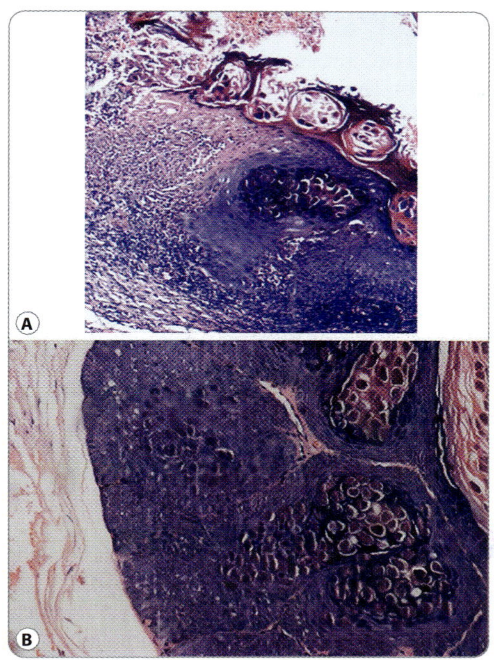

Figs. 3A and B: Molluscum contagiosum bodies in the epidermis.

➲ DERMOSCOPY

Dermoscopic features of MC include central white-yellow amorphous area, peripheral branched vessels, and crown vessels, which do not cross the centers of the lobules.

➲ DIFFERENTIAL DIAGNOSIS

- *Solitary*:
  - Pyogenic granuloma—history of bleeding present
  - Keratoacanthoma—crateriform lesions and no material on curettage
  - Appendageal tumors
- *Multiple*:
  - Plane warts—lack umbilication
  - Milia—lack umbilication, no koebnerization
  - Syringoma—skin-colored papules with watery discharge on puncturing
  - Varicella—vesicles on erythematous base with fever and coryza; multinucleated giant cells on Tzanck smear
  - Folliculitis—follicle-oriented pustules
  - Basal cell epithelioma

In the immunosuppressed, especially in the human immunodeficiency virus (HIV) infected, differential diagnosis can be cutaneous cryptococcosis, histoplasmosis, and penicilliosis.

COMPLICATIONS

Secondary infection, molluscum dermatitis (Meyerson phenomenon), lesions on the eyelid margin, and conjunctiva can cause conjunctivitis or keratitis.

TREATMENT

It is not always necessary to treat all cases of MC since MC resolves spontaneously. Treatment is required to prevent the spread of infection in persistent cases and in cosmetically concerned individuals. A number of therapeutic modalities are available, but the treatment has to be individualized depending on the age of the patient and the number of lesions.

- *Cryotherapy*: Liquid nitrogen spray may be repeated at 3–4-weekly intervals until all lesions disappear.
- *Curettage*: For large lesions. Other surgical methods include expression of contents of the papule by squeezing it with a pair of forceps, superficial curettage, or shaving if the lesions are superficial.
- *Electrodesiccation*: It is effective but may cause slight pain and scarring.
- *Chemical cautery*: Topical application of 50% trichloroacetic acid, liquid phenol, a keratolytic paint containing 16.7% each of salicylic acid and lactic acid, and cantharidin 0.9%.
- *Topical medications*: Tretinoin (0.05%) applied once daily for weeks or months and topical 5% imiquimod cream applied three times per week.
- *Laser*: Pulsed dye laser can be used.
- *Miscellaneous*: Levamisole, griseofulvin, and cimetidine may be tried.

PROGNOSIS

Excellent, as most lesions resolve spontaneously without scarring, and there is no affection of internal organs, as MCV does not enter the bloodstream.

SUGGESTED READINGS

1. Leung AKC, Barankin B, Hon KLE. Molluscum contagiosum: an update. Recent Pat Inflamm Allergy Drug Discov. 2017;11(1):22-31.
2. Gerlero P, Hernandez-Martin A. Update on the treatment of molluscum contagiosum in children. Actas Dermosifiliogr. 2018;109(5):408-15.

149 Mongolian Spot

➲ SYNONYM

Congenital dermal melanocytosis.

➲ HISTORY

Edwin Baez thought it to be a characteristic of Mongolian race and named it Mongolian spot. The Chinese believed that it is a kick given by god to give the baby a start in life.

➲ ETIOLOGY

Mongolian spot is produced by melanocytes deep in the dermis probably as a result of failure to cross the dermoepidermal junction while migrating from the neural crest in fetal life.

➲ EPIDEMIOLOGY

Mongolian spots are commonly seen at birth.

➲ CLINICAL FEATURES

This is the most common congenital pigmented lesion. Mongolian spots are commonly seen over the lumbosacral region and less often on the buttocks, shoulders, and flanks. They are seen as one or more macules, slate gray or blue in color, varying from 3 to 10 cm in size **(Fig. 1)**. Occasionally, Mongolian spots can be very extensive, covering much of the posterior trunk and shoulders. Mongolian spots usually fade within the first 2 years of life, though they occasionally persist into adulthood. Mongolian spots can be associated with inborn errors of metabolism and neurocristopathy.

Variants of Mongolian spot include:

- Common type—regress normally by early childhood
- Extensive type—regress very slowly
- Persistent type—persist into adulthood
- Generalized—involve large areas covering almost entire anterior or posterior trunk and extremities
- Aberrant—involve unusual sites head and neck region
- Superimposed—darker Mongolian spot over lighter one
- Speckled—groups of dotted pigmentation

➲ DERMOSCOPY

Ill-defined greyish green patch can be seen.

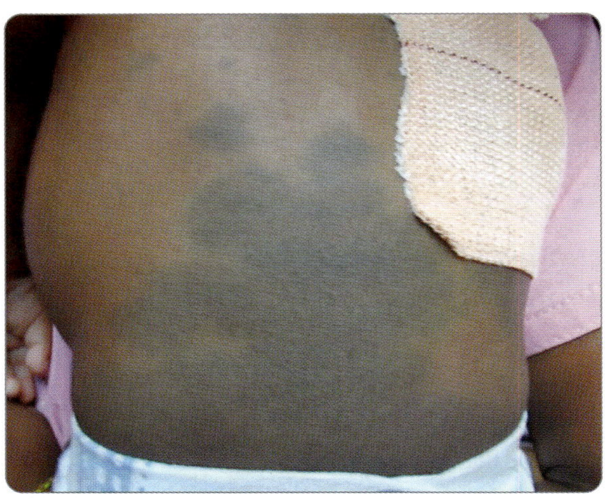

Fig. 1: Dark blue hyperpigmented patches of Mongolian spot over the back.

HISTOPATHOLOGY

Histologically, they consist of bundles of spindle-shaped melanocytes containing fine melanin granules dispersed between collagen fibers.

DIFFERENTIAL DIAGNOSIS

- Nevus of Ito—involvement of the shoulder area predominantly
- Dermal melanocytic hamartoma
- Hori's nevus
- Bruise—color changes with time, resolution of lesions

COMPLICATIONS

Complications can be persistent and atypical. Mongolian spots may be associated with port-wine stains in patients with phakomatosis pigmentovascularis, cleft lip malformation, or type 1 gangliosidosis.

TREATMENT

The condition is usually self-limiting and does not require treatment. Opaque cosmetics may be used as camouflage. Q-switched ruby laser and Q-switched neodymium-doped yttrium aluminum garnet laser can also be used.

SUGGESTED READING

1. Gupta D, Thappa DM. Mongolian spots. Indian J Dermatol Venereol Leprol. 2013;79:469-78.

150 Monilethrix

SYNONYMS

Spindle hair, beaded hair, necklace hair.

HISTORY

It was first described by Walter Smith, later termed as Monilethrix by Radcliffe Crocker.

ETIOLOGY

Monilethrix is a rare genetic disorder associated with increased hair fragility and pathognomonic beaded hair appearance. It is inherited as autosomal dominant trait due to mutation in gene *hHb6*, *hHb3*, and *hHb1* located on chromosome 12p13, which encodes for hair keratin (KRT81, KRT83, and KRT86). Few reports of autosomal recessive pattern of inheritance have also been documented due to mutation in *DSG4* gene encoding desmoglein 4.

EPIDEMIOLOGY

Monilethrix appears in infancy.

CLINICAL FEATURES

Disease becomes apparent within first few months of life when lanugo hairs are shed and replaced with short, dry, lusterless hair. Child presents with sparse hair and increased fragility. Beaded hairs which are hallmark of disease emerge from keratotic follicular papules, primarily seen on occiput. Presentation can vary from mild disease, which affects only scalp to severe form where eyebrows, eyelashes, and body hair can also be involved. Scarring alopecia has also been reported. Scalp hair is fragile at constricted sites, resulting in apparent hypotrichosis.

Gradual improvement occurs with age, pregnancy, and during summertime.

ASSOCIATED CONDITIONS

Associated conditions include follicular papules in nape of neck, keratosis pilaris, nail dystrophy, cataract, teeth abnormalities, syndactyly, oligophrenia, and mental disability.

TRICHOSCOPY

On trichoscopy, hair shaft shows regular uniform elliptical nodes (normal shaft thickness) and intermittent internodes (constrictions), also known as regularly bent ribbon sign.

➲ LIGHT MICROSCOPY

On light microscopy, pearl necklace appearance with areas of knots and narrowing along hair shaft is seen. Nonmedullated elliptical nodes are seen at regular intervals of 0.7–1 mm.

➲ DIFFERENTIAL DIAGNOSIS

Differential diagnoses include pseudomonilethrix, pili torti, trichorrhexis nodosa, alopecia areata, and alopecia secondary to chemotherapy.

➲ TREATMENT

- Oral retinoids and topical minoxidil have been shown to be effective.
- N-acetyl cysteine shows initial improvement but does not persist on long term.

➲ PROGNOSIS

Condition improves with age but can be variable.

➲ SUGGESTED READING

1. Chabchoub I, Souissi A. (2023). Monilethrix. Treasure Island (FL). StatPearls Publishing. [online] Available from https://www.ncbi.nlm.nih.gov/books/NBK539813/ [Last accessed January, 2025].

151 Morphea

SYNONYMS

Localized scleroderma, circumscribed scleroderma.

ETIOLOGY

The cause of morphea is unknown. There is migration of mononuclear leukocytes across endothelial cell monolayers, increased platelet-derived growth factor and receptor expression, and increased transforming growth factor-β (TGF-β) receptor expression. It is postulated that this may lead to increased connective tissue growth factor (*CTGF*) gene expression and ultimately fibrosis.

Strongest genetic association with morphea was found with human leukocyte antigen (HLA) class II allele DRB1*04:04 and class I allele HLA-B37.

EPIDEMIOLOGY

The incidence peaks between 20 and 40 years of age, with F:M ratio of 3:1.

CLINICAL FEATURES (TABLE 1)

There are three stages in morphea—edematous, indurated, and atrophic stages. Morphological variants include:

- *Circumscribed plaque lesions*: These occur as indurated areas of skin, which are purplish initially and later become thickened and ivory in color, with a lilac-colored edge. The surface is usually smooth, shiny, with absence of hair and sweating **(Fig. 1)**.
- *Guttate*: Smaller and more numerous than plaque lesions.
- Bullous
- Subcutaneous morphea/deep morphea/morphea profundus–"groove sign" (a depression along the course of a vein, between muscle groups)
- Linear **(Fig. 2)**

Table 1: Differences between generalized morphea and scleroderma.

Features	Generalized morphea	Scleroderma
Raynaud's phenomenon	Absent	Present
Sclerodactyly	Absent	Present
Nailfold capillaroscopy	Normal	Abnormal
Systemic involvement	Absent	Present

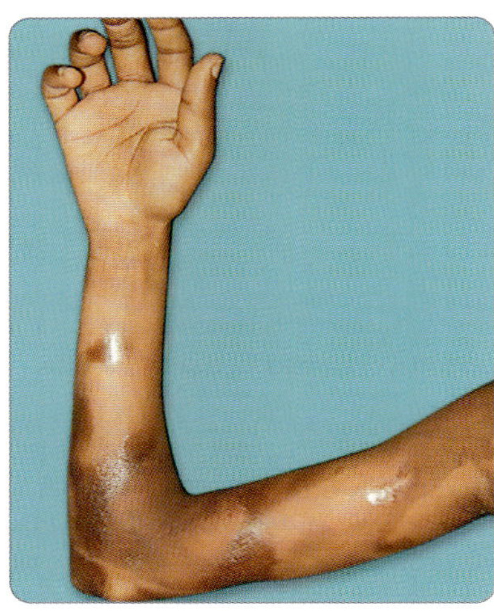

Fig. 1: Multiple atrophic plaques of morphea on the arm and forearm.

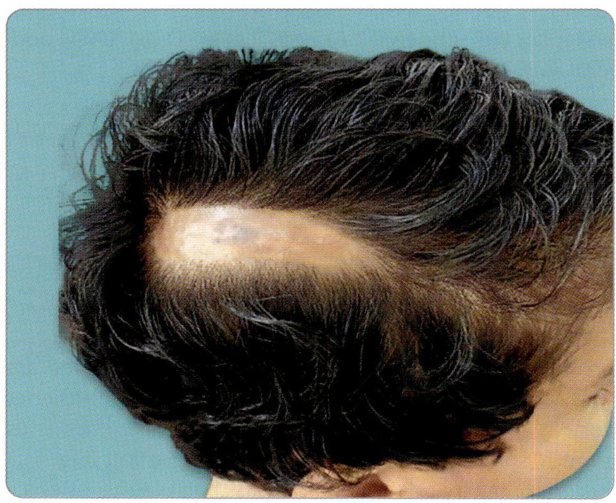

Fig. 2: Linear morphea noted over scalp.

- *Frontoparietal lesions*: "en coup de sabre" (from its resemblance to a sabre cut), with or without hemiatrophy **(Fig. 3)**.
- *Localized scleroderma in childhood*: Childhood onset occurs in 2–3% of all cases of scleroderma. Most present with morphea-type lesions (particularly linear) although systemic sclerosis does occur.
- *Disabling pansclerotic morphea of children*: This is a severe, mutilating form of morphea involving the dermis, fat, fascia, muscle, and even bone, usually starting before the age of 14 years.

➲ DERMOSCOPY

On dermoscopy, white fibrotic beams crossed by linear branching vessels are seen with loss of hair in the involved area.

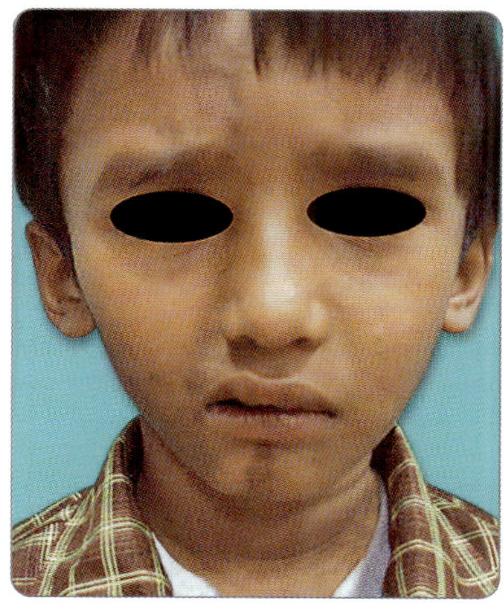

Fig. 3: En coup de sabre, linear morphea over the face extending to the scalp, resulting in facial hemiatrophy.

HISTOPATHOLOGY

The epidermis may be normal, or flattened and atrophic with loss of the rete ridges. Initially dermis is edematous, with swelling and degeneration of the collagen fibrils, which become homogeneous and eosinophilic. There is scanty perivascular lymphocytic infiltrate. The dermal appendages, dermal and subcutaneous fat, are progressively lost. Small dermal blood vessels may show intimal thickening.

DIFFERENTIAL DIAGNOSIS

- Cutaneous polyarteritis nodosa—present more with cutaneous ulceration and vasculitis-like picture
- Macular vascular nevus
- Scleredema of Buschke—usually seen following infection/ inflammation, areas like upper back, nape of neck involved, increased mucin deposition in histopathological examination (HPE)
- Atrophy of Pierini and Pasini—smaller lesions with classical cliff edge-like margins
- Lipodystrophia centrifugalis abdominalis infantilis
- Granuloma annulare—annular lesions, palisading granuloma in HPE
- Lichen sclerosis—differential diagnosis (DD) for guttate variant, patulous follicular opening at center of atrophic macule; follicular plugging and trilayered appearance on HPE
- Eosinophilic fasciitis
- Hypertrophic scar
- Porphyria cutanea tarda
- Atrophoderma
- Nephrogenic fibrosing dermopathy

➲ TREATMENT

Topical or intralesional steroids, topical calcipotriol, alone or in combination with ultraviolet A1 (UVA-1), topical tacrolimus, and 5% imiquimod cream can be tried. Other systemic agents used are phenytoin, *p*-aminobenzoate, griseofulvin, etretinate, methotrexate, vitamin E, chloroquine, and hydroxychloroquine.

➲ PROGNOSIS

The lesions tend to improve with time. Very rarely, patients with localized morphea may subsequently develop classical systemic sclerosis.

➲ SUGGESTED READING

1. Penmetsa GK, Sapra A. (2023). Morphea. Treasure Island (FL): StatPearls Publishing. [online] Available from https://www.ncbi.nlm.nih.gov/books/NBK559010/ [Last accessed January, 2025].

152 Mucormycosis

SYNONYMS

Zygomycosis, phycomycosis.

HISTORY

In 1855, Kurchenmeister isolated *Mucor* from a lung and described zygomycosis.

ETIOLOGY

Causative agents are zygomycete fungi such as Rhizomucor, Absidia, Rhizopus, Cunninghamella, Mortierella, and Saksenaea. Poorly controlled diabetes, lymphoma, severe burns, trauma, multiple myeloma, hepatitis, immunodeficiency states, neutropenia, or renal disease are the risk factors.

CLINICAL FEATURES

Most common route of entry is through respiratory tract. In cutaneous mucormycosis, the spores are introduced directly on to the skin. It can present with a variety of cutaneous lesions varying from firm papules and necrotic papulonodules to hemorrhagic bullae and necrotic ulcers. Initial involvement of facial skin may be subtle, with unilateral facial swelling and slight erythema. Advanced disease is characterized by large areas of necrosis covered by a thick hemorrhagic crust.

HISTOPATHOLOGY

The characteristic feature is the presence of nonseptate broad hyphae that have 90° branching; the hyphae have been likened to ribbons. Periodic acid–Schiff (PAS) staining may be helpful. Suppuration and necrosis, as well as blood vessel invasion by the fungi, are often seen.

COMPLICATIONS

The fungus can invade blood vessels causing widespread infarction.

DIFFERENTIAL DIAGNOSIS

Infection of the site by other organisms, vasculitis.

TREATMENT

Standard management of mucormycosis requires early diagnosis, reversal of risk factors and underlying illness, surgical debridement, and prompt administration of intravenous antifungals.

Intravenous amphotericin B 1–1.5 mg/kg/day is the treatment of choice; total dose given over the course of therapy is usually 2.5–3 g. Posaconazole 400 mg twice daily also results in resolution of lesions.

Other adjuncts include hyperbaric oxygen where increased oxygen pressure improves ability of neutrophils to kill the organism and facilitate wound healing.

➲ PROGNOSIS

Prognosis depends on the timing of therapeutic intervention, as well as the degree of the underlying immunodeficiency of the patient with mortality ranging from 25 to 87%, depending on the site of infection.

➲ SUGGESTED READING

1. Hernández JL, Buckley CJ. (2023). Mucormycosis. Treasure Island (FL): StatPearls Publishing. [online] Available from https://www.ncbi.nlm.nih.gov/books/NBK544364/ [Last accessed January, 2025].

153 Mycetoma

SYNONYMS

Maduramycosis, Madura foot.

HISTORY

Dr John Gill provided the first formal description of mycetoma in 1842, in Madurai, India. The name "Madura foot" was coined by Cole Brook in 1846. Pinoy in 1913 subdivided the disease into actinomycotic and eumycotic mycetoma.

ETIOLOGY

Eumycetoma is caused by fungi, which produce dark grain viz. *Madurella mycetomatis*, *Magnaporthe grisea*, *Leptosphaeria senegalensis*, *Curvularia lunata*, and pale grains viz. *Scedosporium apiospermum*, *Neotestudina rosatii*; *Acremonium* species; and *Fusarium* species. Actinomycetoma is caused by *Actinomadura madurae*, *Actinomadura pelletieri*, *Streptomyces himalayensis*, *Nocardia brasiliensis*, *Nocardia otitidiscaviarum*, and *Nocardia asteroides*.

CLINICAL FEATURES

The typical patient is a man in fourth decade onward.

Most common site is foot, lower leg, or hand, although head or back involvement may also occur. Infection of the chest wall is most characteristic of *Nocardia*. Firm, painless nodules that spread slowly with the development of papules, draining sinus tracts with granules in the discharge or tissue is classical **(Figs. 1 and 2)**. Local

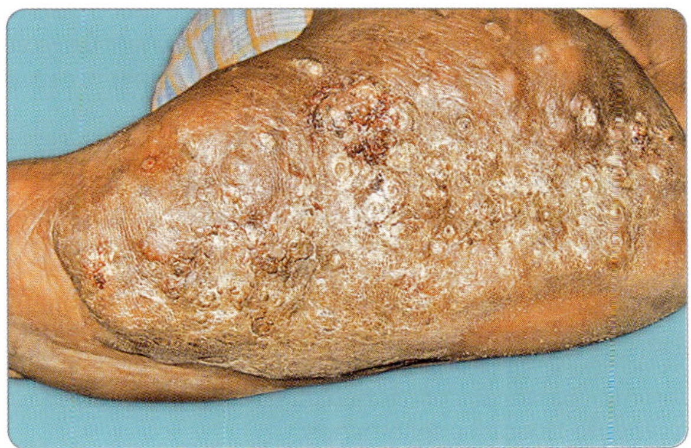

Fig. 1: Mycetoma. Large plaque with multiple papules and discharging sinus on the surface.

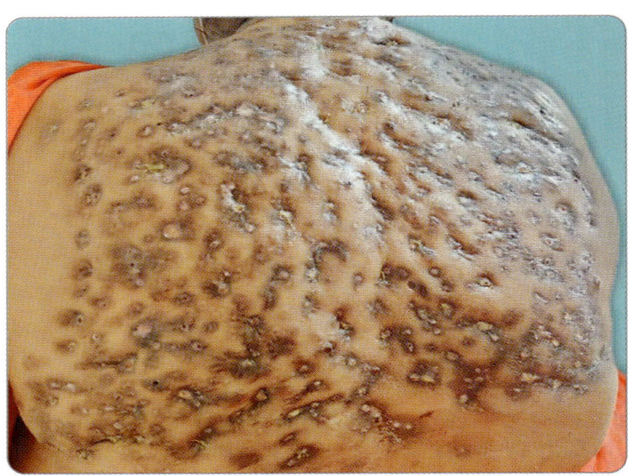

Fig. 2: Multiple discharging sinuses noted over back of patient with actinomycetoma.

tissue swelling, chronic sinus formation, and later bone involvement distort and deform the original site of infection. Lesions are seldom painful.

DERMOSCOPY

On dermoscopy, yellow globules, white superficial scales, telangiectasia and dotted vessels, blood spots, and whitish structureless areas are seen.

HISTOPATHOLOGY

Pseudoepitheliomatous hyperplasia is a common histologic finding that accompanies suppurative and granulomatous inflammation of the dermis and subcutis as well as fibrosis. The characteristic grains represent tightly packed colonies of organisms. Estimation of the diameter of the filaments comprising the grain (compared to the size of the nuclei of surrounding inflammatory cells) allows a distinction between eumycotic (thicker filaments, brown, oval, or irregular granule with radiating hyphae and chlamydospores at the periphery surrounded by eosinophilic precipitate called Splendore–Hoeppli reaction) and actinomycotic (thin, fine filaments) mycetoma. Special stains, e.g., silver (Grocott) and Brown–Brenn can aid in distinguishing the subtype.

Radiological examination and computed tomography (CT) scan are done to assess the extent of the lesion. Bone involvement is diffuse in actinomycotic mycetoma with spicular periosteal reaction, medullary sclerosis and calcification. In eumycetoma, bone changes are localized and osteolytic lesions are common.

DIFFERENTIAL DIAGNOSIS

- Chronic bacterial or tuberculous infection—absence of Splendore-Hoeppli phenomenon
- Osteomyelitis—bony involvement with discharging sinus tracts from the bone
- Soft tissue tumors—no discharge of granules

COMPLICATIONS

Complications can be bone involvement, dissemination (rare), and lymphadenopathy following secondary infection.

TREATMENT

In eumycetoma, a trial of chemotherapy with ketoconazole 400 mg/day, itraconazole 200 mg/day, dapsone, griseofulvin, high-dose terbinafine, miconazole, and potassium iodide has been tried, but the response is poor. Surgery (usually amputation) is the definitive procedure.

Welsh regimen for actinomycetoma consists of injection amikacin 500 mg intravenous (IV) twice daily along with cotrimoxazole BD for 3 weeks followed by continuation of cotrimoxazole alone for further 2 weeks. This 5-week regimen is one cycle. Three such cycles are followed by cotrimoxazole monotherapy for 1–1.5 years. Other drugs include streptomycin, gentamycin, rifampicin, dapsone, and sulfadoxine-pyrimethamine.

In refractory cases or those with allergies to amikacin-cotrimoxazole combination, cotrimoxazole should be replaced by amoxicillin clavulanate, and amikacin should be replaced by netilmicin.

During pregnancy, monotherapy with amoxicillin-clavulanate is indicated.

PROGNOSIS

Actinomycotic mycetoma responds well to treatment, whereas eumycotic mycetoma needs surgical intervention.

SUGGESTED READING

1. Reis CMS, Reis-Filho EG de M. Mycetomas: An epidemiological, etiological, clinical, laboratory and therapeutic review. Anais Brasileiros de Dermatologia. 2018;93(1):8-18.

154 Mycosis Fungoides

➲ SYNONYMS

Alibert–Bazin syndrome, granuloma fungoides.

➲ HISTORY

Mycosis fungoides (MF) was first described in 1806 by French dermatologist Jean-Louis-Marc Alibert.

➲ ETIOLOGY

Genetic, environmental, and immunologic factors have all been considered. Stepwise accumulation of genetic abnormalities may result in clonal proliferation, malignant transformation, and ultimately progressive and widely disseminated disease. Persistent antigenic stimulation has been proposed as an initial event, but the nature of the antigen(s) involved is unknown. Recent studies suggest that CD8+ cytotoxic T cells (CTL) play a crucial role in the antitumor response in MF.

➲ EPIDEMIOLOGY

Mycosis fungoides typically affects older adults (median age at diagnosis: 55–60 years), but may occur in children and adolescents as well. Men are affected more often than women.

➲ CLINICAL FEATURES

Characteristically, patients with classical MF progress from patch stage to plaque stage and finally to tumor stage disease, and they have a protracted clinical course over years or even decades. Early patch stage MF is characterized by the presence of variably sized erythematous, finely scaling lesions, which may be mildly pruritic. These early lesions may show poikiloderma vasculare atrophicans changes. The initial skin lesions have a predilection for the buttocks and other covered sites of the trunk and limbs. It should be stressed that many patients never progress beyond the plaque stage of the disease. However, a number of patients may develop nodules or tumors. These patients with tumor stage MF characteristically show a combination of patches, plaques, and tumors. The later often show ulceration **(Fig. 1)**.

Rare clinical variants—bullous/vesicular lesions, purpuric lesions, poikilodermatous, syringotropic, and hypopigmented lesions.

Sézary syndrome: Triad of erythroderma with pruritus, lymphadenopathy, and atypical circulating lymphocytes.

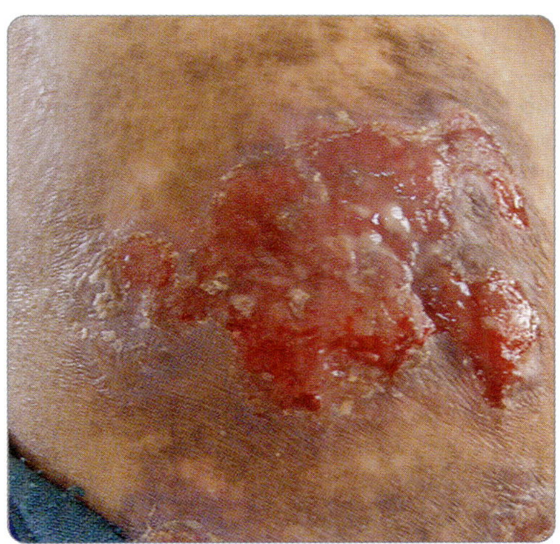

Fig. 1: Ulcerated plaque stage of mycosis fungoides.

CLINICAL VARIANTS DEFINED IN WORLD HEALTH ORGANIZATION (WHO)-EUROPEAN ORGANIZATION FOR RESEARCH AND TREATMENT OF CANCER (EORTC) CLASSIFICATION

Clinical variants include folliculotropic MF, pagetoid reticulosis (Woringer–Kolopp disease), granulomatous slack skin.

DERMOSCOPY OF MYCOSIS FUNGOIDES

- Classic patch stage—shows yellow-orange patch with white scales and fine short linear and spermatozoa-like vessels (highly specific).
- Poikilodermatous MF—shows polygonal structures consisting of lobules of white storiform streaks and fine red dots or hairpin vessels with reticular brown septa, consisting of unevenly distributed pigmented dots over pink white background.
- Folliculotropic MF—early lesions show white perifollicular halos of variable sizes, late lesions show comedo-like openings.

HISTOPATHOLOGY

Early patch lesions in MF show superficial band-like or lichenoid infiltrates, mainly composed of lymphocytes. Atypical lymphocytes with highly convoluted (cerebriform) nuclei, and they are confined to the epidermis (epidermotropism).

In typical plaques, epidermotropism is more pronounced. The presence of intraepidermal nests of atypical cells (Pautrier's microabscesses) is a highly characteristic feature.

With progression to tumor stage, epidermotropism is no longer present, and the tumor cells increase in number and size, blast cells with prominent nuclei, and intermediate forms predominate.

➲ DIFFERENTIAL DIAGNOSIS

- Eczema—history of oozing, spongiosis on histopathological examination (HPE)
- Psoriasis—Munro's neutrophilic abscess in stratum corneum
- Superficial fungal infections—fungal elements on KOH mount
- Large plaque parapsoriasis
- Lymphomatoid contact dermatitis and drug reactions
- Actinic reticuloid
- Other types of cutaneous T-cell lymphoma (CTCL)

➲ COMPLICATIONS

Erythroderma may develop with sparing of areas of skin that are folded, which is called deck chair or folded luggage sign.

➲ TREATMENT

Treatment should be symptom oriented and stage adapted.

- *Premycotic phase*: Topical corticosteroids, ultraviolet B (UVB), and psoralen and UVA (PUVA).
- *Stage IA–IIA (patches/plaques)*: PUVA, topical nitrogen mustard (HN2), topical bexarotene, imiquimod, total skin electron beam (TSEB).
- *Stage IIB (skin tumors)*: Same as stage I. Relapse: PUVA + interferon-alpha (IFN-α), PUVA + retinoids (acitretin; oral bexarotene), and denileukin diftitox
- *Stage III (erythroderma)*: Low-dose chlorambucil and prednisone, low-dose methotrexate. Add skin-targeted therapies (PUVA; HN2; RT), if necessary.
- *Stage IV (nodal, visceral involvement)*: Multiagent chemotherapy (e.g., CHOP). Biological response modifiers (denileukin diftitox; IL-12, etc.).

➲ PROGNOSIS

Overall, patients with MF limited to skin have a 5-year survival rate of 80–100%.

➲ SUGGESTED READING

1. Vaidya T, Badri T. (2023). Mycosis Fungoides. Treasure Island (FL): StatPearls Publishing. [online] Available from https://www.ncbi.nlm.nih.gov/books/NBK519572/ [Last accessed January, 2025].

155 Necrobiosis Lipoidica

➲ HISTORY

The condition was first described in 1929, by Oppenheim, who called it dermatitis atrophicans lipoidica diabetica. Urbach then coined the term necrobiotic lipoidica diabeticorum and as it is not peculiar to diabetes it is now called necrobiosis lipoidica (NL).

➲ ETIOLOGY

The disease has a strong association with diabetes mellitus. It is suggested that the disease develops secondary to diabetic microangiopathy. Smoking and trauma exacerbate the disease.

➲ EPIDEMIOLOGY

Necrobiosis lipoidica is commonly seen in young adults with insulin-dependent diabetes mellitus. It is three times more common in females.

➲ CLINICAL FEATURES

Necrobiosis lipoidica is characterized by collagen degeneration manifesting primarily on the pretibial area. The lesion is a sclerodermatous plaque, round or oval, circumscribed with a slightly elevated rim. New lesions are reddish brown, but with progression the center of the lesion becomes yellowish and the peripheral border may acquire a violaceous hue, with scaling and telangiectasia.

➲ DERMOSCOPY

Dermoscopy shows linear vessels with branches distributed uniformly on the background of yellowish structureless area. White linear streaks can also be seen.

➲ ASSOCIATED CONDITIONS

Associated conditions include diabetes mellitus, ulcerative colitis, Crohn's disease, ataxia telangiectasia, postjejunal bypass, and sarcoidosis.

➲ HISTOPATHOLOGY

Epidermis is normal to atrophic, absent if ulceration is present. Full-thickness dermal changes are present, which may extend into subcutaneous tissue also. As the dermis is firm, biopsy specimens are rectangular than being tapered down. Early lesions show perivascular and interstitial mixed inflammatory cell infiltrate, less well-defined necrobiosis with degeneration of collagen and elastin.

Lipid and cholesterol clefts are present in necrobiotic area. Mucin is present in the dermis but not as abundant as in granuloma annulare. Histiocytes, Langerhans cells, and foreign body giant cells border the areas, while the infiltrate has eosinophils and plasma cells. Old lesions show atrophy and fibrosis of dermis.

COMPLICATIONS

Complications include ulceration and Koebner's phenomenon.

DIFFERENTIAL DIAGNOSIS

- Xanthoma—foam cells, touton giant cells seen on histopathological examination (HPE)
- Morphea—homogenization of collagen in dermis
- Granuloma annulare—degenerated collagen replaced by mucin
- Vasculitis—leukocytoclasia on biopsy
- Lichen sclerosus
- Necrobiotic xanthogranuloma
- Sarcoidosis—naked granulomas on HPE
- Rheumatoid nodule
- Tuberculoid Hansen's—epithelioid cell granuloma with Langhans giant cell
- Stasis dermatitis
- Nodular panniculitis—inflammation of subcutaneous tissue

TREATMENT

Spontaneous resolution has been seen in 17% of cases and may not require treatment in the absence of ulceration or symptoms.

Topical steroids, intralesional steroids, pentoxifylline, ticlopidine, and aspirin are the treatment options.

For atrophic inactive lesions, topical steroids should be avoided as they may exaggerate atrophy and result in ulceration.

Phototherapy can be useful in active inflamed lesions.

Calcineurin inhibitors have been shown to be effective in resolving ulceration.

Tumor necrosis factor alpha (TNF-α) inhibitors are the other options available.

Other systemic agents commonly employed include fumaric acid esters, steroids, and dapsone.

PROGNOSIS

The condition is usually chronic and heals with scarring over a period of time. Squamous cell carcinomas have been reported rarely.

SUGGESTED READING

1. Lepe K, Riley CA, Salazar FJ. (2023). Necrobiosis Lipoidica. Treasure Island (FL): StatPearls Publishing. [online] Available from https://www.ncbi.nlm.nih.gov/books/NBK459318 [Last accessed January, 2025].

156 Netherton Syndrome

➲ SYNONYMS

Bamboo hair syndrome, Comèl–Netherton syndrome.

➲ HISTORY

Netherton syndrome (NS) is named after EW Netherton, who in 1958 described a young girl with generalized scaly dermatitis and fragile nodular hair-shaft deformities, which he termed trichorrhexis nodosa.

➲ ETIOLOGY

Netherton syndrome results from mutation in *SPINK5*, which encodes the serine protease inhibitor LETK1.

➲ CLINICAL FEATURES

Netherton syndrome is an autosomal recessive condition presenting as combination of ichthyosis, atopy, and hair shaft deformities. Infants are often born prematurely, develop the lesions in utero, or during the first week of life. They have generalized scaling erythroderma, but not a collodion baby phenotype. Failure to thrive is profound, requiring hospitalization to support and correct the electrolyte imbalance. Patients may have diarrhea, intestinal villous atrophy, high risk of sepsis, and may have raised immunoglobulin E (IgE). Skin barrier function is poor, affected babies have markedly increased percutaneous absorption.

Ichthyosis linearis circumflexa, the characteristic skin change associated with NS, is characterized by migratory polycyclic scaly lesions with peripheral double-edged scale. Ichthyosis linearis circumflexa is not generally seen before 2 years of age, and occurs eventually in 70% of patients. Ichthyosiform erythroderma tends to improve with increasing age. Partial remissions have been noted, but there is no tendency for spontaneous resolution. Routine histological examination is not helpful, but electron microscopy reveals specific features.

The classic hair shaft abnormality, trichorrhexis invaginata, (bamboo hair, ball, and socket deformity), results from defect in keratinization of internal root sheath. Hair is easily breakable, poorly manageable, dry, and lusterless. Hair from multiple areas should be examined, since only 20–50% may be affected.

Atopic diathesis includes urticaria, angioedema, asthma, and or anaphylaxis.

TRICHOSCOPY

Trichoscopy of scalp reveals invaginating distal portion of hair into proximal part with characteristic bamboo hair and golf-tee hair appearance.

DIFFERENTIAL DIAGNOSIS

- Psoriasis—silvery white scales, positive Auspitz sign
- Hyper-IgE syndrome—absence of hair shaft disorder
- Erythrokeratoderma variabilis
- Erythroderma—diffuse erythema and scaling >90% body surface area
- Nonbullous ichthyosiform erythroderma
- Acrodermatitis enteropathica—only periorificial and intertriginous areas involved with psoriasiform lesions
- Seborrheic dermatitis

TREATMENT

Treatment comprises the use of a humidified incubator in neonates, frequent application of emollients, and proper cleansing of skin. Anemia and hypoalbuminemia necessitate repeated transfusions and albumin infusion in some infants. Topical corticosteroids are ineffective and should be avoided as erythroderma and extensive skin involvement at this age may contribute to rapid absorption and systemic toxicity. Systemic retinoids can exacerbate the disease.

Narrowband ultraviolet B phototherapy, psoralen and ultraviolet radiation are the other treatment options with varying success.

Intravenous immunoglobulin and anti-tumor necrosis factor (TNF) alpha therapy are the therapeutic options for severe illness.

Other biologics tried include dupilumab [interleukin 4 (IL-4) and IL-13 inhibitor] and secukinumab (IL-17 inhibitor).

SUGGESTED READINGS

1. Saleem HMK, Shahid MF, Shahbaz A, Sohail A, Shahid MA, Sachmechi I. Netherton Syndrome: A Case Report and Review of Literature. Cureus. 2018;10(7):e3070.
2. Nouwen AEM, Schappin R, Nguyen NT, Ragamin A, Bygum A, Bodemer C, et al. Outcomes of Systemic Treatment in Children and Adults With Netherton Syndrome: A Systematic Review. Front Immunol. 2022;13: 864449.

157 Neurofibromatosis

SYNONYM

Von Recklinghausen disease.

HISTORY

Von Recklinghausen provided the first description of the clinical and pathologic nature of the neurofibromas in 1882. Lisch described the iris nodules, which more recently have been recognized as an important criterion in the clinical diagnosis of neurofibromatosis (NF).

ETIOLOGY

Gene for NF-1 is located on chromosome 17q11.2 and codes for neurofibromin, a protein that negatively regulates signals transduced by Ras protein. The gene for NF-2 is located on 22q11-q13 and encodes for merlin (schwannomin).

CLINICAL FEATURES

Neurofibromatosis is an autosomal dominant syndrome, characterized by developmental changes in the nervous system, bones, and skin.

Ricardi has classified NF into eight types:

1. Classical
2. Central with acoustic neuromas
3. Mixed with features of both 1 and 2
4. Variant—diffuse café-au-lait macules (CALMs), variable family history
5. Segmental/Dermatomal
6. Cutaneous only with multiple CALM, no neurofibromas, and no family history
7. Onset of features after 30 years
8. Others—not fitting from 1 to 7

TYPE 1 NEUROFIBROMATOSIS

Patients have many neurofibromas, CALMs, axillary freckles (Crowe's sign), giant pigmented hairy nevi, sacral hypertrichosis, cutis verticis gyrata, and macroglossia. Lisch nodules are found in the iris in 25% of patients lesser than 6 years of age and in 94% of adults.

Neurofibromas are soft tumors that can be pushed down into the panniculus by light pressure with the finger and spring back when released (buttonhole sign). Subcutaneous plexiform neurofibromas are virtually pathognomonic of NF-1. They occur as large nodules containing multiple encapsulated neurofibromas **(Fig. 1)**.

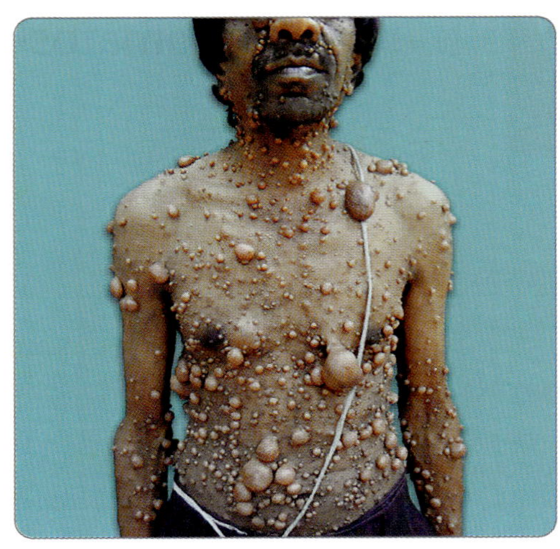

Fig. 1: Multiple neurofibromas of varying sizes over the face and trunk.

The overlying skin is usually hyperpigmented and on palpation gives the bag of worms feeling.

Acromegaly, cretinism, hyperparathyroidism, myxedema, pheochromocytoma, or precocious puberty occurs. Bone changes may produce kyphosis, lordosis, pseudoarthrosis, spina bifida, and atraumatic fractures. Neuromas of spinal nerves may cause paralysis. Patients are four times more likely to develop malignancies than normal population. Cutaneous neurofibromas may develop neurofibrosarcoma. Growing or hardening lesions are the indications for biopsy. Wilm's tumor, rhabdomyosarcomas, leukemia, mental retardation, dementia, epilepsy, and intracranial malignancies can occur.

Hypertelorism indicates brain involvement.

Diagnostic Criteria for Neurofibromatosis Type 1

Two or more of the following criteria have to be present.

- Six or more CALMs > 5 mm in prepubertal individuals and >15 mm in postpubertal individuals **(Fig. 2)**
- Two or more neurofibromas of any type or one plexiform neurofibroma
- "Freckling" in the axillary or inguinal regions **(Figs. 3 and 4)**
- Optic gliomas
- Two or more Lisch nodules (iris hamartomas)
- Osseous lesion, such as sphenoid wing dysplasia or thinning of long bone cortex, with or without pseudoarthrosis
- First-degree relative (parent, sibling, or offspring) with NF-1 by the above criteria

Dermoscopy of Neurofibroma

Dermoscopy shows central white scar-like area with peripheral halo of hyperpigmentation. Fingerprint-like pigmentary lines and peripheral pigment network can be seen.

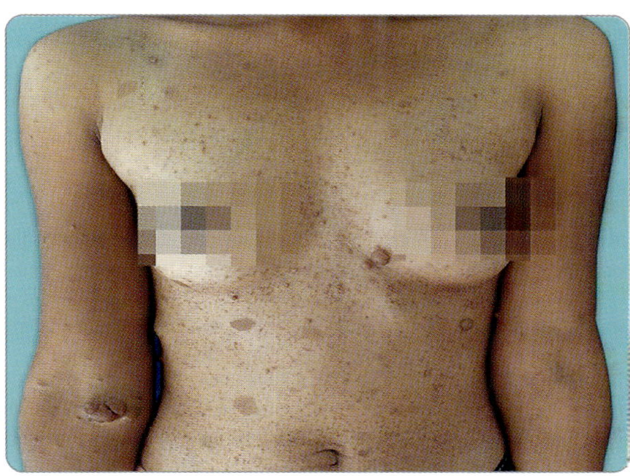

Fig. 2: Multiple café-au-lait macules (CALMs) noted with multiple neurofibromas and freckling of skin over abdomen.

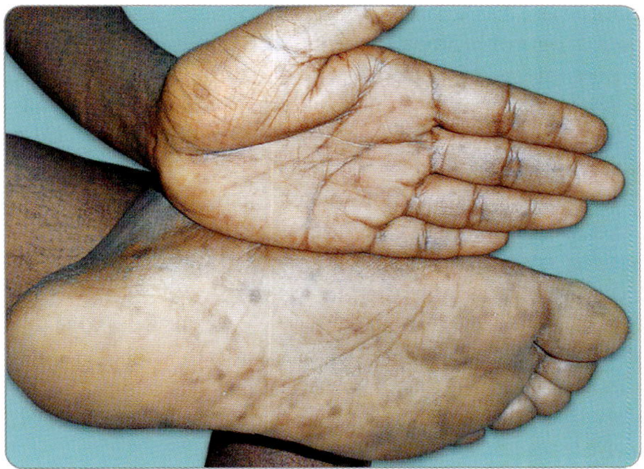

Fig. 3: Palmoplantar freckling—Patrick Yesudian sign.

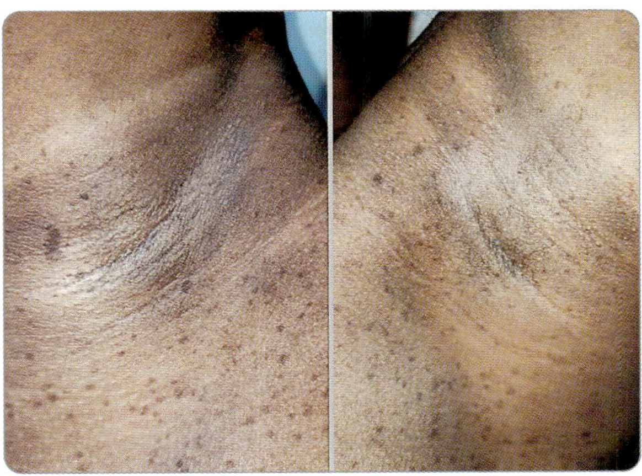

Fig. 4: Axillary freckling noted in a female patient of neurofibromatosis.

➲ TYPE 2 NEUROFIBROMATOSIS

Type 2 neurofibromatosis is distinguished by bilateral acoustic neuromas, usually in the absence of cutaneous lesions, although neurofibromas and schwannomas can occur.

➲ HISTOPATHOLOGY

Neurofibromas are well-circumscribed encapsulated, spindle cell proliferations with a mucinous background and many mast cells.

➲ TREATMENT

The CALMs that are typically present early in life do not require treatment, except for cosmesis. Although Lisch nodules are almost never symptomatic, the child should be followed annually by an ophthalmologist to check for visual field defects that may result from optic gliomas. Children with NF-1 should also have careful monitoring of their blood pressure, as renal artery stenosis can occur in this age group. Simple surgery can be performed on selected neurofibromas. Laser ablation has also been used to eradicate cutaneous neurofibromas. Long-term follow-up is essential, as a small percentage of patients will develop malignant peripheral nerve sheath tumors within their plexiform neurofibromas, and there is also an increased risk for the development of other soft tissue sarcomas.

Pirfenidone which is a farnesyltransferase inhibitor is being tried. It downregulates Ras oncogene and is antifibrotic.

Genetic counseling can be offered with prenatal diagnosis and preimplantation genetic diagnosis. Successful use of multiplex polymerase chain reaction (PCR) for microsatellite markers linked to the *NF1* gene has been reported, obviating the need to detect the mutation itself. Lastly, all patients and families should be referred early on to organizations that offer information, education, and support.

➲ SUGGESTED READING

1. Le C, Bedocs PM. (2023). Neurofibromatosis. Treasure Island (FL): Statpearls Publishing. [online] Available from https://www.ncbi.nlm.nih.gov/books/NBK459329/ [Last accessed January, 2025].

158 Nevus Anemicus

➲ SYNONYM

Pharmacological nevus.

➲ ETIOLOGY

Nevus anemicus is considered to represent an increased vascular reactivity to catecholamines. This is supported by the finding that the pallor can be overcome by local injection of alpha-adrenergic blocker phentolamine.

➲ EPIDEMIOLOGY

The lesions are present at birth.

➲ CLINICAL FEATURES

Nevus anemicus is a congenital localized anomaly of the skin characterized by macular areas of pallor, resulting from reduced blood flow, most often seen on trunk. It is a well-defined hypopigmented macule with an irregular border, often surrounded by smaller white macules beyond the border of the major lesion, and the skin has a normal texture.

On diascopy, it is indistinguishable from the blanched surrounding normal skin. Intradermal injection of histamine produces a flare. Friction, cold, or heat application fails to induce erythema in the involved area. Wood's lamp does not accentuate the lesion.

➲ DERMOSCOPY

Dermoscopy shows structureless white areas with paucity of blood vessels in lesional skin with diffuse erythema and linear telangiectatic vessels in the surrounding skin.

➲ ASSOCIATED CONDITIONS

Associated conditions include port-wine stain, neurofibromatosis, tuberous sclerosis, phakomatosis pigmentovascularis, telangiectatic nevus, and Becker nevus.

➲ HISTOPATHOLOGY

Skin appears normal with normal melanin pigmentation.

➲ DIFFERENTIAL DIAGNOSIS

- Nevus depigmentosus—on diascopy the borders are preserved.
- Tinea versicolor—hypo- or hyperpigmented macules with branny scaling, banana, and grapes appearance on KOH mount

- Vitiligo—no change in lesion on diascopy with absence of melanocytes

TREATMENT

Reassurance and camouflage makeup to hide the lesion.

PROGNOSIS

The lesion persists unchanged throughout life.

SUGGESTED READING

1. Kolb L, Troxell T, Krishnamurthy K. (2023). Nevus Anemicus. Treasure Island (FL): StatPearls Publishing. [online] Available from https://www.ncbi.nlm.nih.gov/books/NBK459139/ [Last accessed January, 2025].

159 Nevus Comedonicus

➲ SYNONYMS

Follicular nevi, comedo nevus.

➲ HISTORY

In 1895, Kofmann described the first case of nevus comedonicus.

➲ ETIOLOGY

Exact etiology is unclear. Majority of the cases are sporadic. Comedo nevus is caused by a defect in the development of pilosebaceous apparatus, characterized by inability to produce properly formed hair matrix cells or sebaceous glands.

➲ EPIDEMIOLOGY

The lesions may develop any time from birth to middle age.

➲ PATHOPHYSIOLOGY

Mutation in fibroblast growth factor receptor 2 (FGFR2) along with increased expression of interleukin-1 (IL-1) alpha is considered important factor in pathogenesis.

Other factors include gamma secretase, filaggrin, and NEK9 mutation.

➲ CLINICAL FEATURES

Large comedones are arranged in linear, segmental, blaschkoid, unilateral or bilateral, extensive or diffuse pattern **(Fig. 1)**. They are asymptomatic, and usually present on face, trunk, neck, and upper extremities. Rarely, they may occur on palms and soles. There is no

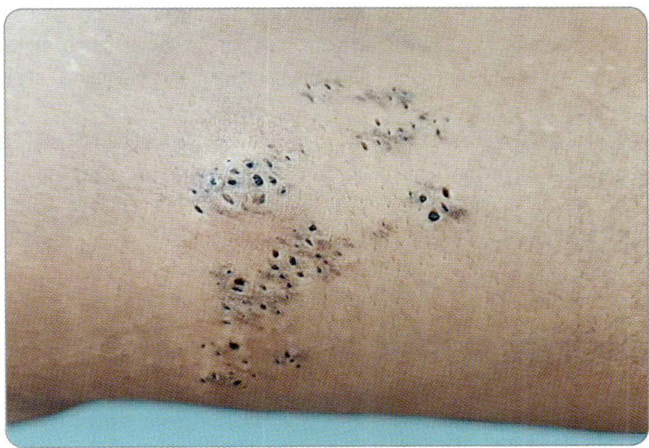

Fig. 1: Nevus comedonicus over the back of an adult male.

change in the lesions with menstruation, pregnancy, or menopause, although postpubertal enlargement may be seen.

Two specific subtypes have been described:

1. Nonpyogenic type
2. Type associate

DERMOSCOPY

Dermoscopy shows multiple well-defined structureless brown homogenous circular areas surrounding keratin plugs.

ASSOCIATED SYNDROMES

Associated syndromes include epidermal nevus syndrome and nevus comedonicus syndrome (nevus comedonicus in combination with systemic abnormalities in central nervous system, skeletal system, another skin manifestation, or ocular and dental abnormalities).

HISTOPATHOLOGY

Rudimentary hair follicles, sebaceous glands, and even trichilemmal cysts are present. Dyskeratosis and epidermolytic hyperkeratosis are seen.

DIFFERENTIAL DIAGNOSIS

- Basal cell nevus with comedones
- Linear basal cell nevus
- Acne
- Acne nevus
- Trichofolliculoma
- Basaloid follicular hamartoma
- Nevus sebaceous

COMPLICATIONS

Complications include bacterial infections, cysts, fistula, abscess formation, and scarring.

TREATMENT

Keratolytic agents (topical retinoids, salicylic acid, and 12% ammonium lactate), manual extraction of comedones, dermabrasion, excision of smaller lesions, CO_2 laser ablation, intralesional steroids, and oral isotretinoin.

Newer treatment avenues being explored include FGFR inhibitors, IL-1 alpha inhibitors, and anti-gamma-secretase drugs.

PROGNOSIS

The lesions persist throughout life.

SUGGESTED READING

1. Kaliyadan F, Troxell T, Ashique KT. Nevus Comedonicus. Treasure Island (FL): StatPearls Publishing. [online] Available from https://www.ncbi.nlm.nih.gov/books/NBK441903 [Last accessed January, 2025].

160 Nevus Depigmentosus

➲ SYNONYM

Nevus achromicus.

➲ ETIOLOGY

In nevus depigmentosus, there is an aggregation of melanosomes within melanocytes due to their defective transport to keratinocytes.

➲ EPIDEMIOLOGY

The lesions are present from birth and occurs equally in both sexes.

➲ CLINICAL FEATURES

Congenital, stable, asymptomatic depigmented macule of variable size with regular or serrated borders, single or multiple commonly found on trunk, neck, face, and proximal parts of extremities. It may be focal, segmental, or generalized in distribution. Lesions may be rounded, circumscribed, dermatomal, in whorls or streaks pattern.

Variants of achromic nevus:

- Isolated achromic nevus
- Segmental achromic nevus
- Linear or systematized achromic nevus

Woods lamp examination: Nevus depigmentosus appears off white compared to chalk-white accentuation seen in vitiligo **(Fig. 1)**.

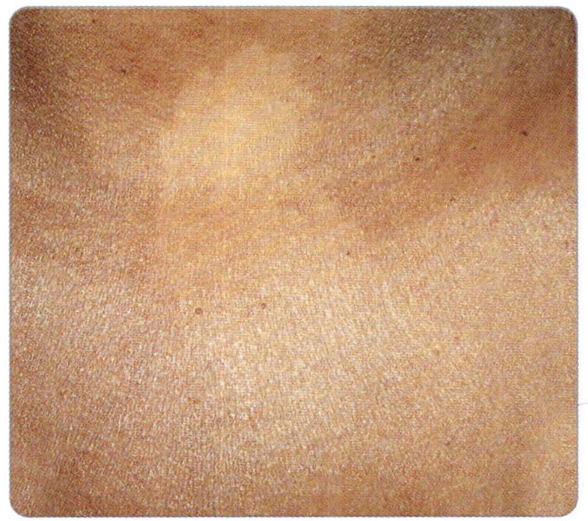

Fig. 1: Hypopigmented lesion of nevus depigmentosus over the chest.

DERMOSCOPY

On dermoscopy, achromic nevus appears as white structureless area with irregular serrated border and pseudopod-like extensions with faint reticulate pigment network. Hairs within lesion are normal with perifollicular pigmentation. Pigmentation in the surrounding skin is normal with no hyperpigmented border.

HISTOPATHOLOGY

There is normal or reduced number of melanocytes, but DOPA reaction shows them to be less reactive. There is no pigmentary incontinence.

DIFFERENTIAL DIAGNOSIS

- Nevus anemicus—borders merge with normal skin on diascopy
- Ash leaf macules—found in association with other classical lesions of tuberous sclerosis
- Vitiligo—absence of melanocytes, negative DOPA reaction, koebnerization seen
- Hypomelanoses of Ito—whorled pattern of hypopigmented macules seen, associated neurological, skeletal deformities
- Incontinentia pigmenti—history of (H/o) evolution of lesions from vesicles, plaques, and pigmentation

TREATMENT

No treatment is necessary. Cosmetic camouflage may be helpful. For small lesions plastic surgery with skin grafting may be considered on cosmetic backgrounds. Other options used to attempt repigmentation include: Excimer laser and phototherapy (PUVA).

PROGNOSIS

The lesions remain unchanged throughout life.

SUGGESTED READING

1. Ankad BS, Shah S. Dermoscopy of Nevus Depigmentosus. Pigment Int. 2017;4:121-3.

161 Nevus Flammeus

SYNONYM

Port-wine stain.

HISTORY

The term is derived from the city of Oporto, the center of Portugal's red port-wine trade.

ETIOLOGY

It represents an error in vascular development occurring during embryogenesis. There is decrease in autonomic innervation of the cutaneous vasculature.

EPIDEMIOLOGY

Lesions are present at birth and have an equal sex distribution.

CLINICAL FEATURES

Flat irregular macule is present at birth, unilateral distribution, varying in size from few millimeters to several centimeters, tend to darken with age **(Fig. 1)** and may develop small nodules (cobblestone appearance), leading to significant disfigurement. Lesions are seen commonly on the face or any part including the mucosae. Soft tissue swelling and bony hypertrophy may develop under a port-wine stain.

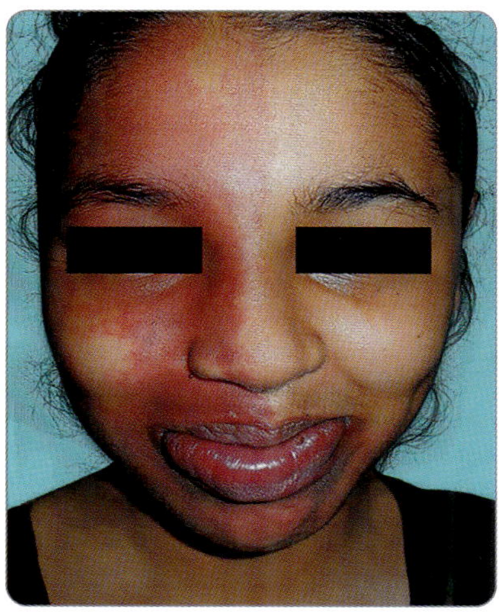

Fig. 1: Erythematous lesion over one half of the face.

Investigations must include ophthalmological examination and brain magnetic resonance imaging (MRI).

ASSOCIATED SYNDROMES

- Sturge–Weber syndrome
- Klippel–Trénaunay syndrome
- Cobb syndrome
- Beckwith–Wiedemann syndrome
- Von Hippel–Lindau syndrome
- Wyburn–Mason syndrome
- Thrombocytopenia-absent radius (TAR) syndrome
- Proteus syndrome
- Phakomatosis pigmentovascularis
- Nevus anemicus
- Nevus oligemicus

HISTOPATHOLOGY

There is developmental defect leading to ectasia of dermal capillaries. There is no proliferation of endothelial cells.

DIFFERENTIAL DIAGNOSIS

- Infantile hemangioma—compressible vascular swelling seen
- Birth trauma—color of lesions change with time and resolve
- Bruise—evolution of lesions
- Salmon patch
- Cherry angioma—multiple small red papules
- Glomus tumor—associated with pain and pulsations
- Lymphocytoma cutis—presence of atypical cells in biopsy

COMPLICATIONS

Complications include glaucoma, choroidal angiomas, pyogenic granuloma, acquired tufted angioma, basal cell carcinoma, and psychological complications.

TREATMENT

Treatment can be tunable dye lasers, flash lamp pulsed dye laser and camouflage for early macular lesions, multiple cryogen spurts with multiple laser pulses, multiple pass laser treatment, alexandrite laser, neodymium:yttrium aluminum garnet laser, KTP (potassium-titanyl-phosphate) laser, intense pulsed light, and photodynamic therapy.

PROGNOSIS

They do not regress spontaneously, but increase in proportion with the growth of child.

SUGGESTED READING

1. Goldberg DJ. Treatment of port wine stains. J Cosmet Laser Ther. 2010;12(1):1.

162 Nevus of Ota and Ito

➲ SYNONYMS

Nevus fuscoceruleus ophthalmomaxillaris (Ota), persistent aberrant Mongolian spots, oculodermal melanocytosis, nevus fuscoceruleus acromiodeltoideus (Ito).

➲ HISTORY

Nevus of Ota was described by Ota and Tanino in Japan in 1939. Nevus of Ito was initially described by Minor Ito in 1954.

➲ ETIOLOGY

The exact etiology is unknown. It may represent melanocytes that have not migrated completely from the neural crest to the epidermis during the embryonic stage.

➲ EPIDEMIOLOGY

Lesions may appear at birth or childhood.

➲ CLINICAL FEATURES

Nevus of Ota presents as persistent, speckled, macular, slate brown or bluish hyperpigmentation in the distribution of ophthalmic **(Fig. 1)** and maxillary division of trigeminal nerve including peri-orbital, temple, forehead, malar area, nose, and oral mucosa. 75% of cases are unilateral. The color may vary from day to day in both sexes and during menstruation. Bluish discoloration of conjunctiva,

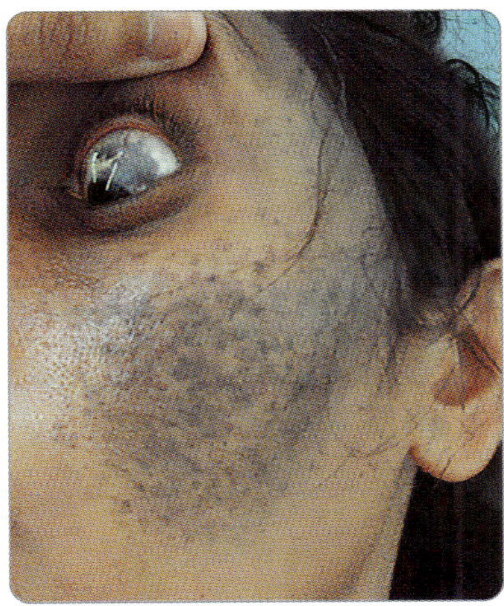

Fig. 1: Bluish pigmentation over the malar area and conjunctiva in nevus of Ota.

sclera, cornea, iris, retina, fundus, optic nerve, hard palate, pharynx, nasal mucosa, buccal mucosa, tympanic membrane, or affected site may be present.

Nevus of Ito are located in the areas supplied by lateral supraclavicular and lateral brachial cutaneous nerves.

Hori's nevus is bilateral acquired nevus of Ota like macules. There is no conjunctival involvement.

HISTOPATHOLOGY

Stellate dermal melanocytes are present in the mid-dermis and around blood vessels and dermal appendages.

DERMOSCOPY

The most common dermoscopic features include brown and gray structureless areas with a patchy distribution and scattered brown-gray dots. Other variable features include terminal hairs, white clods in a "four dots clod" arrangement, perifollicular hypopigmentation, yellowish structureless areas, and serpentine vessels.

DIFFERENTIAL DIAGNOSIS

- Melasma—present bilaterally, no conjunctival involvement
- Pigment demarcation lines—absence of discrete macules
- Melanocytic nevus—presence of nevus cells in sheets/nests
- Becker's nevus—present commonly on shoulder with increased hair growth over the patch
- Mongolian spot—uniform bluish green pigmentation
- Bruise—change in color with time
- Postinflammatory pigmentation
- Melanoma
- Blue nevus

COMPLICATIONS

Complications include ipsilateral sensorineural deafness, glaucoma, malignant melanoma, and malignant blue nevus.

TREATMENT

Treatment includes cosmetic camouflage, CO_2 snow along with dermabrasion, sequential dry ice application, epidermal peeling with argon laser, liquid N_2 cryotherapy, Q-switched ruby laser, and Nd:YAG lasers.

PROGNOSIS

The lesions persist for life without any tendency for remission or spontaneous resolution.

SUGGESTED READINGS

1. Dinulos JG. Dermal melanocytosis and associated disorders. Curr Opin Pediatr. 2015;27:480-5.
2. Harrison-Balestra C, Gugic D, Vincek V. Clinically distinct form of acquired dermal melanocytosis with review of published work. J Dermatol. 2007;34:178-82.

163 Nevus Sebaceous

➲ SYNONYMS

Nevus sebaceus of Jadassohn, organoid nevus.

➲ HISTORY

Nevus sebaceous was described by Jadassohn in 1895. Mehregan and Pinkus preferred the term organoid nevus.

➲ ETIOLOGY

The condition may be familial or sporadic.

➲ EPIDEMIOLOGY

Nevus sebaceous is noticed first at birth or early childhood.

➲ CLINICAL FEATURES

Natural history of sebaceous nevi comprises three stages:

1. Prepubertal—lesions present at birth or later. Solitary, circumscribed, sharply demarcated, yellowish-orange, smooth velvety plaques on scalp or linearly on face
2. Postpubertal—nevus becomes thickened, larger, waxy, greasy, more nodular, and verrucous **(Fig. 1)**
3. Neoplastic changes—benign tumors are syringocystadenoma papilliferum, syringoma, apocrine cystadenoma, trichilemmoma, spiradenoma, nodular hidradenoma, and keratoacanthoma. Malignancy is seen in middle age (5%).

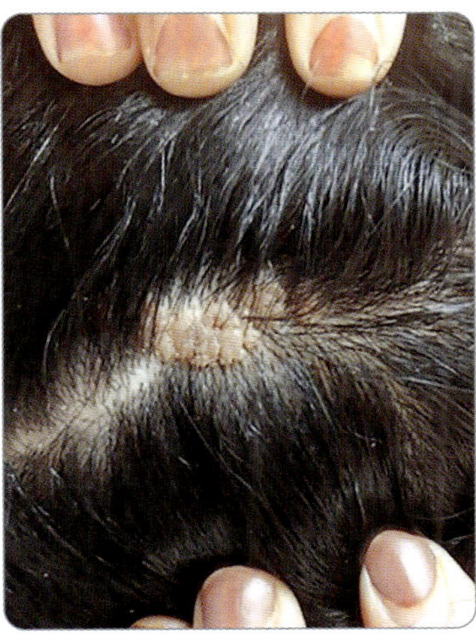

Fig. 1: Nevus sebaceous of scalp.

Basal cell carcinoma, squamous cell carcinoma, sebaceous, apocrine, and eccrine carcinoma are seen. A rapid increase in size, nodulation, or ulceration should lead to suspicion of a malignancy.

➲ SYNDROMES ASSOCIATED

Syndromes associated are nevus sebaceous syndrome, didymosis aplasticosebacea, and SCALP (Sebaceous nevus syndrome, CNS malformations, Aplasia cutis congenita, Limbal dermoid, and Pigmented nevus) syndrome.

➲ HISTOPATHOLOGY (FIGS. 2 AND 3)

- Prepubertal—multiple underdeveloped sebaceous glands, immature lobules with incompletely formed hair follicles
- Postpubertal—hyperkeratosis, hypergranulosis, papillomatosus, well-developed sebaceous glands, and apocrine glands

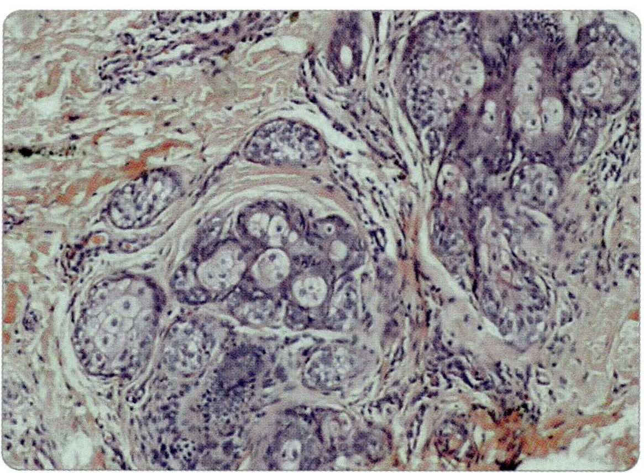

Fig. 2: Nevus sebaceous. Large numbers of mature or nearly mature sebaceous glands and overlying papillomatous hyperplasia of the epidermis are seen.

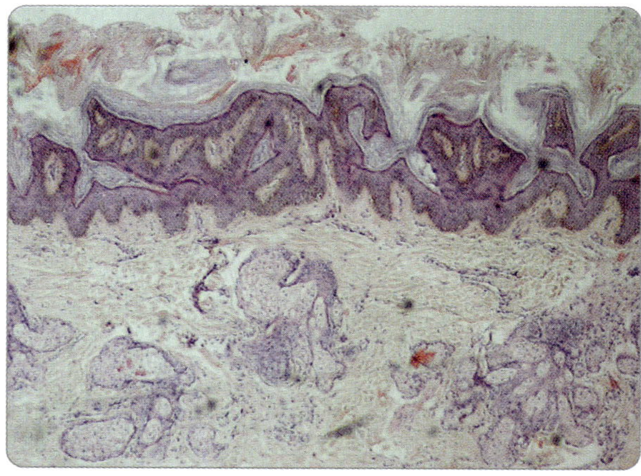

Fig. 3: Masses of sebaceous gland lobules.

DERMOSCOPY

- Patches—yellowish globules aggregated in clusters on a yellow background
- Plaques—brown globules, whitish-yellow lobular aspect, yellow-grayish papillary appearance
- Nodules—homogeneous yellowish, vascularization (linear irregular or arborescent vessels)

DIFFERENTIAL DIAGNOSIS

- Aplasia cutis—absence of hair and absence of plaque
- Syringocystadenoma papilliferum
- Early juvenile xanthogranuloma—presence of foamy cells and touton giant cells
- Solitary mastocytoma—positive Darier's sign

COMPLICATIONS

There is risk of malignant transformation.

TREATMENT

Treatment can be prophylactic surgical excision, Mohs micrographic surgery, CO_2 lasers, photodynamic therapy with aminolevulinic acid (ALA) or methylaminolevulinate (MAL), and tissue expanders.

PROGNOSIS

The lesions tend to recur with metastases, where the outcome may be fatal.

SUGGESTED READINGS

1. Moody MN, Landau JM, Goldberg LH. Nevus sebaceous revisited. Pediatr Dermatol. 2012;29(1):15-23.
2. Kelati A, Baybay H, Gallouj S, Mernissi FZ. Dermoscopic Analysis of Nevus Sebaceus of Jadassohn: A Study of 13 Cases. Skin Appendage Disord. 2017;3(2):83-91.

164 Nevus Spilus

➲ SYNONYMS

Speckled nevus: Nevus on nevus, spotty nevus, speckled lentiginous nevus, speckled zosteriform lentiginous nevus, speckled nevus spilus, cafè-au-lait spot, partial unilateral lentiginosis.

➲ HISTORY

Nevus spilus (NS) was first described by Burkley in 1842 as evenly pigmented patches, and Ito and Hamado in 1952 were the first to apply the term NS to speckled lesions.

➲ ETIOLOGY

Nevus spilus and also congenital nevus are postulated to result from a postzygotic genetic alteration of the melanocytic lineage, which gives rise to a clone of melanocytes predisposed to developing neoplasm; the question whether NS is a congenital or acquired lesion remains controversial to this day.

➲ EPIDEMIOLOGY

Nevus spilus is a relatively common health condition whose prevalence varies from between 0.2 and 2.3% according to the age groups taken into consideration; the prevalence is similar to the occurrence of a congenital nevus among the general public. NS even if not immediately present at birth, it needs to be considered a congenital lesion, or one with close links to a congenital nevus. There do not seem to be significant differences in predominance between people of either sexes, or among ethnic groups even though there tends to be a certain predilection for the Caucasian race.

➲ CLINICAL FEATURES

Nevus spilus starts at birth as a hyperpigmented patch (cafè-au-lait spot), reaches its peak in number between the ages of five and nine, while it reaches its characteristic speckled aspect between the ages of 6 and 39 years.

Nevus spilus can be classified into three distinct clinical types, in relation to the size and location.

Nevus spilus is considered small if >1.5 cm, medium if it varies from 1.5 to 19.9 cm, and large if its diameter exceeds 20 cm.

Nevus spilus can be found anywhere on the body, but the most common location is on the chest and upper limbs.

The speckles within NS are often macules rather than papules, with a variable number of elements. The speckled lesions can be various types of nevi—junctional, compound, intradermal dysplastic, or Spitz nevi, blue nevi, ink spot lentigo, and neurotic nevi.

HISTOPATHOLOGY

Histologically, the hyperchromatic base of the classic NS shows the histological features of lentigo simplex or a cafè-au-lait patch.

The increase of pigmentation is in fact linked to a rise in the number of melanocytes in the basal layer, as well as a rise in melanin content of the basal keratinocytes themselves. In addition, there is a moderate acanthosis and elongation of rete ridges.

DERMOSCOPY

Dermoscopy shows darker brown areas with a reticuloglobular pattern against the background of light brown and reticular pattern pigmentation.

DIFFERENTIAL DIAGNOSIS

Differential diagnosis includes agminated nevus, cafè-au-lait patches, segmental neurofibromatosis, LEOPARD syndrome, Becker nevus, and pigmented spots in Albright's disease.

PROGRESSION/DEVELOPMENT

The risk of malignant change appears to vary from 0.13 to 0.2% and seems higher than for congenital melanocytic nevus.

TREATMENT

Regular monitoring of NS appears to be essential; excision is indicated when surveillance is difficult because of the site or when any clinical modification occurs. Biopsy must be performed in suspect areas. Because the extent of malignant transformation is not clearly defined, excision should be complete and carried out to the fascial level, as the nevus cells extend deep around the hair follicles in similar fashion to congenital nevocellular nevi.

For small lesions excision, closure is done; for larger lesions, serial excision, skin expansion, association, and skin grafting can be done. Mechanical dermabrasion and ablative and nonablative lasers have also been tried. Lasers that have been used to treat cafè-au-lait macules (CALMs) and NS are pulsed dye laser, erbium YAG, QS Nd:YAG, Q-switched ruby laser (QSRL), and Q-switched Alexandrite laser (QSAL).

SUGGESTED READING

1. Corradin MT, Cacitti V, Giulioni E, Patriarca MM, Vettorello A. Nevus Spilus: A Review of the Literature. SM Dermatolog J. 2015;1(1):1003.

165 Nocardiosis

➲ ETIOLOGY

Nocardiosis is an acute or chronic, suppurative, granulomatous disease caused by members of the genus *Nocardia*. *Nocardia* are gram positive, partially acid-fast, aerobic filamentous bacteria. Some are branched, but tend to be shorter and more fragmentary than actinomycetes. *Nocardia* species are aerobic actinomycetes living free in nature. They may gain entry directly into wounds to cause localized actinomycotic mycetoma; inhalation would result in primary pulmonary disease and may result in metastasis to any part of the body. *Nocardia asteroides* complex is the predominant human pathogen; other pathogenic species being *Nocardia brasiliensis*, *Nocardia otitidiscaviarum* (*caviae*.), and *Nocardia farcinica*.

➲ CLINICAL FEATURES

Patient may give a history of local trauma and contact with soil as cellulitis, pustules, pyoderma, ulcerations, and a lymphocutaneous syndrome mimicking sporotrichosis. *N. brasiliensis* is usually associated with this. In normal hosts, the disease is benign and often resolves spontaneously or with iodides or sulfonamides. In a few cases, dissemination has been reported.

Primary Subcutaneous Infection

Nocardia causes mycetoma, a chronic, suppurative, granulomatous disease of the subcutaneous tissues and bones, characterized by localized swellings with multiple sinuses discharging granules that are the microcolonies of the organisms.

Primary Pulmonary Disease

Nocardiosis is primarily a pulmonary disease. The clinical manifestations include malaise, weight loss, fever, night sweats, and cough. The lesion can present as a solitary lung abscess, an acute necrotizing pneumonia, or a progressive fibrosis with extension to the pleura and chest wall with penetration.

➲ LABORATORY DIAGNOSIS

Samples of sputum, bronchial aspirate, pleural fluid, cerebrospinal fluid, and biopsy material should be examined for the presence of Gram positive, partially acid-fast, branching filaments of bacterial width and coccobacillary forms. Tissue sections should be stained by Brown and Brenn modification of Gram and Kinyoun's acid-fast stain or methenamine silver stain in order to visualize the organism. In addition to routine culture on Sabouraud dextrose agar paraffin, bait technique should be used for isolation of *Nocardia* because of their ability and the inability of most commensal microflora to utilize paraffin as the sole source of carbon and grow on it. The isolates are identified on the basis of morphological, cultural, biochemical, antimicrobial sensitivity, and animal pathogenicity tests.

HISTOPATHOLOGY

Suppuration is the most characteristic feature of nocardiosis. Multiple abscess formation with central necrosis and little or no fibrosis are seen. Encapsulation is found in cerebral lesions. In a hematoxylin and eosin stained section, the organism is usually missed. With Brown and Brenn modification of Gram stain, the delicate, gram positive, branching filaments of bacteria fragmenting into bacillary and coccoid forms are seen. They are partially acid-fast when stained with Kinyoun's acid-fast stain. Methenamine silver stains the organism. Periodic acid-Schiff is not useful.

DIFFERENTIAL DIAGNOSIS

- Tuberculosis—presence of epithelioid granulomas with lymphocyte cuff and Langhans giant cells
- Actinomycosis—demonstration of bacterial colonies in the sulfur granules
- Chronic bacterial infections
- Kaposi sarcoma—mostly on the limbs, bluish to violaceous nodules, lack suppuration
- Deep fungal infections—demonstration of fungi in mount and culture

TREATMENT

The most widely used therapy is cotrimoxazole for 6–12 months or sulfadiazine and sodium bicarbonate for 4–6 weeks followed by sulfisoxazole for 12–18 months. Minocycline, amikacin, imipenem, and linezolid are used successfully as primary agents. Amikacin in combination with imipenem, extended spectrum cephalosporins, amoxicillin–clavulanate, newer macrolides, other aminoglycosides, and fluoroquinolones have also been considered as potentially efficacious drug.

SUGGESTED READINGS

1. Ramos-E-Silva M, Lopes RS, Trope BM. Cutaneous nocardiosis: A great imitator. Clin Dermatol. 2020;38(2):152-9.
2. Dodiuk-Gad R, Cohen E, Ziv M, Goldstein LH, Chazan B, Shafer J, et al. Cutaneous nocardiosis: report of two cases and review of the literature. Int J Dermatol. 2010;49(12):1380-5.

166 Nummular Dermatitis

➲ SYNONYMS

Nummular eczema, discoid eczema, microbial eczema.

➲ HISTORY

Nummular (meaning "coin-shaped") dermatitis is a form of endogenous eczema. The term was probably coined by Darier.

➲ ETIOLOGY

The etiology is unknown and likely multifactorial. It is a distinctive primary endogenous form of eczema. Some authors have found a high incidence of atopy. Some have stressed the role of infection, local physical or chemical trauma, dry skin, and contact sensitization (e.g., nickel, chromate, mercury, aloe, balsam of Peru, and fragrances). It is also seen in patients on methyldopa, interferon therapy for hepatitis C, and tumor necrosis factor-alpha blocking therapy. Emotional stress, venous hypertension, and excessive alcohol intake may play a role in some cases.

➲ AGE GROUP

Nummular dermatitis has two peaks of age distribution. The most common is in the sixth to seventh decade of life. This is most often seen in males. A smaller peak occurs in the second to third decade of life, which is most often seen in association with atopic dermatitis. This is more often seen in females. It is uncommon in children.

➲ CLINICAL FEATURES

The diagnostic lesion of discoid eczema is a coin-shaped plaque of closely set, thin-walled vesicles on an erythematous base, most commonly found on the arms and legs. Later it progresses to a more scaly stage, often with central clearing, and peripheral extension, causing ring-shaped or annular lesions. After any period between 10 days and several months, secondary lesions occur, often in a mirror-image configuration on the opposite side of the body. It is very characteristic of this disease that patches which have apparently become dormant may become active again. Pruritus may be intense and excoriations are often prominent. Nummular dermatitis usually takes a very chronic course.

A particularly therapy-resistant variety has been termed "oid-oid disease" (Sulzberger–Garbe syndrome).

➲ HISTOPATHOLOGY

There is a subacute dermatitis indistinguishable from other forms of eczema, with spongiotic vesicles and a predominantly lymphohistiocytic infiltrate. Eosinophils may also be present in the upper dermis.

DERMOSCOPY

Dermoscopic findings show shiny yellow clods, scales, and irregularly distributed brownish-red globules.

DIFFERENTIAL DIAGNOSIS

Differential diagnosis includes asteatotic eczema, atopic dermatitis, contact dermatitis, mycosis fungoides, lichen simplex chronicus, pityriasis rosea, psoriasis, tinea corporis, and Bowen's disease.

COMPLICATIONS

Complications include nummular dermatitis. Lesions may become secondarily infected. Heavily excoriated or infected lesions may leave permanent scars.

TREATMENT

Rule of the 4 R's:

1. *R*ecognition of the culprit irritant/allergen
2. *R*emoval of the irritant/allergen
3. *R*eduction of skin inflammation
4. *R*estoration of the skin barrier

Treatment is aimed at rehydration of the skin and repair of the epidermal lipid barrier, reduction of inflammation, and treatment of any infection.

Medium to high-potency topical corticosteroid ointments, topical tacrolimus or pimecrolimus, and emollients represent topical treatment options. Tar preparations have also been used successfully. Oral, intramuscular, or parenteral steroids may be required in cases of severe, generalized eruptions. When eruptions are generalized and prolonged, phototherapy [generally ultraviolet B (UVB)] may be helpful. Oral antihistamines or sedatives may help reduce itching and improve sleep. Oral antibiotics, such as dicloxacillin, cephalexin, or erythromycin, should be used in cases of secondary infection. Few studies have shown lasting efficacy after the use of methotrexate in children. Recently, dupilumab has also shown promise as a possible emerging treatment.

PROGNOSIS

Patients need to be informed that once nummular dermatitis develops, it is often recurrent. Avoidance of exacerbating factors and close attention to moisturizing the skin may help reduce the frequency.

SUGGESTED READING

1. Robinson CA, Love LW, Farci F. (2023). Nummular Dermatitis. Treasure Island (FL): StatPearls Publishing. [online] Available from https://www.ncbi.nlm.nih.gov/books/NBK565878/ [Last accessed January, 2025].

167 Onychomycosis

➲ SYNONYMS

Tinea unguium, ringworm of the nail.

➲ ETIOLOGY

About 70% of cases are caused by *Trichophyton rubrum*, 20% by *T. mentagrophytes*, and 5% by yeasts, the majority of which is caused by *Candida albicans*. 4% of cases are by nondermatophyte molds like *Acremonium*, *Aspergillus*, *Fusarium*, *Onychocola canadensis*, *Scopulariopsis brevicaulis*, and *Scytalidium dimidiatum*. Diabetes mellitus, frequent trauma, vascular defects, occlusive footwear, improper drying of feet, and use of communal showers are risk the factors.

➲ AGE

Onychomycosis is common between 40 and 60 years. Men are infected more than women.

➲ CLINICAL FEATURES

The five clinical types of onychomycosis are:

1. Distal subungual onychomycosis—invasion through distal nail bed, most common type
2. Proximal subungual onychomycosis (PSO)—invasion through newly formed proximal nail plate.
3. White superficial onychomycosis (WSO)—invasion of the superficial layers of nail plate
4. Total dystrophic onychomycosis (TDO)
5. Endonyx type

Toe nail infections are four to six times more common than finger nails. Affected nail is discolored, dystrophic, and brittle **(Fig. 1)**. The infection spreads proximally up the nail bed to the ventral nail plate. PSO results mainly from infection of the proximal nail fold, and is evident as a white to beige opacity on the proximal nail plate. This opacity gradually enlarges to affect the entire nail, and subungual hyperkeratosis, leukonychia, proximal onycholysis, and destruction of the entire nail unit may be seen. WSO is a direct invasion of the dorsal nail plate, resulting in white to dull yellow sharply bordered patches anywhere on the surface of the toenail. *Candida* species invade via the hyponychial epithelium to affect the entire thickness of the nail plate.

➲ HISTOPATHOLOGY

Hyphae are seen lying between the nail laminae parallel to the surface, with a predilection for the ventral nail and nail bed

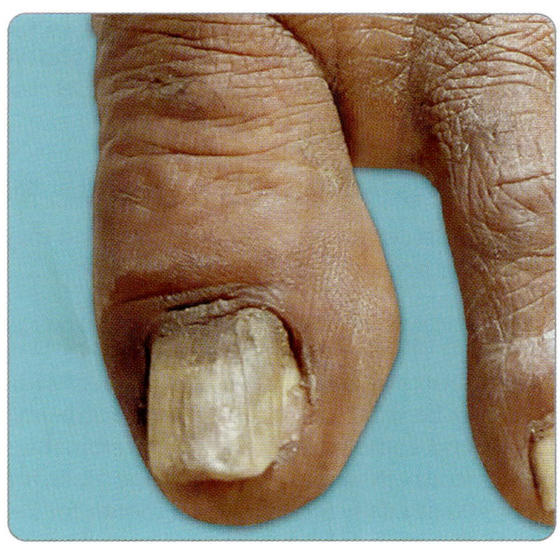

Fig. 1: Discoloration and dystrophy of the nail due to onychomycosis.

stratum corneum. The epidermis may show spongiosis and focal parakeratosis, and there is a minimal dermal inflammatory response. In WSO, the organisms are present superficially on the dorsal nail and display unique "perforating organs" and "eroding fronds." Candidal onychomycosis displays invasion of pseudohyphae throughout the entire nail plate, adjacent cuticle, granular layer and stratum spinosum of the nail bed, and the hyponychial stratum corneum.

DERMOSCOPY/ONYCHOSCOPY

The main dermoscopic signs of onychomycosis are "ruin appearance," "longitudinal striae," and "spikes" on the proximal margin of onycholytic areas; the "aurora borealis" sign had the highest sensitivity and specificity.

- *Ruin appearance*: Ventral indentations of the nail plate caused by dermal debris
- Subungual hyperkeratosis
- *Sulphur nuggets*: Yellow clumping sulfur nugget-like debris under the nail plate
- *Longitudinal striae*: Longitudinal pigmentation of different colors in streaks within the nail plate
- *Onycholysis*: Separation of the nail plate from the nail bed

Jagged edge with spikes/spiked pattern, straight onycholytic edge:

- Distal irregular termination
- Splinter hemorrhage
- Chromonychia
- *Aurea borealis*: Area of various colors associating various degrees of green, bluish-gray, black, white, and yellow in association with onycholysis, striae, and streaks.
- Leukonychia
- Melanonychia

DIFFERENTIAL DIAGNOSIS

Differential diagnosis includes psoriasis, hand eczema, lichen planus, pachyonychia congenital, Darier disease, lichen planus, acquired and congenital leukonychias, onychogryphosis, exfoliative dermatitis, Norwegian scabies, Reiter syndrome, and yellow nail syndrome. All of these conditions show negative KOH mount of the nailbed scrapings and culture of nail clippings.

COMPLICATIONS

It can cause pain, discomfort, and disfigurement and may produce serious physical and occupational limitations.

TREATMENT

In cases without matrix involvement, topical treatment with ciclopirox or amorolfine may be sufficient. In cases with matrix involvement, oral antifungals and combinations are used. Terbinafine 250 mg/day for 12 weeks (toe nails) and 6 weeks for finger nails, itraconazole 200 mg/day or 400 mg daily for 1 week per month for 2–3 months, and fluconazole 150 mg/week for 6–12 weeks can be given.

Sequential therapy combines use of two oral antifungals acting on two different pathways in ergosterol metabolism. Patients are given two pulses of itraconazole followed by one or two pulses of terbinafine. Itraconazole was administered before terbinafine, because the former is barely detectable in plasma 10–14 days after completing a pulse.

Boosted oral antifungal treatment and boosted antifungal topical treatment targets resting fungal cells to produce sensitive hyphae as they are less refractory to antifungals. A piece of a Sabouraud's agar slide is secured onto the affected nail in alternance with oral intake of itraconazole.

Surgical methods can be used to remove part (debridement) or whole (avulsion) of the nail plate.

Newer therapies: Ciclopirox hydro lacquer based on water-soluble biopolymer technology, 1% fluconazole and 20% urea in a mixture of ethanol and water, terbinafine nail solution, and Noveon dual-wavelength (using 870-nm, 930-nm light) near-infrared diode laser.

PROGNOSIS

A disease-free toe nail occurs in 25–50% of patients who take systemic antifungal agents.

SUGGESTED READING

1. Singal A, Khanna D. Onychomycosis: Diagnosis and management. Indian J Dermatol Venereol Leprol. 2011;77:659-72.

168 Oral Hairy Leukoplakia

➲ ETIOLOGY

Epstein–Barr virus (EBV) is the causative agent. Hairy leukoplakia (HL) is seen in severe immunodeficiency, especially human immunodeficiency virus/acquired immunodeficiency syndrome (HIV/AIDS) with CD4 count 200–300 cells/mm^3.

➲ CLINICAL FEATURES

Lesions are typically unilateral or bilateral, adherent, slightly elevated whitish or gray patches, principally located mainly on lateral margins, dorsum, or ventrum of the tongue. Occasionally, they may be observed over the floor of the mouth, palate, or oropharynx. It is usually asymptomatic, and there may be daily variations in morphology. It is not premalignant.

➲ HISTOPATHOLOGY

Histopathology remains the gold standard for diagnosis. It shows hyperkeratosis, parakeratosis, acanthosis, keratinized "hair-like" projections, koilocytosis with pyknotic nuclei, perinuclear halos in the prickle cell layer, intranuclear inclusions, marked decrease or absence of Langerhans cells, and limited or no inflammatory cell infiltrate in the lamina propria.

➲ DERMOSCOPY/MUCOSCOPY

Polarized mucoscopy of leukoplakia shows white-to-pink structureless areas, intervening pink lines, and surface corrugations. The periphery of the lesions showed white clods and dotted vessels with irregular arrangement.

➲ DIFFERENTIAL DIAGNOSIS

Differential diagnosis includes idiopathic leukoplakia, smoker's keratosis, frictional keratosis, acute pseudomembranous candidiasis, chronic hyperplastic candidiasis, plaque-like type of lichen planus, lichenoid reaction, trauma, white sponge nevus, and graft-versus-host disease.

➲ COMPLICATIONS

Complications can be dysesthesia, alteration of taste, and the psychological impact of its unsightly cosmetic appearance.

➲ TREATMENT

Treatment can be topical application of podophyllin 25% resin, retinoids, and gentian violet. Oral acyclovir 800 mg five times per day, valacyclovir 1,000 mg three times a day, and famciclovir 500 mg three times a day gives response in 2–3 weeks. Responds to highly active antiretroviral therapy (HAART).

Cryotherapy and surgical excision can be done.

➲ SUGGESTED READING

1. Greenspan JS, Greenspan D. Oral hairy leukoplakia: Diagnosis and management. Oral Surg Oral Med Oral Pathol. 1989;67(4):396-403.

169 Osler–Weber–Rendu Syndrome

➲ SYNONYM

Hereditary hemorrhagic telangiectasia.

➲ HISTORY

While Henri Rendu (1896), Sir William Osler (1901), and Frederick Parks Weber (1907) emphasized and published detailed observations of the syndrome, which bears their names; it was Sutton (1864) who first described Osler–Weber–Rendu disease and Benjamin Guy Babington (1865) was the first to note its familial nature.

➲ ETIOLOGY

Hereditary hemorrhagic telangiectasia (HHT) is an autosomal dominant disorder identified by the triad of telangiectasia, recurrent epistaxis, and a positive family history for the disorder. HHT type 1 and type 2 are due to defective endoglin (ENG) and activin receptor-like kinase 1 (*ALK1*) genes, respectively. Mutations of *ENG* are located on the long arm of chromosome 9 (9q33-34), whereas *ALK1* mutations are on the long arm of chromosome 12 (12q13). HHT type 3 involves mutations of the long arm of chromosome 5 (5q31.1-32), and type 4 maps to the short arm of chromosome 7 (7p14). An HHT-juvenile polyposis overlap syndrome due to mutations of *SMAD4* has also been described.

➲ AGE GROUP

Hereditary hemorrhagic telangiectasia may begin in childhood or even in infancy, but far more commonly begins at puberty or in early adult life.

➲ CLINICAL FEATURES

Diagnosis is based on the four components of the Curaçao criteria, established by the Scientific Advisory Board of the HHT Foundation International, Inc., viz.

- *Epistaxis*: Spontaneous and recurrent
- *Telangiectasias*: Multiple, at characteristic sites, including lips, oral cavity, fingers, and nose
- *Presence of internal lesions*: Gastrointestinal (GI) telangiectasia, pulmonary, hepatic, cerebral, and spinal arteriovenous malformation (AVMs).
- *Family history*: First-degree relative with HHT according to these criteria.

The diagnosis is considered definite if any three of the mentioned criteria are present and possible if any two of the criteria are present.

➲ DERMOSCOPY

Dermoscopy shows small red clots and thick serpentine and linear vessels with a radial arrangement on a pinkish background.

➲ DIAGNOSIS

It is recommended that patients with HHT have a complete blood count and hematocrit, evaluation of feces for occult blood, brain magnetic resonance imaging (MRI) with and without gadolinium to screen for cerebral AVMs, and contrast echocardiography to screen for pulmonary shunting. Chest computed tomography (CT) is done to characterize pulmonary AVM, if shunting is found.

➲ DIFFERENTIAL DIAGNOSIS

Differential diagnosis includes generalized essential telangiectasia, unilateral nevoid telangiectasia, scleroderma with CREST syndrome, rosacea, actinic keratitis, venous hypertension, and ataxia telangiectasia.

➲ COMPLICATIONS

Complications include asymptomatic pulmonary and central nervous system (CNS) AVM, and their hemorrhagic or embolic complications, viz. brain abscess and stroke are responsible for mortality in most of HHTs.

➲ TREATMENT

The varied treatment modalities include estrogen, ε-aminocaproic acid, cryotherapy, cautery, infrared coagulation, radiofrequency, pulse dye laser, Nd-YAG laser, and surgical ablation.

➲ PROGNOSIS

Rate of mortality due to complications is 10%.

➲ SUGGESTED READING

1. Tokoro S, Namiki T, Ugajin T, Miura K, Tanaka M, Yokozeki H. Hereditary hemorrhagic telangiectasia (Rendu-Osler-Weber's disease): detailed assessment of skin lesions by dermoscopy and ultrasound. Int J Dermatol. 2019;58(11):e224-6.

170 Pachydermoperiostosis

➲ SYNONYMS

Hypertrophic osteoarthropathy, Touraine–Solente–Golé syndrome.

➲ HISTORY

Touraine and Solente, who first characterized pachydermoperiostosis, distinguished its three forms: (1) The "complete" form with pachyderma and pachyperiostosis, (2) the "incomplete" form with face, acral, and bony involvement, (3) the "forms fruste" which may present with only clubbing and thickening of face and/or scalp, but no periosteal ossification.

➲ ETIOLOGY

Primary pachydermoperiostosis is a rare inherited disorder, which occurs predominantly in males. Both autosomal dominant and autosomal recessive inheritance have been demonstrated and mutations in the *HPGD* gene, encoding nicotinamide adenine dinucleotide $(NAD)^+$-dependent 15-hydroxyprostaglandin dehydrogenase, have been identified. Secondary pachydermoperiostosis (synonym secondary hypertrophic osteoarthropathy) is usually provoked by severe pulmonary disease, adenocarcinoma or epidermoid carcinoma of the bronchus, pleural mesothelioma, bronchiectasis, lung abscess or, less often, carcinoma of the stomach, esophagus or thymus.

➲ AGE

Primary pachydermoperiostosis usually begins soon after puberty. Secondary pachydermoperiostosis occurs predominantly in men aged 30–70 years.

➲ CLINICAL FEATURES

- *Primary pachydermoperiostosis*: The skin of the face, forehead, and scalp becomes grossly thickened and thrown into folds **(Fig. 1)**. The folding of the scalp produces one of the forms of cutis verticis gyrata. The skin of the hands and feet is also thickened, but usually not folded. Seborrhea of the face and scalp, and hyperhidrosis of hands and feet may be troublesome. Thickening of the phalanges and of the bones of the limbs produces spade-like hands and feet with increased circumference of arms and legs. The fingers and toes are clubbed **(Fig. 2)**.
- *Secondary pachydermoperiostosis*: The bone changes are the most obvious feature, develop more rapidly, and are often painful. The skin changes may be absent and are often relatively mild.

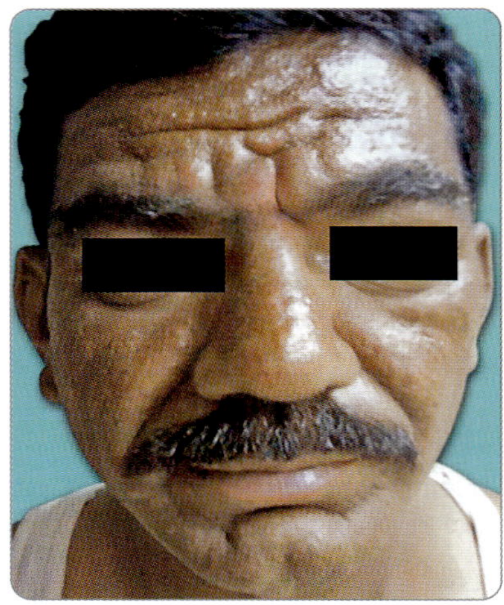

Fig. 1: Thickening of skin over the face; skin is thrown into folds over forehead and chin.

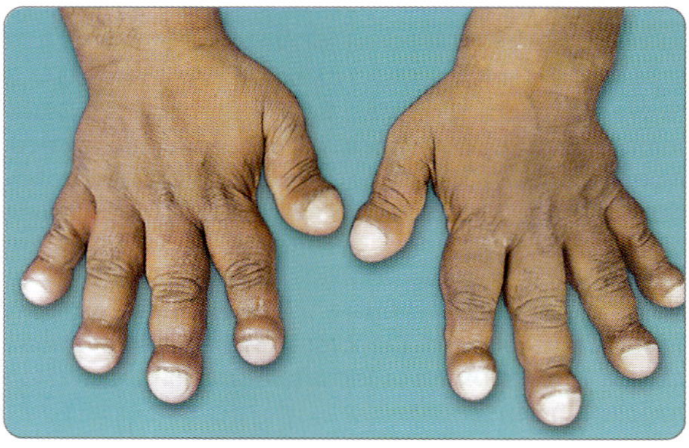

Fig. 2: Thickening of skin over the hands with clubbing.

➲ HISTOPATHOLOGY

The skin shows hypertrophy of collagen and of epidermis and epidermal appendages, and an increase of acid mucopolysaccharide.

➲ DIFFERENTIAL DIAGNOSIS

Differential diagnosis includes acromegaly and thyroid acropachy.

➲ TREATMENT

Nonsteroidal anti-inflammatory drugs, systemic corticosteroids, colchicine, and bisphosphonates can be used to reduce the pain due to osteoarthropathy. Etoricoxib, which inhibits cyclooxygenase-2, was reported to improve both the swelling of joints and the facial coarsening.

➲ SUGGESTED READING

1. Munichandrappa P, Singh N, Thappa DM. Pachydermoperiostosis. Indian J Dermatol Venereol Leprol. 2016;82(1):57-8.

171 Pachyonychia Congenita

➲ SYNONYMS

Congenital pachyonychia, Jadassohn–Lewandowsky syndrome (PC-1), Jackson–Lawler syndrome (PC-2), pachyonychia congenita syndrome.

➲ HISTORY

Pachyonychia congenita (PC) is a rare, heritable disorder of the skin first described by Jadassohn and Lewandowsky in 1906.

➲ ETIOPATHOGENESIS

Mutations of a gene controlling the specific biochemical conversion of normal metabolic precursors could cause changes in the structures of ectodermal origin. A defect probably involves multiple ectodermal cellular structures. These defects account for the inherent structural weaknesses and lowered resistance of the skin and mucous membranes to pressure, irritation, and friction that are responsible for the clinical manifestations.

Clinically, there is the Kumar and Loos classification of 1935, which was later modified by Joseph in 1964:

- *Type I*—symmetric keratoses of the palms and soles with follicular keratoses of the body
- *Type II*—similar to type I but with leukokeratosis oris (Riehl type); most common form
- Type III—includes the characteristics of types I and II and, in addition, corneal dyskeratosis

The abnormality of the nails, being the most consistent clinical feature of this syndrome, is the most suitable marker for following genetic transmission. The syndrome is the expression of a mutant autosomal gene with dominant effect but variable expression and, occasionally, what seems to be incomplete penetrance.

➲ CLINICAL MANIFESTATIONS

In 1943, Ormsby and Montgomery summarized the symptoms of dystrophic nail changes, hyperkeratosis of the hands and feet **(Figs. 1A and B)**, hair anomalies, leukokeratosis of mucous membranes (especially the tongue and oral mucosa), follicular keratosis (especially on the elbows and knees), corneal dyskeratosis, and bullae found usually on the soles but sometimes on the buttocks and ankles, natal and neonatal teeth, cataracts, plantar, and, occasionally, palmar hyperkeratosis, congenital white sponge nevus, diffuse alopecia (which can also be congenital), angular cheilosis, constant or transient hoarseness, laryngeal lesions that may cause acute respiratory distress syndrome and therefore require surgery, and mental retardation **(Figs. 2A and B)**.

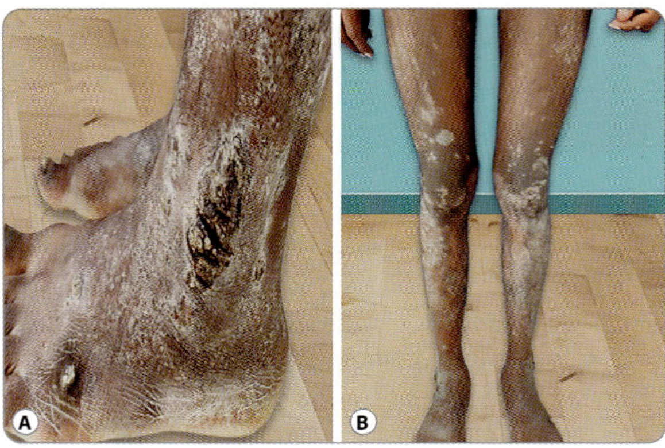

Figs. 1A and B: Clinical images of pachyonychia congenital tarda—hyperkeratotic lesions (A) around ankle joint and (B) over the knees.

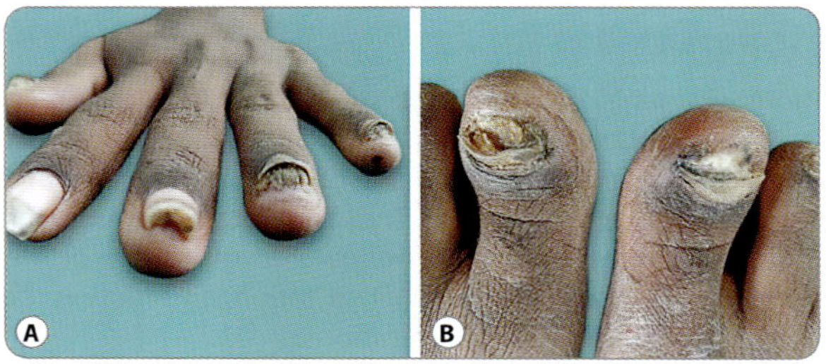

Figs. 2A and B: Dystrophic nail changes in both the fingers and toes.

➲ ASSOCIATED SYNDROME

Associated syndrome are steatocystomas and oral candidiasis.

➲ HISTOPATHOLOGY

The primary histopathologic changes of the skin in PC are marked hyperkeratosis, acanthosis, moderate hypergranulosis of the epidermis, and, occasionally, focal parakeratosis and follicular plugging. If the skin is injured, intraepidermal bullae may develop. A slight lymphocytic infiltrate is usually present in the upper dermis. Melanophages and epidermoid cysts sometimes are also seen within the dermis. The nail plate and proximal nail matrix appear histologically normal, whereas the nail bed shows marked hyperkeratosis. Hard keratin arises irregularly from the nail folds. The distal nail matrix is hyperplastic and papillomatous, producing large quantities of homy material mixed with periodic acid Schiff-positive hyalin. Consequently, the deformed nail resembles a miniature horse's hoof.

➲ TREATMENT

Treatment is palliative; lubricants, keratolytics, and protective footwear were the most beneficial in our patients. Systemic retinoid treatment can be considered for severe cases. Radical excision of the nail, nail bed, and nail matrix with skin implantation at the site of the removed nail can be done. Such surgical treatment must be followed by vigorous curettage and electrofulguration of matrices and nail beds.

➲ SUGGESTED READING

1. Feinstein A, Friedman J, Schewach-Millet M. Pachyonychia congenita. J Am Acad Dermatol. 1988;19(4):705-11.

172 Paederus Dermatitis

SYNONYMS

Rove beetle rash, dermatitis linearis, spider lick, night burn, Nairobi fly rash.

ETIOLOGY

The genus *Paederus* belongs to the family Staphylinidae, order Coleoptera, class Insecta; 622 species are known worldwide, and the most common species in India is *Paederus melampus*.

Paederus is nocturnal, maximum activity is in the spring and summer (May–September) and attracted to fluorescent and bright light sources; they live in moist habitat and feed on debris; although they can fly, they are agile and prefer to run. They are 7–10 mm long and 0.5 mm wide adults.

Once in contact, an attempt to crush the insect causes the release of hemolymph in the skin, containing pederin (latigaza), which is a contact vesicant. Pederin is an amide with tetrahydropyran rings, which blocks DNA and protein synthesis; acantholysis is by the release of epidermal proteases.

CLINICAL FEATURES

Paederus dermatitis may affect any sex, race, and age. The disease depends on patient activities and insect habitat, mostly seen over the exposed sites involving the upper extremities, neck, chest, trunk, and face, usually seen as an irritant contact dermatitis within 24 hours, characterized by burn-like lesions with vesicles, bullae, and pustules. A characteristic kissing lesion can be seen, e.g., flexure of the elbows and adjacent surfaces of the thigh. An atypical erythematous and desquamative variant has also been noted.

DERMOSCOPY

Dermoscopy of early blister beetle dermatitis (BBD) lesions showed multiple discrete and confluent yellowish-white structures, brown dots, roundish white globules, gray structures, and "targetoid pattern," brown areas over intense reddish pink background. Late BBD lesions revealed pinkish-white area, reduced gray structures, and dotted and globular vessels.

HISTOPATHOLOGY

In the early vesicle stage, there are intraepidermal vesicles, floored by the basal layer; inside the vesicle, there is fluid and a weft, formed by degenerated epithelial cells (ghosts). In the dermis, there is perivascular infiltrate, marked in the papilla, and edema may also be noted.

The vesicles change into pustules full of neutrophils; during healing, the pustules are pushed upward by new keratinocytes, resembling the spongiform pustule of Kogoj.

The direct immunofluorescence (DIF) is negative for immunoglobulins.

➲ DIFFERENTIAL DIAGNOSIS

Differential diagnosis includes herpes simplex, herpes zoster, liquid burns, acute allergic or irritant contact dermatitis, millipede dermatitis, and phytophotodermatitis.

➲ TREATMENT

Treat as irritant contact dermatitis. Wash with soap and water, apply cold wet compresses, topical corticosteroids, and antibiotics.

➲ PREVENTION

Learn to recognize the beetle, avoid killing or crushing, cut down surrounding vegetation, and use insect nets. Insecticides (pyrethroid) can be used.

➲ SUGGESTED READING

1. Karthikeyan K, Kumar A. Paederus dermatitis. Indian J Dermatol Venereol Leprol. 2017;83(4):424-31.

173 Paget's Disease of Breast

➲ SYNONYM

Mammary Paget's disease.

➲ HISTORY

The characteristic erythema and eczematous changes of the nipple seen with Paget's disease of the breast were first described by Velpeau in 1856. In 1874, however, Sir James Paget described the association between these characteristic nipple areola changes and carcinoma of the breast.

➲ ETIOLOGY

The majority of the cases of Paget's disease arise from either invasive or in situ ductal carcinoma in the deeper breast tissue. In a minority of cases, no underlying in situ or invasive carcinoma is found. The current view is that Paget's disease arises from the apocrine duct-derived epithelial cells.

➲ AGE GROUP

Paget's disease is rare before the fourth decade and is most frequent in the fifth and sixth decades.

➲ CLINICAL FEATURES

Mammary Paget's disease (MPD) often presents with a long-standing history of pruritic, unilateral, erythematous, scaly patch or plaque involving the nipple and occasionally areola. Ulceration and weeping with an eczematous appearance are frequently present. Retraction of nipple can be seen. Up to one-half of all patients with MPD have a palpable underlying breast mass.

➲ DERMOSCOPY

Dermoscopy of the lesion reveals irregular linear vessels and multiple blue-gray dots (peppering) corresponding to melanophages in the papillary dermis. Shiny white streaks or chrysalis-like structures were recently identified as dermoscopic features of MPD.

➲ HISTOPATHOLOGY

Paget's disease is characterized by the presence of Paget cells: Large, round, and pale-staining cells with large nuclei. Intercellular bridges are absent. The cells appear singly or in small nests between the squamous cells. Usually, acanthosis is present, the granular layer is preserved, and there is no parakeratosis, but atypical cells may be "spat out" into the stratum corneum. Frequently, a layer of basal cells separates the Paget cells from the basement membrane and is seen crushed beneath the nests of Paget cells. In the dermis, an inflammatory reaction is often present.

DIFFERENTIAL DIAGNOSIS

- *Nipple eczema*—can be bilateral and oozing and crusted plaques are seen; absence of Paget's cells
- *Erosive adenomatosis*—absence of Paget's cells
- *Psoriasis*—other classical sites are involved; absence of oozing, and silvery scales are present.
- *Pemphigus*—multiple erosions are seen; acantholytic cells on Tzanck smear
- *Bowen's disease*—full thickness epidermal dysplasia is present; lacks Paget's cells
- *Basal cell carcinoma*—ulceration with rolled out edge, rare site to be present, and basaloid cells in nests
- *Malignant melanoma*—atypical melanocytes in sheets
- *Seborrheic dermatitis*—bilateral involvement is seen, and other seborrheic areas show scaling.
- *Lichen simplex*—lichenification is seen; absence of discharge.

COMPLICATIONS

Failure to identify and treat, which can lead to metastatic disease with poor prognosis.

TREATMENT

Mastectomy and lymph node evaluation remain the standard definitive treatment. Adjuvant treatment with radiation, chemotherapy, or hormonal therapy is recommended based on lymph node status and specific features of primary tumor.

PROGNOSIS

Local recurrence is common, even in cases with a wider excision. Poor prognosis is associated with depth of invasion and with the elevated serum levels of carcinoembryonic antigen (CEA).

SUGGESTED READING

1. Sakorafas GH, Blanchard K, Sarr MG, Farley DR. Paget's disease of the breast. Cancer Treat Rev. 2001;27(1):9-18.

174 Palmoplantar Keratodermas

INTRODUCTION

Palmoplantar keratodermas (PPKs) are a heterogenous group of disorders characterized by abnormal thickening of the palms and soles.

- *Progrediens*: There is progression with age.
- *Transgrediens*: It spreads to the dorsal surface.

The keratodermas are classified into three subgroups **(Table 1)**:

1. Simple keratodermas
2. Complex keratodermas
3. Syndromic keratodermas

HISTOPATHOLOGY

The histological changes are largely nonspecific and/or confined primarily to the epidermis. Skin biopsy is done from the weight-bearing area, the thenar, and the hypothenar eminence. Epidermolytic PPK (EPPK) is characterized by hyperkeratosis, acanthosis, and papillomatosis. Epidermolysis at the spinous, granular cell layer is noted by light microscopy. Thickened granular layer with irregularly shaped keratohyalin granules is present. Electron microscopy shows keratin aggregates and cytolysis.

Nonepidermolytic PPK (NEPPK) is characterized by orthokeratosis, acanthosis, and well-preserved granular layer. All the keratodermas are difficult to distinguish histologically, and clear differential diagnosis is difficult.

DERMOSCOPY

Palmoplantar keratoderma secondary to ichthyosis vulgaris shows light red background with diffused white and yellow patchy scaling and regular linear and patchy glomerular vessels.

TREATMENT

- *General measures*: Wicking socks (absorb sweat), insoles/orthotics, comfortable footwear, podiatry—paring of the calluses, and treating the infection
- *Topical preparations*: Keratolytics, steroids, retinoids, and calcipotriol
- *Systemic treatments*: Oral retinoids—alitretinoin/acitretin and botulinum toxin injections
- *Experimental treatments*: Drug repositioning—rosuvastatin, rapamycin, and erlotinib.
- *Gene targeting therapy*: siRNA, CrispR-Cas9, and topical gentamicin

Table 1: Classification of palmoplantar keratodermas (PPKs).

Type	*Synonyms*	*Inheritance*	*Gene defect*	*Onset*	*Ectodermal features*
Unna–Thost PPK	Nonepidermolytic PPK	AD	*KRT1*	Early infancy	Sharply localized to palms and soles (knuckle pads), hyperhidrosis, and pitted keratolysis
Vörner PPK	Epidermolytic PPK	AD	*KRT9* *KRT1*	Early infancy	Sharply localized to palms and soles (knuckle pads) and no hyperhidrosis
Greither and Sybert PPK	Transgrediens and progrediens PPK	AD	*KRT1*	Infancy	Transgredient PPK, extensor keratosis pseudoainhum, and hyperhidrosis
Mal de Meleda **(Figs. 1A to D)**	Nagashima PPK and recessive Norbotten PPK	AR	*ARS B (SLURP-1)*	Birth or early infancy	Transgredient mutilating extensor keratosis, hyperhidrosis, nail dystrophy, and pseudoainhum
Gamborg–Nielsen PPK	Recessive Norbotten PPK	AR	Unknown	Unknown	Transgredient, knuckle pads, mutilating extensor keratosis, and hyperhidrosis
Olmsted syndrome	PPK with periorificial plaques	AD	Unknown	Birth or early infancy	Transgredient mutilating PPK, hyper- or hypohidrosis, nail dystrophy, alopecia, deafness, dental loss, leukokeratosis, perioral, perianal, and perineal warty hyperkeratotic plaques
Vohwinkel syndrome		AD	*GJB2*	Infancy	Flexion contractures; edges of keratoderma have projections into normal skin showing koebnerization; and nail dystrophy, onychogryphosis, and linear and/or starfish keratosis (warty papules on knuckles that coalesce)

Continued

Continued

Type	*Synonyms*	*Inheritance*	*Gene defect*	*Onset*	*Ectodermal features*
Loricrin keratoderma	Camisa PPK, variant of Vohwinkel PPK	AD	*GJB2*	Infancy	Generalized desquamation at birth (collodion baby), mild ichthyosis, and rugose keratoderma, which confluences with a honeycomb pattern
Huriez syndrome	Sclerotylosis	AD	Unknown	Birth	More marked on the soles and lacks erythema and dermatoglyphics; nail—longitudinal ridging, hypoplasia, clubbing, overcurvature, onychorrhexis, and koilonychia; and SCC in the atrophic skin
Papillon–Lefèvre syndrome	PPK with periodontitis Haim–Munk syndrome	AR		Birth or early infancy	The condition associates three elements: 1. Transgredient PPK 2. Periodontal disease leading to shedding of the primary (by the age of 4 or 5 years) and secondary dentition 3. Recurrent cutaneous and systemic pyoderma
Naxos disease	PPK with woolly hair and cardiomyopathy	AR	*Plakoglobin*	Infancy	Wooly hair and right ventricular cardiomyopathy
Striate PPK	Focal nonepidermolytic PPK or Brünauer–Fuhs–Siemens type	AD	• *Type 1: DSG1* • *Type 2: DSP* • *Type 3: KRT1*	4–10 years	Focal islands of hyperkeratosis on pressure points; striate lesions on the palms, flexor aspects of the fingers, or an even thin hyperkeratosis described as "membranous"; ridging of the nails and cuticular hyperkeratosis; and woolly hair
Focal epidermolytic PPK	Wachter type	AD	*KRT16*		Hereditary painful callosities

Continued

Continued

Type	*Synonyms*	*Inheritance*	*Gene defect*	*Onset*	*Ectodermal features*
Howell–Evans syndrome	Tylosis with esophageal carcinoma	AD		Late infancy to adolescence	Esophageal cancer
Pachyonychia congenita type 1	Jadassohn–Lewandowsky type	AD	*KRT6/16*	Infancy to early childhood	Nail changes, hair abnormalities, oral leukokeratosis, and laryngeal (hoarseness and fatal respiratory obstruction in infancy) follicular hyperkeratosis
Pachyonychia congenita type 2	Jackson–Lawler type	AD	*KRT6/17*	Infancy to early childhood	Epidermal cysts and steatocystoma, natal teeth, unruly hair, and milia; adults have protuberant eyebrow
Richner–Hanhart syndrome	Tyrosinemia type II or oculocutaneous tyrosinemia	AR	*TAT*	Infancy to adolescence	Photophobia and corneal erosions develop within the first few months of life, diagnosed by slit-lamp examination; painful circumscribed callosities making the child walk on the toes; bullous lesions and hyperhidrosis; and corneal ulceration and glaucoma
Carvajal syndrome	Striate PPK with woolly hair and cardiomyopathy	AR	*DSP*	Infancy	Woolly hair and left ventricular cardiomyopathy

(AD: autosomal dominant; AR: autosomal recessive; SCC: squamous cell carcinoma)

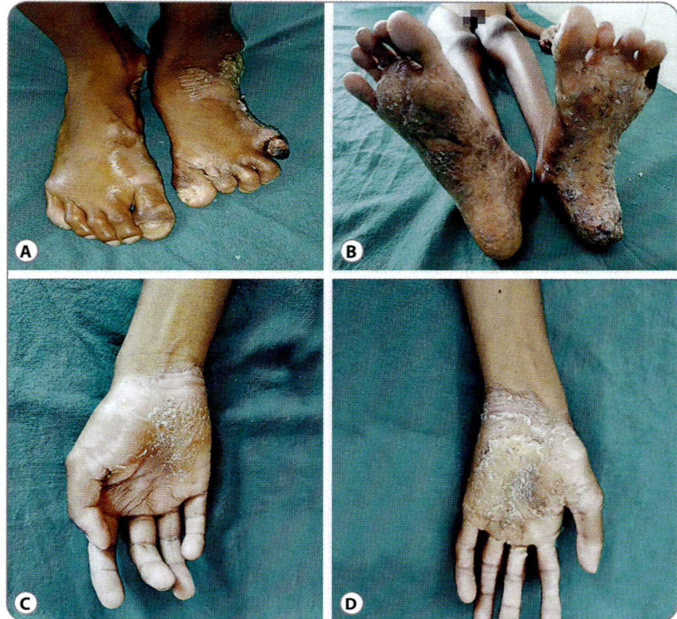

Figs. 1A to D: Clinical images of mal de Meleda type of palmoplantar keratodermas (PPK) showing hyperkeratosis of the palms and soles.

SUGGESTED READING

1. Sakiyama T, Kubo A. Hereditary palmoplantar keratoderma "clinical and genetic differential diagnosis." J Dermatol. 2016;43(3):264-74.

175 Papular Urticaria

➲ SYNONYMS

Lichen urticatus, prurigo simplex.

➲ ETIOLOGY

Papular urticaria is caused by hypersensitivity to a variety of insect bites, including those of mosquitoes, fleas, bedbugs, and mites.

➲ AGE GROUP

Papular urticaria is rare in the first year of life. Incidence increases by 2 years onward and tends to decline after 7 years, as repeated bites tend to induce hyposensitization.

➲ CLINICAL FEATURES

The features are chronic recurrent eruption of irritable urticated papules occurring in patients with an acquired sensitivity to insect bites. The lesions tend to have a characteristic distribution and configuration. There is usually a seasonal incidence depending on the habits of the biting insect. The primary lesions are wheals, papules, or wheals surmounted by papules, often with a central hemorrhagic punctum. The lesions are grouped into clusters or arranged in a straight (breakfast, lunch, and dinner sign) or curved line. They are markedly pruritic, and the tops of the lesions are usually scratched off and crusted. If there is no secondary pyoderma, the lesions heal in about 2–10 days, only to return in a fresh crop after some time.

Geographic variations occur in the species responsible for papular urticaria, but mosquitoes, bedbugs, and fleas are important causes throughout the world. A number of dipterous insects other than mosquitoes may also cause papular urticaria. Mites parasitic on domestic pets and occurring in stored products like flour, grains, and dried food can also produce papular urticaria.

The distribution of lesions depends on the biting habits of the insect and the clothing habits of the host. They are commonly seen on exposed parts. Bedbug bites are seen chiefly on the buttocks, back, and sides of the trunk, where the body comes in contact with the bed or chair **(Figs. 1A to D)**.

➲ HISTOPATHOLOGY

The features include mild subepidermal edema with extravasation of erythrocytes, interstitial eosinophils, and exocytosis of lymphocytes.

➲ DIFFERENTIAL DIAGNOSIS

- *Scabies*—nocturnal itching, involvement of the circle of Hebra, and classical burrow lesions.

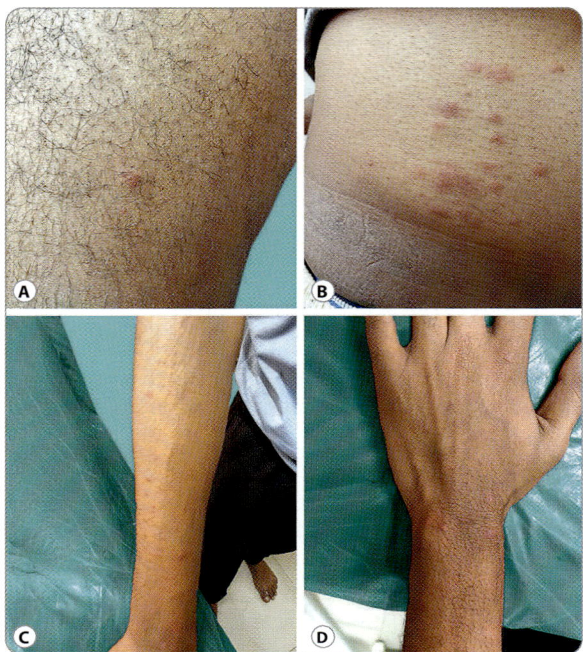

Figs. 1A to D: Papular urticaria: Few of them excoriated over the arms, thighs, and trunk.

- *Varicella*—prodrome of fever, coryza, and vesicles on erythematous base over the whole body.
- Tzanck smear shows multinucleated giant cells.
- *Dermatitis herpetiformis*—biopsy shows papillary tip abscess, granular deposits of immunoglobulin A (IgA) on direct immunofluorescence (DIF).
- *Gianotti–Crosti syndrome*—extensive excoriated and crusted lesions are seen mainly on the extremities, mostly in children.

COMPLICATIONS

Excoriations and secondary eczematization.

TREATMENT

Counsel the parents that precautions should be taken to avoid insect bites.

Three "Ps" of management include *p*rotective clothing, *p*ruritus control, and *p*atience.

Mildly potent topical corticosteroids and antihistamines can be prescribed for symptomatic relief.

Short course of systemic corticosteroid for severe reactions can be started, and management of anaphylaxis can be done if it occurs.

SUGGESTED READING

1. Singh S, Mann BK. Insect bite reactions. Indian J Dermatol Venereol Leprol. 2013;79(2):151-64.

176 Parapsoriasis

SYNONYMS

Small plaque parapsoriasis, persistent superficial dermatitis, chronic superficial scaly dermatitis, chronic superficial spongiotic dermatitis, large plaque parapsoriasis, parapsoriasis en plaque.

HISTORY

In 1902, Brocq proposed the term parapsoriasis for all inflammatory dermatoses. Between about 1950 and 1970, the parapsoriasis group was divided into two categories: Pityriasis lichenoides and parapsoriasis en plaque. The emphasis was on the potential of parapsoriasis en plaque to evolve into mycosis fungoides (MF).

ETIOLOGY

Parapsoriasis appears to bridge chronic dermatitis and MF. It is a cutaneous T-cell lymphoproliferative disorder.

SEX RATIO

Small plaque parapsoriasis is associated with male predominance. The male-to-female ratio is 3:1.

CLINICAL FEATURES

Classification of parapsoriasis:

- *Large plaque parapsoriasis (LPP)*:
    - Variants: Poikilodermatous and retiform
- *Small plaque parapsoriasis (SPP)*:
    - Variant: Digitate dermatosis

Large plaque parapsoriasis lesions are fewer, ill-defined erythematous or brown patches, or very thin plaques that are asymptomatic or mildly pruritic. The size is variable, but typically, most are >5 cm. They are found mainly on the bathing trunk and flexural areas. Extremities and the breasts may be involved in women. The surface is covered with scales that are small and scanty. They may appear finely wrinkled—"cigarette paper" wrinkling. It is a monoclonal lymphocyte disorder and can progress to MF.

Small plaque parapsoriasis is a benign condition characterized by well-defined round, oval, discrete patches over thin, nonindurated plaques, mainly on the trunk. The lesions measure <5 cm in diameter, are asymptomatic, and covered with fine, moderately adherent scales **(Fig. 1)**.

Digitate dermatosis: A distinctive variant of fingerprint shape and is yellowish or fawn in color; it follows lines of cleavage of the skin and often measures >5 cm.

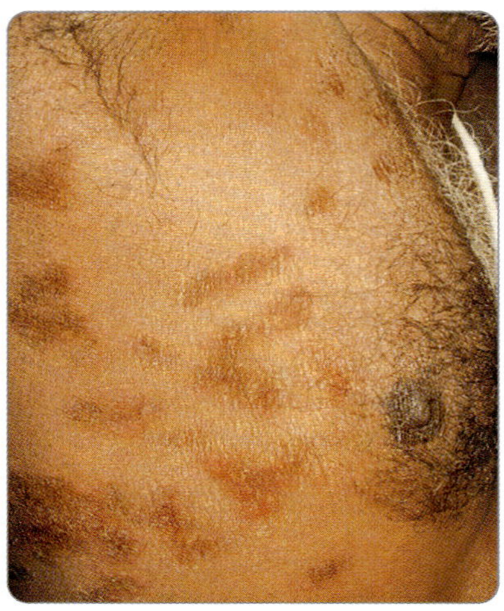

Fig. 1: Well-defined oval patches with fine scaling over the trunk in parapsoriasis.

Xanthoerythrodermia perstans: Digitate lesions with a yellow hue.

DERMOSCOPY

Small plaque parapsoriasis: Diffuse orange structureless areas (orange background) along with white scales localized in the skin furrows; no vessels are visible.

In poikilodermatous variant of LPP, there is whitish scaling and a reddish background, likely due to hyperkeratosis and inflammation, respectively; an orangish-brown background which may be due to extravasation of red blood cells with hemosiderin deposition in the dermis; and relatively blurred branched vessels due to epidermal thinning, making the dermal vessels more evident.

HISTOPATHOLOGY

- *Small plaque psoriasis*: Epidermis shows focal parakeratosis, mild spongiosis, and exocytosis of mononuclear cells. There is mild perivascular lymphohistiocytic infiltrate in the upper dermis. Atypical lymphocytes are never found.
- *Large plaque psoriasis*: Epidermis may be atrophic or psoriasiform with focal basal cell degeneration.

There is a presence of mononuclear cells in the epidermis, especially in the basal layer (epidermotropism) with band-like multifocal lymphohistiocytic infiltrate. Lymphocytes may be large, atypical, with no microabscesses. Superficial perivascular infiltrate in the upper dermis is seen.

DIFFERENTIAL DIAGNOSIS

- *Large plaque parapsoriasis*—patch stage of MF, Pautrier's microabscess, and atypical lymphocytes are seen.
- Genodermatoses (Rothmund–Thomson syndrome, Bloom's syndrome, and dyskeratosis congenita)

- Collagen vascular diseases (dermatomyositis and lupus erythematosus)
- *Lichenoid drug eruptions*—more of parakeratosis and eosinophilic infiltrate is seen.
- *Secondary syphilis*—venereal disease research laboratory (VDRL) test positivity
- Chronic radiodermatitis
- *Small plaque parapsoriasis*—pityriasis lichenoides chronica
- *Psoriasis*—classical Munro's microabscess are seen in the stratum corneum.
- *Mycosis fungoides*—atypical lymphocytes are present.

TREATMENT

Small plaque parapsoriasis should be reassured and may be left untreated. Emollients, topical tar preparations, topical corticosteroids, and ultraviolet B (UVB) phototherapy can be given. Patients should be examined initially every 3–6 months and subsequently every year to ensure that the character of the process is stable.

Large plaque parapsoriasis requires more aggressive therapy. The goal of treatment is to suppress the disorder to prevent possible progression to overt MF. High-potency topical corticosteroids with UVB phototherapy or psoralen and ultraviolet A (PUVA), topical nitrogen mustard particularly for the poikilodermatous type.

Follow up every 3 months initially and every 6 months to 1 year subsequently for the evidence of progression.

PROGNOSIS

Both LPP and SPP may persist for years to decades with little change in appearance, clinically or histopathologically. Approximately 10–30% of cases of LPP progress to overt MF, another cutaneous T-cell lymphoma. LPP does not resolve without treatment.

SUGGESTED READING

1. Sehgal VN, Srivastava G, Aggarwal AK. Parapsoriasis: a complex issue. Skinmed. 2007;6(6):280-6.

177 Paronychia

ETIOLOGY

A paronychial infection usually starts in the lateral nail fold. Cracks, fissures, or trauma to the nail fold allows bacterial entry. Patients at risk include those with dyshidrotic eczema, contact dermatitis, and those with chronic dry, chaffed, or irritated skin such as dishwashers, florists, gardeners, or housekeepers.

Acute paronychia is most commonly caused by *Staphylococcus aureus* or *Streptococcus* species. Others may be *Pseudomonas* species, *Proteus* species, or anaerobes. A mixed bacterial infection is common, particularly in patients with diabetes. Chronic paronychia is commonly caused by *Candida albicans*. Predisposing factors for chronic paronychia include chronic wet work, as seen in housewives, exposure to irritants, or excessive manicuring. Recurrent paronychia may be caused by herpes virus (herpetic whitlow).

AGE GROUP

There is no predilection for age; it is more common in females with M:F ratio of 3:1.

CLINICAL FEATURES

The term paronychia is used for the inflammation of the nail folds, posterior or lateral. It can be acute or chronic. It is characterized by acute or chronic purulent, tender, and painful swellings of the tissues around the nail, caused by an abscess in the nail fold.

The affected digit becomes swollen, red, and painful. Compression of the nail fold may produce pus drainage. Green coloration of the nail may suggest *Pseudomonas* species infection. Vesicles on an erythematous base may be seen in herpetic whitlow. It may subside on its own, or if it spreads, it may cause nail deformity by affecting the matrix.

Candidal paronychia commonly presents as chronic swelling, with hypertrophy of the nail plate and nail dystrophy. Eczematization and subungual abscess formation may complicate the condition **(Fig. 1)**. Difference between acute and chronic paronychia has been tabulated in **Table 1**.

DIFFERENTIAL DIAGNOSIS

- *Herpetic whitlow*—the whole of the finger pulp is involved.
- *Pyogenic granuloma*—reddish outgrowth that bleeds on touch
- *Contact dermatitis*—many fingers are involved; ragged cuticle is seen; and other areas like hands/feet are involved.
- *Dyshidrotic eczema*—deep-seated vesicles mainly over the lateral borders of the fingers

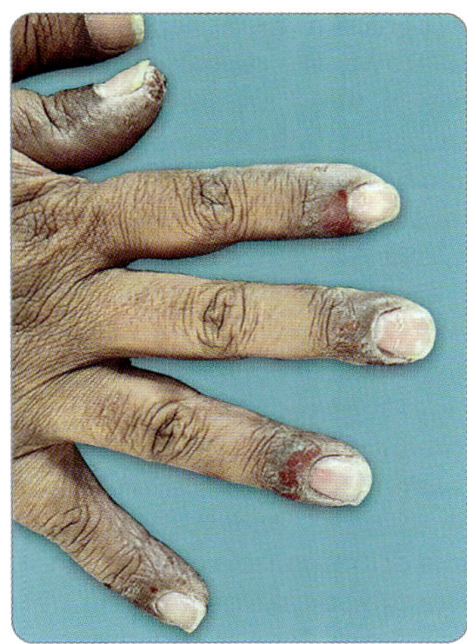

Fig. 1: Swelling over the proximal part of the nail with nail changes in paronychia.

Table 1: Acute and chronic paronychia.

Acute paronychia	*Chronic paronychia*
Affects males and females equally	More common in females: 9:1
Common in children	Seen in fifth to sixth decade
Usually involves only one finger	May involve >1 finger
Usually involves the thumb	Usually involves the middle finger
Most cases resolve in 6–10 days	Untreated cases lead to eventual discoloration and loss of nail

- Fingertip injuries
- *Hand infections*—swelling and erythema of hand are also seen.
- *Onychomycosis*—nail plate changes are also seen.
- *Psoriasis*—nail pitting, salmon patches, and subungual hyperkeratosis are present.
- *Warts*—verrucous growth is present.
- Ganglion
- Squamous cell carcinoma.

COMPLICATIONS

Failure to properly treat a paronychia can result in hand infection and, occasionally, systemic infection from hematogenous extension.

- The abscess initially forms on the lateral nail fold. It can spread to the eponychium, eventually forming a "horseshoe" that includes the opposite nail fold.
- It may spread to the pulp space of the finger, creating a felon.
- An untreated infection can spread to the deep spaces of the hand and beyond, causing osteomyelitis.

TREATMENT

- *Acute paronychia:* Acutely inflamed pyogenic abscesses should be incised and drained. In acute suppurative paronychia, semisynthetic penicillin or a cephalosporin with excellent staphylococcal activity like cephalexin 250–500 mg QID should be given orally. If these are ineffective, methicillin-resistant *Staphylococcus aureus* (MRSA) or a mixed anaerobic bacteria infection should be suspected and treated accordingly. Tincture of iodine 2 drops BID helps to keep the nail and skin dry.

- *Chronic paronychia:* Avoidance of all causative and aggravating factors and to keep the hands dry. For all wet work, the patient should be advised to wear cotton gloves under rubber or plastic gloves and avoid manicure of the proximal nail folds.

Topical therapy requires a combination of steroid and antimicrobial. A potent steroid may be used for short period to decrease inflammation. Topical imidazoles or nystatin ointment may be sufficient to treat *Candida*. If unresponsive to therapy, systemic fluconazole or itraconazole can be tried. If mixed etiology is suspected, then an antibiotic like gentamycin cream may be added. Incision and drainage are done if superimposed acute infection develops.

PROGNOSIS

The prognosis is usually good if treated promptly. The incidence of chronic paronychia is increased among immunocompromised individuals.

SUGGESTED READING

1. Leggit JC. Acute and Chronic Paronychia. Am Fam Physician. 2017;96(1): 44-51.

178 Pediculosis

INTRODUCTION

Pediculosis is lice infestation. Humans can be infested with three kinds of lice—*Pediculosis capitis* (head louse), *Pediculosis corporis* (body louse), and *Pthirus pubis* (crab or pubic louse). Louse feed on human blood and deposit their eggs on the hair shaft or the seams of clothes. Nits hatch in 7–10 days. They are obligate human parasites and cannot survive away from the hosts for >10 days.

PEDICULOSIS CAPITIS

SYNONYMS

Head lice infestation, cooties, nits.

HISTORY

Head lice have infested mankind for thousands of years. Nits have been found on the hair of both Egyptian and Peruvian mummies.

ETIOLOGY

It is caused by *Pediculus humanus variant capitis* (head louse). Head lice are spread by head-to-head contact as well as by fomite transmission.

AGE GROUP

Children between 3 and 11 years of age and girls have the highest incidence.

CLINICAL FEATURES

Scalp pruritus is the classical manifestation of the infestation. Pruritic papular lesions may occur on the nape of the neck, and, occasionally, a generalized nonspecific pruritic eruption develops. In severe, neglected cases, pus and exudate may produce matting of the hair—a state that has been termed "plica polonica." The empty egg cases ("nits") are easily identified and occur in the greatest density on the parietal **(Fig. 1)** and occipital regions called "louse pit." The detection of adult lice and nymphs provides evidence of an "active" infection, whereas the presence of eggs and egg cases alone merely indicates that infection has occurred at some time. The most reliable method of diagnosing current, active infection is by detection combing, which has been shown to be superior to direct visual examination of the hair and scalp. Wood's lamp examination helps in screening large number of cases, as the empty nits give gray fluorescence and nits with unborn louse give white fluorescence.

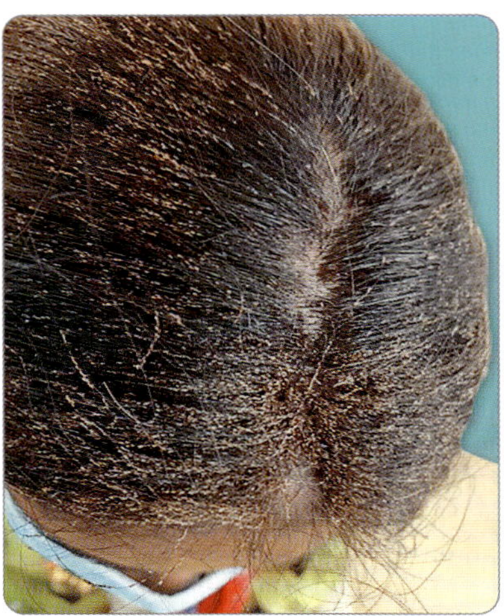

Fig. 1: *Pediculosis capitis* shows nits.

HISTOPATHOLOGY

The epidermis and dermis reveal the signs of inflammation, but these alterations are neither specific nor diagnostic.

DIFFERENTIAL DIAGNOSIS

- *Seborrheic scales*—greasy, cream-to-yellow scales, and the absence of nits
- Artifacts in hair, e.g., hair spray and hair casts (pseudonits)—easily removable from hair
- *Piedra*—fungal spores in a collection are seen, and metallic sound is heard on combing.
- *Delusion of parasitosis*—absence of lice and nits
- *Scabies*—burrows are present, and scrapings on KOH mount show mites.
- *Trichorrhexis nodosa*—mainly axillary and pubic hair involved, nodes can be easily dislodged
- *Monilethrix*—beading is found in the hair, which is evident on trichoscopy.
- Trichonodosis

COMPLICATIONS

Complications include secondary bacterial infections and plica polonica.

TREATMENT

Topical application of permethrin 1%, lindane 1%, and malathion 0.5% should be repeated after 1 week. Oral ivermectin 200 μg/kg can be given. Other treatment options include spinosad 0.9% suspension, benzyl alcohol 5% lotion, dimethicone 4% lotion, and isopropyl myristate 50% rinse.

PEDICULOSIS PUBIS

SYNONYMS

Pthirus pubis, pubic lice, crab lice.

ETIOLOGY

It is transmitted by sexual or close contact and to a lesser extent via contaminated clothing, towels, and bedding. The chance of acquiring pubic louse infestation after a single exposure is >90%. It is the most contagious sexually transmitted disease (STD).

AGE GROUP

Infestation is most frequently observed in those of 15–40 years, correlating with the increased levels of promiscuous sexual activity.

CLINICAL FEATURES

Itching, mainly in the evening and at night, is the principal symptom. Close inspection of affected areas will reveal lice grasping hairs close to the skin surface and louse eggs attached to the hair shafts. Louse feces are often visible as rust-colored speckles on the skin and hair, and the underclothes may be spotted with altered blood. When crab lice are discovered on the pubic area, other hairy areas of the body should be examined, as these lice may colonize the eyebrows, eyelashes, beard, axillae, areolar hair, and the scalp margins. In heavy infections in men, the hair on the trunk and limbs may be extensively colonized. Blue-gray macules (maculae ceruleae) are occasionally seen on the skin. Bullous lesions attributed to crab lice have been reported.

DIFFERENTIAL DIAGNOSIS

- *Scabies infection*—itching is present, no lice present clinging to the hair, and other classical sites are involved.
- *Contact dermatitis*—itchy papulovesicles are seen.
- White piedra
- *Trichomycosis pubis*—yellowish concretions are present in the hair.
- *Hair casts*—cylindrical white to gray structures are seen and can be easily slided along the hair.

COMPLICATIONS

Complications include secondary infection because of excoriation, local lymphadenitis, and fever.

TREATMENT

Sexual partners should be treated simultaneously. Most commonly, 1% permethrin rinse, 5% permethrin cream, or 1% lindane shampoo are utilized, two applications, 1 week apart, Moreover, all hairy areas of the body must be inspected for the existence of lice and then treated if there is any possibility of their presence. Eyelash infestation is treated by rubbing petroleum jelly onto the eyelashes three times a day for 3–7 days.

PEDICULOSIS CORPORIS

➲ SYNONYMS

Body lice, clothing louse, vagabonds' disease, morbus errorum.

➲ ETIOLOGY

It is caused by *Pediculosis humanus variant corporis*. It is common in people with poor hygiene.

➲ AGE GROUP

The prevalence rates of body lice are tied to poor hygiene, poverty, and homelessness. There are no racial, age, or sex restrictions.

➲ CLINICAL FEATURES

In most infected persons, itching is the principal complaint. Pruritus is the result of sensitization to louse salivary antigens. The body is often covered in excoriations. In those who have harbored clothing lice for long periods of time, the skin is often hyperpigmented (so-called "vagabonds' disease"; morbus errorum), and this is probably a postinflammatory phenomenon. Lice and eggs should be sought in the clothing.

➲ HISTOPATHOLOGY

The epidermis has minimal spongiosis with nonspecific infiltrates of eosinophils and neutrophils in the dermis.

➲ DIFFERENTIAL DIAGNOSIS

- *Scabies infestation*—excoriated papules are seen, burrows on web spaces are seen.
- *Atopic dermatitis*—extensors in infants and flexural lichenification in adults are seen, history of (H/o) atopy
- Allergic or irritant contact dermatitis
- *Drug reaction*—other features like fever, hepatomegaly, and lymphadenopathy are seen.
- *Viral exanthema*—blanchable erythematous maculopapular rash is present, and enanthems in mucosal surfaces are associated.
- Renal impairment and hepatic impairment (systemic causes of pruritus)

➲ COMPLICATIONS

Complications include secondary infection with *Staphylococcus aureus*, *Streptococcus pyogenes*, and other bacteria. Worldwide, body lice may act as vectors for *Rickettsia prowazekii, Bartonella quintana* (typhus and trench fevers), and *Borrelia recurrentis* (relapsing fever).

TREATMENT

Preferably, the clothing and bedding of infested individuals are discarded in tightly sealed, plastic biohazard bags and incinerated. Only if the latter is not possible should disinfection be attempted. Fumigation of the clothing and heating it to a temperature of 65°C for 15–30 minutes can be done. Hot ironing of the seams of upholstered furniture and exposure to infested items are strictly avoided for 2 weeks.

DERMOSCOPY

On dermoscopy, empty nits can be seen as translucent, ovoid structure, with a flattened free end attached to the base of the hair shaft. They can be differentiated from pseudonits, which are caused by seborrheic dermatitis and are whitish, easily detachable amorphous structures. In addition, details of nits, nymphs, and adult lice can be appreciated using this method. Sometimes, the louse feeding on blood from the scalp can be seen.

SUGGESTED READING

1. Ko CJ, Elston DM. Pediculosis. J Am Acad Dermatol. 2004;50(1):1-12.

179 Piebaldism

➲ HISTORY

The word piebald is the combination of the "pie" in the magpie (a bird of black and white plumage) and the "bald" of the bald eagle (which has a white feathered head). The first descriptions date to early Egyptian, Greek, and Roman writings. Generation after generation demonstrated a distinctive, predictable familial mark—a white forelock.

➲ ETIOPATHOGENESIS

Piebaldism is a rare autosomal dominant congenital disorder, which results from mutations in the KIT proto-oncogene, located on chromosome 4q11-12. A functioning KIT receptor is required for the normal development of melanocytes, both immediately before melanoblast migration from the neural crest and also postnatally.

➲ CLINICAL FEATURES

The leukoderma has a characteristic distribution pattern that favors the central anterior trunk, the midextremities, the central forehead, and the midfrontal portion of the scalp, with a resultant white forelock. The lesions are present at birth and classically spare the posterior midline. The white forelock, which is present in 80–90% of patients, is the most familiar feature. However, its absence does not exclude the diagnosis. All the hairs of the forelock are white, and the skin beneath the forelock is also amelanotic **(Fig. 1)**. The

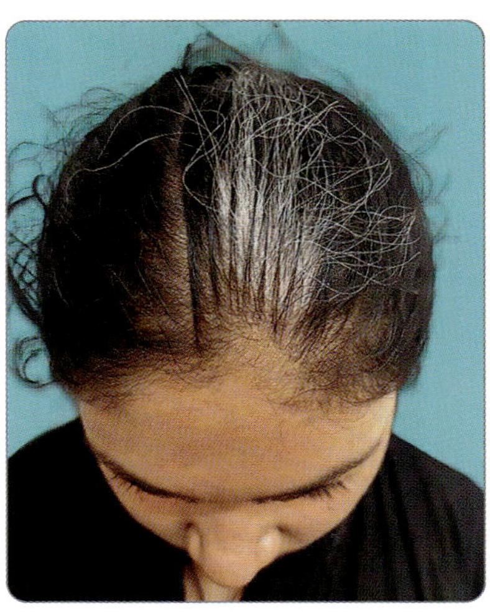

Fig. 1: White forelock with amelanotic skin.

latter is midline in location, triangular or diamond-shaped, and often symmetrical. Posteriorly, the apex can reach the vertex, and anteriorly, it may extend to the root of the nose and include the medial third of the eyebrows; extension to the nose is rare.

The areas of leukoderma are quite distinctive and allow for the diagnosis, even in the absence of a white forelock. They are irregular in shape, well circumscribed, and milk-white in color, and they contain normally pigmented and hyperpigmented macules and patches ranging from a few millimeters to several centimeters in diameter. Hyperpigmented patches also occur within uninvolved skin and should not be misinterpreted as evidence of neurofibromatosis type 1. Poliosis of the eyebrows and eyelashes is a common finding, as are white hairs within the areas of leukoderma.

Except for their cutaneous findings, most patients are otherwise healthy. It has rarely been associated with deafness.

PATHOLOGY

By light and electron microscopy, no melanocytes can be identified in either the interfollicular epidermis or the hair follicles of amelanotic skin. The hyperpigmented macules are characterized by an abundance of melanosomes in the melanocytes and keratinocytes.

DERMOSCOPY

Dermoscopic evaluation of the depigmented lesions reveals distorted melanocytic network with reduced pigment intensity, absence of perifollicular pigment, vast areas of depigmentation, and islands of normal skin or hyperpigmentation.

DIFFERENTIAL DIAGNOSIS

- *Addison's disease*—hyperpigmentation of palmar creases, knuckles, and buccal mucosa
- *Albinism*—generalized depigmentation of the skin and light-colored iris
- *Vitiligo*—generalized patches and not associated with eye changes
- Waardenburg's syndrome—associated with deafness
- Alezzandrini syndrome
- Vogt–Koyanagi–Harada syndrome

TREATMENT

Most treatments used for vitiligo, (e.g., topical corticosteroids or phototherapy) are not efficacious.

Autografts of the normal skin into amelanotic areas, including grafting of autologous melanocytes, are a therapeutic option, but this often requires multiple procedures.

A cosmetic cover-up as a means of camouflage can be recommended.

Protection against sunburn is also necessary. Follicular unit transplantation can be done.

The depigmented areas have been successfully treated using dermabrasion and split-skin grafting, autologous melanocyte transplantation, epidermal sheet grafting, and autologous cell suspension transplantation after superficial full-surface ablation.

SUGGESTED READING

1. Oiso N, Fukai K, Kawada A, Suzuki T. Piebaldism. J Dermatol. 2013;40(5):330-5.

180 Pellagra

➲ SYNONYMS

Alpine scurvy, mal de la rosa, mal rosso, maidism, mayidism, Saint Ignatius' itch.

➲ HISTORY

Gaspar Casal first described pellagra in 1762 and termed it *mal de la rose*, because affected patients had the typical reddish and glossy rash on the dorsum of the hands and feet. Pella = skin, agra = rough. In 1926, Goldberger reported that nicotinamide was a preventive factor of pellagra.

➲ ETIOLOGY

Pellagra represents the classic form of vitamin B3 deficiency. Deficient intake of niacin and tryptophan (a corn-rich diet), alcoholism, gastrointestinal (GI) diseases, drugs (e.g., isoniazid), carcinoid syndrome, human immunodeficiency virus (HIV), and psychiatric disturbances are associated with niacin deficiency. The essential amino acid tryptophan is converted to niacin in the liver, and in the carcinoid syndrome, tryptophan is diverted toward serotonin synthesis. Primary pellagra is due to inadequate niacin or tryptophan in the diet, and secondary pellagra occurs due to conditions where there is an inadequate absorption of niacin, such as chronic diarrhea. Niacin is required for adequate cellular function and metabolism as an essential component in coenzyme I [oxidized form of nicotinamide adenine dinucleotide (NAD)] and coenzyme II [reduced form of nicotinamide adenine dinucleotide phosphate (NADP)], which either donate or accept hydrogen ions in vital oxidation–reduction reactions.

➲ CLINICAL FEATURE

The classic triad of clinical features is dermatitis, diarrhea, and dementia. The dermatitis begins as symmetric erythema in sun-exposed areas that later become scarlet or hyperpigmented with desquamation and crusting **(Figs. 1 and 2)**. A shell-like appearance is the characteristic feature. Painful fissures may appear on the palms and soles. The photosensitive eruption forms a broad band around the neck, known as "Casal's necklace." Pellagra may also present as perianal inflammation and erosions. Mucus membrane findings include edema, cheilitis, and red atrophic glossitis. Buccal and vaginal mucosae are susceptible to ulceration and secondary infection.

In addition to diarrhea, abdominal pain and achlorhydria may be present. GI symptoms always precede cutaneous manifestations.

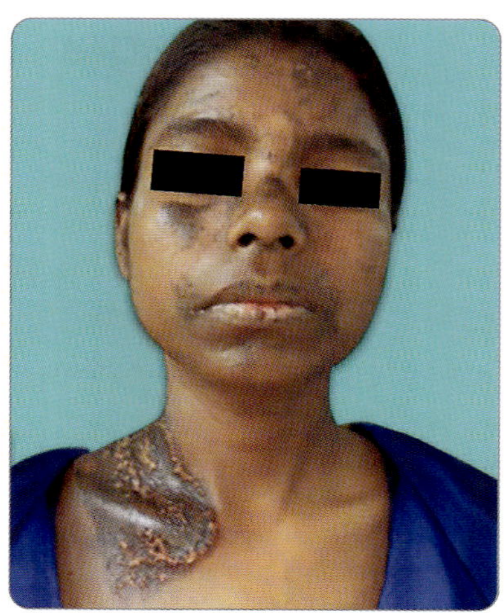

Fig. 1: Hyperpigmented eczematous lesion over face and side of the neck (exposed sites).

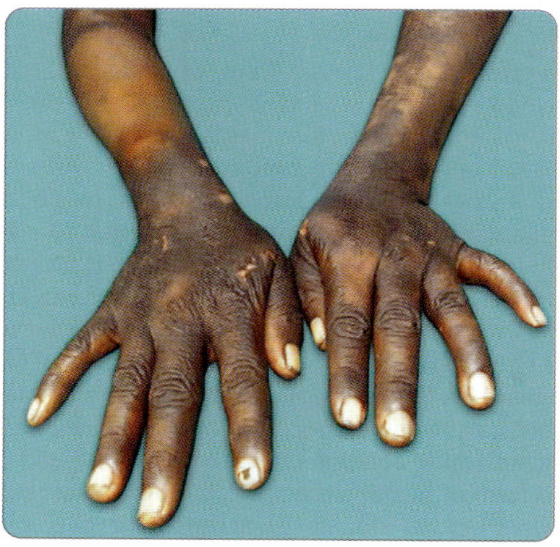

Fig. 2: Symmetric hyperpigmentation and desquamation of the skin over the dorsum of the hands.

Dementia develops in the setting of prolonged niacin deficiency. Patients are depressed, apathetic, irritable, and anxious, and in severe instances, they have frank disorientation. The diagnosis of vitamin B3 deficiency must be considered if glossitis, GI symptoms, and symmetric dermatitis in sun-exposed areas are present.

➲ HISTOPATHOLOGY

The significant histopathological findings include epidermal pallor and some degree of ballooning of the keratinocyte, presence of dilated blood vessels with extravasation, and little or no inflammatory infiltrate.

➲ DERMOSCOPY

Dermoscopy shows white double-edged scales, brown polygonal areas, follicular white dots, and brown dots against a pink background.

➲ DIFFERENTIAL DIAGNOSIS

Patients with Hartnup disease can have similar cutaneous findings. Other differential diagnoses include contact dermatitis (nonphoto-exposed areas are also involved), drug-induced pemphigus, polymorphic light eruption (absence of mucosal inflammation), and porphyria cutanea tarda (presence of bullae, scarring, porphyrin detection in urine, and blood).

➲ DIAGNOSIS

Low serum niacin, tryptophan, NAD, and NADP levels reflect niacin deficiency. Urinary excretion of N1-methyl-nicotinamide or metabolites of niacin is reduced.

➲ TREATMENT

High-protein diet or nicotinic acid or nicotinamide, 100–400 mg/day. Niacinamide is usually tolerated better than nicotinic acid, and it is the preferred agent, because it does not precipitate the flushing, itching, and burning observed after the ingestion of large doses of niacin. Sunscreens and emollients for topical application.

➲ SUGGESTED READINGS

1. Narasimha VL, Ganesh S, Reddy S, Shukla L, Mukherjee D, Kandasamy A, et al. Pellagra and Alcohol Dependence Syndrome: Findings From a Tertiary Care Addiction Treatment Centre in India. Alcohol Alcohol. 2019;54 (2):148-51.
2. Sugita K, Ikenouchi-Sugita A, Nakayama Y, Yoshioka H, Nomura T, Sakabe J, et al. Prostaglandin E2 is critical for the development of niacin-deficiency-induced photosensitivity via ROS production. Sci Rep. 2013;3(1):2973.

181 Pemphigus

HISTORY

Pemphigus is derived from the Greek word, *pemphix, which means* a blister or a bubble. Pemphigus was first used by De Sauvages, but its present meaning was given by Wichmann in 1791. Beutner and Jordon in 1964 discovered circulating antibodies directed against the cell surface keratinocytes in pemphigus vulgaris patients.

TYPES

- *Pemphigus vulgaris*:
  - Variant: Pemphigus vegetans
- *Pemphigus foliaceus*:
  - Variant: Pemphigus herpetiformis
  - Variant: Pemphigus erythematosus
- Induced pemphigus
- Intercellular immunoglobulin A (IgA) dermatosis
- Paraneoplastic pemphigus

ETIOLOGY

Pemphigus is commonly seen in Eastern countries, India, Malaysia, China, and also in Ashkenazi Jews. Genetic factors such as major histocompatibility complex (MHC) genotypes, human leukocyte antigen (HLA)-DRB1, DQB1, and viral DNA have also been implicated. Incidence is higher in patients having other immunological disorders such as thymoma or myasthenia gravis, lupus erythematosus, bullous pemphigoid, and Castleman tumors. Pemphigus vulgaris antibody is the antidesmoglein-3 directed against desmosomal cadherin. It is found mostly in lower epidermis, oral mucosa, and scalp. Pemphigus foliaceus antigen, which is desmoglein-1, on the other hand is found throughout the epidermis but more abundantly in upper parts.

AGE GROUP

Pemphigus is mainly a disease of the middle aged between 40 and 60 years, but affects younger adults more in India.

CLINICAL FEATURES

Mucosal lesions: 50–70% of patients present with oral lesions. These may precede cutaneous manifestations or maybe the only manifestations. Most common lesions are ill defined, irregularly shaped buccal or palatal erosions, fragile, and break easily; intact bullae are rare. Other surfaces involved are conjunctiva, nasal, pharynx, larynx, esophagus, urethra, penis, vulva, and cervix.

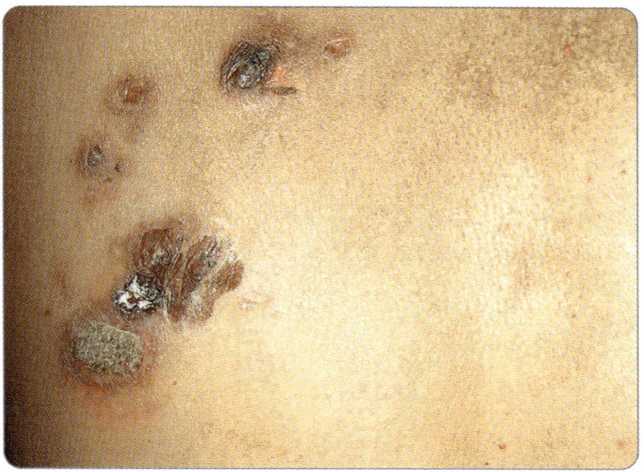

Fig. 1: Crusted lesions of pemphigus vulgaris.

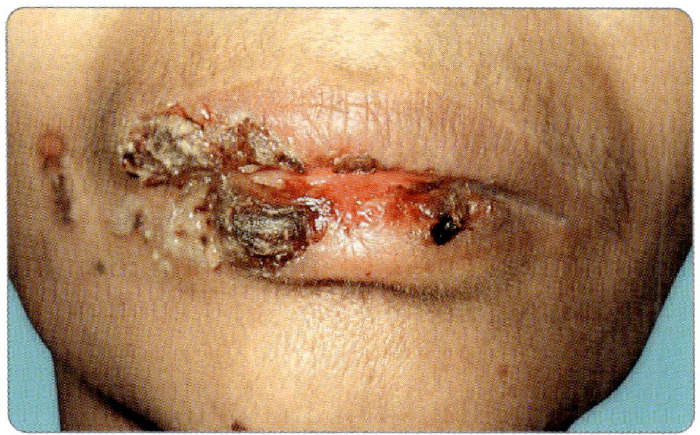

Fig. 2: Crusts and erosions on the lips.

Cutaneous lesions may be localized or more commonly generalized. Predilection for scalp, face, axilla, groin, and pressure points is seen. Palms and soles are usually spared. Lesions appear as flaccid blisters with clear fluid, which may become turbid or later burst to form painful erosions covered with crust with no tendency to heal **(Figs. 1 and 2)**. Nikolsky's sign can be elicited. Healing usually occurs without scarring, but pigmentary changes and acanthomas may occur.

➲ HISTOPATHOLOGY

The earliest change is intercellular edema with loss of intercellular attachments in basal layer. Suprabasal epidermal cells separate from basal layer to form clefts and blisters **(Figs. 3 and 4)**. Cells in basal layer remain attached to basement membrane, but separate from one another to form "row of tombstone" on the floor. Blister cavities contain acantholytic cells. Superficial dermis has a mild, superficial, mixed inflammatory infiltrate. Electron microscopy shows widening of intercellular space followed by splitting of desmosomal junctions.

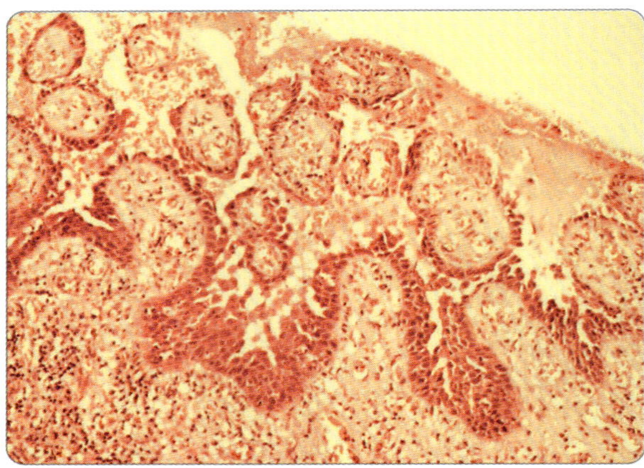

Fig. 3: Suprabasal cleft.

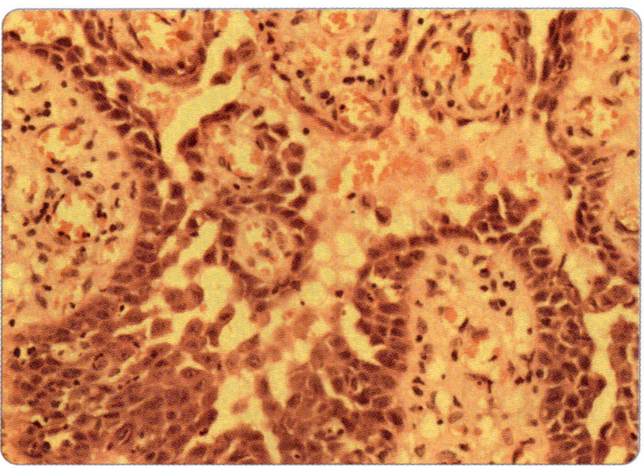

Fig. 4: Basal cells—row of tombstone appearance.

Direct immunofluorescence (DIF) is the "gold standard," which shows deposition of IgG and C3 on surface of keratinocytes throughout the epidermis, in and around lesions giving a fishnet appearance. Indirect immunofluorescence detects circulating pemphigus autoantibodies in 80% patients, especially against Dsg-3.

SEROLOGICAL DIAGNOSIS

A very sensitive and specific method of enzyme-linked immunosorbent assay (ELISA) allows detection of IgG anti Dsg-1 and anti-Dsg-3 in over 90% patients of mucocutaneous and mucosal pemphigus, respectively.

DERMOSCOPY

Dermoscopy of the immediate perilesional area of scalp lesion reveals hair casts encircling hair shafts corresponding with outer root sheath acantholysis. Other frequently observing features of pemphigus lesions are extravasations, yellow hemorrhagic crusts, yellow dots with whitish halo, white polygonal structures in pemphigus foliaceus, and linear serpentine vessels.

DIFFERENTIAL DIAGNOSIS

- *Oral lesions*:
  - Acute herpetic stomatitis—smaller ulcers with yellowish slough on the floor and surrounded by an erythematous halo
  - Erythema multiforme—interface dermatitis is seen on biopsy
  - Aphthous ulcers—lack of acantholytic cells
  - Bullous lichen planus—basal cell degeneration and lichenoid infiltrate are seen
- *Cutaneous lesions*:
  - Pemphigoid—absence of acantholytic cells and sub-epidermal blister with eosinophils are seen
  - Erythema multiforme—target lesions seen, palms and soles involved, no acantholytic cells
  - Hailey–Hailey disease—flexures are mainly involved, oral lesions are rare, and negative DIF

COMPLICATIONS

- *Diseases associated*: Loss of body fluids leading to hypovolemia, shock, and sepsis. Oral lesions may cause decreased food intake and malnutrition.
- *Therapy related*: Immunosuppression, leading to opportunistic infections, steroid toxicity, and other adjunct therapy toxicities.

TREATMENT

- *Topical therapy*: It is sufficient for patients with oral and mild cutaneous involvement. Potent topical or intralesional steroids can be used. Pilocarpine gel has also been used. Good oral hygiene is also important to prevent opportunistic infections. Topical antifungals and antiseptic mouth rinse should be advised.
- *Systemic therapy*: Corticosteroids are the mainstay along with an adjunct. Usually prednisolone in 1.0–1.5 mg/kg/day along with topical steroids is sufficient to control disease in majority patients. Alternate options are giving 60–100 mg prednisolone/day or intravenous (IV) pulses of 100 mg dexamethasone or 1 g methylprednisolone.
- *Adjunctive therapy*: It includes cyclophosphamide in conjunction with steroids. Azathioprine alone or in combination, mycophenolate mofetil, cyclosporine, dapsone, and methotrexate can be given. In resistant cases, rituximab, plasmapheresis, intravenous immunoglobulin (IVIg), psoralen and ultraviolet A (PUVA), and extracorporeal photopheresis may play a role.

➲ PROGNOSIS

With use of steroids, mortality has come down to 5–15%, but some patients succumb to complications of therapy like steroid-associated complications. Disease activity generally decreases with time and relapses mostly occur within first 2 years after diagnosis. Prognosis is severe in Jews and older patients. Pemphigus foliaceus and vegetans have a better prognosis than vulgaris.

➲ SUGGESTED READING

1. Porro AM, Seque CA, Ferreira MCC, Enokihara MMSES. Pemphigus vulgaris. An Bras Dermatol. 2019;94(3):264-7809.

182 Perforating Disorders

➲ INTRODUCTION

The perforating diseases are a group of papulonodular skin disorders, characterized by keratotic plugs or crusts in which dermal connective tissue "perforates" or is eliminated through the epidermis.

➲ HISTORY

In 1916, Kyrle reported hyperkeratosis follicularis et parafollicularis in cutem penetrans. Lutz first described elastosis perforans serpiginosa (EPS) 1953. Though originally described by Pinkus in 1954, the term transepidermal elimination (TEE) disorder was coined by Mehregan. Mehregan, Schwartz, and Livingood reported the first child with reactive perforating collagenosis in 1967. Mehregan and Coskey expanded the concept of perforating disease to include perforating folliculitis in their article in 1968.

➲ CLASSIFICATION (TABLE 1)

- *Major perforating dermatoses*:
  - Primary perforating dermatoses:
    - Kyrle's disease (KD)
    - Reactive perforating collagenosis
    - Elastosis perforans serpiginosa
    - Perforating folliculitis
  - Acquired perforating dermatoses:
    - Perforating disorder of diabetes
    - Perforating disorder of renal failure/dialysis
- *Secondary perforating dermatoses*:
  - Endogenous substances:
    - Chondrodermatitis nodularis helicis
    - Hematomas
    - Perforating pseudoxanthoma elasticum
    - Perforating calcinosis
    - Gout
  - Exogenous foreign material:
    - Silica
    - Wood splinters

➲ DERMOSCOPY

Yellow brown, homogeneous structureless areas, linear and dotted vessels, white halo around the lesion, and pink-, orange-, and red-colored background can be observed on dermoscopy.

Table 1: Classification and clinical features of perforating disorders.

Kyrle's disease: Hyperkeratosis follicularis et parafollicularis in cutem penetrans	• Idiopathic • Associated with • diabetes mellitus • Hepatic abnormalities Congestive heart failure • Renal disease • Primary event is disturbance of epidermal keratinization by formation of dyskeratotic foci and acceleration of the process of keratinization	F > M wide age range exists, third to fifth decade	• Papules, nodules, and plaques with a central keratotic plug **(Fig. 1)** • Koebnerization may be present • *Sites*: Legs and arms • The lesions may be asymptomatic or pruritic	Follicular or extrafollicular cornified plug with focal parakeratosis in epidermal invagination, without demonstrable elastin or collagen. Marked acanthosis seen	• Folliculitis • Flegel's disease • Darier disease • Hypertrophic LP • Other perforating disorders	• Keratolytics, 5-fluorouracil, topical corticosteroids, methotrexate, chloroquine, prednisone • Vitamin A at a dose of 100,000 IU/day • Topical retinoic acid 0.1% cream isotretinoin 1 mg/kg/day • PUVA • Carbon dioxide laser cryosurgery
Reactive perforating collagenosis (RPC)	• Childhood form is inherited • Acquired sporadic form associated with CRF, DM, hypothyroidism, hyperparathyroidism, liver dysfunction. • Malignancies • Focal damage to collagen and its elimination of the through the epidermis	M = F	• Small, keratotic papules develop after minor trauma. Flesh-colored, umbilicated, dome-shaped papules or nodules as large as 10 mm with an adherent, keratinous plug. They heal spontaneously in 6–8 weeks to leave a hypopigmented area or slight scar • Koebner phenomenon may occur; intense pruritus is a feature of the acquired form • *Sites*: Extensor surfaces of the limbs and the dorsa of the hands	The epidermis is perforated by disrupted collagen bundles forming a cup-shaped invagination, lined by acanthotic epithelium along the sides	• Other perforating diseases • Prurigo nodularis • Papular urticaria • Perforating granuloma annulare	• The lesions are self-healing, but usually are recurrent • Topical retinoic acid, isotretinoin, allopurinol, doxycycline, UVB, and PUVA

Continued

Continued

Elastosis perforans serpiginosa (Synonyms: Perforating elastoma, elastoma intrapapillare perforans	• Idiopathic • *Reactive EPS*: Associated regularly with systemic, inherited, fibrous tissue abnormalities, such as Down syndrome, Ehlers–Danlos syndrome, Marfan syndrome, osteogenesis imperfecta, scleroderma, and pseudoxanthoma elasticum • *Drug-induced EPS*: D-penicillamine	M:F = 4:1 second decade	• Eruptive, dome-shaped, umbilicated papules, flesh colored to red, grouped in linear, arciform, circular, or serpiginous patterns, measuring several centimeters reaching up to 15–20 cm. The central core contains a keratotic plug • The sites most commonly affected are the nape of the neck, upper extremities, face, lower extremities, and trunk	Focal development of elastotic staining tissue and basophilic debris in the dermis, overlying epidermis, grows down to engulf the elastotic material	• Porokeratosis of Mibelli • Reactive perforating collagenosis • Perforating granuloma annulare	Isotretinoin, imiquimod, and cryotherapy

(CRF: chronic renal failure; DM: diabetes mellitus; EPS: elastosis perforans serpiginosa; LP: lichen planus; PUVA: psoralen and ultraviolet A)

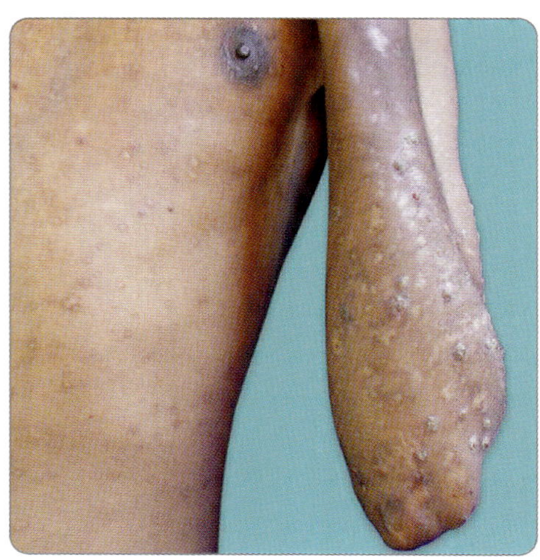

Fig. 1: Multiple hyperkeratotic lesions with central crust in a patient with renal failure.

SUGGESTED READINGS

1. Wang W, Liao Y, Fu L, Kan B, Peng X, Lu Y. Dermoscopy Features of Acquired Perforating Dermatosis Among 39 Patients. Front Med (Lausanne). 2021;8:631642.
2. Harbaoui S, Litaiem N. (2023). Acquired Perforating Dermatosis. Treasure Island (FL): StatPearls Publishing. [online] Available from https://pubmed.ncbi.nlm.nih.gov/30969537/ [Last accessed January, 2025].

183 Perioral Dermatitis

➲ SYNONYM

Periorificial dermatitis.

➲ HISTORY

Perioral dermatitis was first described in 1950s. Initially, it was considered to be a variant of rosacea, but later considered as a distinct entity.

➲ AGE GROUP

Commonly affected age group is 20–45 years with female preponderance. It can also occur in children >6 months of age.

➲ ETIOLOGY

Though exact etiology is not known, use of topical steroids has been implicated. Repeated and chronic usage of potent topical steroids, also nasal steroids, steroid inhalers, and systemic steroids predispose for the development of severe disease.

Other factors in the causation of perioral dermatitis are impaired skin barrier, atopic diathesis, and organisms such as fusiform *Spirilla*, *Candida*, and *Demodex folliculorum*, which have been cultured from the lesions, fluoride content of chewing gum, dental fillings, toothpastes, and cosmetics. Ultraviolet (UV) light, heat, and wind can cause aggravation of lesions. Premenstrual deterioration of symptoms suggest hormonal influence.

➲ CLINICAL FEATURES

Perioral dermatitis presents with multiple, discrete, symmetrically distributed grouped erythematous papules, papulovesicles, and pustules over the perioral area. A clear zone of 5 mm width around the vermillion border is a distinct feature. Lesions can be associated with itching, burning, and scaling. In rare cases, involvement of perinasal and periocular region can also be seen.

➲ HISTOPATHOLOGY

Mild acanthosis, spongiosis, focal perifollicular parakeratosis in epidermis, and lymphohistiocytic infiltrate in perifollicular and perivascular region are seen in the dermis along with plasma cells in nongranulomatous form of perioral dermatitis. Follicular spongiosis and eczematous changes are prominent.

Granulomatous form may show non caseating epithelioid cell granulomas and giant cells.

DIFFERENTIAL DIAGNOSIS

- Rosacea—presents with persistent erythema and telangiectasias
- Facial demodicosis—demodex folliculorum can be isolated.
- Seborrheic dermatitis—accentuating at nasolabial folds, retroauricular area.
- Polymorphous light eruption (PMLE)—usually occur after sun exposure
- Allergic contact dermatitis—perioral clear zone is not seen.
- Lip licking cheilitis—well-demarcated border, and scaling is seen

TREATMENT

First and foremost step is to advice on discontinuation of topical steroids. Also, application of cosmetics, soaps, detergents, abrasives, and astringent should be stopped. Oral antibiotics such as tetracycline, minocycline, and doxycycline should be given for 8–12 weeks and then tapering helps resolve the lesions. Along with systemic antibiotics, topical antibiotic such as metronidazole, clindamycin, and erythromycin can also be started.

Other than the above, topical tacrolimus, pimecrolimus, adapalene, and photodynamic therapy with 5 aminolevulinic acid are promising. For recalcitrant cases, isotretinoin 0.2 mg/kg may be considered.

PROGNOSIS

The disease is usually self-limiting without any sequelae or relapse. However, untreated cases may have waxing and waning course.

SUGGESTED READING

1. Lipozenčić J, Hadžavdić SL. Perioral dermatitis. Clin Dermatol. 2014;32(1):125-30.

184 Periorbital Melanosis

➲ SYNONYMS

Periorbital hyperpigmentation, periocular hyperpigmentation, dark circles, infraorbital darkening, infraorbital discoloration.

➲ AGE GROUP

Most affected age group is 16–25 years old. Female preponderance is observed.

➲ ETIOLOGY

The pathogenesis of periocular hyperpigmentation involves a combination of exogenous and endogenous factors. Genetic predisposition, excessive pigmentation, postinflammatory hyperpigmentation from atopic and allergic contact dermatitis, periorbital edema, increased vascularity, and shadowing due to skin laxity, and tear trough associated with aging are considered causative factors. Lifestyle factors such as lack of sleep, stress, alcohol overuse, and smoking may also contribute. Additionally, ultraviolet (UV) radiation can exacerbate periocular hyperpigmentation. When all other potential causes have been ruled out, the condition is referred to as "physiologic periorbital hypopigmentation".

➲ CLASSIFICATION

Periorbital hyperpigmentation (POH) was classified into pigmented (brown color), vascular (blue/pink/purple color), structural (skin color), and mixed type based on the clinical appearance assessed by the physician. This classification was given by Huang et al.

➲ CLINICAL FEATURES

Asymptomatic, light to dark colored, brownish black pigmentation is seen around the eyes. Infraorbital region is more commonly involved giving a tired look to the patient **(Fig. 1)**.

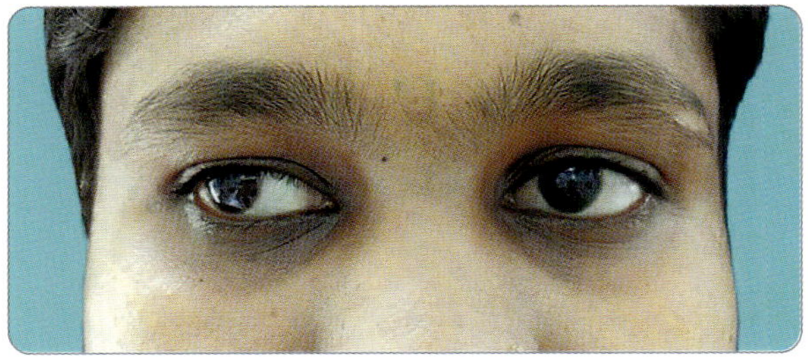

Fig. 1: Periorbital hypermelanosis.

HISTOPATHOLOGY

The hyperpigmentation can be either epidermal or dermal and specialized stains like Fontana Masson can be used to stain melanin.

DERMOSCOPY

On dermoscopy, three different patterns were observed, pigmentary (33%), vascular (15%), and mixed pigmentary vascular (52%). No specific dermoscopic features have been identified.

TREATMENT

The aim of treatment should be to identify and treat the primary cause of hyperpigmentation as well as its contributing factors. Also, different modalities are used according to the cause of POH.

Topical depigmenting agents, such as hydroquinone, kojic acid, azelaic acid, topical retinoic acid, phenolic bleaching agents, triple combination formulations, arbutin, and topical vitamin C can be used. Broad-spectrum sunscreens also help reduce pigmentation.

Physical therapies, including chemical peels such as glycolic acid 20%, lactic acid 15% along with trichloroacetic acid 3.75%, surgical corrections, and laser therapy have also been tried.

Apart from above hyaluronic acid fillers, platelet-rich plasma and carboxytherapy are also used.

SUGGESTED READING

1. Sarkar R, Ranjan R, Garg S, Garg VK, Sonthalia S, Bansal S. Periorbital Hyperpigmentation: A Comprehensive Review. J Clin Aesthet Dermatol. 2016;9(1):49-55.

185 Peutz–Jeghers Syndrome

➲ SYNONYM

Periorificial lentiginosis.

➲ HISTORY

This autosomal dominant disorder was described by Jan Peutz and Harold Jeghers in 1921 and 1947, respectively. The eponym Peutz–Jeghers syndrome was introduced by the radiologist Andre J Bruwer in 1954.

➲ ETIOLOGY

The cause of Peutz–Jeghers syndrome is mutations in tumor suppressor gene *STK11* gene.

➲ CLINICAL FEATURES

Peutz–Jeghers syndrome is an autosomal dominant disorder, showing pigmented macules on the oral mucosa and skin associated with gastrointestinal polyposis. There is no sex or racial preponderance. A family history is found in 60% of cases.

Pigmented macules are present at birth or may appear in infancy, early childhood, or even later in life. The oral mucosa is usually involved; the buccal mucosa, gums, hard palate, and lips are involved. The lesions are irregularly distributed, round, oval or irregular patches, brown or black in color, and 1–5 mm in diameter. They may also be seen on the face, hands, feet, and nails. Facial lentigines are smaller <1 mm, darker and distributed around the nose and mouth. The lesions over the hands and feet are usually larger and more prominent over the palms and soles. The nails may show a diffuse or longitudinal band like pigmentation. Mucosal pigmentation is usually permanent. Skin pigmentation may improve after puberty.

Gastrointestinal polyps are benign hamartomas with relatively less potential for malignant transformation. They may occur throughout the gastrointestinal tract, commonly observed in the small intestine. The symptoms of gastrointestinal polyposis like repeated abdominal colic, rectal bleeding, and hematemesis usually manifest between 10 and 30 years of age.

Sometimes clubbing of fingers, ovarian tumors, and precocious puberty may be seen.

➲ HISTOPATHOLOGY

Pigmented macules show an increased amount of melanin in the basal layer of the epidermis without any associated increase in the number of melanocytes.

DERMOSCOPY

Dermoscopic findings show parallel ridge patterns, which correspond to deposition of melanin, primarily in the *crista profunda intermedia*.

DIFFERENTIAL DIAGNOSIS

- *Addison's disease*: Presents with widespread diffuse hyperpigmentation in addition to mucous membrane pigmentation, freckles, and sun-exposed parts of the body affected, and photo darkening of pigmentation is seen.
- *Cronkite–Canada syndrome*: Shows diffuse pigmentation of the volar aspects of fingers, but mucous membranes are spared.
- *Laugier–Hunziker syndrome*: Melanonychia can be seen and no associated gastrointestinal (GI) polyposis

COMPLICATIONS

Complications include intussusception, GI obstruction, risk of malignancy, rectal bleeding, and anemia.

TREATMENT

Regular endoscopic examination of the upper gastrointestinal tract and the whole colon, and barium follow-through studies of the small intestine every 2 years, along with pelvic examination, have to be done.

Individual polyps may require endoscopic or surgical removal.

In the presence of numerous colonic polyps, a prophylactic colectomy may be performed.

PROGNOSIS

There is 15-fold risk of development of malignancy (colorectal carcinoma followed by CA breast).

SUGGESTED READING

1. Wu M, Krishnamurthy K. Peutz-Jeghers Syndrome. (2023). Treasure Island (FL): StatPearls Publishing. [online] Available from https://pubmed.ncbi.nlm.nih.gov/30570978/ [Last accessed January, 2025].

186 Phrynoderma

➲ HISTORY

The term "phrynoderma" was coined by Nicholls in 1933 to describe the "toad-like" appearance of the skin of undernourished laborers. Frazier and Hu were the ones to claim that cod liver oil produces improvement.

➲ ETIOLOGY

Phrynoderma is seen primarily in Asia and Africa and is rare in developed countries, except in the setting of intestinal malabsorption, anorexia nervosa, or fad diets. Phrynoderma is seen most often in association with vitamin A deficiency, but may be related to severe malnutrition and deficiencies of other vitamins (e.g., vitamin C, E, and B) as well as essential fatty acids.

➲ CLINICAL FEATURES

Follicular papules of various sizes with conical keratotic plugs are seen over extensor aspect of the extremities, especially over the elbows **(Fig. 1)**, neck, knees, thighs, and posterior axillary folds. The lesions may spread to involve the extensor surfaces of the extremities as well as the abdomen, back, and buttocks. The face is the last site to become involved, and the hands and feet are spared. When expressed, the keratotic plugs usually leave pits.

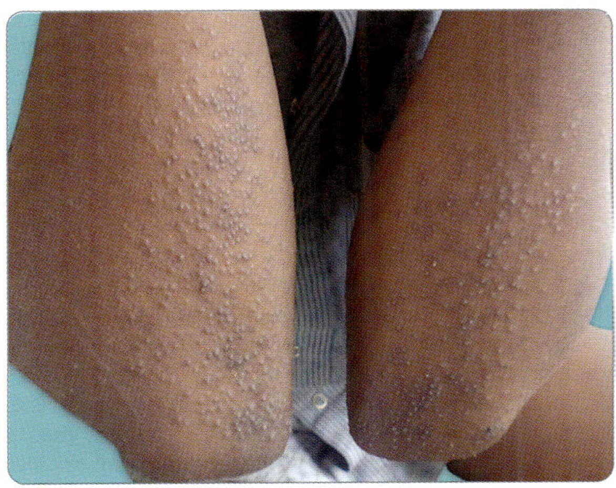

Fig. 1: Horny keratotic papules of phrynoderma on elbows.

Adjunctive symptoms, such as cheilitis, glossitis, blepharitis, diarrhea, muscle weakness and neuritis, may develop when hypovitaminosis A is predominant relative to other vitamin deficiencies. Eye findings are pathognomonic. These include night blindness, xerophthalmia, xerosis cornea, Bitot spots, and keratomalacia. The earliest finding is delayed adaptation to dark nyctalopia.

It can be associated with intestinal malabsorption, anorexia nervous, fad diets, and alcoholism also.

HISTOPATHOLOGY

Biopsy specimens demonstrate moderate hyperkeratosis with distention of the upper portion of the follicle by large, parakeratotic horny plugs. Sebaceous glands are greatly reduced in size and may exhibit epithelial atrophy. When the condition is severe, both eccrine and sebaceous glands may exhibit squamous metaplasia.

DERMOSCOPY

Dermoscopy shows perifollicular white scaling, and keratotic plugs are seen.

DIFFERENTIAL DIAGNOSIS

- Keratosis pilaris—spiny papules with keratin plug, perifollicular erythema, and antenna sign are positive.
- Lichen spinulosus—absence of other features of vitamin deficiencies
- Keratosis circumscripta
- Follicular ichthyosis—any site can be involved, not only knees/elbows
- The diagnosis of classic phrynoderma is confirmed by reduced serum levels of vitamin A (<30 µg/100 mL).

TREATMENT

Treatment is with topical keratolytic ointments (urea 10–30%).

Equilibrated calorie regimen (1,500–2,000 kcal/day) with nutritional supplements. These supplements include vitamin A (50,000 U/day for 1 month, then 5,000 U/day for 2 months), vitamin E (alpha-tocopherol 300 mg/day), and vitamin B complex (thiamine 3 mg/day, nicotinamide 30 mg/day, riboflavin 1 mg/day, calcium pantothenate 1 mg/day, pyridoxine hydrochloride 0.5 mg/day, cyanocobalamin 5 mg/day), as well as vitamin C (500 mg/day) and essential fatty acids (safflower oil 5 mL/day).

Topical keratolytics such as 3% salicylic acid, tretinoin gel, and urea based creams can also be prescribed for scaly plaques for symptomatic relief.

Diets or at least supplements that are rich in vitamins A, B, C, and E, including foods such as yellow vegetables, green leafy vegetables, carrots, whole-milk derivatives, eggs, fish, and oils (e.g., fish-liver oil, soybean oil, safflower oil, sunflower oil, corn oil, palm oil, cottonseed oil), as well as unprocessed cereal grains and nuts are recommended.

➲ PROGNOSIS

The lesions clear in 1–4 months. There may be residual hyperpigmentation and/or scarring.

➲ SUGGESTED READING

1. Maronn M, Allen DM, Esterly NB. Phrynoderma: A Manifestation of Vitamin A Deficiency? the Rest of the Story. Pediatr Dermatol. 2005;22(1):60-3.

187 Piedra

➲ SYNONYMS

Trichomycosis nodularis, trichomycosis nodosa, tinea nodosa, trichosporosis.

➲ HISTORY

In 1865, Beigel first described Piedra, and in 1911, Horta classified Piedra into two types. Piedra means stone in Spanish.

➲ ETIOLOGY

Black piedra is caused by piedraia hortae, and white by *Trichosporon* species—*T. beigelii, T. asahii, T. ovoides, T. inkin, T. mucoides, T. asteroides* and *T. cutaneum*.

➲ AGE AND SEX

Infection is more common in women and preschool children. The mode of transmission could be sharing pillows, bed sheets, and comb.

➲ CLINICAL FEATURES

Black piedra is characterized by firmly attached, hard, brown-black nodules on the hair shaft that vary from microscopic to a few millimeters in size, and are gritty to palpation which produces a metallic sound on brushing the hair. It weakens the hair shaft, often resulting in broken hairs. Scalp hairs are most typically affected, and nodules are most commonly seen on the frontal scalp. In few cases, mustache, beard, and pubic hairs may also get affected. White piedra consists of softer and less adherent whitish to beige nodules that may be discrete or coalesce into sleeve-like structures. Broken hairs are sometimes present but are less common than with black piedra. White piedra can be easily detached from the hair shaft, because it affects the outer lipid layers. This can affect scalp, eyebrows, eyelashes, beard, groin, or axilla.

➲ HISTOPATHOLOGY

In histology or KOH mounts, nodules of black piedra display a periphery of aligned hyphae and a well-organized center of thick-walled cells packed closely together sometimes termed pseudo parenchyma. These nodules are mostly outside of the hair. The nodules of white piedra have a less organized and more intrapilar appearance, with hyphae arranged perpendicularly to the hair shaft.

➲ DERMOSCOPY

Findings are similar to ones on direct examination, but dermoscopy is helpful in differentiating white piedra from pediculosis-induced nits.

➲ DIFFERENTIAL DIAGNOSIS

- Nits—strongly attached to hair shaft, presence of lice
- Hair casts—cylindrical grayish white covering that slided up and down the hair shaft
- Monilethrix—beaded appearance of hair, absence of fungi
- Trichorrhexis nodosa—mainly axillary hair involved
- Trichomycosis

➲ TREATMENT

Shaving the infected hair is often curative and is the best treatment for both black and white piedra. Shaving may be augmented by the use of a topical azole antifungal. Antifungal preparations such as benzoic acid ointment and topical azoles may be used to prevent recurrence. Oral terbinafine 250 mg OD for 6 weeks is also curative.

➲ SUGGESTED READING

1. Pontes ZB, Ramos AL, Lima Ede O, Guerra Mde F, Oliveira NM, Santos JP. Clinical and mycological study of scalp white piedra in the State of Paraíba, Brazil. Mem Inst Oswaldo Cruz. 2002;97(5):747-50.

188 Pilar Cyst

➲ SYNONYMS

Trichilemmal cyst, Wen.

➲ ETIOLOGY

Etiology may be unknown, familial, and inherited by autosomal dominant transmission. A monoallelic mutation in phospholipase C delta 1 (PLCD1) that results in formation of multiple pilar cysts has been proposed. The cyst is known to be derived from external root sheath of the follicular isthmus.

➲ AGE GROUP

Any age group; females more commonly affected, especially in middle age.

➲ CLINICAL FEATURES

Pilar cyst is a cyst arising from external root sheath, containing keratin and breakdown products. It presents as multiple, well-circumscribed, smooth, firm, mobile, flesh-colored, dermal nodules, which may become infected or inflamed after a minor trauma. Commonly located in the scalp, other rare sites are extremities, even pulp of finger. It may also occur along Blaschko's lines and present as trichilemmal cyst nevus. They are slow growing.

➲ HISTOPATHOLOGY

These cysts are well circumscribed in dermis and lined by two or three layers of small, dark keratinocytes. There is an abrupt transition to the center of the lesion, to large pale cells with features of root sheath cells. A granular layer is absent. The peripheral layer shows palisading. The center of the cyst contains keratin debris. A granular layer may be present in hybrid lesions, which have focal changes of epidermoid cyst. Calcification may occur.

➲ DERMOSCOPY

Dermoscopic findings include white shiny rosette-like structure probably caused by horny material in the adnexal opening or by concentric perifollicular fibrosis.

➲ DIFFERENTIAL DIAGNOSIS

- Epidermoid cyst/sebaceous cyst—swelling with central punctum, and white cheesy secretion is present.
- Dermoid cyst—not associated with hair follicle

- Pilomatricoma—ghost cells are seen in biopsy.
- Lipoma—firm, mobile swelling with proliferation of adipose tissue is seen.

COMPLICATIONS

Complications can be infection, calcification, proliferating trichilemmal tumor (PTT), or malignant PTT.

TREATMENT

Excision, usually to obtain a diagnosis.

PROGNOSIS

Shelled out lesions may recur.

SUGGESTED READING

1. Liu M, Han H, Zheng Y, Xiao S, Feng Y. Pilar cyst on the dorsum of hand: A case report and review of literature. Medicine (Baltimore). 2020;99(31):e21519.

189 Pilomatricoma

➲ SYNONYMS

Benign calcifying epithelioma of Malherbe, trichomatricoma, pilomatrixoma.

➲ HISTORY

Pilomatricoma was first described by Malherbe and Chenantais in 1880, later by Forbes and Helwig in 1961, and they also proposed the term pilomatrixoma.

➲ ETIOLOGY

Exact etiology is unknown. Mutation in *CTNNB1* gene pointing at dysregulation in beta-catenin is seen in 75%, and proto-oncogene Bcl-2 is also implicated.

➲ AGE GROUP

Pilomatricoma may occur at any age, but it is most common in <20 years of age; females are more affected. Familial cases are also seen.

➲ CLINICAL FEATURES

Benign tumor is considered to be a hamartoma of hair matrix. Pilomatricoma presents as a solitary, dermal or subcutaneous lesion, usually 3–30 mm in size. Skin over the tumor is normal and has a firm to stone-hard consistency due to calcification within the lesion, and often results in an angulated shape (the "tent" sign).

Sometimes the skin may become inflamed and present as a granulomatous swelling, or it may be ulcerated. The tumor is usually situated in the head and neck region, followed by upper extremities, trunk, and lower extremities **(Figs. 1 and 2)**.

➲ ASSOCIATED SYNDROMES

Associated syndromes include myotonic dystrophy, Turner syndrome, Rubinstein–Taybi syndrome, and *MUTYH* gene mutation-associated polyposis. When associated with these conditions, multiple pilomatricomas can be present.

➲ HISTOPATHOLOGY

Pilomatricoma is situated in the dermis composed of well-circumscribed, rounded islands giving a lobulated contour.

The cells are hair matrix cells maturing toward cortex or root sheath. The outer cells of the tumor are smaller in size and crowded, hence are deeply basophilic. Cytoplasm is scanty, indistinct cell

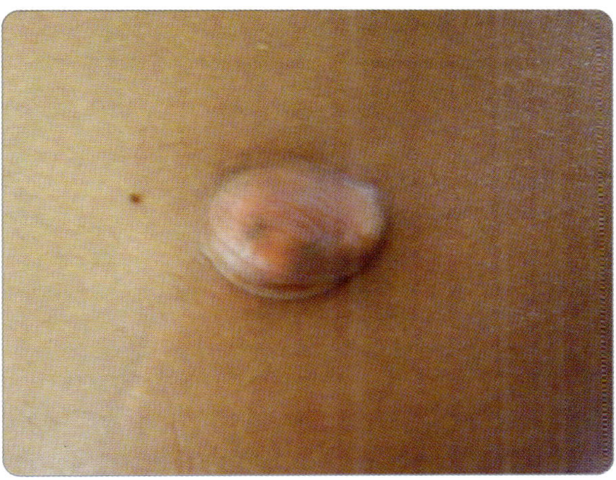

Fig. 1: Solitary nodule with calcification in pilomatricoma.

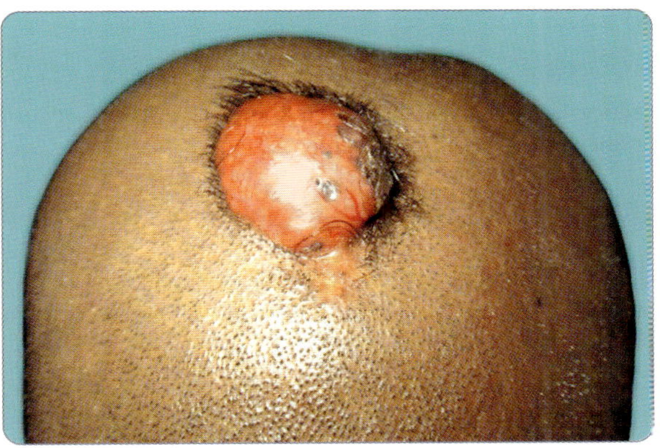

Fig. 2: Solitary nodule on the scalp, which showed changes of malignant transformation on histopathology.

margins but inter cellular connections are seen. Toward the center of the mass, cytoplasm becomes more abundant and eosinophilic. The chromatin is sparse, and clumped in dark granules, and when all basophilic material disappears, a "mummified" ghost cell remains. The central area may get calcified. Melanin may be present. The stroma surrounding the mass may contain inflammatory cells and giant cells.

➲ RADIOLOGICAL IMAGING

Computed tomography (CT) scan picks up a well-demarcated subcutaneous lesion with varying amount of calcification. High signal bands correlating with those formed by basaloid cells are appreciated on magnetic resonance imaging (MRI).

➲ DERMOSCOPY

Dermoscopy shows irregular white structures and polymorphous; atypical vessels are appreciated, although there are no specific dermoscopic features.

DIFFERENTIAL DIAGNOSIS

- Sebaceous cyst—central punctum is seen
- Giant cell tumor
- Chondroma
- Dermoid cyst
- Degenerating fibroxanthoma
- Foreign body reaction
- Osteoma cutis

COMPLICATIONS

Rapid growth, giant tumor formation, overlying striae, or secondary anetoderma may rarely occur. Malignant change may occur rarely, especially in long-standing pilomatricomas and in elderly.

TREATMENT

Complete surgical excision is the treatment. Wide excision in malignant lesions with a margin of 1–2 cyst can be done.

PROGNOSIS

Recurrence is rare after surgery. If there is repeated recurrence, malignancy has to be considered.

SUGGESTED READINGS

1. DeRosa DC, Lin-Hurtubise K. Pilomatricoma: an unusual dermatologic neoplasm. Hawaii J Med Public Health. 2012;71(10):282-6.
2. Zaballos P, Llambrich A, Puig S, Malvehy J. Dermoscopic findings of pilomatricomas. Dermatology. 2008;217(3):225-30.

190 Pitted Keratolysis

SYNONYMS

Keratolysis plantare sulcatum, keratoma plantare sulcatum, ringed keratolysis.

HISTORY

Pitted keratolysis was first named as keratoma plantare sulcatum by Castellani in 1910, but was given its present name, pitted keratolysis, by Taplin and Zaias in 1967.

ETIOLOGY

The causative organism is still debated; the microorganisms commonly implicated are:

- *Micrococcus sedentarius* (now *Kytococcus sedentarius*)
- A species of *Corynebacterium* or *Streptomyces*
- *Dermatophilus congolensis*
- *Actinomyces*

Under appropriate conditions (i.e., prolonged occlusion, hyperhidrosis, and increased skin surface pH), these bacteria proliferate and produce proteinases that destroy the stratum corneum, creating pits. The malodor associated with pitted keratolysis is due to the production of sulfur containing by-products, such as thiols, sulfides, and thioesters.

Occlusive environment, moisture, and warmth are the predisposing factors.

AGE GROUP

Pitted keratolysis can affect patients of any age. No sex or racial predilection. Commonly seen among athletes.

CLINICAL FEATURES

Pitted keratolysis is a superficial infection of the skin characterized by crateriform pitting that primarily affects the pressure-bearing aspects of the plantar surface of the feet [heel, ball of feet **(Fig. 1)**, and toepads] and, occasionally, the palms of the hand.

The primary lesions are pits in the stratum corneum ranging from 0.5 to 7 mm. Larger craters can be formed due to coalescence of adjacent pits. There are numerous superficial erosions of the horny layer of the soles and the undersurfaces of the toes. All parts of both the soles may be affected, but pressure bearing or friction areas are most commonly affected. Hyperhidrosis is often associated, sometimes with maceration, stickiness, and a foul odor.

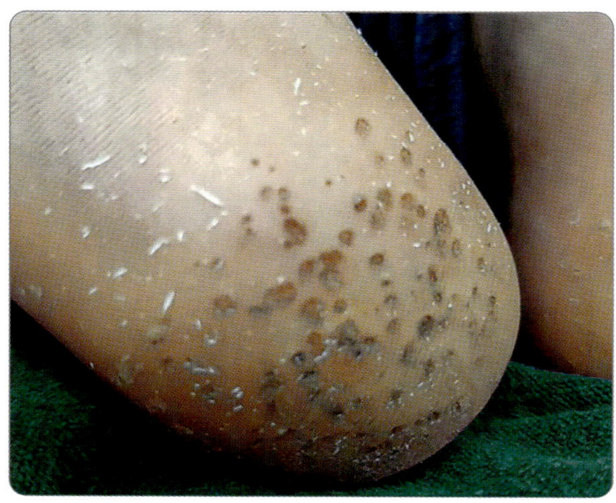

Fig. 1: Multiple, well-defined, grouped pits seen over the ball of foot.

Palms may be rarely affected. A variant of markedly enlarged lesions, called crateriform pitted keratolysis, has also been described.

HISTOPATHOLOGY

Craters are limited to the stratum corneum, and these keratin pits are lined by small cocci as well as filamentous bacteria.

DERMOSCOPY

Dermoscopy shows abundant pits and is very useful in assessing the size, configuration, arrangement, and characteristics of pits.

LABORATORY DIAGNOSIS

It is not always easy to find the organisms in KOH mounts but are more easily detected in Gram-stained scrapings. Culture on brain–heart infusion agar, incubated at 37°C in a mixture of pure nitrogen containing 5–10% carbon dioxide, gives minute, irregular, colorless colonies within 3–5 days.

DIFFERENTIAL DIAGNOSIS

The lesions are easily recognizable, but simple hyperhidrosis, erythrasma, plantar warts and tinea pedis can be considered as differentials.

TREATMENT

Topical erythromycin 1.5% or clindamycin 1% is curative. Effective alternatives are miconazole or clotrimazole cream and Whitfield ointment. Both 5% benzoyl peroxide gel and a 10–20% solution of aluminum chloride hexahydrate may be used. Botulinum toxin can be used if there is associated hyperhidrosis. Aluminum chloride hexahydrate can also be used prophylactically to prevent recurrences.

➲ PROGNOSIS

Pitted keratolysis is cured easily and has an excellent prognosis.

➲ SUGGESTED READING

1. Pattanaprichakul P, Kulthanan K, Bunyaratavej S, Eimpunth S, Rungruang T, Chanyachailert P, et al. The Correlations between Clinical Features, Dermoscopic and Histopathological Findings, and Treatment Outcomes of Patients with Pitted Keratolysis. Biomed Res Int. 2021;2021:3416643.

191 Pityriasis Alba

➲ SYNONYMS

Pityriasis sicca faciei, pityriasis alba faciei, erythema streptogenes, impetigo furfuracea, impetigo sicca, pityriasis simplex, pityriasis maculata.

➲ HISTORY

Pityriasis alba (PA) was described by Fox in 1923.

➲ ETIOLOGY

Pityriasis alba is a minor sign of atopic dermatitis. Sun exposure, poor socioeconomic status, and *Staphylococcus epidermidis* are the proposed triggering factors.

➲ AGE GROUP

Pityriasis alba is commonly seen in children >5 years to early adolescence.

➲ CLINICAL FEATURES

Lesions are asymptomatic, initially erythematous, but generally skin-colored to hypopigmented with a fine overlying scale, few to multiple in number with indistinct borders. Hypopigmentation is accentuated with tanning. Common sites are the cheek **(Fig. 1)**,

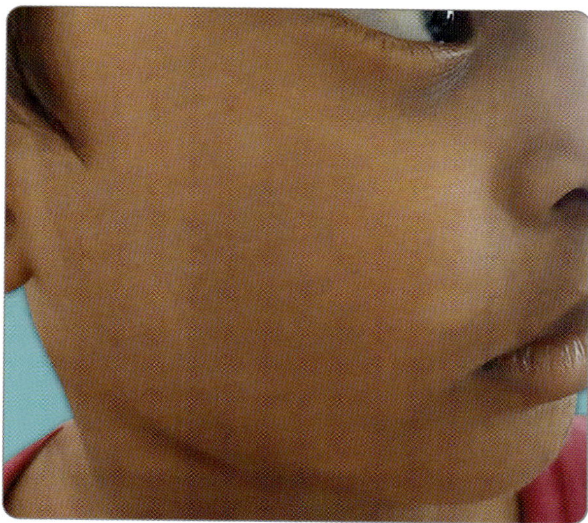

Fig. 1: Multiple, ill-defined, hypopigmented patches with mild scaling noted over the right cheek.

perioral area, forehead, trunk, and proximal arms. Three clinical variants are described, i.e., classical, extensive, and pigmented PA.

HISTOPATHOLOGY

Early lesions show nonspecific abnormalities, including follicular spongiosis, focal parakeratosis, superficial perivascular lymphocytic infiltrate, melanophages, acanthosis, exocytosis, irregular pigmentation, and reduced melanin.

DERMOSCOPY

White structureless areas with ill-defined margins, fine white scales at the center of the lesion, and light brown pigment network are seen.

DIFFERENTIAL DIAGNOSIS

- *Postinflammatory hypopigmentation*—history of (H/o) previous inflammatory lesion and the absence of scaling
- *Tinea versicolor*—spaghetti and meatball appearance in KOH mount of scrapings
- *Indeterminate Hansen's*—lymphocytic infiltrates around the appendages and neurovascular bundles
- *Vitiligo*—lack of melanocytes on biopsy
- *Nevus anemicus*—enhanced vascularity around the lesion
- *Photodermatosis*—H/o aggravation on sun exposure
- Chemical leukoderma
- *Eczema*—oozing and crusting may be seen.
- *Psoriasis*—silvery white scales are seen, and Auspitz sign is positive.

TREATMENT

None are universally effective. Sun protection is recommended. Low potency topical corticosteroid and topical calcineurin inhibitors can be given.

PROGNOSIS

Variable and recurrent lesions may develop. They can persist for >1 year and resolve spontaneously over time. Most lesions disappear before puberty.

SUGGESTED READINGS

1. Miazek N, Michalek I, Pawlowska-Kisiel M, Olszewska M, Rudnicka L. Pityriasis Alba--Common Disease, Enigmatic Entity: Up-to-Date Review of the Literature. Pediatr Dermatol. 2015;32(6):786-91.
2. Ankad BS, Mukherjee SS, Nikam BP. Dermoscopy - Histopathology Correlation: a conspectus in the skin of colour, 1st edition. Singapore: Springer Verlag; 2021.

192 Pityriasis Lichenoides Chronica

HISTORY

Pityriasis lichenoides chronica (PLC) was first described by Juliusberg in 1899.

ETIOLOGY

The etiology is unknown. A hypersensitivity reaction to an infective organism (e.g., toxoplasma, cytomegalovirus, parvovirus, adenovirus, Epstein–Barr virus, and *Streptococci*) leading to allergic vasculitis is the main hypothesis. Alternatively, it may indicate that PLC is primarily a lymphoproliferative disorder that belongs to the cutaneous T-cell lymphoproliferative spectrum.

AGE

Young adults.

CLINICAL FEATURES

It is characterized by a pleomorphic eruption of asymptomatic, red-brown, oval to round, firm lichenoid papules from 3 to 10 mm in diameter with centrally adherent mica-like scales that can be detached by gentle scraping to reveal a shiny brown, pigmented surface. The papules usually appear on the trunk and proximal extremities and spare the palms and soles. The face, scalp, and mucous membranes may be affected in severe cases. Rarely, papules may be present in a segmental pattern or may show the isomorphic phenomenon. They typically leave hypopigmented or hyperpigmented macules, which gradually fade. Scarring is unusual.

HISTOPATHOLOGY

The papules of PLC show psoriasiform changes of epidermal hyperplasia and a sparse infiltrate of lymphocytes and histiocytes around dermal blood vessels.

DERMOSCOPY

Dermoscopy shows orange-yellowish structureless areas with focally distributed nondotted vessels, milky-red globules, and linear vessels. White scales detaching inward in the center of the lesion and few brown dots on bright pink background are also observed.

DIFFERENTIAL DIAGNOSIS

- *Guttate psoriasis*—mainly erythematous scaly papules
- *Pityriasis rosea*—herald patch followed by lesions with collarette of scales is seen.

- Secondary papulosquamous syphilis
- *Lichen planus*—classical lichenoid reaction pattern is seen.
- Small plaque parapsoriasis

TREATMENT

Broad-spectrum antibiotics, such as tetracycline 2 g daily for 2–4 weeks in adults or erythromycin 2 g/day in adults and 30–50 mg/kg body weight per day in children, may be effective. Oral antihistamines may be helpful if significant itching is present.

Psoralen and ultraviolet A (PUVA) can be tried.

PROGNOSIS

The course of pityriasis lichenoides cannot be predicted. The disease may regress in a few months or, sometimes, persist for years.

SUGGESTED READING

1. Khachemoune A, Blyumin ML. Pityriasis lichenoides: pathophysiology, classification, and treatment. Am J Clin Dermatol. 2007;8(1):29-36.

193 Pityriasis Rosea

➲ SYNONYMS

Gilbert's disease, pityriasis circinata, roseola annulata, herpes tonsurans maculosus.

➲ HISTORY

Pityriasis rosea (PR) was first described by Robert Willan and named by Camille Gilbert in 1860 from the Greek word pityriasis (fine scale) and the Latin word rosea (rose-red).

➲ ETIOLOGY

Unclear, infectious cause suspected, probably human herpesvirus (HHV)-6 and HHV-7; some drugs can cause PR-like lesions viz. arsenic, bismuth, gold, omeprazole, metronidazole, and isotretinoin.

➲ AGE GROUP

Pityriasis rosea occurs between the age group of 10 and 35 years, with equal incidence in both sexes; peak incidence is seen in the spring and winter.

➲ PATHOPHYSIOLOGY

A lack of natural killer (NK) cell and B-cell activity in PR lesions has been noted, suggesting a predominantly T cell-mediated immunity.

➲ CLINICAL FEATURES

A single herald patch precedes the exanthematous phase, which develops over a period of 1–2 weeks. Pruritus can be an associated feature. Herald patch is oval, slightly raised plaque 2–5 cm, salmon-red, with fine collarette scale at the periphery **(Fig. 1)**. This is followed by the eruption of fine scaling papules and plaques with marginal collarette, with a central cigarette paper appearance, which develops after 5–15 days. The long axes of the oval lesions follow the lines of cleavage in a "Christmas tree" pattern **(Fig. 2)**. Lesions are usually confined to the trunk and the proximal aspects of the arms and legs. Rarely, lesions are seen on the face. When the skin is stretched across the long axis of a medallion lesion, the scale, being finer and lighter and attached at one end, tends to fold across the line of the stretch-hanging curtain sign.

Oral lesions in the form of erythematous plaques, hemorrhagic puncta, and ulcers occur.

Atypical PR: Lesions may be present only on the face and neck. The primary plaque may be absent, may be the sole manifestation of the disease, or may be multiple. Most confusing are the examples of PR

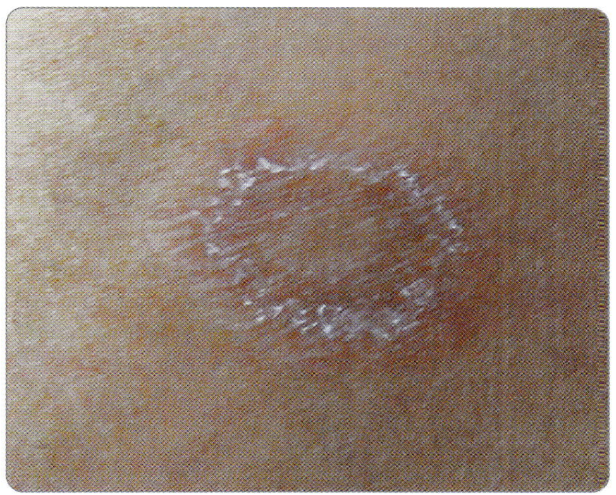

Fig. 1: Herald patch of pityriasis rosea with collarette scale.

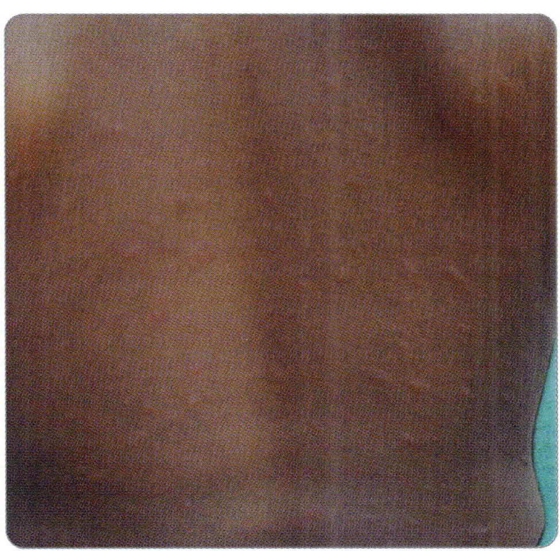

Fig. 2: Christmas tree distribution of erythematous papules over the back.

with vesicles or simulating erythema multiforme. This usually results from irritation and sweating, often as a consequence of inadequate treatment. Various types of PR include papular, vesicular, inverse, localized, flexural, lichenoid, medallion, bullous, hemorrhagic, urticarial, pustular, purpuric, erythema multiforme-like, gigantean type, exfoliative dermatitis, and pityriasis amiantacea-like.

HISTOPATHOLOGY

Histopathology shows patchy or diffuse parakeratosis, absence of granular layer, slight acanthosis, focal spongiosis, and microscopic vesicles. Occasional dyskeratotic cells with an eosinophilic homogeneous appearance, with edema of the dermis and homogenization of the collagen are seen. Small mounds of angulated parakeratosis are attributed to the teapot lid sign, and perivascular mild lymphocytic infiltrates give rise to the coat sleeve appearance. The four characteristic histological findings are eczematoid Unna's sign (eczematoid pattern), Sabouraud's sign (erythrocytes in the papillary dermis and epidermis), Lowenbach's sign (decrease or absence of granular layer), and homogenization of papillary collagen.

➲ DERMOSCOPY

Dermoscopy of herald patch and daughter patches demonstrates similar features and shows diffuse and structureless yellow-orange areas (less appreciable in the skin of color) and characteristic focal whitish peripheral scaling, which is referred to as "collarette scaling."

➲ DIFFERENTIAL DIAGNOSIS

Drug eruptions (e.g., captopril and barbiturates), secondary syphilis, guttate psoriasis (no marginal collarette), erythema migrans with secondary lesions, erythema multiforme (target lesions classical), tinea corporis (fungal hyphae are seen on KOH mount), tinea versicolor, lichen planus, and nummular eczema.

Lesions with a Christmas tree pattern of distribution include PR, secondary syphilis, ashy dermatosis, and seborrheic keratosis.

➲ TREATMENT

Oral antihistamines and/or topical antipruritic lotions for relief of pruritus can be given. Topical glucocorticoids, ultraviolet B (UVB) phototherapy, and short course of systemic glucocorticoids have been tried.

➲ PROGNOSIS

Spontaneous remission occurs in 6–12 weeks or less. Recurrences are uncommon.

➲ SUGGESTED READINGS

1. Leung AKC, Lam JM, Leong KF, Hon KL. Pityriasis Rosea: An Updated Review. Curr Pediatr Rev. 2021;17(3):201-11.
2. Ankad BS, Mukherjee SS, Nikam BP. Dermoscopy - Histopathology Correlation: a conspectus in the skin of colour, 1st edition. Singapore: Springer Verlag; 2021.

194 Pityriasis Rubra Pilaris

SYNONYMS

Devergie's disease, lichen ruber acuminatus, lichen ruber pilaris.

HISTORY

Pityriasis rubra pilaris (PRP) was first described in 1828 by Tarral and by Marie–Guillaume–Alphonse Devergie in 1856 and was named by Besnier in 1889.

AGE

Bimodal onset, early childhood, and fifth decade.

ETIOLOGY

The etiology of PRP is not known. Familial occurrence has been recorded in up to 6.5% of patients. A disorder of vitamin A metabolism has been suggested, since histologically, the changes in PRP are similar to those in hypovitaminosis A, and PRP has been successfully treated with high doses of vitamin A. The association of PRP with autoimmune disorders and human immunodeficiency virus (HIV) infection points to an underlying immunological abnormality. Bacterial superantigens have been blamed, and it has been suggested that juvenile acute PRP is a reactive exanthem. The inherited form of PRP is linked to *CARD14* gene mutation.

GRIFFITH'S CLASSIFICATION

- *Type 1*: Classic adult type
- *Type 2*: Atypical adult type
- *Type 3*: Classic juvenile type
- *Type 4*: Circumscribed juvenile type
- *Type 5*: Atypical juvenile type
- *Type 6*: HIV-associated PRP

CLINICAL FEATURES

Pityriasis rubra pilaris is characterized by reddish orange scaly plaques, palmoplantar keratoderma, and keratotic follicular papules **(Fig. 1)**. The papules are widespread, small, follicular, acuminate, and pinkish yellow, with scaling that coalesces to form plaques of various sizes and shapes distributed symmetrically on the trunk and limbs. The scale is branny, and a reddish orange erythema is present. On the scalp, diffuse erythema and scaling simulating seborrheic dermatitis occur. Horny follicular papules on the back of the proximal phalanges of the fingers may feel like a nutmeg grater. PRP often

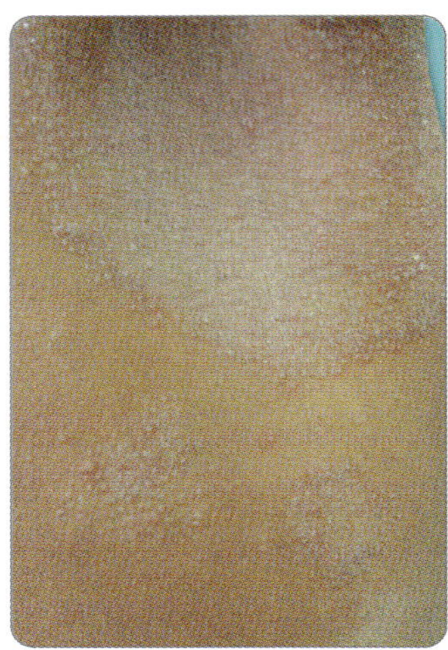

Fig. 1: Grouped horny papules with erythema with normal skin in between lesions.

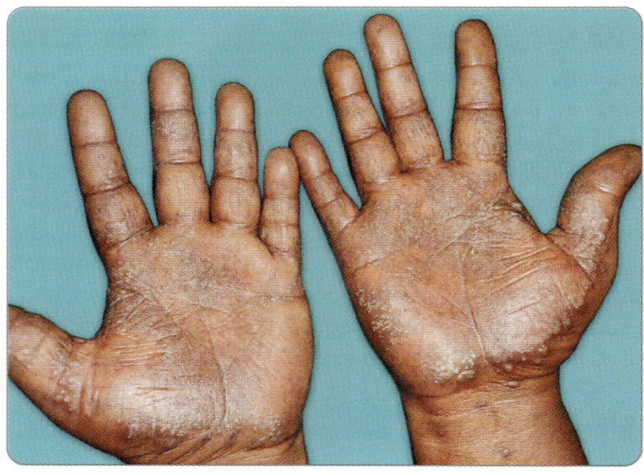

Fig. 2: Thickening of skin over the palms in pityriasis rubra pilaris (PRP).

begins on the scalp and progresses caudally, sometimes resulting in erythroderma with islands of normal skin (nappes claires) within the affected areas, which is diagnostic. There is gross hyperkeratosis, often with painful fissures, of the palms and soles that can extend to their sides. The yellowish hyperkeratosis involving the palms and soles is often called as "PRP sandal" **(Fig. 2)**.

➲ HISTOPATHOLOGY

There is hyperkeratosis with follicular plugging, alternating orthokeratosis, and parakeratosis in both vertical and horizontal directions (checkerboard) or confluent hypergranulosis, thick suprapapillary plates, broad rete ridges, narrow dermal papillae, and sparse superficial perivascular infiltration, mostly of lymphocytes.

DERMOSCOPY

Papular lesions reveal a central keratin plug and round yellowish areas surrounded by linear and dotted vessels. White areas surrounded by brownish rim and brownish white globules can be seen in darker skin.

DIFFERENTIAL DIAGNOSIS

- *Psoriasis*—positive grattage test and Auspitz sign, and Munro's microabscess is seen.
- Erythrokeratodermas
- *Follicular ichthyosis*—hypogranulosis is seen on biopsy.
- *Lichen scrofulosorum*—epitheloid granulomas are seen, and Mantoux test is positive.
- Other follicular keratoses

COMPLICATIONS

Prolonged erythema results in peripheral edema and may precipitate high-output cardiac failure in the elderly.

TREATMENT

Topical emollients and mild keratolytics like 3% salicylic acid ointment or 20% urea may be beneficial. Topical steroids may decrease pruritus, scaling, and erythema. Topical pimecrolimus cream and calcipotriol may be beneficial when limited areas of the body are involved. Systemic drugs used include oral vitamin A (50,000 IU tid), isotretinoin (40 mg bid for adults and 1–2.2 mg/kg body weight per day for children), and etretinate (0.4 mg/kg/day). Clinical improvement with retinoids usually takes 4–6 weeks and sometimes many months. Phototherapy may exacerbate PRP, but narrow band ultraviolet B (UVB) has been reported to be effective. Phototherapy may be combined with acitretin. Methotrexate may also improve the condition in 6 weeks. For resistant cases, cyclosporine, azathioprine, etanercept, and infliximab can be used.

SUGGESTED READING

1. Wang D, Chong VC, Chong WS, Oon HH. A Review on Pityriasis Rubra Pilaris. Am J Clin Dermatol. 2018;19(3):377-90.

195 Pityriasis Versicolor

➲ SYNONYMS

Dermatomycosis furfuracea, liver spots, tinea flava, chromophytosis.

➲ HISTORY

Malassezia species was isolated and characterized by Morris Gardi.

➲ ETIOLOGY

The causative organisms of pityriasis versicolor are the lipophilic yeasts of the *Malassezia* species: *Malassezia globosa*, *M. sympodialis*, *M. furfur*, *M. restricta*, *M. slooffiae*, *M. obtusa*, *M. pachydermatis*, *M. nana*, *M. japonica*, *M. dermatis*, *M. yamotoensis*, *M. caprae*, and *M. equina*.

➲ AGE GROUP

Pityriasis versicolor affects adolescent males.

➲ PATHOPHYSIOLOGY

Genetic predisposition, environmental conditions such as heat and humidity, immunodeficiency, and oily skin predisposed to the conversion of the yeast form of fungi into a pathogenic filamentous form.

➲ CLINICAL FEATURES

Pityriasis versicolor affects the trunk, neck, and/or arms and is uncommon on the other parts of the body. Hypopigmented or hyperpigmented macules/patches with bran-like/furfuraceous scales are seen **(Fig. 1)**. Pale patches may be more common in darker skin; this appearance is known as pityriasis versicolor alba and is less likely to itch. Sometimes, the patches start scaly and brown and then resolve through a nonscaly and white stage. A normal-colored/hypopigmented skin is visualized when scales are removed en masse as a sheet by scraping with a glass slide and scalpel/scotch-type stripping of palpable lesion; this is called coup d'ongle sign.

Stretching the skin of hypopigmented/hyperpigmented scaly macule/patch reveals fine scaling—Besnier sign/stroke of nail sign/cat scratch sign.

A yellow-green fluorescence may be observed on examination of affected areas with a Wood's lamp (long wave ultraviolet A).

Pityriasis versicolor is more common in hot, humid climates or in those who sweat heavily, so it may recur each summer. Pityriasis versicolor does not appear to predispose affected areas to sunburn even when it causes pale white marks.

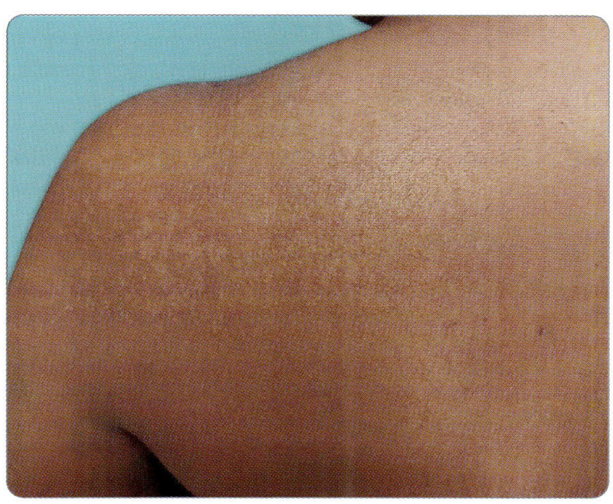

Fig. 1: Multiple, well-defined confluent, hypopigmented patches noted over the shoulder and back.

Hypopigmentation is due to tyrosinase inhibition by azelaic acid that is synthesized by the action of an enzyme present in *Malassezia* on unsaturated fatty acids in skin, the sun protective effect of the scale. Hyperpigmentation is due to the presence of giant melanosomes.

DIFFERENTIAL DIAGNOSIS

- *Vitiligo*—absence of scaling
- *Pityriasis alba*—usually seen only on the face
- *Secondary syphilis*—negative KOH mount
- *Pityriasis rosea*—herald patch is seen, and lesions have typical collarette of scales.
- *Seborrheic dermatitis*—greasy scales are seen.

DIAGNOSIS

- *10% KOH examination*—hyphae and spores are seen in spaghetti and meatball appearance (banana and grapes appearance).
- *Culture on SDA*—colonies are yeast-like, buff-colored on the surface, and reverse dome-shaped.
- Wood's lamp examination shows coppery orange fluorescence.

HISTOPATHOLOGY

Histopathology shows hyperkeratosis with basket weave stratum corneum and increased pigment in the basal layer. Spherical spores/ blastospores and short nonseptate hyphae of *Malassezia* are seen as blue elements in the outer two-thirds of the stratum corneum.

DERMOSCOPY

White structureless areas with faint brownish pigment network and indistinct borders having fine, white scales predominantly on skin creases, which become "double-edged" scales on stretching the skin, are characteristic dermoscopic findings.

TREATMENT

- *Localized lesion*—topical ketoconazole (2%), clotrimazole (1%), miconazole lotions, and selenium sulfide (2.5%)
- *Extensive lesion*—systemic therapy: fluconazole 400 mg single dose and second dose after 2 weeks or 50 mg once daily for 14 days. Other drugs include ketoconazole and itraconazole.

SUGGESTED READINGS

1. Karray M, McKinney WP. (2023). Tinea Versicolor. Treasure Island (FL): StatPearls Publishing. [online] Available from https://www.ncbi.nlm.nih.gov/books/NBK482500/ [Last accessed February, 2025].
2. Ankad BS, Mukherjee SS, Nikam BP. Dermoscopy - Histopathology Correlation: a conspectus in the skin of colour, 1st edition. Singapore: Springer Verlag; 2021.

196 Pityrosporum Folliculitis

➲ SYNONYM

Malassezia folliculitis.

➲ HISTORY

Pityrosporum folliculitis was described first by Weary et al. in 1969.

➲ ETIOLOGY

Pityrosporum folliculitis is caused by *Pityrosporum ovale*.

➲ AGE GROUP

Pityrosporum folliculitis usually affects adult males during the second and third decades of life.

➲ CLINICAL FEATURES

Lesions are associated with severe dandruff or seborrheic dermatitis, mildly pruritic. The lesions are erythematous follicular papules or pustules in the upper trunk, face **(Figs. 1A and B)**, and shoulders, which may be associated with itching. Presentation is very similar to that of acne vulgaris. More commonly seen in patients with acquired immunodeficiency syndrome (AIDS) or Down syndrome.

➲ HISTOPATHOLOGY

Pityrosporum ovale is found in the follicles, usually in the yeast form. A perifollicular mononuclear infiltrate is seen.

➲ DIFFERENTIAL DIAGNOSIS

Differential diagnosis is recalcitrant acne—does not reveal spores on KOH mount unlike pityrosporum folliculitis.

➲ TREATMENT

Treatment of any predisposing factor. Topical 2% ketoconazole or ciclopirox creams. Oral ketoconazole 200 mg daily for 7 days. Oral itraconazole may be required in recurrent cases.

➲ PROGNOSIS

Recurrence is common.

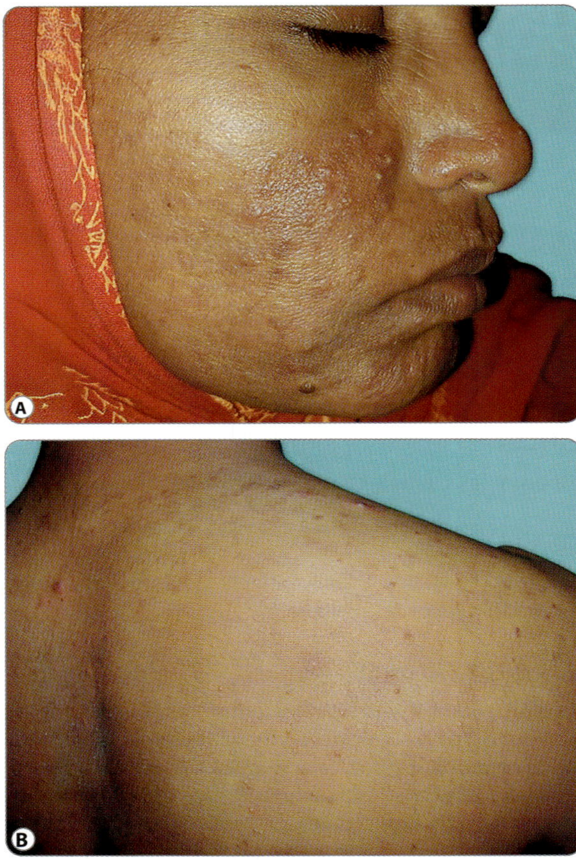

Figs. 1A and B: (A) Erythematous papules of pityrosporum folliculitis over the (A) face and (B) back.

➲ SUGGESTED READING

1. Green M, Feschuk AM, Kashetsky N, Maibach HI. Clinical characteristics and treatment outcomes of Pityrosporum folliculitis in immunocompetent patients. Arch Dermatol Res. 2023;315(6):1497-509.

197 Pityriasis Lichenoides Et Varioliformis Acuta

SYNONYM

Mucha–Habermann disease.

ETIOLOGY

The exact cause of pityriasis lichenoides et varioliformis acuta (PLEVA) is still not fully understood. Several hypotheses have been proposed to explain its origin, including an abnormal immune response to infections, an inflammatory reaction triggered by certain medications, and a lymphoproliferative disorder. PLEVA has been observed to develop after certain infections, such as the Epstein–Barr virus, human immunodeficiency virus (HIV), varicella–zoster virus, *Toxoplasma gondii*, group A *Streptococcus*, and herpes simplex virus type 2.

AGE GROUP

Children and young adults are affected. Males are affected more.

PATHOPHYSIOLOGY

Evidence suggests that in the skin lesions of individuals with PLEVA, there is a presence of deposited immunoglobulin M (IgM) and C3, as well as elevated levels of immune complexes in the bloodstream. These findings indicate the involvement of immune complex deposition or a hypersensitivity reaction in the development of PLEVA.

CLINICAL PRESENTATION

The rash in PLEVA typically emerges in clusters, resulting in a diverse range of lesion types. Initially, an edematous pink papule forms, which then develops central vesiculation and hemorrhagic necrosis **(Fig. 1)**. While new lesions may cause irritation or a burning sensation upon appearance, they often manifest without any noticeable symptoms. The eruption primarily affects the trunk, thighs, and upper arms, particularly the flexor areas, although it can also spread more widely. Additionally, erythematous or necrotic lesions may be present on the mucous membranes. The healing process of these lesions often leads to scarring, which can take on a varioliform appearance.

In some cases, there may be a progression from PLEVA to a condition known as febrile ulceronecrotic Mucha–Habermann disease (FUMHD). This progression occurs after a prior diagnosis of PLEVA. Constitutional symptoms such as fever, headache, malaise, and joint pain may precede or accompany the onset of the skin lesions.

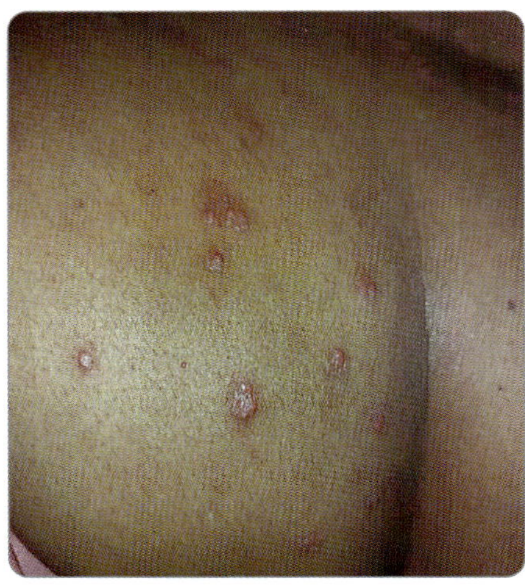

Fig. 1: Edematous pink papule of pityriasis lichenoides et varioliformis acuta (PLEVA) over the trunk.

HISTOPATHOLOGY

Histopathological examination of PLEVA reveals epidermal necrosis, hyperkeratosis, acanthosis, spongiosis, basal cell degeneration, dermal microhemorrhages, and extravasation of red blood cells and melanin. The dermis exhibits edema, lymphohistiocytic inflammatory infiltrate, lymphocyte and erythrocyte extravasation, subepidermal vesicles, and potential dermal sclerosis. Vascular changes include papillary dermal blood vessel dilation, engorgement, and endothelial proliferation.

DERMOSCOPY

Perifollicular amorphous brown area, rim of white scale and red dotted vessels at the periphery, and vessels around white structureless area—"targetoid" appearance.

DIFFERENTIAL DIAGNOSIS

Langerhans cell histiocytosis, Gianotti–Crost syndrome, disseminated herpes simplex virus, varicella–zoster virus, cutaneous small vessel vasculitis, arthropod bite, secondary syphilis, polymorphous light reaction, pityriasis lichenoides chronica, papular eczematous dermatitis, urticaria pigmentosa, and exanthematous drug eruption could be the differentials for PLEVA.

TREATMENT

Systemic antibiotics with anti-inflammatory properties such as doxycycline, minocycline, and azithromycin, as well as corticosteroids and phototherapy, are the first-line drugs. Antihistamines can be used for symptomatic relief.

In case of associated ulceration, local wound care should be advised.

➲ PROGNOSIS

Pityriasis lichenoides et varioliformis acuta has a benign course.

➲ SUGGESTED READINGS

1. Teklehaimanot F, Gade A, Rubenstein R. (2023). Pityriasis Lichenoides Et Varioliformis Acuta (PLEVA). Treasure Island (FL): StatPearls Publishing [online] Available from https://pubmed.ncbi.nlm.nih.gov/36256784/ [Last accessed February, 2025].
2. Ankad BS, Mukherjee SS, Nikam BP. Dermoscopy - Histopathology Correlation: a conspectus in the skin of colour. Springer; 2021.

198 Poikiloderma

➲ ETIOLOGY

Injury to cold, heat, ionizing radiation, exposure to photosensitizing chemicals, and inflammatory dermatoses such as lichen planus, dermatomyositis, lupus erythematosus, systemic sclerosis, and lymphomas are some causes of acquired poikiloderma. Poikiloderma of Civatte (PC) is mediated by photosensitizing chemicals in cosmetics. Defective gene repair and various gene involvements with X-linked and autosomal inheritance patterns are identified.

➲ CLINICAL FEATURES

Poikiloderma refers to the combination of reticulate telangiectasias, pigmentation, atrophy, and depigmentation, which are the primary characteristic features. Petechiae, papules, and mild desquamation are other cutaneous features. They are classified into congenital and acquired poikiloderma. Apart from skin involvement and nail dystrophy, variable photosensitivity can also be observed.

➲ ASSOCIATED SYNDROMES

Congenital poikilodermas include:

- Rothmund–Thomson syndrome
- Dyskeratosis congenital
- Mendes da Costa syndrome
- Hereditary sclerosing poikiloderma of Weary
- Weary–Kindler syndrome
- Kindler syndrome
- Diffuse and macular atrophic dermatosis
- Degos–Touraine syndrome
- Bloom syndrome

➲ POIKILODERMA OF CIVATTE

Poikiloderma of Civatte is a chronic dermatosis presenting with triad of atrophy, hypopigmentation/hyperpigmentation, telangiectasia on the central chest, sides of the neck, and the face in Fitzpatrick skin phototypes I and II. Most commonly, it affects females of menopausal age with low estrogen levels and genetic predisposition.

➲ DERMOSCOPY

Dotted/globular and linear irregular vessels ("spaghetti and meatballs" aspect), perifollicular whitish (spared) areas; additional findings included follicular keratotic plugs (25%), delicate reticular (25%), or structureless brownish areas (12.5%).

➲ HISTOPATHOLOGY

Nonspecific features such as thinning of basal and spinous layers, basal vacuolar degeneration, presence of melanophages in the papillary dermis, and dilatation of superficial blood vessels.

➲ TREATMENT

- No definitive cure
- Treat the underlying condition
- Strict photoprotection with sunscreen
- Depigmenting agents and LASERS have been tried in nonsyndromic cases with variable results.

➲ SUGGESTED READING

1. Rayinda T, van Steensel M, Danarti R. Inherited skin disorders presenting with poikiloderma. Int J Dermatol. 2021;60(11):1343-53.

199 Polyarteritis Nodosa

SYNONYMS

Panarteritis nodosa, periarteritis nodosa.

HISTORY

In 1866, Kussmaul and Maier first described "periarteritis nodosa." The name was revised to "polyarteritis nodosa" in 1903, when Ferrari recognized that the inflammatory process involved the full thickness of the blood vessel wall. A skin-limited form termed "cutaneous PAN" was recognized in 1931.

ETIOLOGY

Polyarteritis nodosa (PAN) has been associated with a number of infections and inflammatory diseases. Hepatitis B infection is thought to be an etiologic trigger in approximately 7% of patients with classic PAN. Cutaneous PAN has been associated with other infections, including streptococcal (especially in children), parvovirus B19, and human immunodeficiency virus (HIV). Inflammatory conditions associated with both classic and cutaneous PAN include inflammatory bowel disease, systemic lupus erythematosus (SLE), and familial Mediterranean fever. Hairy cell leukemia has also been observed in association with classic PAN. Loss of function mutation in CECR1 has also been linked to PAN.

AGE GROUP

Polyarteritis nodosa can occur at any age but typically affects middle-aged to older adults (40–60 years). Cutaneous PAN represents approximately 10% of all cases of PAN, and it is the most common form of PAN in children. It affects men more frequently than women.

CLINICAL FEATURES

Approximately 50% of patients with classic (systemic) PAN have cutaneous involvement. The most common findings are livedo reticularis and "punched-out" ulcers **(Figs. 1A and B)**. Extracutaneous disease is the rule in classic PAN, and patients often present with constitutional symptoms and multiple organ involvement. Common manifestations include abdominal pain, arthralgias, myalgias, mononeuritis multiplex, and congestive heart failure. Involvement of the kidneys occurs at the level of the interlobar renal arteries, resulting in renovascular hypertension and renal failure, but not glomerulonephritis.

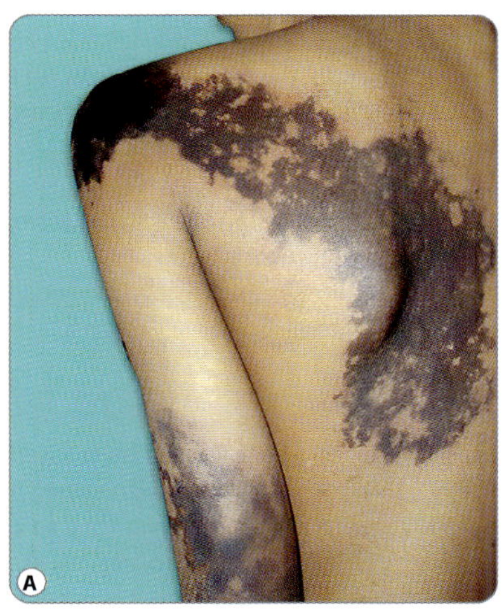

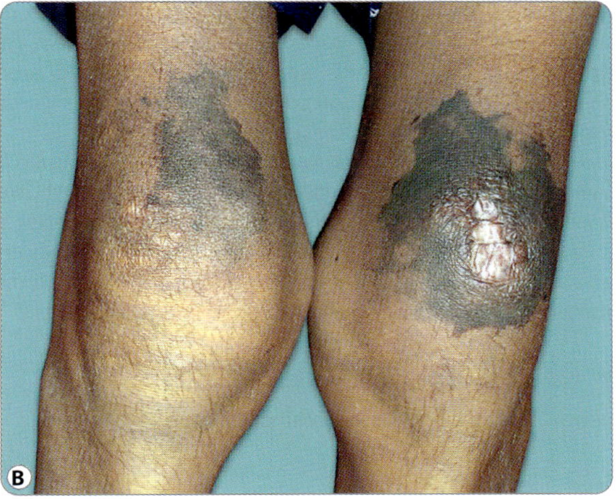

Figs. 1A and B: Polyarteritis nodosa.

Cutaneous PAN presents as painful subcutaneous nodules on the lower extremities, cutaneous necrosis, ulcers, and a starburst pattern of livedo reticularis. A chronic, relapsing clinical course is typical.

➲ HISTOPATHOLOGY

The histopathology of PAN is characterized by a segmental necrotizing vasculitis of medium-sized arteries and fibrinoid necrosis. Focal areas of involvement result in vessel wall weakening and necrosis, leading to aneurysmal dilation and/or stenosis. Direct immunofluorescence (DIF) may show deposits of C3, immunoglobulin M (IgM), and fibrin within vessel walls or perivascularly. The "gold standard" for the diagnosis of PAN is the demonstration of focal, segmental panmural necrotizing inflammation of medium-sized or small arteries with a predilection for bifurcations and branch points.

DIFFERENTIAL DIAGNOSIS

- *Cryoglobulinemic vasculitis*—raised cryoglobulin levels are seen.
- *Autoimmune connective tissue disease*—antinuclear antibody (ANA) profile diagnostic
- Microscopic polyangiitis
- *Wegener's granulomatosis*—granulomatous lesions are seen in the upper and lower respiratory tracts.
- *Churg–Strauss syndrome*—nasal polyps, eosinophilia, and asthma may be associated.

TREATMENT

Patients with idiopathic classic PAN should be treated with systemic corticosteroids (e.g., 1 mg/kg/day of prednisone), with the dose tapered over the course of 6 months. Refractory to corticosteroids, cyclophosphamide (0.5–1.0 g/m^2/month intravenously or 2 mg/kg/day orally) should be added to their regimen for up to 6–12 months. Hepatitis B virus (HBV)-associated PAN is treated with antivirals, interferon 2α, and, recently, lamivudine is used. Topical or intralesional corticosteroids are given for localized areas of cutaneous involvement, but oral corticosteroids may be warranted for progressive or extensive disease.

Successful therapies include intravenous immunoglobulin (IVIg), sulfapyridine (associated Crohn's disease), low-dose methotrexate (7.5–15 mg/week), and pentoxifylline (400 mg orally three times daily). Patients with evidence of a streptococcal infection should be treated with penicillin. Digital necrosis has been reported to improve with intravenous prostaglandins or calcium channel blockers.

PROGNOSIS

Cutaneous PAN follows a benign clinical course.

SUGGESTED READING

1. De Virgilio A, Greco A, Magliulo G, Gallo A, Ruoppolo G, Conte M, et al. Polyarteritis nodosa: A contemporary overview. Autoimmun Rev. 2016;15(6):564-70.

200 Polymorphic Light Eruption

➲ HISTORY

Polymorphic light eruption (PLE) was initially described in the 19th century as eczema solare by Bateman.

➲ ETIOLOGY

Polymorphic light eruption is caused by repeated exposure to ultraviolet (UV) radiation. Both UVA and UVB can induce the lesions.

➲ AGE GROUP

Polymorphic light eruption is most frequent in women <30 years of age. Up to 50% of patients have a positive family history.

➲ CLINICAL FEATURES

Polymorphic light eruption is characterized by a polymorphic eruption ranging from papulovesicular lesions to large plaques, localized predominantly in a photoexposed distribution **(Figs. 1A and B)**. In the same patient, however, the lesions are monomorphic. Lesions develop more commonly in early summer and gradually improve as summer progresses because of a "hardening effect." Typical sites affected are the bridge of the nose, cheeks, and chin; the back; the sides; the "V" area of the neck; the dorsal aspect of the hands; the dorsolateral aspect of the arms; and, sometimes, the dorsal aspect of the feet. Clinical variants include photosensitive lichenoid eruption and juvenile spring eruption.

➲ HISTOPATHOLOGY

Polymorphic light eruption is characterized by dense perivascular T-cell infiltrate in the upper and mid-dermis. Immunohistochemistry shows an increase in Langerhans cells (OKT6) in the epidermis.

➲ DERMOSCOPY

Ring scales—white-colored circular scales that are continuous, arranged in a ring-shaped manner with central clearing against an ochre to light brown background—are observed.

➲ COMPLICATIONS

Complications can be eczematization and lichenification.

➲ DIFFERENTIAL DIAGNOSIS

Differential diagnosis includes lupus erythematosus, hydroa vacciniforme, actinic prurigo, solar urticaria, chronic actinic dermatitis, actinic reticuloid, contact dermatitis, atopic dermatitis,

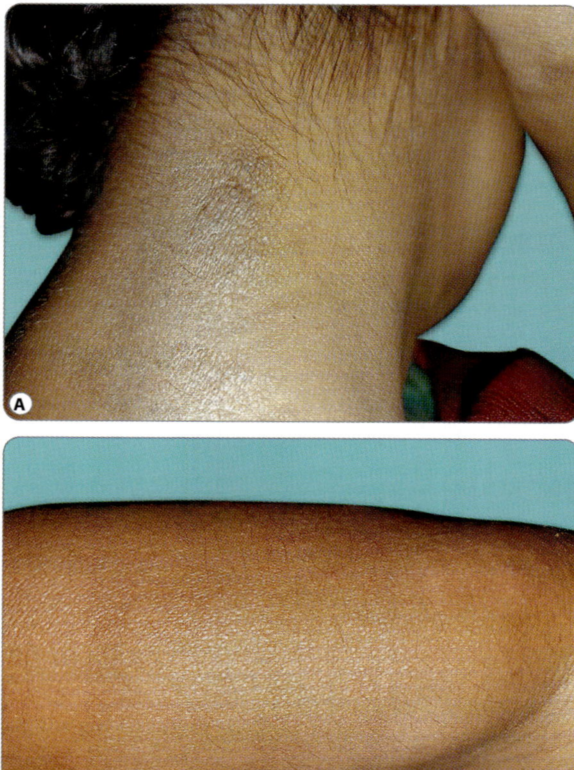

Figs. 1A and B: Multiple papules of polymorphic light eruption (PLE) noted over the posterior aspect of the neck and the extensor aspect of the forearm.

reticular erythematous mucinosis, and genetic and metabolic diseases (xeroderma pigmentosum, porphyrias, pellagra, and Hartnup disease).

➲ TREATMENT

Prophylactic photoprotection is necessary and includes advice regarding the avoidance of the sun and the use of broad-spectrum sunscreens and appropriate clothing. Prophylactic low-dose narrowband UVB or psoralen and UVA (PUVA) therapy is helpful in preventing recurrences. In mild cases, topical steroids and gradually increasing doses of UVB or PUVA may be adequate. In moderate to severe cases, hydroxychloroquine and omega-3 fatty acids have been found useful. Oral steroids, azathioprine, cyclosporine, and thalidomide are useful in severe unremitting PLE.

➲ SUGGESTED READINGS

1. Guarrera M. Polymorphous Light Eruption. Adv Exp Med Biol. 2017;996:61-70.
2. Malakar S, Mehta P. Ring Scales: A New Dermoscopic Sign in Polymorphous Light Eruption. Int J Dermoscop. 2017;1(2):62-4.

201 Pompholyx

➲ SYNONYM

Dyshidrotic eczema.

➲ ETIOLOGY

Contact allergens like nickel sulfate, potassium dichromate, phenylene diamine, nitrofurazone, fragrance mix, cobalt chloride, aspirin, and oral contraceptives have been implicated.

➲ AGE GROUP

Pompholyx is commonly seen in adolescents and young adults <40 years.

➲ CLINICAL FEATURES

Pompholyx constitutes 5–20% of all hand eczema cases, occurs often in the spring, and is also associated with stress. There are two clinical types: Podopompholyx (soles) and cheiropompholyx (palms). They present with vesicles on the palms and soles, which are deep-seated and itchy. On examination, they look like sago grains. Blisters may coalesce, desiccate, and resolve without rupture with desquamation. Lesions are self-limited over 2–3 weeks but may recur. Rubbing and inappropriate treatment cause spread to the volar surface. Nails can become dystrophic.

➲ HISTOPATHOLOGY

Epidermis is spongiotic with intraepidermal vesicles; there is infiltration of epidermis by lymphocytes. Sweat ducts are pushed aside by tense vesicles or passed between them.

➲ DIFFERENTIAL DIAGNOSIS

- *Contact dermatitis*—other areas are involved (the dorsae of the hands and feet).
- *Pustular psoriasis*—previous history of (H/o) psoriasis lesions
- *Inflammatory tinea*—demonstration of fungal hyphae
- *Id reaction*—primary source of infection/inflammation is seen.
- *Bullous pemphigoid*—subepidermal blister is seen; positive direct immunofluorescence (DIF) findings

➲ COMPLICATIONS

Secondary bacterial infection, if not treated, leads to cellulitis and lymphangitis.

➲ TREATMENT

Severe cases can be treated with soaks and compresses of potassium permanganate 1:8,000 dilution or a solution of aluminum subacetate, 1% Burow's solution. Calamine lotion, zinc cream, topical corticosteroids, coal tar preparations, topical tacrolimus 0.1% ointment, and systemic steroids in severe cases can be used. Local photochemotherapy [psoralen and ultraviolet A (PUVA)], intradermal botulinum toxin, azathioprine, and methotrexate are also effective. Alitretinoin (9-cis-retinoic acid) is a retinoid for systemic use. Radiotherapy might be an option for refractory cases. Atopic cheiropompholyx can be treated with subcutaneous injections of the tumor necrosis factor-α inhibitor etanercept 25 mg twice weekly.

It has a prolonged and relapsing course.

➲ SUGGESTED READING

1. Wollina U. Pompholyx: a review of clinical features, differential diagnosis, and management. Am J Clin Dermatol. 2010;11(5):305-14.

202 Porokeratosis

➲ ETIOLOGY

In porokeratosis, there is clonal proliferation of atypical keratinocytes with abnormal differentiation leading to the formation of the cornoid lamella. This expands peripherally and forms the raised boundary between abnormal and normal keratinocytes. Risk factors for the development of porokeratosis are genetic inheritance, ultraviolet radiation, and immunosuppression.

➲ AGE AND SEX

Porokeratosis palmaris et plantaris (PPP) and linear porokeratosis may be seen at any age, from birth to adulthood. Porokeratosis of Mibelli (PM) usually develops in childhood. Disseminated superficial porokeratosis (DSP) develops in the third or fourth decade of life. PM and PPP affect men twice as often as women. Disseminated superficial actinic porokeratosis (DSAP) is twice as likely to develop in women compared to men.

➲ CLINICAL FEATURES

The following types of porokeratosis have been described:

- *Disseminated superficial actinic porokeratosis* is the most common type, with multiple lesions predominantly in sun-exposed sites. The lesions are asymptomatic annular macules with raised thread-like peripheral ridges, developing predominantly on the distal extensor surfaces of the legs and the arms. Palms and soles are spared. Facial lesions are seen in approximately 15% of patients. Family history is usually present, and there is no known risk of malignant transformation.
- *Disseminated superficial porokeratosis (nonactinic):* Lesions are very similar to DSAP, except in a generalized distribution.
- *Disseminated superficial porokeratosis of immunosuppression* is recognized after renal, hepatic, cardiac, and bone marrow transplantation and in acquired immunodeficiency syndrome (AIDS). The distribution is similar to DSAP.
- *Disseminated superficial porokeratosis of childhood* may be inherited as an autosomal dominant condition. Palmoplantar lesions may be associated.
- *Porokeratosis of Mibelli/classic/plaque type of porokeratosis:* It is the second most common type of porokeratosis. Single or few larger annular dry plaques surrounded by a raised, fine keratotic wall with a thin furrow in the center of the ridge, causing a "Great Wall of China effect," is seen **(Fig. 1)**. Lesions are most common on the limbs, and by centrifugal spread, they may achieve several centimeters in diameter. The center is usually atrophic **(Fig. 2)**

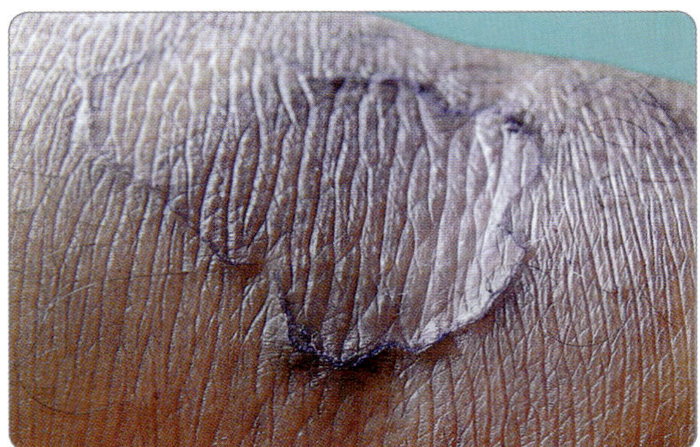

Fig. 1: Porokeratosis of Mibelli. Note the groove in the margins—the Great wall of China effect.

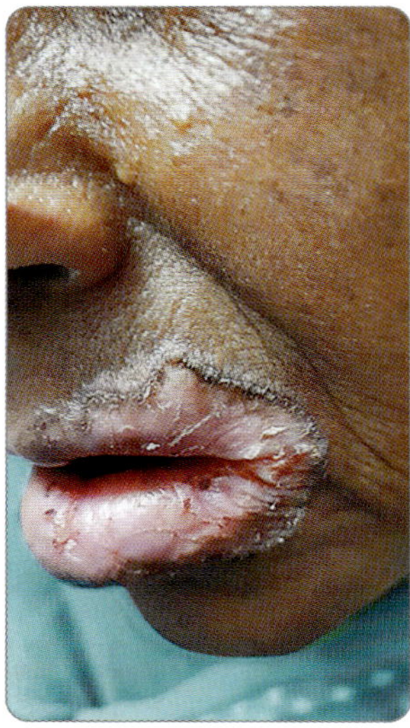

Fig. 2: Porokeratosis over the perioral area.

but may be hyperkeratotic. Autosomal dominant inheritance has been reported.

- *Giant porokeratoses:* These are very rare and are most often found on the foot. Large lesions are said to have the highest malignant potential. The lesions may extend up to 20 cm in diameter with a surrounding wall of 1 cm.
- *Palmoplantar porokeratosis (of Mantoux)/PPP:* The lesions are small, superficial, and relatively uniform, with a slightly hyperpigmented, atrophic center, and a minimally raised peripheral ridge is present since childhood.
- *Linear porokeratosis* following the lines of Blaschko **(Fig. 3)** usually appears in childhood. Malignant degeneration and metastasis have been reported.
- *Punctate porokeratosis:* It presents as multiple, asymptomatic, tiny, hyperkeratotic papules with thin, raised margins developing on the palms and the soles during adulthood.

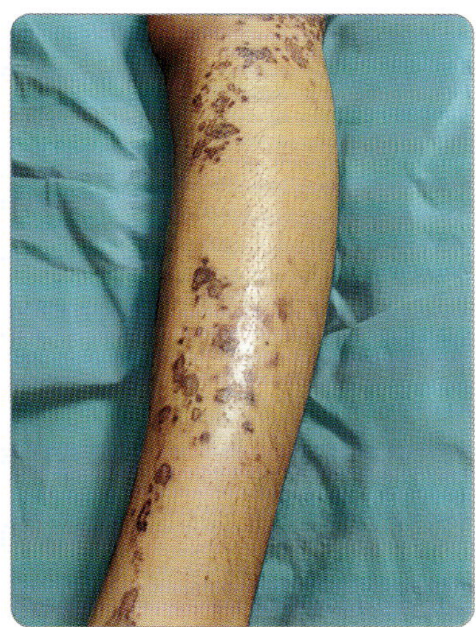

Fig. 3: Linear porokeratosis.

- *Porokeratosis ptychotropica*: It is a verrucous variant localized to the buttocks.
- Hypertrophic type of DSAP
- Porokeratoma/Porokeratotic acanthoma
- Bullous and pruritic variants of DSP
- *Porokeratotic adnexal ostial nevus (PAON)*—incorporate porokeratotic eccrine ostial and dermal duct nevus (PEODDN) and porokeratotic eccrine and hair follicle nevus (PEHFN)
- Pruritic papular porokeratosis

HISTOPATHOLOGY

Biopsy should be taken from the edge of the lesion. Parakeratotic stratum corneum (cornoid lamella) is seen running through the surrounding normal-staining cells. Other features include spongiosis, dermal lymphocytic infiltrate under the lamella, and lichenoid reaction pattern. The central area of a lesion is usually atrophic but may occasionally show hyperkeratosis.

DERMOSCOPY

The keratin rim is the dermoscopic hallmark of porokeratosis. Pigmentation or erosions along the keratin rim, vascular structures, as well as scales, pigmentation, or shiny white structures within the keratin rim are additional dermoscopic clues.

DIFFERENTIAL DIAGNOSES

- *Linear verrucous epidermal nevus*—nevus cells are seen.
- *Psoriasis*—scaling is present, and Munro's microabscess is seen.
- *Discoid lupus erythematosus*—positive carpet tack sign and follicular plugging are present.
- Actinic keratosis
- *Cornoid lamella*—viral warts, ichthyosis, and nevoid hyperkeratoses

➲ COMPLICATIONS

Malignancies, typically squamous cell carcinomas, may develop within lesions of porokeratosis. Giant and linear porokeratosis show maximum malignant potential.

➲ TREATMENT

Treatment of disseminated superficial porokeratoses is usually unnecessary, but topical tacalcitol, 5-fluorouracil ointment, imiquimod cream, etretinate, cryotherapy, carbon dioxide, pulsed dye laser therapy, and photodynamic treatment can be tried. Topical steroids and topical diclofenac may provide symptomatic relief even if no lasting benefit occurs. In a small study, topical lovastatin was used to improve porokeratosis symptoms. Excision is most appropriate when malignant degeneration develops.

➲ PROGNOSIS

Patients with immunosuppression and giant and linear porokeratosis should be monitored for the development of malignancy.

➲ SUGGESTED READING

1. Williams GM, Dreyer MA, Fillman EP. (2023). Porokeratosis. Treasure Island (FL): StatPearls Publishing. [online] Available from https://pubmed.ncbi.nlm.nih.gov/30335323/ [Last accessed February, 2025].

203 Porphyrias

INTRODUCTION

Porphyrias are a group of disorders caused by defects in the biosynthesis of heme, resulting in the accumulation of porphyrins, which are phototoxic.

CLASSIFICATION (TABLE 1)

- *Cutaneous disease only*:
  - Porphyria cutanea tarda (PCT)
  - Congenital erythropoietic porphyria (CEP)
  - Erythropoietic protoporphyria (EPP)
- *Cutaneous disease and acute attacks*:
  - Hereditary coproporphyria (HC)
  - Variegate porphyria (VP)
- *Acute attacks only*: Acute intermittent porphyria (AIP)

HISTOPATHOLOGY

In all cutaneous porphyrias, homogenous material is deposited within the vessel walls of the upper dermal capillaries. It is periodic acid–Schiff (PAS)-positive and diastase-resistant. Bullae in porphyrias are subepidermal with the split occurring in the lamina lucida, leaving the dermal papilla protruding into the blister cavity, an appearance called festooning. There is little or no inflammatory infiltrate.

Table 1: Classification and clinical features of porphyria.

Disease	*Enzyme-deficient*	*Clinical features*	*Investigations*	*Treatment*
Congenital erythropoietic porphyria (Gunther disease)	Autosomal recessive uroporphyrinogen III cosynthase enzyme	Hydrops fetalis, pink/brown staining of nappies, severe photosensitivity, mutilating scarring of the face **(Fig. 1)** and hands, hypertrichosis, erosion of terminal phalanges, sclerodactyly-like changes **(Fig. 2)**, keratoconjunctivitis, cataract, corneal ulcers, teeth stained brown, decreased bone density, hemolytic anemia, and pink to burgundy red teeth **(Fig. 3)** on Wood's lamp	• U—uroporphyrin I-E—coproporphyrin I-E • F—coproporphyrin I-E • R—uroporphyrin I-E coproporphyrin I-E • Zinc and free protoporphyrin—E • P—615–620 nm	Photoprotection, β-carotene, hypertransfusion, hydroxyurea, splenectomy, intravenous hematin, allogenic bone marrow transplantation
Porphyria cutanea tarda (PCT)	• Uroporphyrinogen decarboxylase (UROD) • Type I—acquired deficiency restricted to hepatocytes • Type II—familial, all tissues of the body • Type III—hereditary deficiency localized to the liver • Type IV—toxic porphyria halogenated aromatic hydrocarbons inhibit UROD enzyme	Increased fragility on light-exposed skin, crust, and resolve over few weeks, leaving atrophic scars, milia, mottled hypo/hyperpigmentation, scarring alopecia, hypertrichosis, photo-induced onycholysis, and morphea-like plaques	• U—uroporphyrin III • E—heptacarboxyporphyrin • F—heptacarboxyporphyrin • P—615–620 nm	Photo protection, venesection, desferrioxamine, chloroquine 125–250 mg taken twice a week, and erythropoietin

Continued

Continued

Disease	***Enzyme-deficient***	***Clinical features***	***Investigations***	***Treatment***
Erythropoietic protoporphyria	Ferrochelatase	Presents at 3–5 years, immediate pain on exposure to bright sunlight, and the only physical sign is edema of the dorsae of the hands and face. Erythema is less common. Waxy scarring on the nose, small scar over the cheeks and forehead, mild hypochromic, and microcytic anemia	• U—N • F—protoporphyrin • P—633 nm • R—free protoporphyrin	Photo protection, oral β-carotene (180 mg OD), psoralens and PUVA, narrowband UVB afamelanotide, and an alpha-melanocyte-stimulating hormone (α-MSH) analog improve skin photosensitivity
Acute intermittent porphyria	PBG deaminase. Precipitated by drugs—barbiturates and estrogens, progesterones, sulfonamides, methyldopa, danazol, diazepam, phenytoin, carbamazepine, smoking, and alcohol	Acute attacks are five times more common in females, severe abdominal pain, vomiting, and constipation due to partial ileus, dehydration, hyponatremia, tachycardia, hypertension, motor neuropathy, confusion, abnormal behavior, hallucinations, and agitations	Urinary PBG excretion is elevated	Early diagnosis, avoidance of precipitating factors, and supportive treatment

Continued

Continued

Disease	*Enzyme-deficient*	*Clinical features*	*Investigations*	*Treatment*
Variegate porphyria (VP)	Autosomal dominant protoporphyrinogen oxidase	Begins in adolescence and young adulthood. Skin fragility in sun-exposed skin, painful tense bullae, scarring, pigmentary abnormalities, mild hypertrichosis, and photo-onycholysis; 17% suffer from acute attacks	• U—coproporphyrin III • F—protoporphyrin Coproporphyrin • P—626 nm	Photo protection, avoidance of precipitating factors, β-carotene, canthaxanthin, narrow band UVB, glucose loading, and hematin infusions
Hereditary coproporphyria	Autosomal dominant coproporphyrinogen oxidase	• Fragility and blistering of sun-exposed areas, i.e., indistinguishable from PCT or VP • Skin disease may be exacerbated by intercurrent liver disease	• U—coproporphyrin III • ALA and PBG • F—coproporphyrin III • P—615–620 nm	Avoidance of inducing drugs, glucose loading, and hematin infusions may be helpful

(ALA: aminolevulinic acid; E: elevated; F: feces; P: peak at plasma spectrofluorometry; PBG: porphobilinogen; PUVA: psoralen and ultraviolet A; R: red blood cell; U: urine; UVB: ultraviolet B)

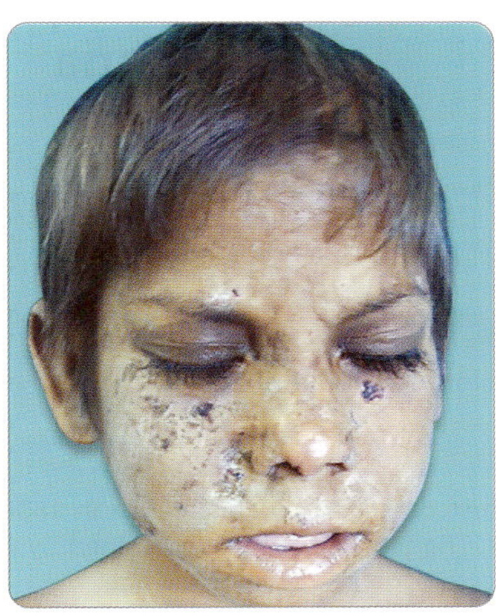

Fig. 1: Congenital erythropoetic porphyria. Scarring and cruts seen over the face.

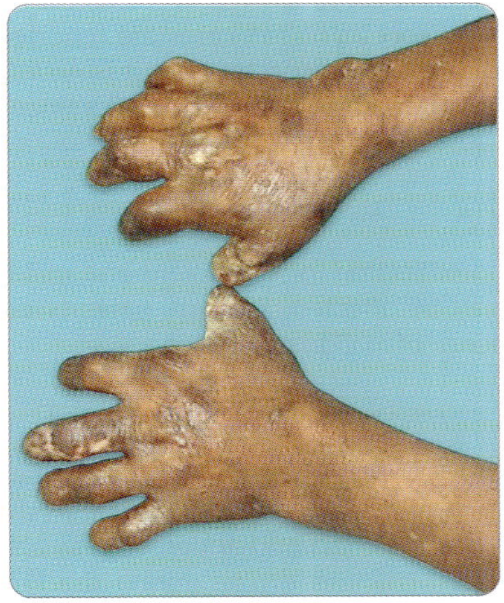

Fig. 2: Sclerodactyly and shortening of fingers.

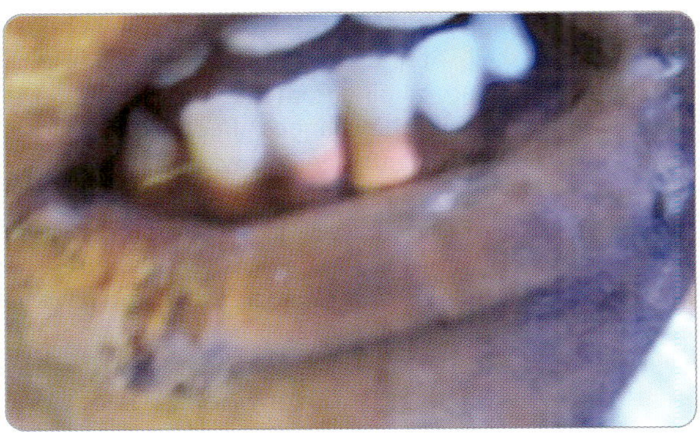

Fig. 3: Pink fluorescence in the teeth on Wood's lamp examination.

➲ SUGGESTED READING

1. Dawe R. An overview of the cutaneous porphyrias. F1000Res. 2017;6:1906.

204 Progeria

SYNONYM

Hutchinson–Gilford syndrome.

HISTORY

Progeria was first described by Hutchinson in 1886 and then by Gilford in 1897. The term "progeria" was coined by Gilford in 1904 from the Greek word "geras," meaning old age.

ETIOLOGY

The incidence is thought to be 1 in 8 million, but it is probably closer to 1 in 4 million, as not all cases are reported. Originally, a recessive inheritance was suspected, but it is now known to be a single nucleotide mutation with autosomal dominant expression in approximately 90% of patients.

AGE GROUP

Progeria has a predilection for Caucasians and males, but all races and females may be affected. Progeria patients do not have an increased incidence of malignancy.

CLINICAL FEATURES

Clinical features are not present at birth. The cutaneous features include midfacial cyanosis, and sclerodermoid changes usually affect the legs, but the chest and abdomen may also be involved. Other typical facial changes evolve during the first 2 years and include frontal bossing, progressive prominence of superficial veins, especially of the scalp, a glyphic (chiselled) nose, thin lips, and micrognathia. Loss of subcutaneous fat enhances the appearance of the veins of the scalp, and a chipmunk appearance results. Hair loss is a consistent finding, ranging from the presence of thin, sparse gray hairs to total alopecia. The changes affect both the scalp and eyebrows. Fingertip tufting and sleeping with open eyes are also often seen.

Patients may have wide-based gait, osteoporosis, and hip dislocation. Affected individuals have short stature, normal intelligence, lack secondary sexual characteristics, and have a high-pitched voice.

Severe cardiovascular disease with atherosclerosis and hypertension results in death from myocardial infarction or a cerebrovascular accident. Death usually occurs in the second decade, but survival into the 20s has occasionally been reported.

➲ TREATMENT AND PROGNOSIS

The prognosis is dismal, and the management is currently supportive and symptomatic. Treatment of atherosclerosis, hypertension, diabetes, and other diseases is achieved through the standard conventional monitoring and medical therapy, but the disorder will continue to progress. It has been reported that bosentan, which is an endothelin receptor antagonist, can be used to treat severe cutaneous ulcers. Sodium etidronate can help improve symptomatic calcifications in the soft tissue.

➲ SUGGESTED READING

1. Sickles CK, Gross GP. (2022). Progeria. Treasure Island (FL): StatPearls Publishing. [online] Available from https://pubmed.ncbi.nlm.nih.gov/29939574/ [Last accessed February, 2025].

205 Prurigo

HISTORY

The term was originally introduced in the 19th century by Hebra to denote papules induced by scratching. Prurigo nodularis was first described by Hyde in 1909. Prurigo gestationis was first described by Besnier in 1904.

ETIOLOGY

Insect bites, stress, atopy, summer, pregnancy, malignancy, hepatitis C virus infection, gluten diet, and few cases may be idiopathic.

CLINICAL FEATURES

Itchy skin eruptions that are dome-shaped with a small transient vesicle on top, followed by crusting or lichenification **(Fig. 1)**.

TYPES

Types of prurigo include simple acute prurigo, subacute prurigo, chronic prurigo, dermographic prurigo, prurigo pigmentosa, Besnier's prurigo, Hebra's prurigo, Hutchinson's summer prurigo, prurigo gestationis, tick bite prurigo, prurigo-like lesions in human immunodeficiency virus (HIV) infection.

ASSOCIATED SYNDROME

Gluten enteropathy.

HISTOPATHOLOGY

Prurigo nodularis shows marked acanthosis with long, thickened rete ridges and round cell infiltration in the dermis. Prurigo pigmentosa

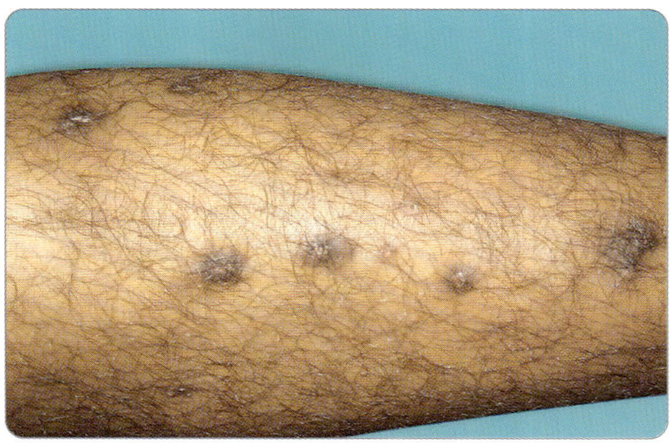

Fig. 1: Linear hyperkeratotic lesions over the shin in prurigo simplex.

shows epidermal spongiosis, liquefaction degeneration of the basal layer, and perivascular round cell collection.

DERMOSCOPY

Dermoscopy of prurigo nodularis shows "white starburst pattern" surrounding brown-reddish/brown-yellowish crust, erosion, and/or hyperkeratosis/scales.

DIFFERENTIAL DIAGNOSIS

Differential diagnosis includes atopic eczema and insect bites reaction.

COMPLICATIONS

Complications can be lichenification, postinflammatory hyperpigmentation, and scarring.

TREATMENT

Treatment includes oral antihistamines, topical steroids, dapsone, minocycline, isotretinoin, thalidomide, metronidazole, intralesional steroids, cryotherapy, bath psoralen and ultraviolet A (PUVA), azathioprine, and cyclosporine.

Tofacitinib, a JAK1, 3 inhibitor, would inhibit T helper 2 (Th2) and Th17 expression and specifically inhibit the signaling of interleukin 4 (IL-4) (JAK1, JAK3, and STAT6) and IL-31 (JAK1, STAT3, and STAT5), making it a justifiable and cost-effective treatment option in prurigo nodularis.

PROGNOSIS

Prurigo nodularis runs a protracted course.

SUGGESTED READING

1. Sardana K, Mathachan SR, Agrawal D. Treatment of recalcitrant paediatric prurigo nodularis with tofacitinib, an exquisite example of bench-to-bedside translation of JAK-STAT expression. Indian J Dermatol Venereol Leprol. 2023;1-3.

Pruritic Urticarial Papules and Plaques of Pregnancy

➲ SYNONYMS

Polymorphic eruption of pregnancy, toxemic rash of pregnancy, toxic erythema of pregnancy, late-onset prurigo of pregnancy.

➲ AGE GROUP

Pruritic urticarial papules and plaques of pregnancy (PUPPP) typically occurs in primigravidae during the last trimester.

➲ ETIOLOGY

The exact cause is still unknown, although the condition has been correlated with or attributed to abnormal weight gain in the mother and the newborn and to multiple pregnancies. Familial cases have been reported.

➲ CLINICAL FEATURES

The initial lesions of PUPPP are small (<2 mm), erythematous papules on the abdomen, mostly in the later part of the last trimester. They are often located along the striae **(Fig. 1)**. They soon coalesce to form larger plaques, mostly periumbilical in location. Lesions are extremely pruritic and disturb the sleep of the patients, but excoriations are very uncommon. The lesions gradually spread to involve the buttocks and thighs and may occasionally involve the arms, forearms, and legs. The breasts and the areas above them are rarely affected, while the face is always spared. Rarely, target lesions may be seen. The erythematous papules, on closer look,

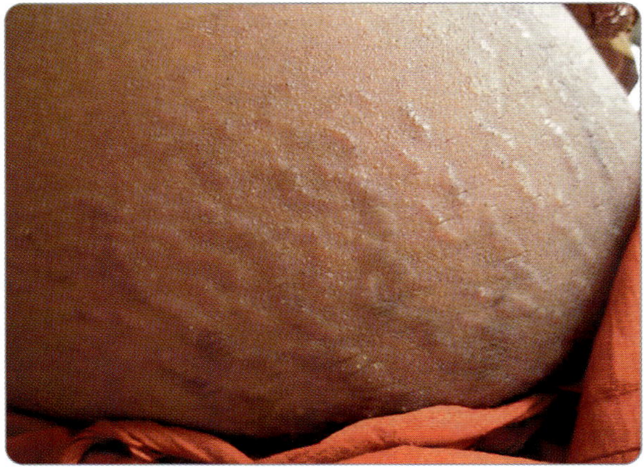

Fig. 1: Erythema and edema over the striae in pruritic urticarial papules and plaques of pregnancy (PUPPP).

reveal a narrow pale halo surrounding them. Primigravidae are most affected. Almost all cases have their onset after the 35th week. Postpartum onset is very uncommon.

➲ HISTOPATHOLOGY

The histopathology of the lesions varies with the clinical stage of the eruption. The early urticarial papule shows epidermal and dermal edema and a perivascular infiltrate consisting of lymphocytes, histiocytes, and occasionally eosinophils. The fully developed plaque has, in addition, spongiosis and rarely vesicle formation. Eosinophils are seen in about one-fourth of the biopsy samples. Healing lesions show only acanthosis and parakeratosis.

➲ DIFFERENTIAL DIAGNOSIS

- Cholestasis of pregnancy
- Prurigo of pregnancy
- Pruritic folliculitis of pregnancy

➲ TREATMENT

General measures, such as cool, soothing baths, frequent application of emollients, and light cotton clothing, offer additional symptomatic relief. Recently, intramuscular injection of autologous whole blood has been suggested as an alternative treatment option in the case of postpartum PUPPP. Topical corticosteroids are effective and provide symptomatic relief in all cases. Most women do not require topical corticosteroids near term. In severe cases, a brief tapering course of systemic corticosteroids provides relief. H1 antihistamines are not useful in controlling the pruritus.

➲ PROGNOSIS

The disease remits after delivery, generally within a few days. It is not associated with high maternofetal morbidity or mortality.

➲ SUGGESTED READING

1. Chouk C, Litaiem N. (2023). Pruritic Urticarial Papules and Plaques of Pregnancy. Treasure Island (FL): StatPearls Publishing. [online] Available from https://www.ncbi.nlm.nih.gov/books/NBK539700/ [Last accessed February, 2025].

207 Pseudofolliculitis Barbae

➲ SYNONYMS

Pili incarnati, ingrown hair, shaving bumps, barber's itch, folliculitis barbae, razor bumps.

➲ HISTORY

Pseudofolliculitis barbae was accurately described, and its pathogenesis delineated in 1956 by Strauss and Kligman.

➲ ETIOLOGY

Pseudofolliculitis barbae occurs mainly in men with curly hair, especially Blacks. The process of shaving tightly curled hair creates a residual point. This retracts under the skin and gets embedded or curls over and ingrows, thus producing a foreign body inflammatory reaction. Close shaving will worsen this condition, as the retracted tip may come out through the follicular wall rather than the actual follicular opening.

➲ CLINICAL FEATURES

They present as erythematous follicular papules and pustules. Mild cases are transient, but severe cases lead to scarring. Initially, the pustules are sterile, but later, secondary infection may occur. This condition is generally seen in men in the beard area, but any area that is frequently shaved can be affected. Similar condition occurring in the genital area is termed pseudofolliculitis pubis.

Pseudofolliculitis barbae can be divided into two types of ingrown hairs: Transfollicular (hair never exits the follicle) and extra-follicular (hair that has exited the follicle and re-entered the skin).

➲ DERMOSCOPY

Dermoscopy shows structureless pattern with a gray-blue, thick, curved line and adjacent red lines.

➲ COMPLICATION

Complication can be keloids.

➲ DIFFERENTIAL DIAGNOSIS

- *Acne vulgaris*—comedones are seen.
- *Bacterial folliculitis*—pustules show organisms on gram-stain.
- *Tinea barbae*—fungal elements are isolated.
- *Rosacea*—erythema, papulopustules, and telangiectasias are seen.

TREATMENT

- Treatment is mainly supportive and allows the hair to grow. Most lesions resolve if shaving is avoided for 3–4 weeks. If patients have to shave, a length of 0.5–1 mm should be left to prevent ingrowth of hair.
- Topical corticosteroids and retinoids can be used to reduce the inflammation.
- Secondary infection can be controlled with either oral or topical antibiotics.
- Topical application of glycolic acid lotion is an effective therapy for pseudofolliculitis barbae and allows the patient to resume a daily shaving regimen.
- A permanent solution can be obtained by laser hair reduction. This reduces the density of hair and makes hair fine and soft.

SUGGESTED READING

1. Perricone NV. Treatment of pseudofolliculitis barbae with topical glycolic acid: a report of two studies. Cutis. 1993;52(4):232-5.

208 Pseudoxanthoma Elasticum

➲ SYNONYMS

Darier–Grönblad–Strandberg syndrome, Grönblad–Strandberg–Touraine syndrome, Marchesani–Weill syndrome, Touraine syndrome I.

➲ HISTORY

In 1884, French dermatologist Felix Balzer described the skin manifestations.

➲ ETIOLOGY

Pseudoxanthoma elasticum (PXE) is an autosomal recessive multisystem disorder, exhibiting progressive calcification of elastic tissue. Clinically, the most significant changes occur in the skin, eye, and systemic vasculature (e.g., gastrointestinal and coronary vessels). It occurs due to mutation of *ABCC* gene, which encodes an ABC-cassette transporter.

➲ AGE AND SEX

Pseudoxanthoma elasticum appears to be more severe in female patients. The average age of diagnosis in patients with a positive family history is 8–12 years.

➲ CLINICAL FEATURES

Patients with PXE show marked clinical heterogeneity, with some patients displaying lesions of the skin, eye, and cardiovascular system, while others in the same family (presumably the same gene) show only the involvement of one system. Typically, the skin in PXE demonstrates yellowish, flat-topped discrete, and confluent papules in the skin creases of the sides and the nape of the neck, perineum, axillae, umbilicus, and flexural folds, with skin redundancy that increases with advancing age. These changes are often termed "plucked chicken skin," "cobblestone," or "Moroccan leather." Calcification of affected skin is common. Perforating periumbilical PXE has also been described. Infiltrative oral, anal, and vaginal mucosal lesions may also occur. The dermatologic features generally begin in the second decade but are often subtle and overlooked. More commonly, a visual or vascular complication, such as a gastrointestinal tract bleed, prompts the patient to seek medical care.

The most common ophthalmologic finding is the angioid streak (87% of patients).

- *Major criteria*:
  - Flexural yellow cobblestone lesions
  - Characteristic histological features of lesional skin, using elastic tissue and calcium stains (e.g., van Gieson and von Kossa)
  - Angioid streaks in the retina
- *Minor criteria*:
  - Characteristic histological changes in nonlesional skin
  - Family history of PXE in the first-degree relatives

COMPLICATIONS

Calcification of the degenerated elastic tissue of the internal lamina of blood vessels results in hypertension from resultant renal artery stenosis, and gastrointestinal bleeding may occur during adolescence. Late vascular sequelae in PXE include cerebrovascular accidents, intermittent claudication, and myocardial infarction. Severe coronary artery disease has been noted in adolescents with PXE; coronary artery bypass surgery may be ameliorative. Physical signs may include diminished peripheral pulses, hypertension, murmurs consistent with mitral valve prolapse and congestive heart failure, and peripheral gangrene. Rectovesical prolapse may also occur.

HISTOPATHOLOGY

The histologic changes on biopsy of lesional skin from patients with PXE are diagnostic, showing distinctive broken curls of basophilic elastic fibers, with routine hematoxylin and eosin or Verhoeff van Gieson staining. Calcium deposition on elastic fibers can be easily detected with von Kossa stain. Similar dystrophic fibers have been noted histologically as an incidental finding in inflammatory skin diseases in patients who do not have PXE. Soft tissue radiographs of the upper and lower extremities may reveal vessel wall calcification.

DERMOSCOPY

Multiple irregular yellowish areas alternating with multiple linear vessels. These yellowish plaques coalesced to form parallel strands.

DIFFERENTIAL DIAGNOSIS

Differential diagnosis includes actinic elastosis (mainly sun-exposed areas and less systemic features), late-onset focal dermal elastosis, elastoderm, perforating periumbilical calcific elastosis, PXE-like papillary dermal elastolysis, white fibrous papulosis of the neck, and cutis laxa.

➲ TREATMENT

There is no cure for this genetic alteration of elastic tissue. Plastic surgery may improve the appearance of sagging skin, although extrusion of calcium particles through the surgical wound may result in delayed healing and unsightly scars.

The suggested role of oxidative stress in PXE has prompted an ad hoc attempt at antioxidant therapy, with daily doses of tocopherol acetate and ascorbic acid.

➲ SUGGESTED READING

1. Germain DP. Pseudoxanthoma elasticum. Orphanet J Rare Dis. 2017;12(1):85.

209 Psoriasis

HISTORY

The term "lepra" was applied to various cutaneous disorders, including psoriasis, vitiligo, eczema, boils, and alopecia areata. The Roman sage Aurelius Cornelius Celsus gave the first clinical description of psoriasis. Galen used the term psoriasis, and Robert Willan (1808) specifically distinguished and described it as a recognizable entity.

AGE GROUP

Psoriasis can present at any age and can appear just after birth or in old age. There is a bimodal age of onset, the first peak at 15–20 years of age and a second one at 55–60 years.

ETIOLOGY

Hypotheses of psoriasis pathogenesis have changed over the decades, but its etiology is still not known. It is believed to be a multifactorial disease where both genetic and environmental factors act together. With the availability of monoclonal antibodies, the evidence suggests that psoriasis is a T-cell mediated autoimmune chronic inflammatory disease. Patients with psoriasis have an increased frequency of human leukocyte antigen (HLA)-B13, HLA-B17, and HLA-Bw16.

HISTOPATHOLOGY

The histopathological features of a fully developed psoriatic lesion are as follows:

- Parakeratosis, which is usually uniform.
- Presence of "microabscesses of Munro" in the horny layer. They consist of pyknotic nuclei of neutrophils that have migrated from the "squirting papillae" to the spongiform pustules and then to the horny layer.
- Absence of a granular layer
- Regular elongation of rete ridges. Their lower portion is thickened, sometimes showing a camel foot-like shape.
- Regular elongation of the dermal papillae that are clubbed at their upper portions. There are dilated and tortuous capillaries in the papillae, with edema and perivascular mononuclear cell infiltration. There is no papillomatosis in the strict sense of the word.
- There is thinning of the suprapapillary parts of the stratum malpighii, with the occasional presence of small spongiform pustules. In pustular psoriasis, these abscesses are large and prominent.

➲ CLASSIFICATION

Psoriasis can be clinically classified as follows:

- Guttate psoriasis
- Chronic plaque psoriasis
- Exfoliative psoriasis
- Pustular psoriasis
- Psoriasis unguis
- Mucus membrane psoriasis
- Arthropathic psoriasis
- *Regional variations in psoriasis*: Scalp, face, eyes, body flexures, scrotum, napkin area, palms, and soles

➲ CLINICAL FEATURES

The disease presents as chronic, symmetrical, erythematous, well-defined, dry, red, scaly papules, and plaques **(Fig. 1)**. The scales are abundant, loose, dry, and silvery white or micaceous. Whiteness is due to the presence of air trapped in between the layers of scales. On grattage, characteristic coherence of the scales can be seen as if one scratches a wax candle. When the scales are completely scraped off, the stratum mucosa (basement membrane) is exposed and is seen as a moist red surface (membrane of Bulkeley) through which dilated capillaries can be seen as red spots. On further scraping, these capillaries at the tips of elongated papillae are torn, leading to multiple bleeding points. Occasionally, a surrounding zone of hypopigmentation ("Woronoff's ring") is seen, usually associated with treatment due to the deficiency of prostaglandin E2 (PGE2). Another feature seen in psoriasis is the Koebner phenomenon. Nail changes include irregular pitting **(Fig. 2)** salmon patch and subungual hyperkeratosis.

➲ HISTOPATHOLOGY (FIG. 3)

- *Parakeratosis*: Retention of nuclei in the stratum corneum
- *Acanthosis*: Thickening of the epidermis

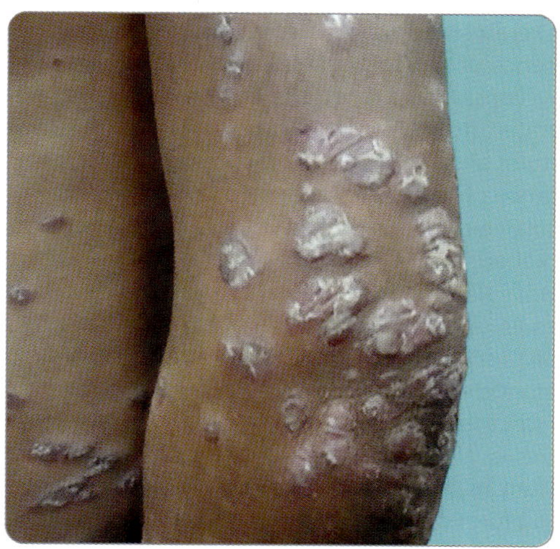

Fig. 1: Well-defined scaly plaques of chronic plaque psoriasis.

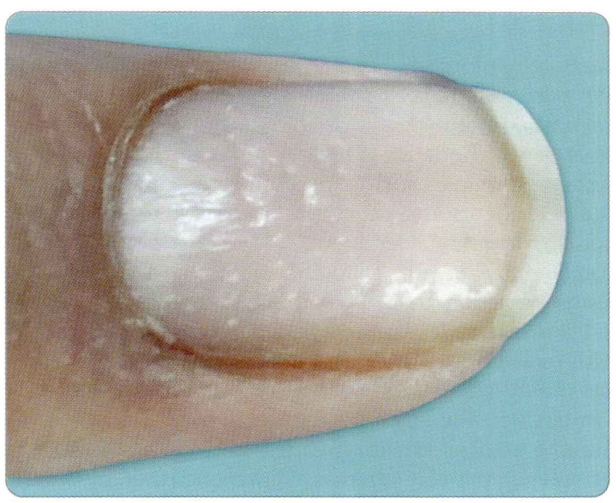

Fig. 2: Irregular pitting of nails in psoriasis.

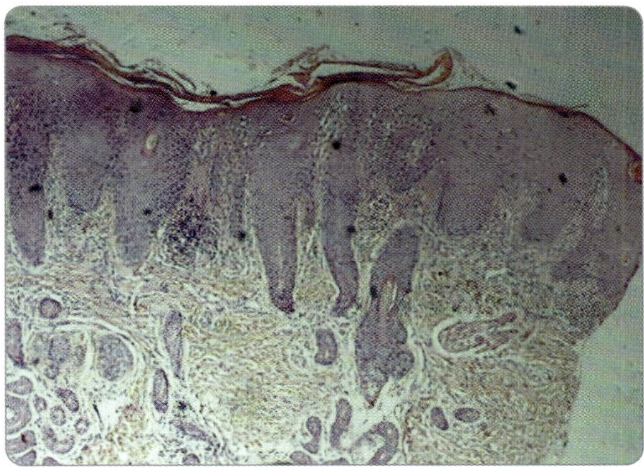

Fig. 3: Psoriasis—thin granular layer, moderate acanthosis, focal spongiosis, and elongated rete ridges.

- Absent or reduced granular layer
- Thinning of the suprapapillary plates
- Dilated blood vessels in the papillary dermis
- Perivascular inflammation of lymphocytes and neutrophils
- *Munro microabscesses*: Collections of neutrophils in the epidermis
- *Spongiform pustules*: Pockets of neutrophils in the epidermis

DERMOSCOPY

Dermoscopy shows regularly distributed dotted vessels in a reddish-pinkish background and white scales.

ASSOCIATED CONDITIONS

Associated conditions include atherosclerosis, cardiovascular morbidities, type 2 diabetes mellitus, and lymphoma.

➲ TREATMENT

Topical treatment for mild psoriasis includes the use of emollients, topical corticosteroids, calcipotriene, tazarotene, topical tars, anthralin, and keratolytics.

Treatment of moderate to severe psoriasis includes phototherapy and systemic therapies, such as methotrexate, acitretin, cyclosporine, and biologic agents. Treatment can be effected using combination, rotational, or sequential regimens.

- *Combination therapy:* Different agents have different mechanisms of action that allow them to be combined at lower individual dosages to provide synergistic or additive efficacy, with reduced toxicity or side effects. Once the psoriatic lesion has been effectively cleared or sufficiently reduced with combination therapy, one agent is typically removed (usually the one associated with greater safety risks or cost), and the second agent is continued as maintenance therapy.
- *Rotation therapy:* The main goal of rotational therapy is to minimize the risk of cumulative toxicity by switching from one therapy to another before the initial agent has a chance to build to potentially toxic levels.
- *Sequential therapy:* Sequencing specific therapies to maximize the rate of initial improvement, minimize long-term toxicity, and improve overall outcomes. Sequential therapy typically entails three phases:
    i. The clearing phase, which utilizes a rapidly acting therapy, often has greater side effects
    ii. The transitional phase, which once the patient shows improvement, introduces maintenance therapy while gradually tapering the initial therapy
    iii. The maintenance phase, consisting of treatment with the maintenance regimen alone for as long as needed

The systemic drugs commonly used for the treatment of psoriasis include oral retinoids (viz., acitretin) and antimetabolites (viz., methotrexate, mycophenolate mofetil, azathioprine, and hydroxyurea).

Apremilast, a phosphodiesterase-4 inhibitor, inhibits the hydrolyzation of the second messenger cAMP. This leads to the reduced expression of proinflammatory cytokines. It has anti-inflammatory effects on keratinocytes, fibroblasts, and endothelial cells.

➲ PROGNOSIS

Psoriasis vulgaris is usually a lifelong disease, with variable periods of spontaneous remissions (ranging from 1 year to decades) and exacerbations.

➲ SUGGESTED READING

1. Rendon A, Schäkel K. Psoriasis Pathogenesis and Treatment. Int J Mol Sci. 2019;20(6):1475.

210 Psoriatic Arthritis

➲ HISTORY

The association of arthritis with psoriasis was first formally described in 1818 by Alibert.

➲ ETIOLOGY

Psoriatic arthritis (PsA) is an inflammatory arthritis associated with psoriasis. Arthritis occurs in about 5–10% of patients with psoriasis. Like cutaneous psoriasis, PsA also is a genetically determined disorder. Human leukocyte antigen (HLA) studies reveal that the B27, DR3, A26, and B38 haplotypes are significantly associated with PsA. Environmental factors like trauma may precipitate arthritis.

➲ AGE GROUP

It occurs commonly between the ages of 30 and 55 years.

➲ MOLL AND WRIGHT CLASSIFICATION

- Classic type
- Rheumatoid arthritis (RA) type
- Arthritis mutilans
- Oligoarticular type
- Psoriatic spondylitis

➲ ASSOCIATED SYNDROMES

Associated syndromes include the SAPHO (synovitis, acne, pustulosis, hyperostosis, and osteomyelitis) syndrome, POPP (psoriatic onycho-pachydermo-periostitis) syndrome, ocular lesions like conjunctivitis, iritis, scleritis, and keratoconjunctivitis sicca, ulcerative colitis, Reiter's disease, Behçet's syndrome, myopathy, aortic incompetence, amyloidosis, and Crohn's disease.

➲ CLINICAL FEATURES

The classic form of arthritis involves the distal interphalangeal joints of the fingers and toes **(Fig. 1)**. In the acute stage, the involved joint is swollen and tender; the swelling often includes juxta-articular tissues, leading to the so-called "sausage" appearance of the affected fingers and toes. The nails of the affected fingers are usually involved. If there are >30 pits on the fingernail of a patient with chronic inflammatory arthritis, the diagnosis of PsA is confirmed.

Radiological features of PsA: The changes are asymmetric and oligoarticular in psoriasis. The peripheral joints as well as the spine may be involved. Important changes in the peripheral joints are

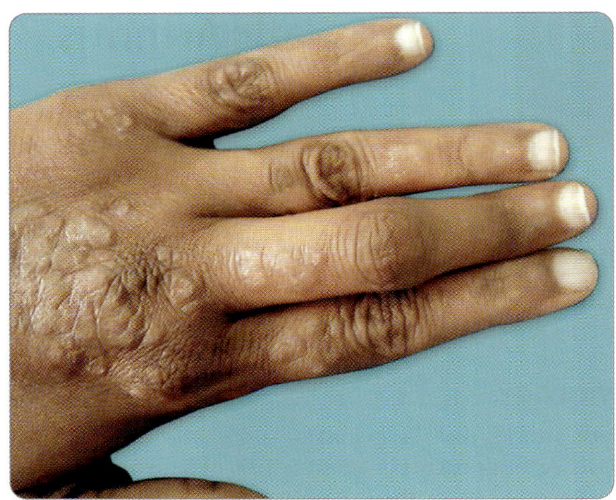

Fig. 1: Psoriatic arthritis.

osteolysis, which results in the whittling away of the phalanges, metacarpals, and metatarsals. Due to this, the phalanges show splaying of their bases, causing "fish-tail" deformity or, more commonly, "pencil-in-cup" deformity.

DIFFERENTIAL DIAGNOSIS

Differential diagnosis includes rheumatoid arthritis, ankylosing spondylitis, and Reiter's disease.

TREATMENT

Patients are managed with nonsteroidal anti-inflammatory drugs (NSAIDs) alone or in combination with the first-line disease-modifying antirheumatic drugs (DMARDs), sulfasalazine, or methotrexate, or both, depending on the severity. Local treatment involves the administration of local steroids into one or a few sites of enthesitis or synovitis. Other modes of treatment include cyclosporines, leflunomide, and tumor necrosis factor (TNF) alpha blockers.

- *Interleukin 17 inhibitors (IL-17i)*: These are useful for patients with moderate-severe active PsA with peripheral and axial joint disease and skin disease.
- *IL-12/23i and IL-23i*: These are useful for patients with moderate-severe active PsA with peripheral joint disease and skin disease; check the tuberculosis (TB) test before starting and check the complete blood count (CBC) and comprehensive metabolic panel (CMP) every 3–4 months.
- *T-cell costimulatory inhibitors*: These are useful for patients with mild-moderate PsA with peripheral joint disease, minimally effective for psoriasis, check TB test before starting, and check CBC and CMP every 3–4 months.
- *Abatacept*: Cytotoxic T lymphocyte associated antigen-4 immunoglobulin G (CTLA4-IgG) Fc fusion protein; the dose is

125 mg subcutaneously (SC) every week or 500–1,000 mg every month after loading (depending on weight); the United States Food and Drug Administration (FDA) approved it for PsA and RA.

- *Phosphodiesterase-4 (PDE-4) inhibitors*: These are useful for patients with mild PsA with peripheral joint disease and skin disease; no laboratory testing is needed to monitor therapy.
- *Apremilast*: Dose is 30 mg bid after titration.

PROGNOSIS

For most patients with PsA, the musculoskeletal manifestations are relatively milder than those of RA. After 8 years of the disease, half of the patients develop significant deformity of one or more joints. In some cases, the prognosis is good, and in some, there is waxing and waning; some patients may progress to fibrosing or bony ankylosis.

SUGGESTED READING

1. Tiwari V, Brent LH. (2023). Psoriatic Arthritis. Treasure Island (FL): StatPearls Publishing. [online] Available from https://pubmed.ncbi.nlm.nih.gov/31613490/ [Last accessed February, 2025].

211 Pterygium Unguis

➲ ETIOPATHOGENESIS

An inflammatory destructive process is followed by fusion of the nail fold and underlying nail bed and matrix. The fibrotic band then obstructs normal nail growth.

➲ CLINICAL FEATURES

The term pterygium describes the winged appearance achieved when a central fibrotic band divides a nail proximally in two. However, the fibrotic tissue may not always grossly alter the nail and can extend from the lateral nail fold as well as the more typical proximal nail fold origin. A large pterygium may destroy the whole nail.

There are two types described further.

Dorsal Pterygium

Dorsal pterygium results from the nail matrix destruction and appears as a V-shaped extension of the skin of the proximal nail fold that adheres to the nail bed **(Fig. 1)**. Superficial abnormal vessels may be seen, and there are no skin markings. It is seen in trauma, lichen planus, graft-versus-host disease, and leprosy, where it may represent scarring secondary to neuropathic damage and secondary purulent infection.

Other uncommon causes of pterygium unguis include sarcoidosis, onychotillomania, peripheral vascular disease, radiotherapy, Raynaud's phenomenon, systemic lupus erythematosus, pemphigus

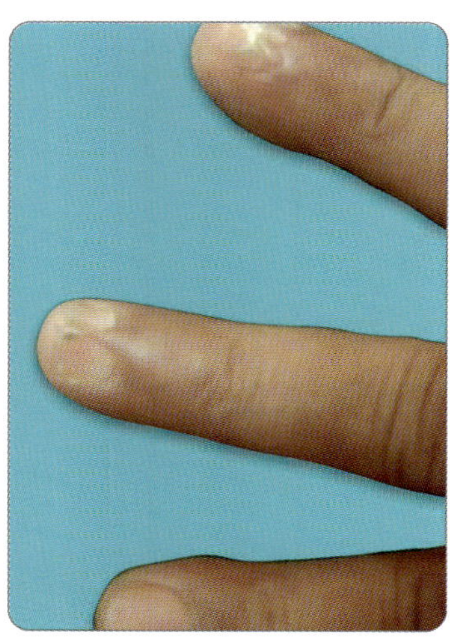

Fig. 1: V-shaped extension of the proximal skin fold attached to the nail bed.

foliaceous, dyskeratosis congenita, toxic epidermal necrolysis, and cicatricial pemphigoid.

Ventral Pterygium

Ventral pterygium, or pterygium inversum unguis, occurs on the distal undersurface of the nail, with forward extension of the nail bed epithelium dislocating the hyponychium and obscuring the distal groove. The overlying nail may be normal, but adjacent soft tissues can be painful. It may be secondary to trauma, systemic sclerosis, Raynaud's phenomenon, lupus erythematosus, familial, and infective.

ONYCHOSCOPY

Onychoscopic examination of one of the nails shows dilated and tortuous proximal nail fold capillaries, with red dots suggestive of glomerular dilated capillaries in the exposed nail bed.

DIFFERENTIAL DIAGNOSIS

Differential diagnosis includes trauma, bullous diseases, digital ischemia, dyskeratosis congenita, and graft-versus-host disease.

TREATMENT

There is no effective treatment.

Treatment with systemic corticosteroids may be required to avoid pterygium formation. Anecdotally, methotrexate or acitretin may be needed to eliminate the corticosteroid.

PROGNOSIS

Pterygium is permanent.

SUGGESTED READING

1. Grover C, Singal A, Bhattacharya SN. Pterygium Complicating Nail Psoriasis and Trachyonychia: Is It Rare? Skin Appendage Disord. 2021;7(4): 298-305.

212 Purpura Fulminans

➲ SYNONYM

Purpura gangrenosa.

➲ HISTORY

Purpura fulminans (PF) was first described by Guelliot in 1884.

➲ ETIOLOGY

- Neonatal PF is due to hereditary deficiency of protein C, protein S, and antithrombin III (ATIII).
- Idiopathic or chronic PF follows a bacterial or viral illness after a variable latent period.
- Acute infectious PF occurs along with meningococcal, varicella, gram-negative *Bacilli*, *Staphylococci*, *Rickettsia* species, *Streptococci*, and measles septicemia.

➲ CLINICAL FEATURES

Purpura fulminans due to homozygous protein C deficiency manifests from 2 hours to 2 weeks after birth. The life-threatening thrombotic event involves the skin, central nervous system, eyes, and kidneys. The clinical manifestation is characterized by a sudden onset of widespread purpura commonly involving extremities, though any parts of the body may be affected. Soon the lesions enlarge and vesiculate, forming hemorrhagic bullae. Subsequently, the skin undergoes necrosis, resulting in black eschar formation **(Figs. 1 and 2)**. The margins of the lesions are well-demarcated,

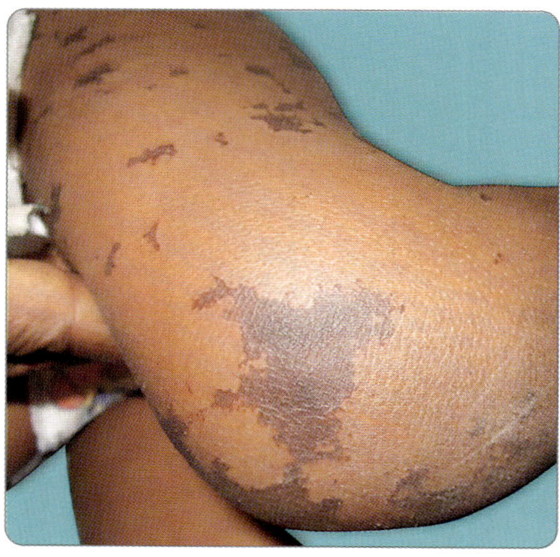

Fig. 1: Purpura over the knees in purpura fulminans.

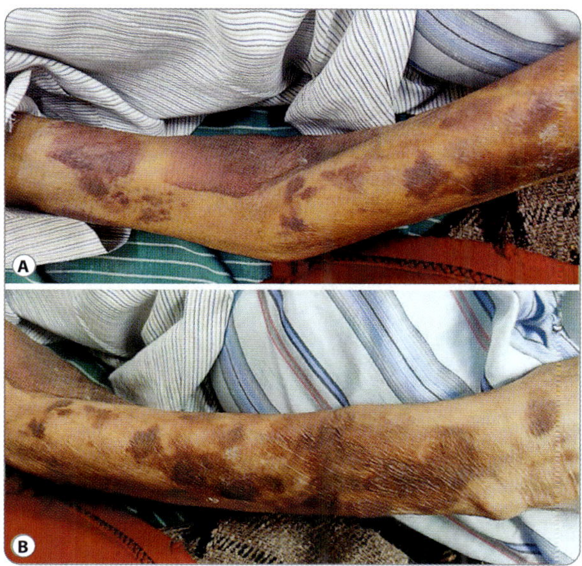

Figs. 2A and B: Purpura over the bilateral forearms in purpura fulminans.

erythematous, and indurated. The cutaneous manifestations culminate in disseminated intravascular coagulation (DIC) with associated internal bleeding. In acute infectious PF, the characteristic lesions occur in a neonate with associated signs of septicemia.

DIAGNOSIS

The estimation of protein C activity is a reliable test to diagnose hereditary protein C deficiency; blood culture should be done to identify the causative organism for septicemia.

TREATMENT

Irrespective of the underlying cause, the neonatal PF must be diagnosed and treated rapidly and aggressively. Acute infectious PF can be managed with immediate heparinization and infusion of fresh frozen plasma (FFP) (15 mL/kg every 12 hours) along with the resuscitation measures for septic shock. Prostacyclin, a thromboxane A2 antagonist, in the initial dose of 5 ng/kg/min, then increased and maintained at 15 ng/kg/min for 48 hours, has been used successfully in the treatment of acute infectious PF. It has beneficial effects on pulmonary hypertension and thromboxane-induced platelet aggregations, which occur in septicemia.

In the acute infectious form, broad-spectrum antibiotics should include coverage of *Neisseria meningitidis*, *Streptococcus*, *Staphylococcus*, and *Clostridia* species. Often, carbapenem or vancomycin with beta-lactamase inhibitors combinations are used. In all forms of the disease, repeated tissue assessments with debridement of affected areas are carried out as needed. Repeated surgeries are often required.

PROGNOSIS

The mortality is almost 100% in untreated hereditary neonatal PF, whereas acute infectious PF is associated with 50% mortality.

SUGGESTED READING

1. Perera TB, Murphy-Lavoie HM. (2023). Purpura Fulminans. Treasure Island (FL): StatPearls Publishing. [online] Available from https://pubmed.ncbi.nlm.nih.gov/30422460/ [Last accessed February, 2025].

213 Pustular Psoriasis

ETIOLOGY

Pustular psoriasis is precipitated by overtreatment with topical tar, anthralin, or potent steroids or by systemic therapy with progesterone or corticosteroids. The foci of infection, pregnancy, and hypocalcemia may also precipitate it.

CLASSIFICATION

- *Localized pustular psoriasis*:
  - Palmoplantar pustulosis
  - Acrodermatitis continua
- *Generalized pustular psoriasis (GPP)*:
  - Acute
  - Pregnancy
  - Infantile and juvenile
  - Circinate
  - Localized (not hands and feet)

CLINICAL FEATURES

In psoriasis vulgaris, the surface of a plaque is dry with silvery white, loose scales. When it is studded with tiny, superficial, sterile pustules, it is called pustular psoriasis.

GENERALIZED TYPE (VON ZUMBUSCH TYPE)

This is the most severe form of GPP. The skin lesions start abruptly as multiple erythematous, tender plaques that soon become studded with pinhead-sized, tiny sterile pustules that may coalesce to form lakes of pus **(Fig. 1)**. Features of systemic toxicity, such as fever, chills, polyarthralgia, and malaise, may be associated. Each pustule dries up in 2–3 days and is exfoliated as thin scales or as brown crusts. At the same time, fresh crops of pustules erupt on the shiny underlying skin, and the cycle is thus repeated. The disease may last for weeks or even months.

Differential Diagnosis

- *Acute generalized exanthematous pustulosis*—usually follows drug intake, and nonfollicular blisters arise over the normal skin; no other signs of psoriasis are seen.
- *Subcorneal pustular dermatosis*—waves of pustules are seen with desquamation, and subcorneal blister is seen on histopathological examination (HPE).
- *Reiter's disease*—presence of circinate balanitis, arthritis, and conjunctivitis; macropustules on biopsy are seen.

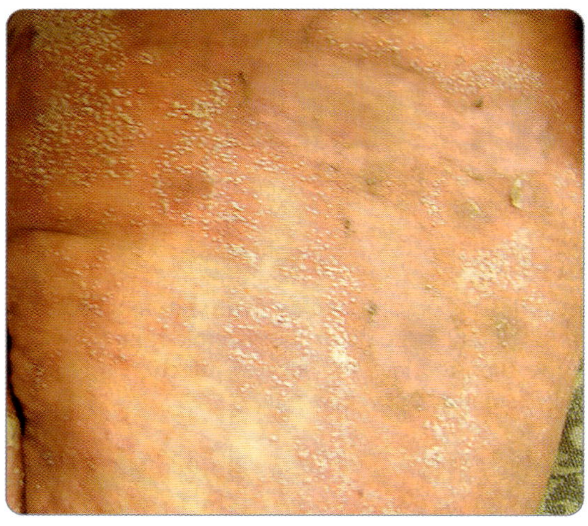

Fig. 1: Multiple pustules on an erythematous base in pustular psoriasis.

➲ PALMOPLANTAR PUSTULOSIS

Erythematous, scaly, well-defined plaques with numerous sterile, tiny, yellow pustules are distributed bilaterally symmetrically on the thenar and hypothenar eminences of the palms, soles, and the sides of the heels.

Differential Diagnosis

Tinea is usually asymmetrical or unilateral. The toe clefts may be involved. Secondary infection of eczema may be pustular but is more painful, and gram stains and culture of pustule contents will establish the diagnosis.

➲ HISTOPATHOLOGY

In acute GPP, there is intense inflammation. The earliest infiltrate is lymphocytic. Intense papillary and epidermal edema causes spongiosis. The arrival of masses of neutrophils leads to spongiform pustule formation (Kogoj) and abscesses that quickly become macroscopic. There is acanthosis, with elongation of rete ridges. The stratum corneum soon becomes parakeratotic, and the subcorneal pustule is shed as epidermal turnover is accelerated.

➲ DERMOSCOPY

Dermoscopy shows red-dotted vessels with milky globules on reddish background.

➲ COMPLICATIONS

Hypoalbuminemia, hypocalcemia, acute tubular necrosis, secondary infection, and inflammatory polyarthritis are the complications.

TREATMENT

Treatment can be withdrawal of provocative factors like tar and dithranol. Treatment of any underlying infection, bland topical application, and fluid and protein replacement. Systemic treatment—oral retinoids are the treatment of choice (acitretin 1 mg/kg/day). Psoralen and ultraviolet A (PUVA), methotrexate, cyclosporine, colchicine, dapsone, and biologicals such as infliximab, adalimumab, etanercept, and anakinra are also effective.

SUGGESTED READING

1. Mirza HA, Badri T, Kwan E. (2022). Generalized Pustular Psoriasis. Treasure Island (FL): StatPearls Publishing. [online] Available from https://pubmed.ncbi.nlm.nih.gov/29630241/ [Last accessed February, 2025].

214 Pyoderma Faciale

➲ SYNONYM

Rosacea fulminans.

➲ ETIOLOGY

Etiology is unknown. Despite the severity, there are no systemic symptoms or evidence of any infection.

➲ AGE

Pyoderma faciale affects women commonly in their 20s and 30s.

➲ CLINICAL FEATURE

Pyoderma faciale is an uncommon eruptive facial disorder with intense reddish or cyanotic erythema, combined with superficial and deep abscesses, cystic lesions, and sometimes sinus tracts, often containing purulent material.

➲ HISTOPATHOLOGY

The epidermis shows hyperkeratosis with follicular plugging and rectification of interpapillary cones. Papillary dermis showed dilated vessels and hair follicles surrounded by a mixed inflammatory process, consisting of neutrophils and lymphocytes in periadnexal and perivascular disposition.

➲ DIFFERENTIAL DIAGNOSIS

Pyoderma faciale has to be differentiated from acne by the absence of comedones and rapid onset, fulminating course. Unlike rosacea, it is not associated with flushing and has no eye symptoms.

➲ COMPLICATIONS

The lesions may rarely heal with scarring.

➲ TREATMENT

Tablet minocycline (100–200 mg/day), oral isotretinoin (0.5 mg/kg) for 4–6 months, and intralesional steroids for cystic lesion can be given. To minimize exacerbations, oral prednisolone (0.5–1 mg/kg) for 2–3 weeks can be given.

Other drugs include oral metronidazole and dapsone.

Dapsone can be used in cases of therapeutic failure or treatment-resistant cases.

➲ PROGNOSIS

The disease rarely persists for more than a year. No recurrences are seen.

➲ SUGGESTED READING

1. Coutinho JC, Westphal DC, Lobato LC, Schettini AP, Santos M. Rosacea fulminans: unusual clinical presentation of rosacea. An Bras Dermatol. 2016;91(5 suppl 1):151-3.

215 Pyoderma Gangrenosum

➲ HISTORY

Pyoderma gangrenosum (PG) was described by Brocq in 1916 and Brunsting in 1930.

➲ ETIOLOGY

The exact etiology is not fully known. 50% of the cases are associated with systemic diseases such as inflammatory bowel diseases, arthritis, hematological malignancies, and monoclonal gammopathies.

➲ AGE

Pyoderma gangrenosum is seen commonly in 20–50 years of age.

➲ CLINICAL FEATURES

Pyoderma gangrenosum is a primarily sterile inflammatory neutrophilic dermatosis characterized by recurrent cutaneous ulcerations with a mucopurulent or hemorrhagic exudate.

Onset occurs with sterile pustules that rapidly progress and turn into very painful ulcers of variable depth and size, with undermined bluish or violaceous borders and surrounding erythema **(Fig. 1)**. The legs are most commonly affected, but parts of the skin and mucus membranes may also be involved. The clinical course can be mild or malignant, chronic or relapsing with significant morbidity. In many cases, PG is associated with an underlying disease, most commonly

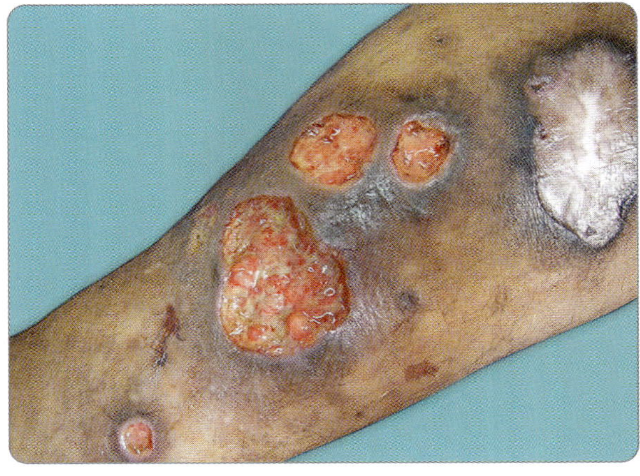

Fig. 1: Multiple ulcers with undermined edges and scar of pyoderma gangrenosum.

Table 1: Clinical variants of pyoderma gangrenosum.

Type	*Histopathology*	*Clinical features*
Ulcerative	Massive epidermal and neutrophilic infiltrate and abscess formation	Classical type, legs and trunk, inflammatory bowel disease (IBD), arthritis, and monoclonal gammopathies
Pustular	Perifollicular neutrophilic infiltrate and subcorneal pustule formation	Painful pustules with surrounding erythema and extensor aspect of the limbs
Bullous/ Atypical	Neutrophilic infiltrate and intraepithelial vesicle formation	Superficial hemorrhagic bullae; ulcerates and heals with scarring; arms are a common site; and associated with myeloproliferative diseases
Vegetative	Granulomatous reaction with peripheral palisading histiocytes and giant cells	Nonpainful ulcers on nonpurulent base

inflammatory bowel disease, rheumatic or hematological disease, or malignancy **(Table 1)**. The pathergy test is positive.

There is also a rare peristomal variant.

➲ DERMOSCOPY

Dermoscopy shows ulcers, background color yellow indicative of necrotic tissue, red or purple hue indicative of inflammation and vascular changes, polymorphic vessels with both dotted and linear vessels.

➲ INVESTIGATIONS

It is a diagnosis of exclusion.

➲ DIFFERENTIAL DIAGNOSIS

This condition is a disease by exclusion of arterial insufficiency, Sweet's syndrome, blastomycosis, factitial disease, traumatic ulceration, tuberculous gumma, atypical mycobacterial infections, Churg–Strauss syndrome (allergic granulomatosis), ecthyma, ecthyma gangrenosum, impetigo, insect bites, sporotrichosis, malignancy, venous insufficiency, and Wegener granulomatosis.

➲ TREATMENT

- *Mild*: Wet compresses, hydrophilic occlusive dressing, antimicrobial agents, topical steroids, and topical tacrolimus
- *Severe*: Oral steroids, dapsone, clofazimine, minocycline, azathioprine, cyclosporine, infliximab and etanercept, plasmapheresis, intravenous (IV) immunoglobulin, and thalidomide

➲ PROGNOSIS

The prognosis is good. The disease may recur and result in scarring. Death is due to an associated disease.

➲ SUGGESTED READINGS

1. George C, Deroide F, Rustin M. Pyoderma gangrenosum - a guide to diagnosis and management. Clin Med (Lond). 2019;19(3):224-8.
2. Langan SM, Groves RW, Card TR, Gulliford MC. Incidence, mortality, and disease associations of pyoderma gangrenosum in the United Kingdom: a retrospective cohort study. J Invest Dermatol. 2012;132:2166-70.

216 Pyogenic Granuloma

➲ SYNONYMS

Eruptive hemangioma, lobular capillary hemangioma, band-aid disease, granuloma telangiectaticum, granuloma pyogenicum.

➲ HISTORY

Pyogenic granuloma was described by Poncet and Dor in 1897. The term granuloma pyogenicum was coined by Hartzell, and it is a misnomer.

➲ ETIOLOGY

The exact etiology is unknown, and it may follow penetrative injury. Drugs like retinoids, capecitabine, 5-fluorouracil (5-FU), and indinavir have been implicated.

➲ AGE GROUP

Second decade and increases during pregnancy (granuloma gravidarum and pregnancy tumor).

➲ CLINICAL FEATURES

Benign circumscribed polypoidal vascular lesion, usually solitary, with a tendency to bleed **(Fig. 1)**. The lesions grow over the weeks and then persist. Common sites are gingiva, fingers, face, and labia. Multiple lesions are common over the trunk. Variants include

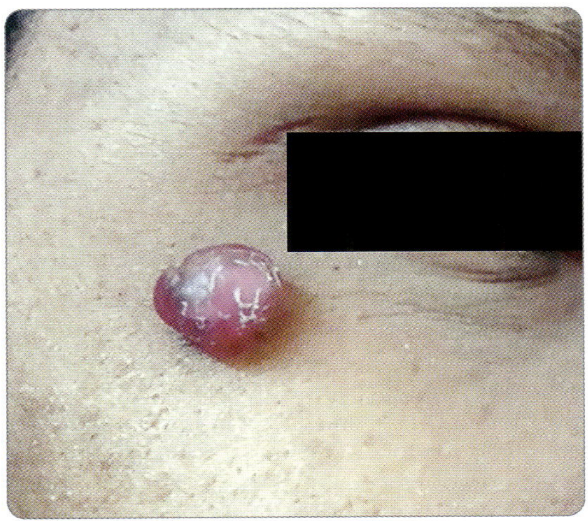

Fig. 1: Circumscribed polypoidal vascular lesion of pyogenic granuloma.

multiple lesions, satellite, subcutaneous, intravenous, giant, and recurrent.

ASSOCIATED SYNDROMES

Sturge–Weber syndrome and POEMS (polyneuropathy, organomegaly, endocrinopathy, M-protein, and skin changes) syndrome are the associated syndromes.

HISTOPATHOLOGY

Lobule of capillaries and venules separated by fibrous septa, and the epidermis forms a collarette at the base. Feeding vessels extend to adjacent dermis.

DERMOSCOPY

The most frequent dermoscopic pattern of pyogenic granuloma consists of reddish homogenous areas separated by white lines resembling rails and surrounded by a white collarette.

DIFFERENTIAL DIAGNOSIS

- *Amelanotic melanoma*—absence of bleeding and atypical melanocytes
- *Kaposi sarcoma*—mainly over the legs, seen in immunocompromised people, thick endothelial cells in vascular channels, and promontory sign is positive
- *Glomus tumor*—painful, pulsating tumor mainly in the nailbed or fingertips, and collection of glomus cells
- *Bacillary angiomatosis*—ulcerated nodules/plaques and demonstration of bacteria by Warthin–Starry stain in tissue specimen
- *Hemangioma*—proliferation of capillaries/veins, present usually at birth or during infancy; spontaneously involute/leave behind pigmentation
- *Verruca*—skin-colored/hyperpigmented, verrucous surface, and koilocytes on biopsy
- Irritated seborrheic keratosis

COMPLICATIONS

Complications include ulceration and recurrent intrapapillary endothelial hyperplasia.

TREATMENT

Shave removal, surgical excision, curettage, cryotherapy, imiquimod 5%, intralesional steroids, and sclerosants such as ethanolamine oleate, sodium tetradecyl sulfate, polidocanol, and bleomycin have shown sporadic patient benefits. The Multinational Association for Supportive Care in Cancer (MASCC) Skin Toxicity Study Group has published guidelines preventing and treating lobular capillary hemangiomas, recommending weekly chemical cauterization, electrodesiccation, or nail avulsion.

For small lesions in cosmetically sensitive areas or lesions in children, practitioners may consider nonoperative management with pulsed dye laser, CO_2 laser ablation, or electrocautery if laser therapies are not available.

➲ PROGNOSIS

Recurrent.

➲ SUGGESTED READING

1. Sarwal P, Lapumnuaypol K. Pyogenic Granuloma. (2022). Treasure Island (FL): StatPearls Publishing. [online] Available from https://pubmed.ncbi.nlm.nih.gov/32310537/ [Last accessed February, 2025].

217 Raynaud's Phenomenon

➲ HISTORY

Raynaud's phenomenon is named after French physician Maurice Raynaud (1814–1881).

➲ ETIOLOGY

Raynaud's phenomenon is an exaggeration of vasomotor response to cold or emotional stress. More specifically, it is a hyperactivation of the sympathetic system causing extreme vasoconstriction of the peripheral blood vessels, leading to tissue hypoxia.

➲ RAYNAUD'S DISEASE ("PRIMARY RAYNAUD'S PHENOMENON")

Idiopathic.

➲ ALLEN AND BROWN CRITERIA FOR RAYNAUD'S DISEASE

- Intermittent attacks of discoloration of the acral parts
- Bilateral involvement
- Absence of clinical arterial occlusion
- Gangrene or atrophic changes are rare
- Symptoms present for 2 years
- Absence of other diseases, which could explain the symptoms
- Predominance in women

➲ RAYNAUD'S SYNDROME ("SECONDARY RAYNAUD'S PHENOMENON")

Secondary to connective tissue disorders, drugs (beta-blockers, cytotoxic drugs—particularly bleomycin, ciclosporin, bromocriptine, ergotamine, and sulfasalazine), jobs involving vibration, particularly drilling, Lyme's disease, hypothyroidism, cryoglobulinemia, malignancy, reflex sympathetic dystrophy, carpal tunnel syndrome, and vaso-occlusive diseases.

➲ AGE

Raynaud's phenomenon usually presents in the third decade, mostly in women.

➲ CLINICAL FEATURES

It is a vasospastic disorder causing discoloration of the fingers and occasionally toes. When exposed to cold temperatures, the blood supply to the fingers or toes, and in some cases, the nose or earlobes, is markedly reduced; the skin turns pale or white (called pallor) and becomes cold and numb. When the oxygen supply is depleted, the skin color turns blue (called cyanosis).

These events are episodic, and when the episode subsides or the area is warmed, the blood flow returns, and the skin color first turns red (rubor) and then back to normal, often accompanied by swelling, tingling, and a painful "pins and needles" sensation.

INVESTIGATIONS

- Digital artery pressure. Pressures are measured in the arteries of the fingers before and after the hands have been cooled. A decrease of at least 15 mm Hg is diagnostic (positive).
- Doppler ultrasound
- Full blood count
- Blood test for urea and electrolytes
- Thyroid function tests
- An autoantibody screen
- Nail-fold vasculature

COMPLICATIONS

Chronic, recurrent cases of Raynaud's phenomenon can result in atrophy of the skin, subcutaneous tissues, and muscle. In rare cases, it can cause ulceration and ischemic gangrene.

TREATMENT

General Care

- Environmental triggers should be avoided, e.g., cold and vibration.
- Emotional stress is another recognized trigger.
- Extremities should be kept warm.
- Smoking should be avoided.
- Consumption of caffeine and other stimulants and vasoconstrictors must be prevented.

Raynaud's disease may be aggravated by hormones and hormone regulators, such as hormonal contraception. Contraception that is low in estrogen is preferable, and the progesterone-only pill is often prescribed for women with Raynaud's disease.

Drug Therapy

- Calcium channel blockers (nifedipine) or diltiazem.
- Angiotensin II receptor antagonists (losartan) reduce the frequency and severity of attacks.
- Alpha-1 adrenergic blockers such as prazosin.
- Sildenafil (Viagra) improved both microcirculation and symptoms in patients with secondary Raynaud's phenomenon resistant to vasodilatory therapy.
- If tissue ischemia is present in the digits and symptoms are severe, then intravenous infusion of prostaglandin is used. Different intravenous prostaglandins include iloprost, epoprostenol, treprostinil, and alprostadil. Prostaglandin functions as a strong vasodilator and also prevents platelet cell aggregation.

- Fluoxetine, a selective serotonin reuptake inhibitor, and other antidepressant medications may reduce the frequency and severity of episodes if caused mainly by psychological stress.
- RayVa is a topical cream for the treatment of Raynaud's phenomenon. It contains prostaglandin E1 as the active ingredient and a permeation enhancer, DDAIP, which facilitates the delivery of the drug into the bloodstream.

Surgical Intervention

- In severe cases, a sympathectomy procedure can be performed. Here, the nerves that signal the blood vessels of the fingertips to constrict are surgically cut. Microvascular surgery of the affected areas is another possible therapy. Infusions of prostaglandins, e.g., prostacyclin, may be tried, with amputation in exceptionally severe cases.
- A more recent treatment for severe Raynaud's phenomenon is the use of botox.

SUGGESTED READING

1. Musa R, Qurie A. (2023). Raynaud Disease. Treasure Island (FL): StatPearls Publishing. [online] Available from https://pubmed.ncbi.nlm.nih.gov/29763008/ [Last accessed February, 2025].

218 Reactive Arthritis

➲ SYNONYMS

Reiter's syndrome, arthritis urethritica, venereal arthritis, polyarteritis enterica.

➲ HISTORY

In 1916, Hans Conrad Julius Reiter, who was a Nazi war criminal, described the triad of reactive arthritis.

➲ ETIOLOGY

Reactive arthritis usually follows a bout of urethritis or diarrheal illness. Implicated organisms are *Chlamydia trachomatis*, *Shigella*, *Salmonella*, *Yersinia*, *Campylobacter*, *Ureaplasma*, *Borrelia*, *Cryptosporidium*, *Gonococci*, Bacillus Calmette–Guérin (BCG) vaccine, and *Ureaplasma urealyticum*. It is associated with human leukocyte antigen (HLA)-B27 genotype.

➲ AGE GROUP

The disease occurs chiefly in young men of age 15–35 years. The M:F ratio in postvenereal disease is 10:1.

➲ CLINICAL FEATURES

The syndrome is characterized by a clinical triad of urethritis, conjunctivitis, and arthritis of >1 month duration. Patient presents with painful urination and pyuria. Cystitis, prostatitis, and seminal vestibulitis may be present. Vulval ulceration and circinate balanitis are seen. About a third of patients develop conjunctivitis, which may be bulbar, tarsal, or angular. Keratitis is usually superficial and extremely painful. Iritis is common, especially in recurrent cases. An asymmetric arthritis affects peripheral joints, especially those of weight-bearing, i.e., the knee, ankle, and metatarsophalangeal joint (sausage toes). Its onset is usually sudden. Pain in one or both heels due to enthesitis of the Achilles tendon is a frequent symptom. Sacroiliitis may develop in up to two-thirds of patients, most of whom are of HLA-B27 genotype.

Skin involvement commonly begins with small guttate, hyperkeratotic, crusted, or pustular lesions of the genitals, palms, or soles. Involvement of the glans penis occurs in 25% of patients. Lesions on the soles and trunk often become thickly crusted or hyperkeratotic. The eruption on the soles is called keratoderma blennorrhagicum. The buccal and lingual mucosa may show painless, shallow, red erosions. The nails become thick and brittle, with heavy subungual keratosis. Children are much more likely to have the postdysenteric form, often with conjunctivitis and arthritis as the most prominent complaints.

HISTOPATHOLOGY

Histopathology of keratoderma blennorrhagicum shows hyperkeratosis, hyperplasia, elongation of rete pegs, parakeratosis, neutrophilic infiltration forming microabscess, and spongiform pustules.

Leukocytosis and elevated sedimentation rate are the most consistent findings. There is no specific test for Reiter's syndrome.

DERMOSCOPY

Dermoscopy shows closely placed islands of brownish plate surrounded by flaccid pustules simulating double-edged scale. Glomerular and dotted vessels are seen underneath the crust. Older lesions show silvery scale.

DIFFERENTIAL DIAGNOSIS

Differential diagnosis includes rheumatoid arthritis (positive RA), ankylosing spondylitis, gout (podagra seen, raised serum uric acid), psoriatic arthritis [distal interphalangeal joint (DIPJ) involved classically], gonococcal arthritis, acute rheumatic fever, chronic mucocutaneous candidiasis, sarcoidosis, Lyme's disease (presence of erythema chronicum migrans), syphilis, and serum sickness. The presence of associated mucocutaneous lesions establishes the diagnosis.

COMPLICATIONS

Complications can be carditis, cardiac valvular disease, severe arthritis disabling work, amyloidosis, and death.

TREATMENT

Mucocutaneous lesions are generally self-limited and clear with topical steroids, calcipotriol, or tazarotene. Joint disease is managed with rest and nonsteroidal anti-inflammatory drugs (NSAIDs). If an infectious agent has been identified as a trigger for reactive arthritis, antimicrobial therapy is strongly recommended, often for a long-term of 3–6 months. It can significantly shorten the time to remission. Antibiotics, such as doxycycline, are effective in some cases. Methotrexate, acitretin, cyclosporine, and infliximab are used for refractory diseases. Disease-modifying antirheumatic drugs (DMARDs), mainly sulfasalazine, are effective in both acute and chronic reactive arthritis.

PROGNOSIS

Few cases resolve by 6 months, rest by 12 months. HLA-B27 positive, family history, and chronic gut lesions are likely to have prolonged duration of disease.

SUGGESTED READING

1. Cheeti A, Chakraborty RK, Ramphul K. (2023). Reactive Arthritis. Treasure Island (FL): StatPearls Publishing. [online] Available from https://pubmed.ncbi.nlm.nih.gov/29763006/ [Last accessed February, 2025].

219 Rosacea

SYNONYMS

Acne rosacea, curse of the Celts.

ETIOLOGY

The cause of rosacea remains unknown. Most patients have an abnormal vasomotor response to thermal and other stimuli. Chronic solar damage is an important contributor. *Demodex folliculorum* and *Helicobacter pylori* have been found to be causative.

AGE GROUP

Women within the age range of 36–50 years are commonly affected. The M:F ratio is 1:3.

CLINICAL FEATURES

Rosacea is a chronic disorder affecting the facial convexities (nose, forehead, cheeks, and chin), the scalp, upper chest, back, and even the limb, characterized by frequent flushing, persistent erythema, and telangiectasia. During episodes of inflammation, patients develop swelling, papules, and pustules, persisting tissue thickening due to edema, fibrosis, and glandular hyperplasia, leading ultimately to a *peau d'orange* appearance and phymas. It is more common in fair-skinned people. Factors which trigger flushing include emotion and stress, hot drinks, alcohol, and spicy food. Aggravating factors include the use of topical steroids. Sun exposure may worsen or improve rosacea. There are four subsets of rosacea, viz. erythematotelangiectatic rosacea, papulopustular, phymatous, and ocular rosacea.

ASSOCIATED SYNDROMES

Haber syndrome is a genodermatosis characterized by a rosacea-like facial dermatosis and multiple verrucous lesions on nonsun-exposed skin.

HISTOPATHOLOGY

Telangiectasia is indicated by the presence of dilated superficial capillaries. Lymphatic channels may also be dilated deeper in the mid-dermis. Solar elastosis is prominent, and mild perivascular lymphohistiocytic infiltrate is seen in erythematotelangiectatic cases, an intense infiltration which may be perifollicular, interfollicular, and perivascular in papular rosacea. Mast cell density is reported to be increased. Some lesions contain palisading granulomas. Foreign body-type giant cells may be observed in the upper parts of hair follicles. *D. folliculorum* has been observed in up to 51% of cases.

DERMOSCOPY

Common dermoscopic findings in rosacea include telangiectasia, erythema, follicular plugs, and perifollicular erythema.

DIFFERENTIAL DIAGNOSIS

- *Polycythemia vera*—erythromelalgia
- *Carcinoid*—flushing attacks with hypotension, diarrhea, and bronchospasm
- *Mastocytosis*—generalized flushing and Darier's sign positive
- *Acne vulgaris*—comedones are pathognomonic.
- Connective tissue disease (lupus erythematosus, dermatomyositis, and mixed connective tissue disease)
- *Sarcoidosis*—raised serum angiotensin-converting enzyme (ACE) levels
- Idiopathic flushing
- Seborrheic dermatitis
- Phytodermatitis

COMPLICATIONS

- *Chronic lymphedema*: A characteristic pattern of lymphedema of the upper half of the face has been termed chronic upper facial erythematous edema or Morbihan's disease.

  Thickening of affected skin and rhinophyma are late complications.

  Phymatous rosacea **(Fig. 1)** can also affect the chin (gnathophyma), forehead (metaphyma), cheeks, eyelids (blepharophyma), and ears (otophyma).
- *Eye complication:* Sensation of grittiness, irritability of the eyes, conjunctival congestion, blepharitis, episcleritis, rosacea keratitis, chalazion, and hordeolum are also common.

  Reduction in tear secretion associated with ocular rosacea would suggest involvement of the lacrimal glands.

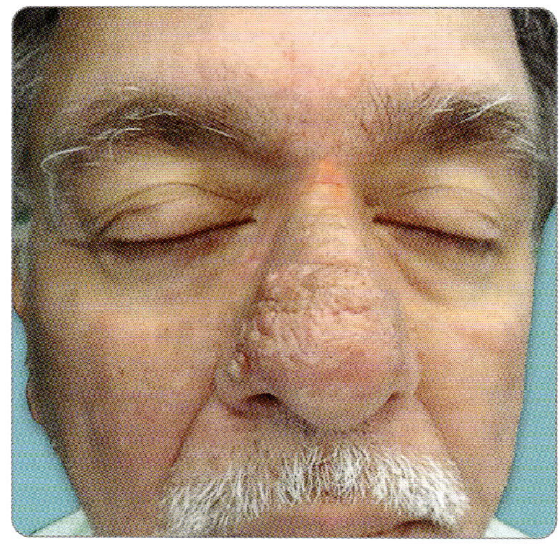

Fig. 1: Erythema over the face with rhinophyma in rosacea.

TREATMENT

Oral tetracycline antibiotics (tetracycline, doxycycline, and minocycline) and topical antibiotics such as metronidazole and permethrin 5% are usually the first line of defense. Isotretinoin is used to treat severe cases of papulopustular and phymatous rosacea. For flushing and blushing, centrally acting α-2 agonist clonidine, beta-blockers nadolol and propranolol, and silymarin have been tried.

Octreotide

Level of evidence 3, grade of recommendation D: A single anecdotal observation has reported clearance of rosacea lesions in three of four treated patients with octreotide, a somatostatin analog.

Zinc Sulfate

Level of evidence 1–, grade of recommendation B: Two randomized control trials have been found dealing with zinc sulfate; in one randomized control trial, significant improvement was seen in 19 patients with zinc sulfate (100 mg thrice daily) compared to placebo, while the other study did not show any significant advantage over placebo (220 mg twice daily for 3 months; 44 patients).

Serine Protease Inhibitors

Patients suffering from rosacea possess higher levels of the serum protease kallikrein 5 compared to the general population, which cleaves the cathelicidin precursor into LL-37, a key molecule involved in the pathogenesis of rosacea. Thus, serum protease inhibitors are being evaluated for the treatment of rosacea. Topical epsilon-aminocaproic acid, a serine protease inhibitor, has been found to improve the erythema significantly in patients suffering from papulopustular rosacea within 6 weeks of starting therapy.

Mast Cell Stabilizers

Mast cells have been suggested to play a key role in the pathogenesis of rosacea by releasing cathelicidins, LL-37, matrix metalloproteinases, and other inflammatory cytokines. Thus, agents blocking mast cell degranulation may have a beneficial role, at least theoretically. With this idea, a topical mast cell stabilizer, cromolyn sodium (4%), has been compared with a placebo to obtain modest symptomatic improvement.

Laser treatment can be done for telangiectasia and rhinophyma.

PROGNOSIS

The persistence of rosacea may result in chronic thickening and induration of the face (leonine facies), and rhinophyma is common in males. Eye involvement is usually mild and reversible. Most symptoms of rosacea can usually be controlled, but the flushing is often impossible to suppress.

SUGGESTED READING

1. Sarkar R, Podder I, Jagadeesan S. Rosacea in skin of color: A comprehensive review. Indian J Dermatol Venereol Leprol. 2020;86:611-21.

220 Roseola Infantum

➲ SYNONYMS

Exanthema subitum (means sudden rash), sixth disease, rose rash of infants, baby measles, 3-day fever, wind measles.

➲ ETIOLOGY

Human herpesvirus 6 (HHV-6)B strains are almost always the cause of human disease, with HHV-6A strains rarely being implicated. After the initial infection, the virus persists and can be detected in saliva from a high percentage of healthy subjects, which is the likely mode of spread.

➲ AGE GROUP

Roseola infantum is seen in children <2 years, with peak incidence between 6 and 9 months.

➲ CLINICAL FEATURES

The incubation period is from 10 to 15 days. Fever ranges between 39.5° and 40°C, begins abruptly, and persists for 3–5 days. Irritability, inflamed tympanic membranes, ulcers at the posterior palate and uvula, periorbital edema, and hematuria are early manifestations. As the temperature falls, an eruption of discrete rose-pink maculopapules develops on the neck and trunk; it may later spread to the arms, face, and legs. The lesions may rarely become vesicular. After 1 or 2 days, the rash fades, leaving no scaling or pigmentation. The patient's cervical and occipital lymph nodes are usually enlarged.

Febrile convulsions are not uncommon. The eruption of primary HHV-6 infection is almost restricted to the first 3 years of life. If primary infection occurs in adults, there may be a mononucleosis-like illness, fever, rash, and mainly cervical lymphadenopathy, which may persist for up to 3 months, or an acute but self-limiting hepatitis.

Reactivation of HHV-6 in immunosuppression causes a variety of symptoms like fever, rash, hepatitis, encephalitis, pneumonitis, and bone marrow suppression.

➲ ASSOCIATED SYNDROMES

Multiple sclerosis, Guillain–Barré syndrome, chronic fatigue syndrome, lymphoproliferative disorders, pityriasis rosea, and Kikuchi–Fujimoto disease.

➲ DIAGNOSIS

Confirmation is by demonstrating a rise in antibody titer to HHV-6, typically by indirect immunofluorescence using cells infected with

HHV-6 antigen. Immunoglobulin M (IgM) antibody is usually present 5–7 days after the rash, maximal 2 weeks after infection, and persists for about 2 months, with a rise in anti-IgG titers. Molecular detection of viral RNA by reverse transcription polymerase chain reaction (RT-PCR) or DNA by PCR is possible, but only quantitative PCR reliably distinguishes primary from latent infection.

➲ DIFFERENTIAL DIAGNOSIS

Rubella, measles, and the picture of roseola infantum can also be caused by HHV-7 infection. The lack of symptoms during the febrile phase and the appearance of the eruption as the fever subsides should suggest the diagnosis.

➲ COMPLICATIONS

Fatal encephalitis, thrombocytopenia, hemophagocytic syndrome, leukocytosis, and leukopenia with a relative lymphopenia are usual.

➲ TREATMENT

Only symptomatic measures are usually required. Treatment is supportive with rest, maintaining fluid intake, and antipyretics such as acetaminophen or ibuprofen to control the fever. Antiviral therapy with ganciclovir, cidofovir, or foscarnet in severe forms can be given.

➲ PROGNOSIS

It is a self-limiting disease, and treatment is required only in atypical and immunocompromised states.

➲ SUGGESTED READING

1. Mullins TB, Krishnamurthy K. (2023). Roseola Infantum. Treasure Island (FL): StatPearls Publishing. [online] Available from https://www.ncbi.nlm.nih.gov/books/NBK448190/ [Last accessed February, 2025].

221 Rubella

➲ SYNONYM

German measles.

➲ HISTORY

Friedrich Hoffmann, a German physician, made the first clinical description of rubella in 1740. Henry Veale coined the name "rubella" (from the Latin, meaning "little red").

➲ ETIOLOGY

Rubella virus is a member of the genus *Rubivirus* and family *Togaviridae*; it does not require an insect vector. Epidemics occur in the spring, and transmission is by droplets. It is infective from the end of the incubation period to the fourth day of the rash.

➲ AGE GROUP

Rubella affects older children and young adults.

➲ CLINICAL FEATURES

The rash appears after an IP of 14 days (range: 12–21 days). Adolescents and adults have a brief prodromal illness lasting 1–5 days, consisting of fever up to 39°C, headache, malaise, sore throat without coryza, and suffusion of the conjunctivae with a gritty sensation. The symptoms subside as the rash develops. An exanthem of dull-red macules or petechiae confined to the soft palate (Forchheimer sign) is present in 20% of patients during the prodromal period or on the first day of the rash.

Tender lymphadenopathy begins 5–7 days before the rash and characteristically involves the suboccipital, postauricular, and cervical glands.

The rash appears first on the face and spreads rapidly downward to the trunk and limbs. It consists of pink macules, discrete initially, but soon becomes confluent on the face as a diffuse erythema. During the second day, the face begins to clear, and the macules on the trunk show some coalescence, and those on the limbs remain discrete. By the third day, the trunk has cleared, and by the fourth day, the eruption on the limbs also fades. The rash may be absent in some (40%).

The blood count may be normal, or leukopenia with an inconstant increase in plasma cells.

➲ ASSOCIATED SYNDROMES

Associated syndromes include congenital rubella syndrome—microcephaly, ventricular septal defect (VSD), patent ductus arteriosus (PDA), sensory neural deafness, and cataract.

RUBELLA IN PREGNANCY

The prenatal damage produced by rubella in early pregnancy was the first noted by Gregg in Australia in 1941. The risk of fetal damage is 85% for infection during the first 11 weeks. Infection at this stage results in multiple defects. Between weeks 12 and 16, the risk of a rubella defect is about 35%.

DIFFERENTIAL DIAGNOSIS

Differential diagnosis includes drug hypersensitivity reaction, Kawasaki disease, rubeola, other viral infections [*Enterovirus*, parvovirus, and human herpesvirus 6 (HHV-6)], and streptococcal scarlet fever.

COMPLICATIONS

- *Arthritis*—more in females and resolves within a month
- *Thrombocytopenic or nonthrombocytopenic*—purpura and encephalitis

DIAGNOSIS

- Hemagglutination inhibition test is diagnostic.
- The presence of specific immunoglobulin M (IgM) antibody is also diagnostic.
- In neonates, the presence of IgM and continued antibody production are indicative of congenital infection. Molecular diagnosis can be done by using reverse transcription polymerase chain reaction (RT-PCR) on swab samples.

TREATMENT

There is no specific treatment. Isolation and supportive therapy are recommended.

PROPHYLAXIS

Active immunization by inoculation with live attenuated rubella virus is employed in infants aged 1–2 years old, together with measles, mumps, and rubella vaccine (MMR vaccine). A preschool booster of MMR is also recommended. A quadruple vaccine including varicella is available.

Pregnancy is a contraindication to the vaccine and should be avoided for 4 weeks after its administration.

PROGNOSIS

Rubella is a self-limiting disease; infants with congenital rubella syndrome are infectious till they shed viruses, and mothers caring for them are also prone to infections.

SUGGESTED READING

1. Winter AK, Pramanik S, Lessler J, Ferrari M, Grenfell BT, Metcalf CJE. Rubella vaccination in India: identifying broad consequences of vaccine introduction and key knowledge gaps. Epidemiol Infect. 2018 146(1): 65-77.

222 Rubeola

SYNONYMS

Measles, English measles, morbilli.

HISTORY

The Antonine plague of AD 165–180 was probably measles or smallpox. The scientific description of measles and its differentiation from smallpox was made by a Persian physician, Muhammad Zakariya al-Razi.

ETIOLOGY

Measles is caused by paramyxovirus of the genus *Morbillivirus,* which is a single-stranded RNA virus. Measles infection spreads in humans via the upper respiratory tract, where the initial replication occurs before wide dissemination throughout the body.

AGE GROUP

Measles is common in children of 5–9 years.

CLINICAL FEATURES

The incubation period is 10 days, and the prodromal symptoms include fever, malaise, upper respiratory catarrh, and photophobia. From the second day, Koplik's spots appear on the buccal mucous membrane opposite the premolar teeth as bluish-white spots with bright-red areolae.

The exanthema characteristically develops on the fourth day on the forehead and behind the ears and spreads within 24 hours to the rest of the face, the trunk, and the limbs. The rash is at first macular, soon forms dull-red papules, which tend to coalesce. From the 6th to the 10th day, the rash fades to leave some brownish staining and fine scale. In very severe forms, it may be hemorrhagic. Extensive bullous eruption may rarely develop during the acute stage. In some cases, this eruption has the features of Stevens–Johnson syndrome, but in others, the features are those of toxic epidermal necrolysis.

DIAGNOSIS

Specific measles antibodies are usually detectable 3 or 4 days after the appearance of the rash, and maximum titers are reached 2–4 weeks later. Viral antigen can be detected by immunofluorescence in cell smears prepared from nasopharyngeal aspirates taken early during the illness and in skin biopsy of the exanthem.

DIFFERENTIAL DIAGNOSIS

Drug hypersensitivity reaction (fever with lymphadenopathy, hepatitis, and rash following drug intake), rubella, Henoch–Schönlein purpura (palpable purpura over the buttocks and lower limbs; abdominal pain, bleeding per rectum, and hematuria), other viral exanthems, graft-versus-host disease, and Kawasaki disease are the differential diagnoses.

COMPLICATIONS

Complications are more common in young children and the malnourished. Bronchopneumonia, enteritis, and otitis media are less frequent. The most serious complication is encephalitis (subacute sclerosing panencephalitis).

DIAGNOSIS

Diagnosis can be made by virus isolation or detection via reverse transcription polymerase chain reaction (RT-PCR) in nasopharyngeal secretions or urine.

TREATMENT

Treatment is symptomatic. In areas of high mortality, vitamin A (two doses of 200,000 IU) should be given. Measles pneumonia may be treated with ribavirin. Antibiotics may be required to control secondary bacterial complications. Passive protection by normal human immunoglobulin (Ig) is given within 5 days of exposure, which prevents or attenuates the infection in contacts and is reserved for children at special risk. Active immunization with live attenuated viral vaccine has reduced the incidence of measles infections.

PROGNOSIS

Uncomplicated measles is self-limiting. Malnutrition, inadequate treatment, and immunosuppression will worsen the prognosis.

SUGGESTED READING

1. Gupta SN, Gupta N, Gupta S. Modified measles versus rubella versus atypical measles: One and same thing. J Family Med Prim Care. 2015;4(4):566-9.

223 Sarcoidosis

➲ SYNONYMS

Mortimer's malady, Besnier–Boeck disease, Besnier–Boeck–Schaumann disease.

➲ HISTORY

Sarcoidosis was described initially by Sir Jonathan Hutchinson in 1875 and cutaneous sarcoidosis (lupus pernio) by Besnier in 1889.

➲ ETIOLOGY

Sarcoidosis is a multisystem granulomatous disease characterized by hyperactivity of the cell-mediated immune system. There is upregulation of $CD4^+$ T helper (Th) cells of the Th1 subtype. The identity of the antigen responsible for the cascade of events leading to granuloma formation in patients with sarcoidosis is uncertain. Genetic susceptibility is associated with human leukocyte antigen 1 (HLA-1), HLA-B8, and HLA-DR3 alleles.

➲ AGE GROUP

Bimodal distribution—it peaks between 25 and 35 years and 45 and 65 years.

➲ CLINICAL FEATURES

- *Systemic manifestation*: Lung disease occurs in approximately 90% of patients, ranging from alveolitis to granulomatous infiltration of the alveoli, blood vessels, bronchioles, pleura, and fibrous septa. Hilar and/or paratracheal lymphadenopathy, usually asymptomatic, occurs in 90% of patients. Granulomatous inflammation of the liver, spleen, and bone, as well as the kidney, gastrointestinal tract (upper and lower), and peripheral lymph nodes is seen. Ocular sarcoidosis involves granulomatous inflammation of the iris, ciliary body, choroid, retina, optic nerve, conjunctiva, or lacrimal glands.
- *Cutaneous manifestation*: Most commonly manifests as papules **(Fig. 1)** and plaques, often red-brown in color. Most common sites are the face, lips, neck, upper trunk, and extremities and are fairly symmetric in distribution. Upon diascopy, in which pressure induces blanching ("apple jelly") color is seen. Individual plaques can develop central clearing, leading to an annular configuration, or they can contain prominent telangiectasias (angiolupoid sarcoidosis). A classical finding is the development of cutaneous sarcoidosis within preexisting scars or at the sites of prior trauma.

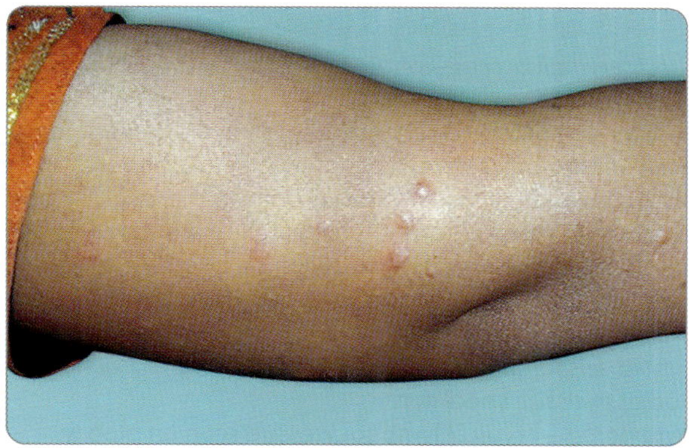

Fig. 1: Multiple papules over the forearm in papular sarcoid.

Less common presentations include hypopigmentation, subcutaneous nodules, ichthyosis, alopecia, ulcerations, erythroderma, and erythema multiforme.

- *Nonspecific cutaneous manifestation* is erythema nodosum, which is associated with subacute, transient sarcoidosis, usually resolves spontaneously, and generally does not require systemic corticosteroid therapy.
- *Nails*: Clubbing, subungual hyperkeratosis, and onycholysis.
- *Oral sarcoidosis*: It may involve mucosa, gingiva, hard palate, and major salivary glands.

SUBSETS

- Darier–Roussy disease
- *Lupus pernio*—papulonodules and plaques, primarily affecting areas most affected by cold (i.e., pernio), including the nose, ears, and cheeks; there is often a beaded appearance along the nasal rim.
- *Löfgren syndrome*—erythema nodosum with hilar adenopathy, fever, migrating polyarthritis, and acute iritis
- *Heerfordt syndrome*—parotid gland enlargement, uveitis, fever, and facial nerve palsy

HISTOPATHOLOGY

The histopathologic hallmark is the presence of superficial and deep dermal epithelioid cell granulomas, with minimal or absent associated lymphocytes or plasma cells ("naked tubercles"). Central caseation is usually absent. Multinucleated histiocytes ("giant cells") are usually of the Langhans type, may contain eosinophilic stellate inclusions known as asteroid bodies, or rounded laminated basophilic inclusions known as Schaumann bodies.

DERMOSCOPY

Small, grouped, translucent orange, globular structures associated with linear vessels of variable diameter and central scar-like areas are observed under dermoscopy.

DIFFERENTIAL DIAGNOSIS

- *Lupus erythematosus*—photosensitivity and follicular plugging on biopsy
- *Papular forms of secondary syphilis*—absence of granulomas and positive serological tests for syphilis
- *Acne agminata*—it usually occurs only on the face.
- *Tuberculoid leprosy*—anesthetic patches are seen; epithelioid granulomas with lymphocyte collar
- *Lupus vulgaris*—granulomas with lymphocyte cuffs are found in the dermis.
- *Lupoid leishmaniasis*—presence of *Leishmania donovani* (LD) bodies in tissue specimen
- *Lymphoma*—atypical lymphocytes are seen on biopsy.

COMPLICATIONS

Associated infections, e.g., cryptococcal infection, aspergillosis, and tuberculosis, are common. Infiltration due to granuloma leads to hypothyroidism, diabetes insipidus, and Cushing's syndrome. It may precede the onset of lymphoma (sarcoidosis–lymphoma syndrome).

TREATMENT

Corticosteroids, either in topical, intralesional, or systemic form, are the mainstay of therapy for systemic sarcoidosis. Oral prednisone 1 mg/kg/day for 4–6 weeks, followed by a slow tapering, is done. Hydroxychloroquine (200–400 mg/day) and chloroquine (250–500 mg/day) can be effective in controlling skin lesions. Other reported therapeutic agents for cutaneous disease include methotrexate (10–25 mg weekly), thalidomide (50–300 mg/day), isotretinoin (1 mg/kg/day for 3–8 months), minocycline (200 mg/day), and allopurinol (100–300 mg/day). Infliximab and adalimumab may be used. Benefit from leflunomide has also been reported.

PROGNOSIS

Females, less severe pulmonary involvement at the onset, patients with positive tuberculin test, and normal globulin levels have good prognosis. HLA-8 is associated with spontaneous resolution.

SUGGESTED READING

1. Jadotte YT, Abdel Hay R, Salphale P, Mocellin S, Kumar S, Niazi A, et al. Interventions for cutaneous sarcoidosis. Cochrane Database Syst Rev. 2018;2018(8):CD010817.

224 Scabies

➲ SYNONYMS

Itch mite infestation, seven-year itch.

➲ HISTORY

In 1687, Bonomo and Cestoni rediscovered the itch mite and established its etiological role in the disease.

➲ ETIOLOGY

Sarcoptes scabiei variant hominis, the causative agent of human scabies, belongs to the suborder Astigmata and family *Sarcoptidae*. Transmission occurs via direct close contact with an infested person; fomite transmission may also occur.

➲ AGE GROUP

Children—the prevalence is the highest in the age group <5 years.

➲ CLINICAL FEATURES

Itching is the predominant symptom. The itching of scabies is characteristically described as "worse at night."

Scabies characteristically involves the webs of the fingers **(Fig. 1)**, flexor aspects of the wrists, elbows, anterior axillary folds, umbilicus and periumbilical region, genitalia, upper thighs, knees, and ankles. In females, the nipple and areola are also involved. The

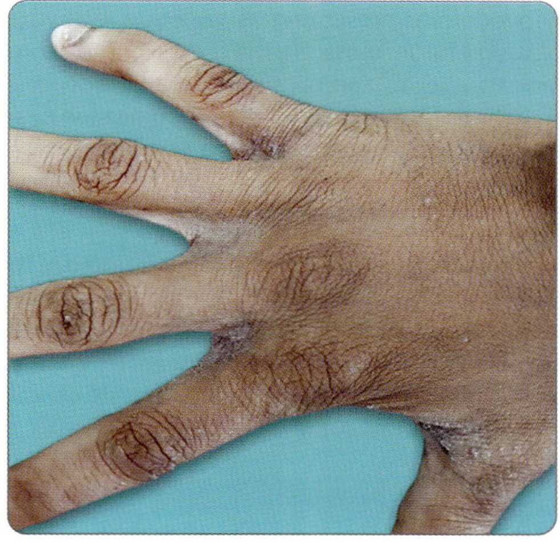

Fig. 1: Multiple excoriated papules in the web spaces.

back is rarely affected. The lower parts of the buttocks and natal cleft are common sites.

An imaginary line intersecting the main sites of involvement—the axilla, elbow, flexures, wrists and hand, and crotch—is called the circle of Hebra. The burrow is the pathognomonic lesion of scabies. It is a serpentine, threadlike, grayish, or dark line, varying in length from a few millimeters to a centimeter or more. The open end is marked by a minute papule or papulovesicle. The mite may be discerned as a whitish dot at the closed end. They are more easily seen in the thin skin of infants and children, where they tend to occur commonly on the palms and soles.

VARIANTS OF SCABIES

- *Scabies in infants*—have florid manifestations of excoriations, crusting, secondary pyoderma, and eczematization
- *Nodular scabies*—persistent dull-red nodules in the elbows, anterior axillary folds, genitalia, and gluteal folds
- *Scabies in clean*—moderate itching with few scattered wheals and papules
- *Crusted/Norwegian scabies*—hyperkeratotic, crusty, scaly lesions with a large number of mites associated with malnutrition, lepromatous leprosy, Down syndrome, diabetes, beriberi, and senile dementia
- *Scabies incognito*—scabies is treated with topical/systemic corticosteroids.
- *Animal-transmitted scabies*—dogs are a major source; when contracted, it is termed pseudoscabies. Burrows are absent. The classical sites are not involved.

DERMOSCOPY

On dermoscopy, "jet with contrail" appearance and "hang glider sign" are seen.

COMPLICATIONS

Secondary pyodermas presenting as impetigo, ecthyma, cellulitis, lymphangitis, and furunculosis are the most common complications. Apart from the local complications, the incidence of acute glomerulonephritis (AGN) occurring as a complication of secondarily infected scabies is probably not appreciated fully.

HISTOPATHOLOGY

A patchy to diffuse infiltrate with eosinophils is noted in the reticular dermis. On transection, a scabies mite may occasionally be seen within the epidermis. Pink "pigtail"-like structures attached to the stratum corneum (which represent fragments of the adult mite exoskeleton) can serve as a clue to the diagnosis of scabies when mites, scybala, or eggs are not identified.

DIFFERENTIAL DIAGNOSIS

Unless skin burrows are noted clinically, all diseases associated with pruritus and infected lesions have to be considered in the differential diagnosis. In particular, atopic, contact, or nummular dermatitis, autosensitization ("id" reaction), pyoderma, dermatitis herpetiformis, bullous pemphigoid, syphilis, pediculosis, and other insect bites should be considered.

PROGNOSIS

Pruritus and lesions can persist for 2–4 weeks after successful treatment. This is often referred to as "postscabetic pruritus." They do not imply treatment failure but rather represent the body's response to dead mites that are eventually sloughed off (within 2 weeks) along with natural epidermal exfoliation. The second application of topical medication is performed in order to reduce the potential for reinfestation from fomites as well as to ensure the killing of any nymphs that may have hatched as a result of the semiprotective environment within the egg that allowed them to survive.

TREATMENT

Permethrin 5% should be applied overnight and repeated after 7 days; also used are benzyl benzoate 25% (three nights), lindane 1% lotion, and sulfur 6% ointment in petrolatum (three nights), crotamiton 10%, and malathion 0.5%. Oral ivermectin 200 μ/kg body weight can be used in children >5 years of age. Persistent nodular scabies clears with topical corticosteroids or intralesional steroids. In refractory cases, systemic methotrexate has been successfully used. The upcoming effective single-dose treatment for scabies is oral moxidectin.

SUGGESTED READING

1. Sunderkötter C, Wohlrab J, Hamm H. Scabies: Epidemiology, Diagnosis, and Treatment. Dtsch Arztebl Int. 2021;118(41):695-704.

225 Scarlet Fever

➲ SYNONYM

Scarlatina.

➲ HISTORY

Scarlet fever was first described in the medical literature by the Sicilian anatomist and physician Giovanni Filippo Ingrassia. The association of streptococci and disease was first described in 1874 by Billroth.

➲ ETIOLOGY

An acute infection caused by the strains of *Streptococcus pyogenes* producing three antigenically unrelated types A, B, and C exotoxin. Toxin production is exclusive to group A streptococci.

➲ AGE GROUP

Scarlet fever occurs in the age of 1–10 years, and is rare in infancy and old age.

➲ CLINICAL FEATURES

Incubation period is 2–5 days. Initially, fever, anorexia, and vomiting occur. If the portal of entry is the throat, then acute follicular or membranous tonsillitis with painful lymphadenopathy occurs. If the portal of entry is a wound, then there is increased tenderness with serous discharge. Rash appears on the second day, initially on the upper trunk. It is a finely punctate erythema, which has been likened to "sunburn with goose pimples." The area around the mouth is spared.

Transverse red streaks in skin folds due to capillary fragility are called Pastia's lines. Oral mucous membrane is bright red, and deeper red puncta are seen on the palate (Forchheimer spots are fleeting small red spots on the soft palate). By the second or third day, scattered, swollen, red papillae give "white strawberry tongue"/raspberry tongue appearance.

There is marked leukocytosis, with neutrophilia and eosinophilia. Erythrocyte sedimentation rate (ESR) is elevated.

The Dick test was invented in 1924 and was used as a test to identify those susceptible to scarlet fever. It is obsolete now.

➲ COMPLICATIONS

Local complications include peritonsillar and retropharyngeal abscesses. Myocarditis, hepatitis, arthritis, meningitis, osteomyelitis, rheumatic fever, and glomerulonephritis may also occur.

DIFFERENTIAL DIAGNOSIS

Differential diagnosis includes rubella, smallpox—early stage, staphylococcal infections, Kawasaki disease, toxic shock syndrome, and drug rash.

TREATMENT

Penicillin 250 mg PO QID for 10 days and benzathine penicillin 1–2 million units intramuscularly (IM) can be given. Clinical response can be expected within 24–48 hours.

PROGNOSIS

Prognosis is good; the mortality of treated cases is <1%.

SUGGESTED READING

1. Basetti S, Hodgson J, Rawson TM, Majeed A. Scarlet fever: a guide for general practitioners. London J Prim Care (Abingdon). 2017;9(5):77-9.

226 Schamberg Disease

➲ SYNONYMS

Progressive pigmented purpuric dermatitis, progressive pigmentary dermatosis of Schamberg, purpura pigmentosa progressive, Schamberg's purpura.

➲ HISTORY

Jay Frank Schamberg described it in 1901.

➲ AGE AND SEX

This disease is more common in males and may occur at any age from childhood onward.

➲ ETIOLOGY

Schamberg's disease is caused by leaky capillaries near the surface of the skin, which allow red blood cells to slip through into the skin, which disintegrate and release their iron that causes a rust color, and this accounts for the orange tint of the rash. Gravity and increased venous pressure are important localizing factors in many cases. Exercise may be a provoking factor. Few common drugs implicated in etiology are nonsteroidal anti-inflammatory drugs (NSAIDs), amlodipine, and injection medroxyprogesterone acetate. It constitutes 50% of cases of capillaritis. Others include itching purpura (eczematid-like purpura of Doucas and Kapetanakis) (about 10%), pigmented purpuric lichenoid dermatosis of Gougerot and Blum (about 5%), lichen aureus (about 10%), and purpura annularis telangiectoides (Majocchi's disease).

➲ CLINICAL FEATURES

The condition affects the legs and often spreads slowly. The lesions are most frequent on the lower limbs but may occur anywhere on the body, including the hands. They may vary in number. Punctate purpuric macules develop on the lower extremities **(Fig. 1)**, particularly around the ankle and on the pretibial region. Widespread lesions with the involvement of the trunk or upper extremities may rarely occur. The confluence of lesions produces irregularly shaped larger macules that may have a brownish color. They may appear as irregular patches of orange or brown pigmentation due to hemosiderin (iron), with characteristic "cayenne pepper" spots appearing within and at the edge of old lesions. There are usually no symptoms, although there may be some slight itching. The eruption may persist for many years. The pattern of the eruption changes, with slow extension and often some clearing of the original lesions.

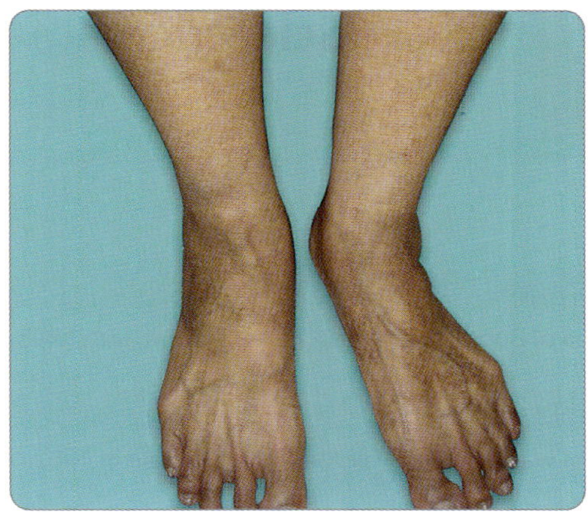

Fig. 1: Punctate purpuric macules over the lower limbs.

➲ HISTOPATHOLOGY

Pathologically, these disorders are characterized by narrowing of the lumen and endothelial swelling of superficial small vessels, accompanied by perivascular T-lymphocytic infiltration, extravasation of erythrocytes, and hemosiderin deposits in macrophages.

➲ DIFFERENTIAL DIAGNOSIS

Differential diagnosis includes venous stasis, postinflammatory hyperpigmentation, drug reactions, and viral exanthema.

➲ TREATMENT

- There is no cure for Schamberg's disease; however, the itching can be controlled by a cortisone cream. Colchicine and vitamin C have been tried.
- First line—nonpharmacological interventions (wearing support stockings) and topical steroids
- Second line—pentoxifylline, narrowband ultraviolet B (NB-UVB), ascorbic acid, and colchicine 0.5 g BD
- Thioglycolic peel, which chelates iron, has shown promising results in improving cosmetic appearance.

➲ SUGGESTED READING

1. Sardana K, Sarkar R, Sehgal VN. Pigmented purpuric dermatoses: an overview. Int J Dermatol. 2004;43(7):482-8.

227 Scleredema

➲ SYNONYMS

Scleredema of Buschke, scleredema adultorum, Buschke's disease.

➲ HISTORY

Scleredema was described by Abraham Buschke in 1902.

➲ ETIOLOGY

Most children and adolescents develop this condition after an upper respiratory tract infection. Streptococcal infection is most commonly identified. In adulthood, the association with adult-onset diabetes mellitus is the second most common presentation. It can also be associated with paraproteinemia or multiple myeloma.

➲ AGE AND SEX

Female-to-male ratio is 2:1.

Although scleredema is referred to as scleredema adultorum, 50% of scleredema cases occur in individuals <20 years.

➲ CLINICAL FEATURES

There is an acute onset of nonpitting induration of the neck, shoulders, and upper back skin **(Fig. 1)**, followed by the involvement of the face and arms. The affected skin appears smooth and waxy, with tense dermal induration and prominent follicular ostia, at times giving a peau d'orange appearance. Scleredema involving the esophagus, bone marrow, nerve, liver, or salivary glands is found rarely. There is an absence of Raynaud's phenomenon, differentiating it from scleroderma.

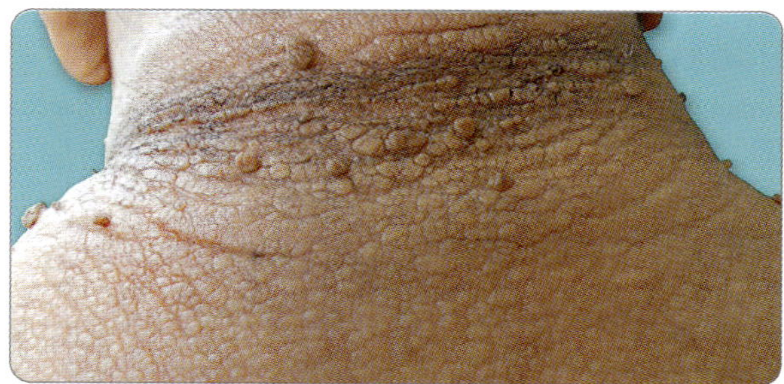

Fig. 1: Nonpitting induration over the neck and shoulders in a diabetic male with scleredema diabeticorum. Note the associated acanthosis nigricans and skin tags.

There are three clinical subgroups:

- *Group 1*—follows acute respiratory infection, usually clears spontaneously in 6 months to 2 years. The duration is not affected by the use of antibiotics.
- *Group 2*—disease occurs insidiously, with no preceding illness, and encompasses cases with monoclonal gammopathy.
- *Group 3*—associated with diabetes mellitus (scleredema diabeticorum)

HISTOPATHOLOGY

The proportion of the dermis is very significantly increased in comparison to adjacent nonaffected skin. There is deposition of mucin between dermal collagen bundles. The deposition is the greatest in the deep dermis. Fibroblasts are normal in number and morphology.

DIFFERENTIAL DIAGNOSIS

- *Primary systemic amyloidosis*—deposition of homogenous masses of amyloid in dermal papillae, which show apple green fluorescence on Congo red stain and polarized microscopy
- *Dermatomyositis*—other systemic involvement and antibody profile
- *Scleroderma*—homogenization of dermal collagen, absence of mucin deposition, and positive antibody profile
- *Cellulitis*—erythema, edema, and local rise in temperature are seen.
- *Sclerema neonatorum*—areas of thick skin are seen in babies with poor general condition.
- Subcutaneous fat necrosis of the newborn.

TREATMENT

Treatment of the associated disease (improved glucose control and treatment of paraproteinemia); ultraviolet A1 phototherapy has been proved effective in a few adult patients. Scleredema has responded to local radiotherapy or electron-beam irradiation, and that associated with monoclonal gammopathy showed a response to extracorporeal photophoresis. Other tried treatment modalities are steroids, methotrexate, cyclosporine, prostaglandin E1, factor XIII, high-dose penicillin, and D-penicillamine.

PROGNOSIS

Postinfectious scleredema usually abates in 1–2 years. Scleredema associated with adult-onset diabetes tends to be more protracted, but some patients appear to improve with better glucose control. Gammopathy-associated disease is more chronic.

SUGGESTED READING

1. Shrestha B, Neopane AK, Panth R. Scleredema-an uncommon cause of swelling in a child-a case report and review of the literature. BMC Res Notes. 2014;7:571.

228 Sclerema Neonatorum

➲ SYNONYM

Sclerema adiposum.

➲ HISTORY

Underwood described sclerema neonatorum in 1784 and termed it "skinbound disease." In 1817, Alibert introduced the term sclerema, derived from the Greek word *skleros*, meaning hard.

➲ ETIOLOGY

Sclerema neonatorum is the inflammation of the subcutaneous fat. Infants have a higher saturated-to-unsaturated fatty acid ratio and, thus, a higher melting point. Prematurity, hypothermia, shock, and metabolic abnormalities further increase this ratio, possibly as a result of enzymatic alteration allowing precipitation of fatty acid crystals within the lipocytes.

➲ AGE GROUP

Sclerema neonatorum affects neonates.

➲ CLINICAL FEATURES

The affected baby is severely ill, and cutaneous lesions appear during the first few days of life. Lesions usually begin on the buttocks and thighs as diffuse, yellow-white woody induration of the skin that rapidly expands to involve large areas of the body. This results in immobility of the body.

➲ HISTOPATHOLOGY

The inflammatory infiltrate is sparse or even absent in the subcutaneous fat, reflecting the poor immunologic response of the severely ill infant. The most characteristic feature is the presence of radially arranged, needle-shaped clefts in adipocytes.

➲ COMPLICATIONS

Flexion contractures at the elbows, knees, and hips; temperature instability; restricted respiration; difficulty in feeding; and decreased spontaneous movement.

➲ DIFFERENTIAL DIAGNOSIS

Differential diagnosis includes Hutchinson–Gilford progeria, scleredema, and subcutaneous fat necrosis of the newborn.

➲ TREATMENT

Underlying disease should be treated. Repeated exchange transfusions may reduce mortality.

➲ PROGNOSIS

Prognosis is poor. Most infants die within a few days.

➲ SUGGESTED READINGS

1. Dorjay K, Dolker S, Arif T, Adil M, Ganju S. Sclerema Neonatorum. Indian J Paediatr Dermatol. 2019;20(4):302-5.
2. Nakalema G, Egesa WI, Kumbakulu PK, Nduwimana M, Anaya AD, Kizito MS, et al. Sclerema Neonatorum in a Term Infant: A Case Report and Literature Review. Case Rep Pediatr. 2020;2020:8837064.

229 Scleroderma

SYNONYM

Systemic sclerosis.

HISTORY

The first definite description was by Carlo Curzio. Scleroderma is derived from the Greek words skleros (hard or indurated) and derma (skin).

ETIOLOGY

Major facets of the disease include inflammation, vasculopathy, and connective tissue-producing cell. The first inflammatory infiltrates in lesional skin are predominantly cells of monocyte lineage. Later, T lymphocytes predominate, and these demonstrate subpopulations of memory cells. Deposition of excessive extracellular matrix in specialized organs causes much of the morbidity and mortality of the disease.

AGE AND SEX

Incidence is 4–9 times higher in women than in men with the peak onset at 30–50 years.

CLINICAL FEATURES

Localized cutaneous systemic sclerosis (SSc):

- Long preexisting history of Raynaud's phenomenon
- Skin sclerosis spares proximal sites **(Figs. 1 and 2)**.
- Anticentromere antibodies positive.
- Includes classic CREST (Calcinosis cutis, Raynaud phenomenon, Esophageal dysfunction, Sclerodactyly, Telangiectasia)
- Low frequency of scleroderma renal crisis

Diffuse cutaneous SSc:

- Proximal skin sclerosis (upper arms, thighs, chest, and abdomen)
- Close temporal relationship between onset of Raynaud and skin sclerosis
- High frequency of pulmonary fibrosis, cardiac involvement, and scleroderma renal crisis
- Often Scl-70 or anti-RNPIII positive.

Systemic sine scleroderma—lacks skin changes, but has systemic manifestations.

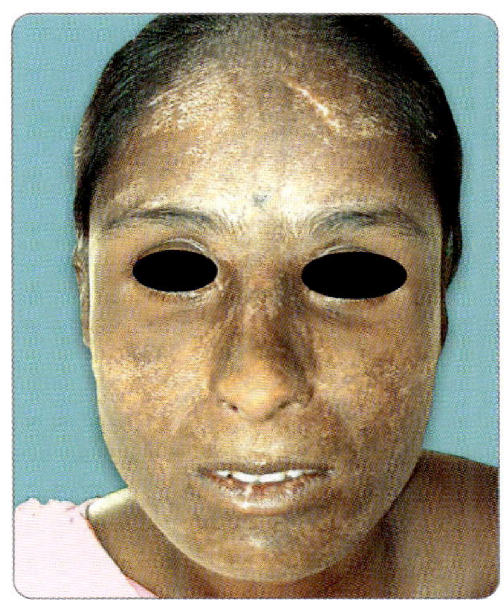

Fig. 1: Mask-like face with loss of skin creases, radial furrowing around the mouth, and salt and pepper pigmentation.

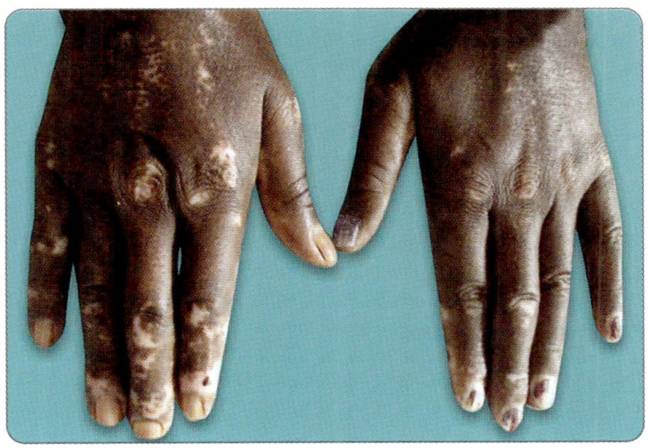

Fig. 2: Hidebound skin over the digits with sclerodactyly.

The American College of Rheumatology (ACR) criteria for the classification of systemic sclerosis require one major criterion or two minor criteria, as follows:

- *Major criterion*: Scleroderma proximal to the metacarpophalangeal or metatarsophalangeal joints
- *Minor criteria*:
  - Sclerodactyly
  - Digital pitting scars or a loss of substance from the finger pad
  - Bibasilar pulmonary fibrosis

➲ HISTOPATHOLOGY

Histopathology shows fibrosis of the lower two-thirds of the dermis and the subcutaneous fibrous trabeculae. Panniculitis may also be prominent. The subcutaneous fat is replaced by fibrous connective tissue. In the dermis, collagen bundles appear pale, homogenous, and swollen, and there may be a sparse perivascular lymphocytic infiltrate **(Figs. 3 and 4)**.

➲ DERMOSCOPY

Active lesions show white clouds and linear branching vessels. Brownish structureless areas were seen in inactive lesions of limited cutaneous scleroderma. Erythematous areas, linear branching vessels, dotted vessels, and crystalline structures were seen in pressure locations.

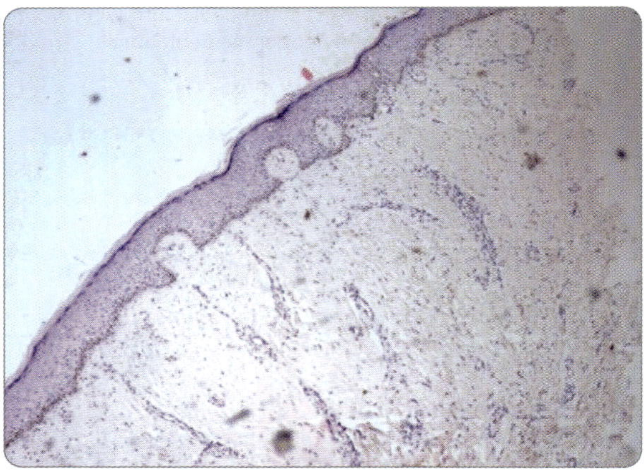

Fig. 3: The epidermis is normal. The collagen bundles are thickened, closely packed, and hypocellular. The appendages are atrophic, lying higher in the dermis.

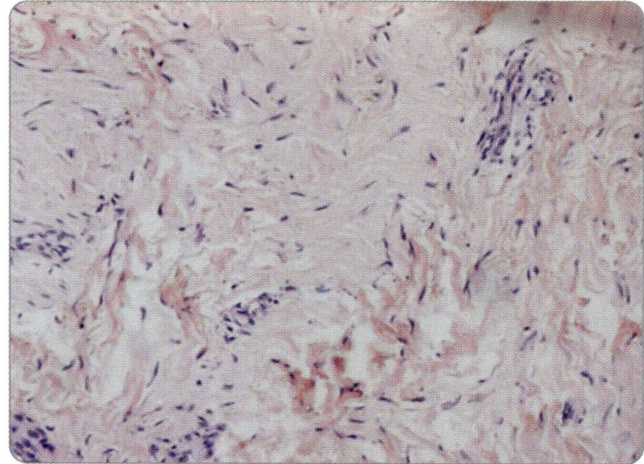

Fig. 4: Dermis showing pale homogenous collagen bundles, sparse inflammatory infiltrate.

DIFFERENTIAL DIAGNOSIS

Differential diagnosis includes generalized and multiple plaque morphea (absence of systemic features), primary Raynaud's phenomenon, systemic lupus erythematosus (presence of malar rash, photosensitivity, oral ulcers and other systemic features, positive ANA, anti-dsDNA), rheumatoid disease (positive RA factor, absence sclerosis), dermato/polymyositis (presence of muscular pain, tenderness, associated classical cutaneous signs), cryoglobulinemia (raised cryoglobulin levels), cold agglutinin disease, hyperviscosity syndromes, macrovascular disease, amyloidosis, acromegaly, mycosis fungoides, porphyria cutanea tarda, and eosinophilic fasciitis.

COMPLICATIONS

Complications include digital vasculopathy and its complications, renal disease, pulmonary arterial hypertension, pulmonary fibrosis, gastrointestinal complications, myositis, and cardiac complications.

TREATMENT

Immunomodulatory treatment includes cyclosporine A, methotrexate, D-penicillamine, cyclophosphamide, immuno-ablation/stem cell transplantation, extracorporeal photopheresis, antithymocyte globulin, and mycophenolate mofetil. Ultraviolet A (UVA) therapy, narrow band (NB) UVB therapy, vitamin D derivatives, and antimalarials such as chloroquine and hydroxychloroquine have been tried.

PROGNOSIS

The prognosis is good for limited cutaneous scleroderma, but is worse for those with the diffuse cutaneous disease, particularly in older age, and for males. Death occurs most often from pulmonary, heart, and kidney complications.

SUGGESTED READING

1. Albuquerque JV, Andriolo BN, Vasconcellos MR, Civile VT, Lyddiatt A, Trevisani VF. Interventions for morphea. Cochrane Database Syst Rev. 2019;7(7):CD005027.

230 Scrofuloderma

➲ SYNONYM

Tuberculosis colliquativa cutis.

➲ ETIOLOGY

Scrofuloderma is a subcutaneous tuberculosis leading to cold abscess formation and a secondary breakdown of the overlying skin. Scrofuloderma represents contiguous involvement of the skin overlying another site of infection.

➲ AGE GROUP

Prevalence is higher among children, adolescents, and the aged.

➲ CLINICAL FEATURES

Scrofuloderma mainly occurs in the parotid, submandibular, and supraclavicular regions and may be bilateral. It first presents as a firm, subcutaneous nodule, usually well defined, freely movable, and asymptomatic. Later liquefaction and perforation occurs, causing ulcers and sinuses. The ulcers are linear or serpiginous with undermined, inverted, bluish edges and soft, granulating floors **(Fig. 1)**. Sinusoidal tracts undermine the skin. Scar tracts develop and bridge ulcerative areas or even stretches of normal skin. Tuberculin sensitivity is usually pronounced.

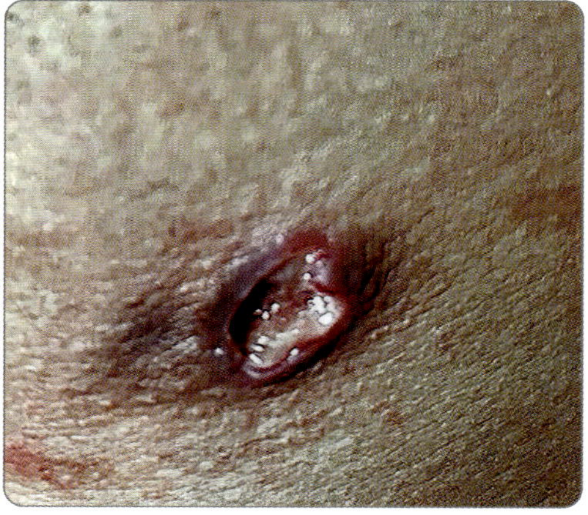

Fig. 1: Scrofuloderma.

HISTOPATHOLOGY

Massive necrosis and abscess formation in the center of the lesion are nonspecific. The periphery of the abscesses or the margins of the sinuses contain tuberculoid granulomas.

DERMOSCOPY

Dermoscopy shows yellow orange structureless areas, linear vessels with or without branches, serosanguineous crust, white structureless areas, and orange-brown scale. Ulceration have been described.

DIFFERENTIAL DIAGNOSIS

Mycobacterium avium—intracellulare lymphadenitis, *Mycobacterium scrofulaceum* infection, syphilitic gummas, sporotrichosis, actinomycosis, severe forms of acne conglobata, and hidradenitis suppurativa are the differential diagnoses.

COMPLICATIONS

Lupus vulgaris may develop at or near the site of scrofuloderma.

TREATMENT

Chemotherapy is the mainstay. Rifampicin 10 mg/kg, isoniazid 5 mg/kg, pyrazinamide 30 mg/kg, ethambutol 15 mg/kg, and streptomycin 15 mg/kg can be given. Surgical intervention is also quite helpful.

SUGGESTED READING

1. Khadka P, Koirala S, Thapaliya J. Cutaneous Tuberculosis: Clinicopathologic Arrays and Diagnostic Challenges. Dermatol Res Pract. 2018;2018: 7201973.

231 Sebaceous Cyst

➲ SYNONYM

Epidermal cyst.

➲ ETIOLOGY

Sebaceous cyst results from damage to pilosebaceous unit. It can also occur due to penetrating trauma to the skin. So, it is a retention cyst, also called epidermal cyst as cyst is lined by superficial squamous cells.

➲ AGE GROUP

Sebaceous cyst may occur in any age group, anywhere in the body but most commonly seen in scalp, face, neck, shoulders, chest, and scrotum.

➲ CLINICAL FEATURES

Sebaceous is a typical cystic swelling, spherical in shape, nontender, smooth surface, and a punctum, which indicates blocked opening of the duct **(Fig. 1)**. Cyst is usually fixed to the skin, and there is indentation on pressure with fingertip with negative trans-illumination test.

Scrotal sebaceous cysts are usually multiple, feel solid, and punctum is often not visible.

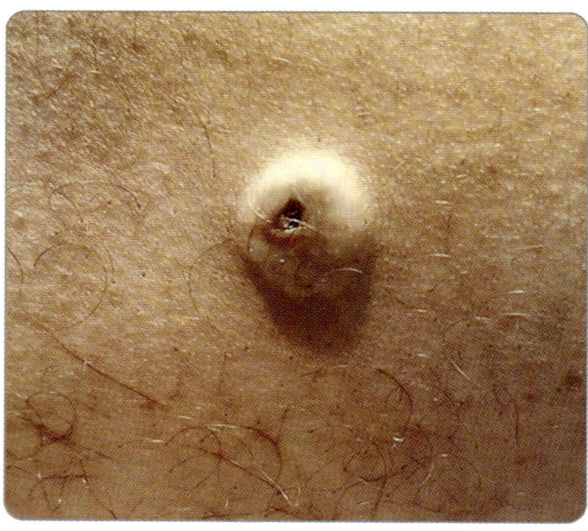

Fig. 1: A spherical, smooth surfaced cystic swelling with a punctum.

HISTOPATHOLOGY

The cysts are lined by an epidermis like epithelium including a granular cell layer. The cysts contain laminated keratin.

DIFFERENTIAL DIAGNOSIS

- Lipoma—firm mobile swelling, slip sign positive
- Dermoid cyst—mostly at midline or paramedian location, absence of secretion
- Neurofibroma—buttonhole sign positive
- Fibroma—lack of punctum and cheesy secretion
- Pilar cyst—lack the punctum
- Milia—white smooth shaped papules, smaller, no secretion

COMPLICATIONS

Complications can be infection, ulceration, sebaceous horn, calcification, and malignancy. When the sebaceous cyst of the scalp ulcerates, excessive granulation tissue forms resembling fungating epithelioma, and is called Cock's peculiar tumor. Slow discharge of the sebum from a wide punctum sometimes hardens and forms sebaceous horn.

DIAGNOSIS

Ultrasonography shows round to oval structure, well-circumscribed, avascular mass located in the dermis and subcutaneous tissue along with the phenomena of dorsal acoustic amplification and lateral shadowing.

PROGNOSIS

Persistent cyst wall leads to recurrence.

TREATMENT

Total excision of the cyst is the treatment of choice, which can be done by dissection method or incision–avulsion technique.

SUGGESTED READING

1. Hoang VT, Trinh CT, Nguyen CH, Chansomphou V, Chansomphou V, Tran TTT. Overview of epidermoid cyst. Eur J Radiol Open. 2019;6:291-301.

232 Seborrheic Keratosis

➲ SYNONYMS

Senile keratosis, basal cell papilloma, senile wart.

➲ HISTORY

In 1927, Frudenthal delineated their clinical and histologic features.

➲ ETIOLOGY

An apparent familial predisposition with a postulated autosomal dominant inheritance with incomplete penetrance, aggravated by sun exposure.

Androgen receptor polymorphism, alteration in distribution of epidermal growth factor (EGF) receptors, and somatic activating mutations in gene that codes fibroblast growth factor FGF receptor 3 are implicated.

➲ AGE GROUP

Seborrheic keratosis (SK) affects elderly individuals.

➲ CLINICAL FEATURES

Seborrheic keratoses arise spontaneously and are most concentrated on the trunk, although the extremities, head, and neck may be involved. They appear as round to oval, variably verrucous, coin-like plaques that vary in size from several millimeters to centimeters **(Fig. 1)**. They exhibit a uniform tan to dark-brown color and usually have a velvety to granular surface with a stuck on appearance.

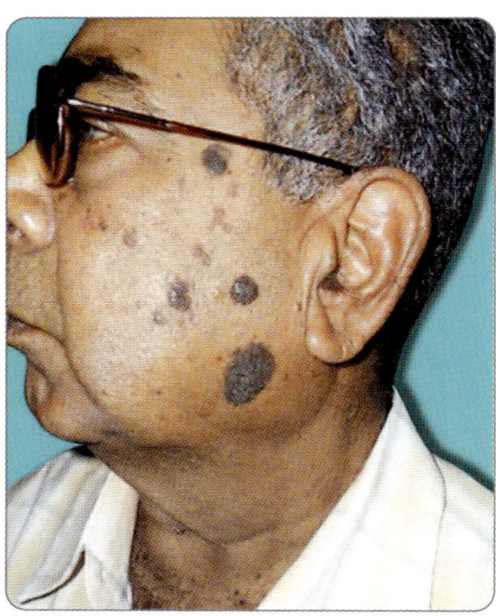

Fig. 1: Coin-shaped hyperkeratotic plaques of seborrheic keratosis.

The explosive onset of multiple SKs in association with internal malignancy is known as the sign of Leser–Trélat, most commonly adenocarcinoma of the stomach. Recently, this rare paraneoplastic syndrome has been linked to an overproduction of alpha-transforming growth factor (α-TGF) by the primary malignant tumor.

HISTOPATHOLOGY

The architecture of most SKs is exophytic, and lesions tend to be sharply demarcated from the adjacent epidermis. They are composed of sheets of small cells that resemble basal cells of the normal epidermis. Often exuberant keratin production occurs at the surface of SKs, and small keratin-filled cysts (horn cysts) and cystic keratin-filled downgrowths from the surface of the lesion into the main tumor mass (pseudo-horn cysts) are characteristic features. Borst–Jadassohn phenomenon can be seen in SK.

Histopathological variants of SK include classical exophytic/acanthotic type, adenoid/reticulate type, hyperkeratotic variant, irritated SK, flat SK, pigmented SK, and melanoacanthoma.

DERMOSCOPY

- *Milia-like cysts—there are two types*:
  1. Tiny white starry
  2. Larger yellowish cloudy
- Irregular crypts
- Fissures/Ridges
- Blue-gray globules
- Light brown fingerprint-like parallel structures
- "Fat fingers" (the gyri of a cerebriform surface)

DIFFERENTIAL DIAGNOSIS

- Epidermal nevi—proliferation of nevus cells
- Acrochordon—fibroepithelial polypoid structure which is pedunculated
- Verruca vulgaris—verrucous surface, koebnerization seen, and koilocytes on biopsy
- Acrokeratosis verruciformis—flat hypo- to hyperpigmented macules on dorsum of hands
- Eccrine poroma—raised lesion associated with pain, serosanguineous discharge
- Bowens disease—larger patches to plaques with areas of crusting, full-thickness epidermal dysplasia is seen
- Squamous cell carcinoma (SCC)—plenty of horn pearls on biopsy
- Actinic keratosis

COMPLICATIONS

None if not manipulated.

TREATMENT

The primary reason for treatment of SKs is cosmetic. Curettage, cryosurgery, excision, and laser ablation are the various treatment modalities available. 40% hydrogen peroxide topical solution and an aqueous nitric–zinc complex solution containing nitric acid, zinc and copper salts, and organic acids (acetic, lactic, and oxalic acid) are under trial for treatment of SKs.

➲ PROGNOSIS

Seborrheic keratoses demonstrate an indolent biologic course characterized by slow enlargement followed by long-term stability. The incidence of malignant degeneration is exceedingly small, although rare instances of associated basal and squamous cell carcinoma have been observed.

➲ SUGGESTED READING

1. Wollina U. Recent advances in managing and understanding seborrheic keratosis. F1000Res. 2019;8:F1000 Faculty Rev-1520.

233 Seborrheic Melanosis

➲ INTRODUCTION

Seborrheic melanosis describes the localized darkening on some seborrheic areas of the face, such as the alar grooves, angles of the mouth, and labiomental crease.

It commonly affects dark individuals from Asia, Africa, and Hispanic population.

➲ CLINICAL FEATURES

Brownish-black pigmentation typically is seen over the seborrheic areas **(Fig. 1)**, forehead, beard areas, retroauricular, neck, upper part of chest, and interscapular areas. It is usually accompanied by erythema and itching especially in patients with seborrheic diathesis (seborrhea and pityriasis capitis). Hyperpigmentation is of melanotic and postinflammatory type.

➲ DERMOSCOPY

Whitish yellow excrescences of sebum coating the vellus hair shafts and prominent follicle openings were common to call. Apart from this, three patterns—vascular, pigmented, and mixed—have been described. Vascular pattern shows a light pink background with out of focus linear and arborizing vessels. Pigment pattern shows prominent hyperpigmented pseudonetwork and annular granular structures. Mixed pattern shows a combination of pigmentation and erythema.

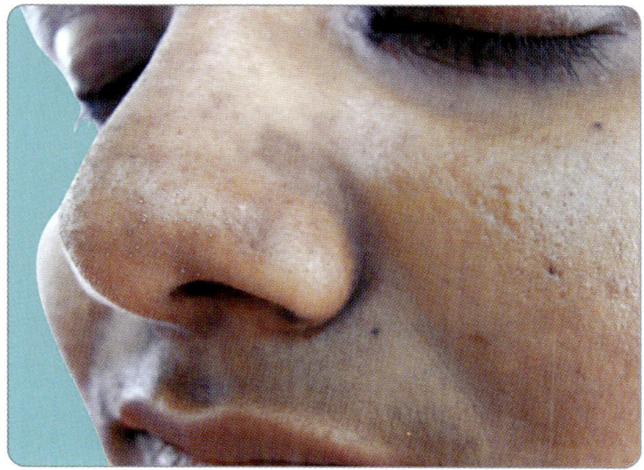

Fig. 1: Pigmentation over nasolabial area in seborrheic melanosis.

DIFFERENTIAL DIAGNOSIS

Differential diagnosis includes tar melanosis, which usually involves the dorsa of hands unlike seborrheic melanosis.

TREATMENT

Topical anti-inflammatory/fungistatic agents effective in seborrheic dermatitis (SD) such as topical calcineurin inhibitors, mild topical steroids, and 2% ketoconazole cream should be tried initially, to allow any inflammatory component to subside, following this, skin-lightning agents such as kojic acid, azelaic acid, and arbutin can be used.

Topical therapy, with hydroquinone, benzoyl peroxide, azelaic acid, etc., can be used.

Sun protection, as it intensifies pigmentation, can be recommended.

PROGNOSIS

Chronic and resistant to therapy.

SUGGESTED READING

1. Vashisht KR, Garg S. Seborrheic Melanosis: A Unique Under-recognized Entity in Ethnic Skin. J Clin Aesthet Dermatol. 2022;15(1):15-6.

234 Seborrheic Dermatitis

➲ SYNONYMS

Pityrosporum dermatitis, dermatitis of the sebaceous areas.

➲ ETIOLOGY

Malassezia species has been implicated. Sebaceous glands become active during puberty and after, which correlates with the increased incidence in this age group. In seborrheic dermatitis of infancy, maternal androgens stimulate the sebaceous glands in first few months of life. It has also been established as an early marker of human immunodeficiency virus (HIV) infection. It is common in Parkinsonism, myocardial ischemia, malabsorption, epilepsy, obesity, and alcoholism.

➲ AGE GROUP

Most common age group is between 18 and 40 years. It is also seen in first few months of infancy. It is also more common in males.

➲ CLINICAL FEATURES

Commonly involves the hairy areas of scalp, face, presternal areas, and interscapular areas. In the scalp, dandruff is the earliest manifestation. They present as sharply marginated patches with greasy scales and may extend beyond the frontal hairline as "corona seborrheica". Erythema, greasy scales, and crusted fissures can develop behind the ears. On the face, lesions develop usually over medial part of eyebrows, glabella, and nasolabial folds. Blepharitis can develop. Precipitation can occur by stress, fatigue, or exposure to sunlight. On the trunk, the most common presentation is of the "petaloid" form, seen in interscapular area or front of chest as small reddish brown papules covered with a greasy scale. A rare variety, pityriasiform, can also occur, having a generalized erythematosquamous eruption. Psoriasiform lesions may also occur **(Fig. 1)**. Flexural variety involves the groins, anogenital, and umbilical areas manifests as an intertrigo with diffuse sharply marginated erythema and greasy scaling. Erythroderma can also occur.

➲ ASSOCIATED SYNDROMES

Associated syndromes include human immunodeficiency virus infection, atopy, and psoriasis.

➲ HISTOPATHOLOGY

Histopathology shows features of both psoriasis and chronic dermatitis. Stratum corneum shows parakeratosis, slight acan-

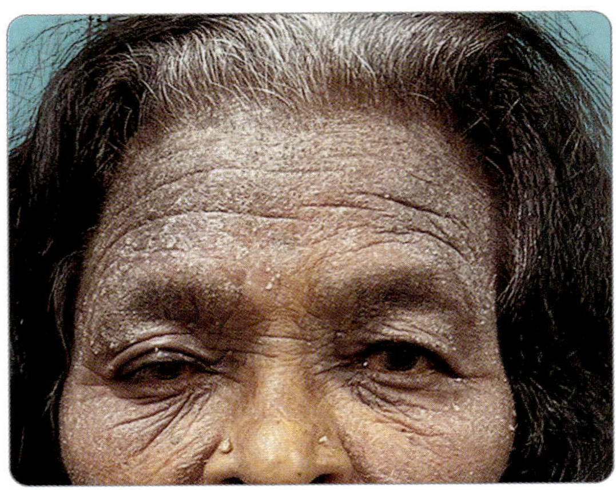

Fig. 1: Extensive seborrheic dermatitis in an immunocompromised patient.

thosis, and spongiosis, which differentiate it from psoriasis. Initial event is a "squirting papilla", capillary dilatation of papillae followed by migration of inflammatory cells through epidermis, leading to spongiosis. Epidermal proliferation is increased and so is desquamation. *Malassezia* yeasts are more prominent in patients with HIV infection.

➲ DERMOSCOPY

Dermoscopy shows arborizing vessels, atypical vessel, and yellowish interfollicular scaling.

➲ DIFFERENTIAL DIAGNOSIS

- Psoriasis—nongreasy white scales, well-defined plaques on the body with classical nail changes
- Infective dermatitis complicating pediculosis—nits and lice can be seen.
- Contact allergy—erythema, papules, and vesiculopustules are seen.
- Trichophyton tonsurans infection (scalp)—demonstration of fungal elements in the scales
- Lichen simplex (nape of neck)
- Pityriasis rosea—collarette of scales is present; herald patch is also seen.
- Tinea corporis—central clearing and peripheral scaling characteristic; fungal hyphae are seen in KOH mount.
- *Candida* infections in flexures
- Pityriasis versicolor—banana and grapes appearance on KOH mount
- Darier's disease—dirty, warty, greasy papules; V-nicking of nail plate; cobblestoning of mucosa; corps ronds and grains in histopathological examination (HPE)
- Zinc deficiency

➲ COMPLICATIONS

Fissuring can lead to eczematization; superadded infections, and erythroderma.

➲ TREATMENT

There is no permanent cure; it can only be suppressed.

Antidandruff formulations against *Malassezia* species such as selenium sulfide, zinc pyrithione, ketoconazole, and tar shampoos can be used. For extensive scaly lesions, 5% salicylic acid ointment can be used. Acute lesions on face and trunk respond to mild steroid ointments, and 2% ketoconazole creams. Topical tacrolimus 0.03% ointment can also be used as a steroid-sparing agent. Other topical therapies used are metronidazole, ciclopirox olamine, and tacalcitol. Unresponsive cases may respond to ultraviolet B (UVB) therapy, oral itraconazole, or oral steroids. Salts like lithium succinate are found helpful.

➲ PROGNOSIS

Suppression can occur, no permanent cure.

➲ SUGGESTED READING

1. Saunte DML, Gaitanis G, Hay RJ. *Malassezia*-Associated Skin Diseases, the Use of Diagnostics and Treatment. Front Cell Infect Microbiol. 2020;10:112.

235 Sjögren's Syndrome

SYNONYMS

Sicca syndrome, Gougerot–Houwer–Sjögren syndrome, Mikulicz disease.

HISTORY

In 1933, Swedish ophthalmologist Henrik Sjögren first gave the features of this syndrome. The first case was described in 1888.

ETIOPATHOGENESIS

The etiology is multifactorial. Certain environmental factors are said to trigger inflammation in individuals who are genetically predisposed [human leukocyte antigen (HLA) B8, DR3, Dw4, tumor necrosis factor (TNF), interleukin 10 (IL-10), and SSA1].

AGE AND SEX

Females are more commonly affected (95%), presenting in their fourth and fifth decades.

CLINICAL FEATURES

Two types of Sjögren's syndrome are described:

1. *Primary:* Here, the symptoms are very severe. They are further divided into two types—benign and those associated with malignancies.
2. *Secondary:* These are associated with underlying connective tissue disease. They are less severe.

The triad consists of xerostomia (dry mouth), xerophthalmia (dry eyes), and lymphocytic infiltration of the exocrine glands.

Cutaneous features include xerosis, pruritus, scaling, subacute cutaneous lupus erythematosus (SCLE)-like rashes, annular erythema, Sweet's-like lesions and papular erythema, Raynaud's syndrome, hyperglobulinemic purpura, inflammatory vasculitis, vitiligo, abnormalities of sweating, and alopecia—diffuse and generalized.

- *Ear, nose, and throat (ENT) problems:* Sinusitis and hearing problems, including deafness. Systemic involvement in the form of fatigue, arthralgia, arthritis, myalgia and myositis, esophageal reflux, interstitial pneumonitis, pulmonary fibrosis, pulmonary hypertension, interstitial nephritis, primary biliary cirrhosis, migraine, neuropathies, and cerebral vasculitis may be seen.
- *Associated conditions*: Connective tissue disease [rheumatoid arthritis (RA) (26%)], systemic sclerosis (22%), Sweet's syndrome, lymphoproliferative disorders—B and T cell, and mucosa-associated lymphoid tissue (MALT)-associated, primary biliary

cirrhosis, chronic hepatitis, lipodystrophy, granulomatous panniculitis, Behçet's disease, coeliac disease, hypothyroidism and thyroiditis, myasthenia gravis, hemochromatosis, dermatitis herpetiformis, Darier's disease, multicentric reticulohistiocytosis, sarcoidosis, and Waldenström's hyperglobulinemic purpura.

Most patients have elevated RA factor, >1:320, antinuclear antibody (ANA) >1:320 with the presence of anti-Ro and anti-La antibodies.

HISTOPATHOLOGY

Histopathology shows lymphocyte and plasma cell infiltration of the exocrine glands, connective tissue proliferation, glandular cell apoptosis, followed by atrophy of glandular structures in affected tissues (salivary glands, sebaceous glands, sweat glands, etc.).

DERMOSCOPY

Dermoscopic features of the filiform papillae of the tongue show completely flattened papillae, which is suggestive of Sjögren's syndrome.

DIFFERENTIAL DIAGNOSIS

Chronic fatigue syndrome, fibromyalgia, drug-induced dryness (anticholinergics), age-related exocrine gland dysfunction, mouth breathing, anxiety, sarcoidosis [raised serum angiotensin-converting enzyme (ACE) levels], radiation injury, amyloidosis, human immunodeficiency virus (HIV) infection, scleroderma, and polymyositis are the differential diagnoses.

COMPLICATIONS

The complications include the emergence of systemic lupus erythematosus (SLE) and RA, infection of the parotid gland, pseudolymphomas, and parotid tumors; pregnant patients with anti-Ro/SS-A antibodies are at risk for fetal loss.

TREATMENT

The mainstay of treatment is local therapy. Keratoconjunctivitis sicca is managed with the frequent use of artificial tears during the day and the use of a lubricating ointment at night for the eyes. Cyclosporine and pilocarpine ocular drops seem to be of some benefit.

Treatment of oral manifestations includes oral hygiene, prevention and treatment of oral infections, use of artificial saliva, and local and systemic stimulation of salivary secretion.

Systemic therapy includes hydroxychloroquine, steroidal and nonsteroidal agents, disease-modifying agents, and cytotoxic therapy to address the extraglandular manifestations.

SUGGESTED READING

1. Both T, Dalm VA, van Hagen PM, van Daele PL. Reviewing primary Sjögren's syndrome: beyond the dryness - From pathophysiology to diagnosis and treatment. Int J Med Sci. 2017;14(3):191-200.

236 Solar Elastosis

➲ SYNONYM

Actinic elastosis.

➲ ETIOLOGY

Solar elastosis results from prolonged exposure to sunlight or infrared radiation. Fair skin, porphyria cutanea tarda, and smoking are risk factors. Ultraviolet B (UVB) wavelengths are the most likely to cause solar elastosis.

➲ AGE AND SEX

Solar elastosis usually presents in the fourth decade, and it is slightly more common in males.

➲ CLINICAL FEATURES

The condition is characterized by degenerative changes in the dermis caused by prolonged exposure to electromagnetic (usually solar) radiation. The affected skin is diffusely thickened and yellowish, and on the neck, it may be divided by well-defined furrows into an irregular rhomboidal pattern (cutis rhomboidalis nuchae). They may also show sharply marginated, thickened plaques on the face or neck **(Figs. 1A and B)**.

When the skin around the orbits is affected, it is often studded with numerous comedones, and this has been called the Favre–Racouchot syndrome. Other signs of sun damage, including irregular pigmentation, wrinkling, scaling, solar keratoses, and malignancy, may be present. This range of changes due to chronic sun damage has been called dermatoheliosis.

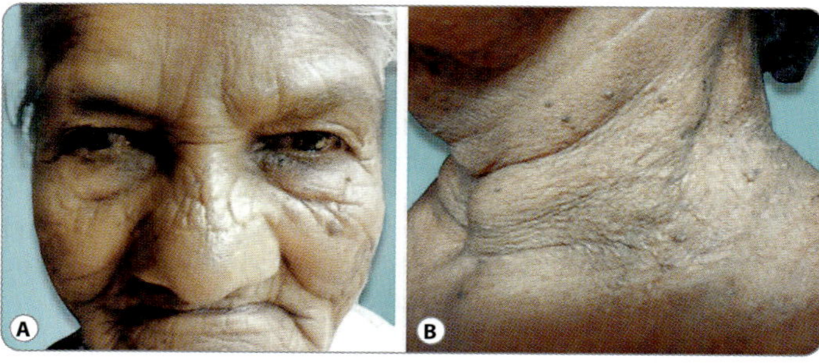

Figs. 1A and B: (A) Sharply marginated, yellowish, thickened plaques over the face; and (B) Cutis rhomboidalis nuchae.

➲ HISTOPATHOLOGY

A biopsy shows a lymphohistiocytic infiltrate around veins. The vessel walls are thickened due to the deposition of basement membrane-like material. The elastic fibers of the upper and mid-dermis become curled and fibrillar, forming irregular masses. In the later stages, swollen bands with finely granular elastin are seen. The fibrous network degenerates into an amorphous elastotic mass.

➲ DERMOSCOPY

Dermoscopy shows yellow-orange hue and telangiectasia.

➲ COMPLICATIONS

Actinic granuloma.

➲ DIFFERENTIAL DIAGNOSIS

- *Plane xanthoma*—foamy cells with Touton giant cells are seen.
- *Pseudoxanthoma elasticum*—fragmented elastic fibers with dystrophic calcification of dermal vessels are seen.
- *Colloid milium*—smooth white-colored papules are seen.

➲ TREATMENT

Strict sun protection with physical or chemical sunscreen. Topical hydroxy acids ("fruit acids"), that is, lactic, glycolic, and citric acids, tretinoin 0.1% cream, and ortazarotene creams have been tried. Nonablative lasers, including the 1320-nm neodymium:yttrium–aluminum–garnet (Nd:YAG) and 1540-nm erbium glass lasers, are claimed to wound the upper dermis without epidermal damage. Newer treatment modalities include topical imiquimod and fluorouracil to reduce the lines and furrows of solar elastosis.

➲ SUGGESTED READING

1. Widgerow AD, Napekoski K. New approaches to skin photodamage histology-Differentiating 'good' versus 'bad' Elastin. J Cosmet Dermatol. 2021;20(2):526-31.

237 Solar Lentigo

➲ SYNONYMS

Lentigo senilis, liver spot, senile freckle.

➲ ETIOLOGY

In response to chronic exposure to ultraviolet (UV) radiation, there is epidermal hyperplasia, proliferation of melanocytes, and accumulation of melanin within keratinocytes. Other hypothesized etiological factors are the activation of somatic mutations in FGFR3 (fibroblast growth factor receptor 3), PIK3CA (phosphatidylinositol-4,5-bisphosphate 3-kinase catalytic subunit alpha), and melanocortin-1 receptor genes.

Psoralen and ultraviolet A (PUVA) lentigo is the development of lentigo in individuals undergoing long-term PUVA photochemotherapy.

➲ CLINICAL FEATURES

Lentigines present as well-circumscribed, round, oval, or irregularly shaped macules that vary in color from tan to dark brown or black. Their size usually ranges from 3 mm to 2 cm and can become confluent, predominantly occurring on sun-exposed areas **(Fig. 1)**.

Solar lentigines have been shown to be an independent risk factor for the development of cutaneous melanoma.

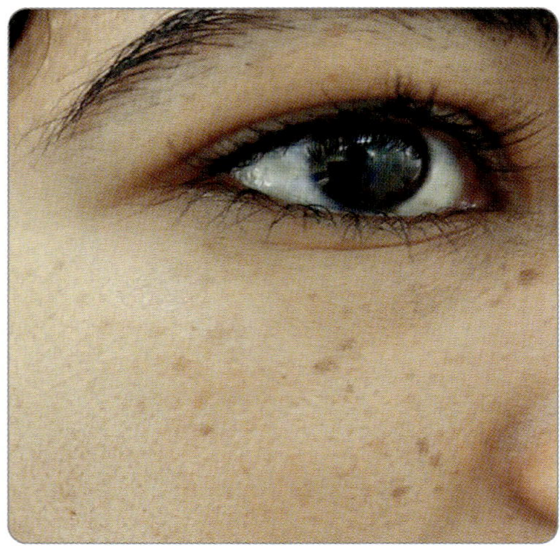

Fig. 1: Multiple round, oval, or irregularly shaped brown macules.

DERMOSCOPY

A diffuse light brown structureless area, sharply demarcated or moth-eaten borders, fingerprinting, and a reticular pattern with thin lines that are sometimes short and interrupted. Ink spot solar lentigo has striking jet-black color with stellate outline.

HISTOPATHOLOGY

Rete ridges often have club-shaped or bud-like extensions, and the epidermis in between the rete is thinned out. There is increased basal layer pigmentation in basaloid cells. The superficial dermis contains melanophages and occasionally a mild perivascular infiltrate of lymphocytes.

DIFFERENTIAL DIAGNOSIS

Differential diagnosis includes ephelides, macular seborrheic keratosis, pigmented actinic keratosis, lentigo maligna, simple lentigo, junctional melanocytic nevus, and large cell acanthoma.

TREATMENT

Treatment options available are dermabrasion, intense pulsed light, cryotherapy, peelings, and laser therapy.

SUGGESTED READING

1. Arginelli F, Greco M, Ciardo S, Josse G, Rossi AB, Le Digabel J, et al. Efficacy of D-pigment dermocosmetic lightening product for solar lentigo lesions of the hand: A randomized controlled trial. PLoS One. 2019;14(5):e0214714.

238 Spider Angioma

➲ SYNONYMS

Spider telangiectasia, arterial spider, spider nevus, nevus araneus.

➲ ETIOLOGY

Spider angioma occurs in 15% of normal persons. They occur in large numbers and increase in size during pregnancy; they are found in two-thirds of all pregnant patients and disappear within 6 weeks of delivery. It is also seen in patients with liver disease. Multiple spider nevi usually indicate the presence of progressive hepatic fibrosis and advanced liver disease. It is said to be associated with estrogen levels.

➲ AGE GROUP

Adults are commonly affected.

➲ CLINICAL FEATURES

They vary in size and shape and may reach up to 1.5 cm in size. The central body may be raised and is pulsatile on diascopy. Radiating vessels are just visible to the naked eye. They occur more commonly on the upper half of the body, especially on the face, neck, and hands. They are usually solitary but may be multiple. They may develop at sites of trauma and may be unilateral. Similar lesions can also occur on mucus membranes of the lips and nose.

➲ DERMOSCOPY

Dermoscopy of a spider angioma shows a central red dot with radiating fine red lines.

➲ HISTOPATHOLOGY

The main vessel of an angioma is an arteriole. The blood flows from this to the periphery and then passes into a capillary network. The pressure in spider telangiectasia can rise up to 40 mm Hg. The lesions consist of a central, ascending, spiral thick-walled arteriole, which ends in a thin-walled ampulla just beneath the epidermis. From the ampulla, thin-walled branching channels radiate peripherally in the papillary dermis. Glomus bodies have also been described. These resemble microarteriovenous malformations.

➲ DIFFERENTIAL DIAGNOSIS

Differential diagnosis includes hereditary hemorrhagic telangiectasia (mucosal lesions may be present, and nailfold capillary changes are noticed), cherry angioma (multiple erythematous papules are present, with no radiating arterioles), and insect bite reaction (central punctum/excoriation/crust are seen).

TREATMENT

- Underlying cause like liver cirrhosis should be treated.
- Only cosmetic, central arteriole may be ablated by diathermy.
- *Other available treatment modalities:* 585-nm pulsed dye laser, 532-nm potassium titanyl phosphate (KTP) laser, and fine-needle electrocautery
- Spider nevi in healthy individuals usually disappear spontaneously.

SUGGESTED READING

1. Samant H, Kothadia JP. (2023). Spider angioma. Treasure Island (FL): StatPearls Publishing. [online] Available from https://www.ncbi.nlm.nih.gov/books/NBK507818/ [Last accessed February, 2025].

239 Spitz Nevi

SYNONYMS

Spitz juvenile melanoma, benign juvenile melanoma.

HISTORY

In 1948, Sophie Spitz gave a publication on Spitz lesions, the source of the eponym. She initially described it as juvenile melanomas, which lacked aggressive metastatic behavior.

ETIOLOGY

These are benign melanocytic proliferations, characterized by spindled nevomelanocytes with no specific etiological factors. Widespread eruptive Spitz nevi have been associated with human immunodeficiency virus (HIV) infection, Addison's disease, chemotherapy, puberty, and pregnancy.

AGE GROUP

Spitz tumors occur usually between 10 and 20 years.

CLINICAL FEATURES

Classical Spitz nevi present as pink to red or rarely hyperpigmented, well-defined, demarcated, dome-shaped papules, frequently occurring on the head and neck region and lower limbs. Agminated or grouped Spitz nevi are characterized by varying numbers of raised nevi occurring in a localized or segmental distribution. Atypical Spitz shows more than one feature deviating from classic Spitz, like size >5 mm, asymmetry, lack of maturation, and high melanocyte density.

HISTOPATHOLOGY

Histopathology shows dome-shaped with sharply demarcated and symmetric proliferation of spindled and epithelioid melanocytes at the dermal–epidermal junction and within the papillary dermis, with regular epidermal hyperplasia. Intraepidermal eosinophilic globules (Kamino bodies) are usually encountered **(Fig. 1)**.

DERMOSCOPY

Dermoscopy shows uniform rounded structures with prominent punctate or rounded blood vessels. A pigmented Spitz nevus may show starburst or globular pattern of pigmentation but later evolves to a homogenous or structureless.

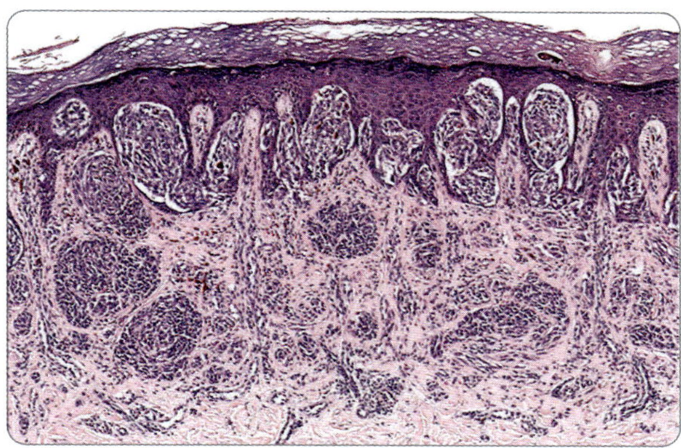

Fig. 1: Histopathology of Spitz nevus.

➲ DIFFERENTIAL DIAGNOSIS

Differential diagnosis can be melanocytic nevi, particularly intradermal nevi, hemangiomas, pyogenic granulomas, verrucae, mollusca contagiosa, juvenile and adult xanthogranulomas, dermatofibromas, mastocytomas, and adnexal tumors.

➲ TREATMENT

Complete excision with margins free of tumor is recommended for all Spitz nevi.

➲ SUGGESTED READING

1. Luo S, Sepehr A, Tsao H. Spitz nevi and other Spitzoid lesions part I. Background and diagnoses. J Am Acad Dermatol. 2011;65(6):1073-84.

240 Sporotrichosis

➲ SYNONYM

Rose gardener's disease.

➲ HISTORY

In 1898, Bernard Schenck first isolated and described *Sporothrix schenckii*.

➲ ETIOLOGY

Sporothrix schenckii is a dimorphic fungus.

➲ AGE AND SEX

Sporotrichosis is seen usually in young adults and has a slightly higher incidence among males.

➲ CLINICAL FEATURES

- *Lymphocutaneous sporotrichosis*: A small subcutaneous nodule or pustule develops at the site of initial injury a few days to 3 weeks after trauma, which breaks down to form a small ulcer, followed by the development of new nodules along the lymphatics at intervals of a few days, which also ulcerate and are frequently connected by lymphatic cords **(Fig. 1)**. The regional lymph nodes become enlarged and may suppurate. The initial lesion tends to heal with scarring after weeks or months.

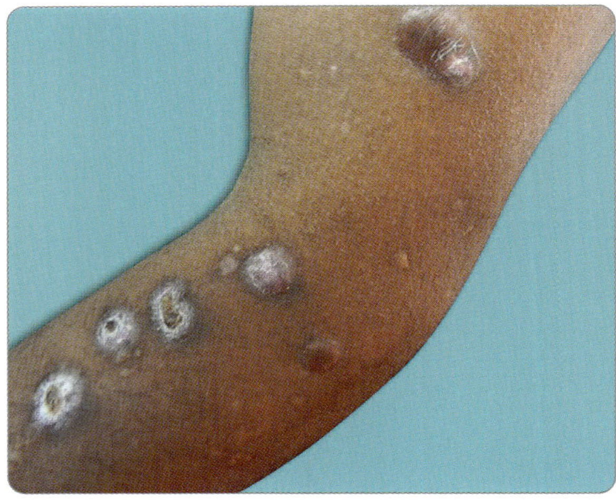

Fig. 1: Multiple well-defined nodules along the lymphatics.

- *Fixed cutaneous sporotrichosis*: In highly endemic areas, the population is sensitized, and primary infection in such a person is restricted to the site of injury.
- *Mucocutaneous sporotrichosis*: In the mouth, pharynx, vocal cords, or nose, the lesions present as painful erythematous, ulcerative, suppurative nodules, which later become granulomatous and heal with scarring.
- *Extracutaneous and disseminated sporotrichosis*: The common sites include joints, especially the knees, ankles, wrists, and small joints of the hands and feet, and bones such as the tibia. The central nervous system may be involved.
- *Pulmonary sporotrichosis*: Infection results from inhalation of conidia and presents as chronic cavitary fibronodular disease.

➲ HISTOPATHOLOGY

Histopathology shows suppurative granuloma. Sporotrichotic, tuberculoid, or foreign body type of granuloma may be seen. The asteroid body consists of a round or oval basophilic yeast-like body (3–5 µm), surrounded by radiating elongation of a homogenous eosinophilic material (7–20 µm). In chronic lesions, extensive pseudoepitheliomatous hyperplasia may occur. *S. schenckii* can be demonstrated in tissue sections by diastase method or fluorescent antibody techniques.

Laboratory diagnosis: Sputum examination stained by periodic acid–Schiff (PAS) or on a calcofluor preparation, isolation of *S. schenckii* on Sabouraud's dextrose agar, demonstration of yeast phase in Brain Heart Infusion Agar, and animal inoculation may show characteristic gram-positive "cigar bodies."

➲ DERMOSCOPY

Dermoscopy shows general erythema, focal structureless white areas, microulcerations, central ulcer, hyperkeratosis, fiber sign, pustule, focal structureless yellow areas, and white perilesional circle.

➲ DIFFERENTIAL DIAGNOSIS

Differential diagnosis includes atypical mycobacterial infection [positive acid-fast bacillus (AFB) culture], cutaneous tuberculosis (epitheloid granulomas surrounded by lymphocytes), cutaneous leishmaniasis [*Leishmania donovani* (LD) bodies are seen], anthrax, gummatous syphilis, staphylococcal lymphangitis, yaws, sarcoidosis, other deep mycosis, and bromoderma.

➲ TREATMENT

The treatment of choice is a saturated solution of potassium iodide administered orally in milk. The initial dose is five drops (1 mL) three times a day after meals. This is increased by one drop/dose until 40 drops three times a day.

Amphotericin B intravenously, itraconazole (200 mg/day), fluconazole, terbinafine (500 mg/day), voriconazole, and posaconazole have been tried. All drugs should be continued for 1 week after clinical resolution.

SUGGESTED READINGS

1. Orofino-Costa R, Macedo PM, Rodrigues AM, Bernardes-Engemann AR. Sporotrichosis: an update on epidemiology, etiopathogenesis, laboratory and clinical therapeutics. An Bras Dermatol. 2017;92(5): 606-20.
2. Mahajan VK. Sporotrichosis: an overview and therapeutic options. Dermatol Res Pract. 2014;2014:272376.

241 Squamous Cell Carcinoma

➲ SYNONYMS

Epidermoid carcinoma, squamous cell epithelioma.

➲ ETIOLOGY

Squamous cell carcinoma (SCC) is a malignant tumor of the skin arising from the epithelium. It is the second most common cutaneous malignancy. Sun exposure, trauma, albinism, burn scars, ionizing radiation, chronic inflammation, chronic discoid lupus erythematosus (DLE), chronic exposure to thermal radiation, long-standing chronic granulomas like venereal granulomas, syphilis, lupus vulgaris, leprosy, lupus erythematosus, chronic ulcers, osteomyelitis sinuses, and hidradenitis suppurativa may predispose to the development of SCC.

➲ AGE AND SEX

Male–female ratio is 2:1, and the incidence increases with age. It is seen commonly after the fifth decade.

➲ CLINICAL FEATURES

Common sites are the sun-exposed areas like the back of the hands and forearms, the upper part of the face, especially in males, on the lower lip, and the pinna. The lesion is indurated, plaque-like, verrucous, tumid, or ulcerated, and firm in consistency; the tissue around is inflamed, and the edge is an opaque yellowish red color. Most lesions are exophytic **(Fig. 1)**. Regional lymph nodes may

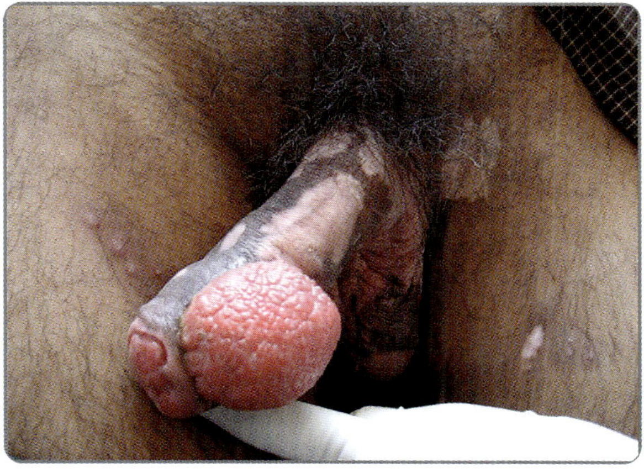

Fig. 1: An exophytic verrucous growth over the shaft of the penis.

become enlarged, either as a result of infection of ulcer or from metastases.

HISTOPATHOLOGY

The tumor may appear as single cells, small groups or nests of cells, or a single mass. The inferior border may broadly impose on the dermis or be represented by individual foci of microinvasion. The aberrant cells have increased mitoses, mitotic figures, nuclear hyperchromasia, and loss of intercellular bridges. Squamous differentiation is seen as foci of keratinization in concentric rings of squamous cells called horn pearls.

DERMOSCOPY

The common dermoscopic features of SCC are white circles, white structureless areas, looped vessels, central keratin, and pink or red background.

DIFFERENTIAL DIAGNOSIS

Wart, seborrheic keratoses, actinic keratoses, melanocytic nevus, pyogenic granuloma, eccrine poroma, chromomycosis, erosive pustular dermatosis of the scalp, atypical fibroxanthoma, basal cell carcinoma (BCC), Bowen's disease, verrucous melanoma, Merkel cell carcinoma, metastatic SCC, and keratoacanthoma are the differential diagnoses.

TREATMENT

Nonexcisional ablative techniques like electrodessication or curettage can be done for small lesions <2 cm, intralesional 5-fluorouracil (5-FU), and interferon alfa. For larger lesions, Mohs' surgery, conventional surgical excision, and radiation therapy can be tried.

Pembrolizumab is the newly Food and Drug Administration (FDA)-approved drug for recurrent, metastatic, locally advanced, treatment-resistant SCC.

PROGNOSIS

Survival depends on the size, location, degree of differentiation, immune status, depth of invasion, and presence of metastasis. Tumors which penetrate through the dermis or are >8 mm thick have an increased risk of recurrence. Most common metastatic locations are the lungs and lymph nodes. The risk of metastasis is 10–20% on tumors' arising on the lip and pinna.

SUGGESTED READING

1. Fania L, Didona D, Di Pietro FR, Verkhovskaia S, Morese R, Paolino G, et al. Cutaneous Squamous Cell Carcinoma: From Pathophysiology to Novel Therapeutic Approaches. Biomedicines. 2021;9(2):171.

242 Staphylococcal Scalded Skin Syndrome

SYNONYMS

Ritter's disease, pemphigus neonatorum, staphylococcal epidermal necrolysis.

HISTORY

The clinical features were first described in 1878 by Baron Gottfried Ritter von Rittershain from Czechoslovakia.

ETIOPATHOGENESIS

Staphylococcal scalded skin syndrome (SSSS) is caused by phage group II strains (types 3A, 3C, 55, and 71) of *Staphylococcus aureus*. Epidermolysins, which are secreted by both methicillin-resistant and methicillin-sensitive strains of *S. aureus*, play an integral role in pathogenesis. *S. aureus* uses these exfoliative toxins (ETs) to disrupt the barrier of the human epidermis in order to survive and proliferate. Specifically, the exfoliative toxins A (ETA) (chromosomally encoded) and B (ETB) (plasmid-encoded) act at the granular layer of the epidermis to cause a split and sterile bullae. ETA and ETB are serine proteases with a very high specificity for human desmoglein 1 (Dsg1). They bind Dsg1 directly, causing a conformational change in the toxin, which cleaves the extracellular domain of Dsg1. As the toxins are excreted via the kidneys, premature infants and adults with chronic renal insufficiency are most commonly affected.

AGE AND SEX

Staphylococcal scalded skin syndrome is primarily a disease of children. Children are more affected due to an immature renal system and immune system. It is more common in nonbreastfed children. It can occur as outbreaks in nurseries.

CLINICAL FEATURES

Staphylococcal scalded skin syndrome is a condition of infants and children (more commonly than adults), involving cleavage of the epidermis through the granular layer, resulting in the formation of tender, flaccid bullae. SSSS is primarily a disease of children <6 years of age. Occasionally, adults with chronic renal insufficiency or immunosuppression can be affected. The disease begins with a prodrome of malaise, fever, irritability, sore throat, and severe tenderness of the skin. Scarlatiniform erythema often first appears on the head, with generalization within 48 hours with the development of wrinkled skin due to the formation of flaccid bullae, which rupture and lie on eroded skin **(Figs. 1A and B)** (wet newspaper sign). Patients demonstrate "sad man" facies, perioral crusting, and radial fissuring with mild facial edema. The Nikolsky

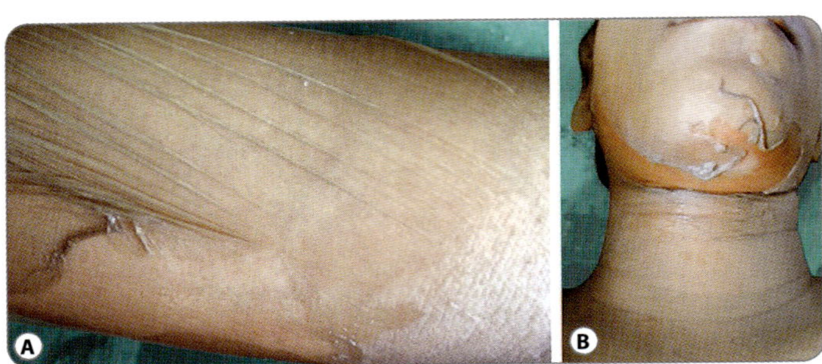

Figs. 1A and B: (A) Peeling of the skin with underlying erythema; and (B) Vesicles are seen on the chin.

sign is positive. The patient may have purulent rhinorrhea or conjunctivitis. Scaling and desquamation continue for the next 3–5 days, with re-epithelialization in 10–14 days. In severe cases, there may be hypothermia and hemodynamic instability. Lesional skin heals without scarring.

HISTOPATHOLOGY

Histological examination shows a sharply demarcated zone of cleavage at or below the stratum granulosum.

DIFFERENTIAL DIAGNOSIS

Differential diagnosis includes sunburn (only on photoexposed areas; the general condition of the baby is normal), drug reaction, Kawasaki disease (conjunctival injection, cervical lymphadenopathy, strawberry tongue, and palmar desquamation are seen), extensive bullous impetigo, viral exanthema (absence of blisters/peeling of skin), toxic shock syndrome, graft-versus-host disease (GVHD), and pemphigus foliaceus (acantholytic cells are seen).

TREATMENT

Patients with extensive, generalized forms of SSSS require hospitalization and parental antibiotics. Oral treatment with a β-lactamase-resistant antibiotic (e.g., dicloxacillin, cloxacillin, and cephalexin) for a minimum of 1 week is usually sufficient for localized disease. Adequate intravenous (IV) fluids to treat dehydration. Emollients and nonadherent dressings to promote skin healing. Avoid silver sulfadiazine, as increased absorption can cause toxicity.

PROGNOSIS

The prognosis is good in children, and if antibiotics are administered early, the mortality rate is low. In adults, the overall mortality rate seems to be higher. Those patients without underlying disease recover more rapidly.

SUGGESTED READING

1. Ross A, Shoff HW. (2023). Staphylococcal Scalded Skin Syndrome. Treasure Island (FL): StatPearls Publishing. [online] Available from https://www.ncbi.nlm.nih.gov/books/NBK448135/ [Last accessed February, 2025].

243 Stasis Dermatitis

➲ SYNONYMS

Stasis eczema, gravitational dermatitis, gravitational eczema, varicose eczema, varicose eczema, hypostatic eczema, dermatitis veineuse.

➲ HISTORY

The term "stasis dermatitis" was introduced by Pillsbury, and the term "gravitation dermatitis" was introduced by Belisario.

➲ RISK FACTORS

The risk factors include older age, female sex, pregnancy, obesity, prolonged sitting or standing, heart failure, and family history of venous disease.

➲ ETIOPATHOGENESIS

Venous hypertension, due to the upright position or incompetence of the valves, slows the blood flow, distends the capillaries, and damages the capillary permeability barrier, allowing the passage of fluid and plasma proteins into the tissue and extravasation of erythrocytes. Proteins (fibrin) are deposited around the vessels as hyaline cuffs, with interstitial edema inhibiting oxygen diffusion and metabolic exchange, which induces upregulation of intercellular adhesion molecule 1 (ICAM-1) and vascular cell adhesion molecule 1 (VCAM-1) on endothelia, expression of L-selectin on neutrophils, and activation of neutrophils and macrophages. Release of inflammatory mediators, free radicals, and proteases by neutrophils leads to pericapillary inflammation. Free iron ions released from hemosiderin deposits activate matrix metalloproteinases via the Fenton reaction. The subsequent imbalance in the capillary network can produce fibrosis and tissue remodeling, lipodermatosclerosis, dysfunction of the lymphatics, and stellate sclerotic areas depleted of capillaries with the formation of peripheral giant capillaries ("atrophie blanche").

➲ CLINICAL FEATURES

The first sign is usually a pitting edema of the medial aspects of the shin followed by inflammation that may mimic cellulitis ("pseudoerysipelas"; acute lipodermatosclerosis).

Later, the skin, subcutaneous adipose tissue, and deep fascia become progressively indurated and mutually adherent (chronic "lipodermatosclerosis"). A firm circular cuff is formed, creating an inverted wine bottle appearance. Later, venous ulcers develop, either spontaneously or by scratching or trauma **(Fig. 1)**.

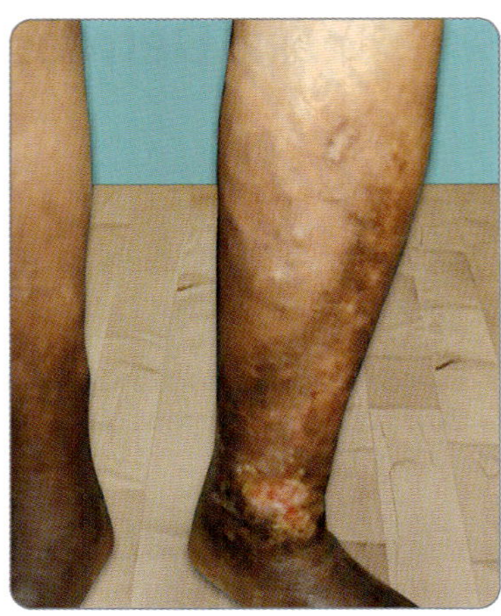

Fig. 1: Varicose veins with pigmentation (hemosiderin deposition) and lipodermatosclerotic changes in the surrounding skin.

➲ COMPLICATION

Contact sensitization to components of topical therapies may lead to secondary dissemination. Due to the disruption of the epidermal barrier, secondary infections may also occur, leading to superficial infections such as impetiginization, cellulitis, and erysipelas. Venous ulcers can occur if underlying chronic venous insufficiency is not treated. It may also develop into acroangiodermatitis (pseudo-Kaposi sarcoma).

➲ PATHOLOGY

Depending on the stage, features of acute, subacute, or chronic eczema are seen. In addition, there are signs of venous hypertension like dilated capillaries surrounded by cuffs of fibrin, hemosiderin deposits, and hyperplastic venules. In later stages, there is fibrosis of the dermal connective tissue and sclerosis of the adipose tissue.

➲ DERMOSCOPY

Dermoscopy shows glomerular-like vessels at high magnification (30×) or red globules at low magnification (10×) and a scaly surface.

➲ DIFFERENTIAL DIAGNOSIS

Differential diagnosis can be asteatotic eczema (mainly over the shins and not the gaiter area, cracked porcelain plate appearance), irritant or allergic contact dermatitis, nummular eczema (localized well-defined scaly/crusted plaque/patch), psoriasis, mycosis fungoides (epidermotropism and Pautrier's microabscess are seen), Kaposi sarcoma, dermatophytic infections (positive KOH mount), and lichen simplex chronicus (lichenification is present, and vertically oriented collagen bundles are seen in the dermis).

➲ TREATMENT

The aim of therapy is the management of venous hypertension. Regular use of adequate compression bandages or stockings to improve venous return, lifestyle changes, and exercise of the calf muscles should be advised. Topical corticosteroids and calcineurin inhibitors are added in patients with refractory disease. Sclerotherapy and ligation of incompetent communicating veins or the removal of insufficient saphenous veins are performed.

➲ SUGGESTED READING

1. Yosipovitch G, Nedorost ST, Silverberg JI, Friedman AJ, Canosa JM, Cha A. Stasis Dermatitis: An Overview of Its Clinical Presentation, Pathogenesis, and Management. Am J Clin Dermatol. 2023;24(2):275-86.

244 Steatocystoma Multiplex

➲ SYNONYMS

Sebocystomatosis, hereditary epidermal polycystic disease.

➲ ETIOLOGY

Etiology is unknown. It may be inherited as an autosomal dominant condition.

➲ AGE GROUP

Steatocystoma multiplex begins in adolescence or early adult life. Both sexes are affected equally.

➲ CLINICAL FEATURES

Multiple, smooth, compressible nodules are present within the dermis, varying in size from a few mm to 20 mm or more **(Fig. 1)**. They usually first appear and become larger during puberty. The disease commonly involves the trunk and proximal parts of the limbs, especially the presternal area and scrotum **(Fig. 2)**. No punctum over the lesion is seen, but comedones may be present. If pricked, an oily fluid can be expressed.

➲ MUTATIONS

KRT17, N92S, R94C, and R94H.

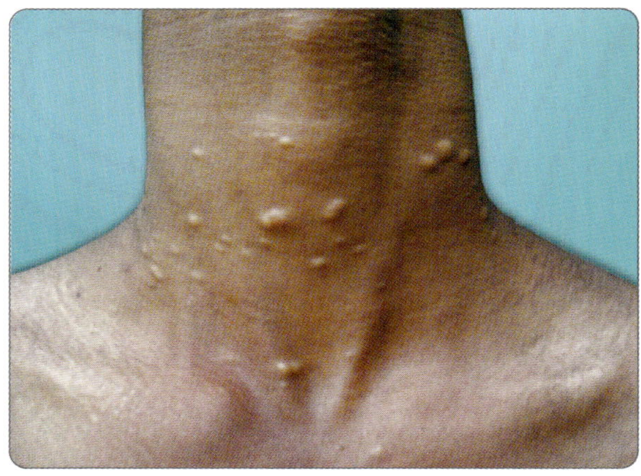

Fig. 1: Smooth compressible nodules over the neck and upper chest.

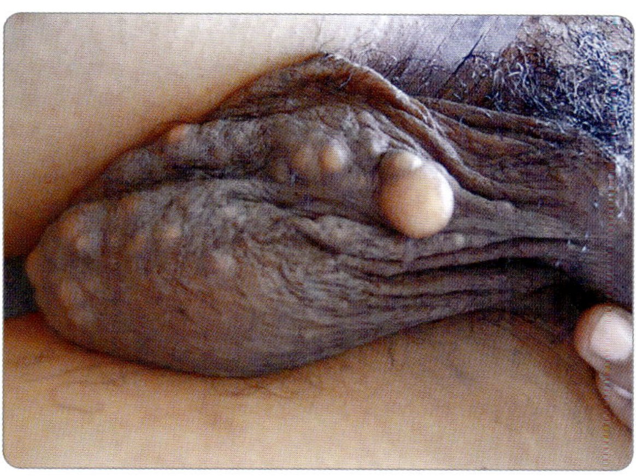

Fig. 2: Multiple nodular swellings over the scrotum.

➲ ASSOCIATIONS

Steatocystoma multiplex is associated with hidradenitis suppurativa (HS), pachyonychia congenita, ichthyosis, koilonychia, acrokeratosis verruciformis of Hopf, hypotrichosis, hypohidrosis, hypothyroidism, hypertrophic lichen planus, multiple keratoacanthomas, rheumatoid arthritis, preauricular sinus, pili torti, pili canaliculi, neurofibromatosis 1, and polycystic kidney disease.

➲ ASSOCIATED SYNDROMES

Pachyonychia congenita, X-linked recessive Lowe syndrome, Gardner syndrome, Noonan syndrome, Alagille–Watson syndrome, and Favre–Racouchot syndrome are the associated syndromes.

➲ HISTOPATHOLOGY

The cysts are situated in the mid-dermis, having sebaceous gland lobules in their walls and containing sebum. The wall is thin and is composed of keratinizing epithelium. Contents are oily and composed of unsplit esters of sebum. Sometimes hairs, hair roots, or even sweat glands may be found connected with the cyst, and the whole complex is joined to the epidermis by a short band of undifferentiated cells.

➲ DERMOSCOPY

Nonpolarized dermoscopy shows a yellowish structureless area with diffuse margins, and on polarized dermoscopy, a distinctive yellowish glow, surrounded by a darker rim, over a backdrop of a pseudoreticular pigmentary pattern. The yellow structureless area corresponds to sebum contained in the cyst cavity. Trapped vellus hairs impart a greenish tinge to the yellow area.

➲ COMPLICATIONS

Inflammation may occur, leading to suppuration and scarring.

➲ TREATMENT

The treatment is excision, mainly for cosmetic purposes. Systemic retinoids have been tried with variable success. Radiofrequency ablation and extrusion of contents are also the treatment options. Lasers like erbium-doped yttrium-aluminum-garnet (Er:YAG) and fractional CO_2 have been tried with good efficacy.

➲ PROGNOSIS

Surgery is curative.

➲ SUGGESTED READING

1. Palaniappan V, Karthikeyan K. Steatocystoma Multiplex. Indian Dermatol Online J. 2023;15(1):105-12.

245 Stevens–Johnson Syndrome

➲ HISTORY

Stevens–Johnson syndrome (SJS) is named for Albert Mason Stevens and Frank Chambliss Johnson, American pediatricians who described the condition in 1922.

➲ ETIOLOGY

Stevens–Johnson syndrome is an immune-mediated delayed hypersensitivity reaction. Drugs (phenytoin, penicillin, phenobarbitone, and sulfonamides) are the most common cause. Upper respiratory tract infections and viral infections have also been implicated.

➲ CLINICAL FEATURES

The cutaneous eruption is preceded by vague, nonspecific symptoms like fever and fatigue occurring 1–14 days before the skin lesions. Bullae are seen on the skin, conjunctiva, oral cavity, nares, and genitalia, involving <10% of body surface area (BSA) **(Fig. 1)**. Ulcerative stomatitis due to hemorrhagic crusting occurs. Flat atypical target lesions or purpuric macules are seen on the trunk. New crops of lesions occur over a period of 10 days to 3–4 weeks.

➲ SCORING SYSTEM

The severity of Stevens–Johnson syndrome/toxic epidermal necrolysis is assessed using SCORTEN. One point is scored for each of the

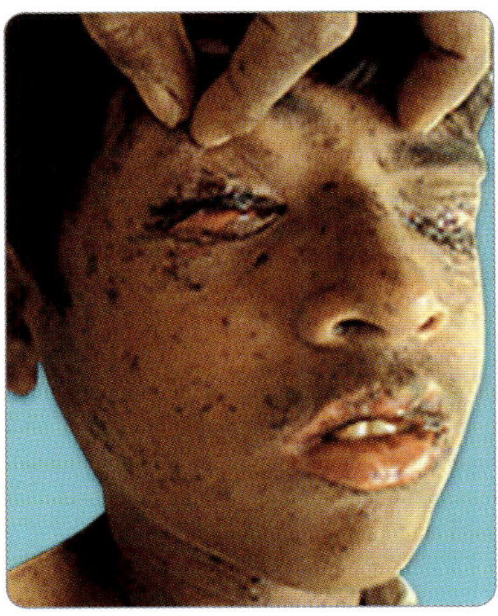

Fig. 1: Stevens–Johnson syndrome (SJS) involving the oral mucosa and conjunctiva.

following seven criteria at admission:

1. Age >40 years
2. Presence of a malignancy
3. Heart rate of >120 beats/min
4. Initial percentage of epidermal detachment >10%
5. Serum urea level >10 mmol/L
6. Serum glucose level >14 mmol/L
7. Serum bicarbonate level <20 mmol/L

A SCORTEN range with their associated mortality (in %) is as follows: Score 0–1 (3.2%), score 2 (12.1%), score 3 (35.3%), score 4 (58.3%), and score 5 (>90%).

➲ COMPLICATIONS

Eye involvement can lead to corneal scarring and blindness, inverted eyelashes, photophobia, and watery eyes; thick mucopurulent sputum and oral lesions may interfere with breathing.

➲ DIFFERENTIAL DIAGNOSIS

Differential diagnosis includes toxic epidermal necrolysis (>30% BSA involved with more severe mucosal lesions), urticaria, cicatricial pemphigoid (subepidermal blister is seen, with positive antibodies), pemphigus vulgaris [acantholytic cells are seen on Tzanck smear; intraepidermal blister and fishnet pattern are seen on direct immunofluorescence (DIF)], paraneoplastic pemphigus, serum sickness, staphylococcal scalded skin syndrome (SSSS) (less frequent mucosal lesions), porphyria cutanea tarda, epidermolysis bullosa acquisita (bullae at trauma-prone areas), Behcet's syndrome, and toxic shock syndrome.

➲ TREATMENT

The offending drug must be withdrawn. Symptomatic treatment with cool compresses, analgesics, and soft diet can be given. Secondary infections should be appropriately treated. Corticosteroids are given until new lesions no longer appear.

Other drugs such as cyclosporine, tumor necrosis factor (TNF) alpha inhibitors, and intravenous immunoglobulin (IVIG) can also be used. Adequate sterile dressing helps in wound healing. Hydration and temperature should be maintained.

➲ PROGNOSIS

Prognosis varies with the severity of the disease. Oral lesions may continue for several months. The risk of recurrence is 30–40%.

➲ SUGGESTED READING

1. Oakley AM, Krishnamurthy K. (2023). Stevens-Johnson Syndrome. Treasure Island (FL): StatPearls Publishing. [online] Available from https://www.ncbi.nlm.nih.gov/books/NBK459323/ [Last accessed February, 2025].

246 Stiff Skin Syndrome

➲ SYNONYM

Congenital fascial dystrophy.

➲ HISTORY

Stiff skin syndrome was first described by Esterly and McKusick in 1971.

➲ ETIOPATHOGENESIS

Stiff skin syndrome may be congenital or develop during early childhood. Familial occurrences have been described, and the mode of inheritance is autosomal dominant. The underlying genetic defect is a mutation in the *FBN1* gene. The presence of giant "amianthoid-like" collagen fibrils in affected fascia has been postulated to reflect a disturbance in the organization of collagen and glycosaminoglycans in the extracellular matrix.

➲ CLINICAL FEATURES

Stiff skin syndrome is characterized by "rock hard" induration and thickening of the skin and subcutaneous tissues, which is most pronounced on the buttocks and thighs, with characteristic sparing of the inguinal folds. The hands and feet are not involved. Mild hypertrichosis is often observed in affected areas. Restricted joint mobility leads to a characteristic posture of hip and knee flexion and prominent lumbar lordosis while standing, and patients may have short stature. The condition is stable or slowly progressive, and abnormalities of internal organs are not typically observed. Patients with unilateral involvement have been reported, some with features that overlapped with scleredema and deep morphea.

➲ HISTOPATHOLOGY

Histologic examination demonstrates markedly thickened, hyalinized fascia without an associated inflammatory infiltrate. Thickened collagen bundles and mucin deposition may or may not be present in the overlying dermis.

➲ DIFFERENTIAL DIAGNOSIS

Differential diagnosis includes sclerema neonatorum, scleredema, scleromyxedema, sclerodermatomyositis, and scleroderma.

➲ TREATMENT

Stiff skin syndrome has a chronic course, and no effective treatments have been reported. Physical therapy can help to prevent progressive joint contractures.

➲ SUGGESTED READING

1. Myers KL, Mir A, Schaffer JV, Meehan SA, Orlow SJ, Brinster NK. Segmental stiff skin syndrome (SSS): A distinct clinical entity. J Am Acad Dermatol. 2016;75(1):163-8.

247 Striae

➲ SYNONYMS

Striae distensae, striae atrophicans, stretch marks, linear atrophy, vergetures, striae cutis distensae, striae gravidarum (in cases where it is caused by pregnancy), lineae atrophicae, linea albicante, or simply striae.

➲ HISTORY

Striae were first described by Roederer in 1773, and the first histologic descriptions were made by Troisier and Ménétrier in 1889.

➲ AGE AND SEX

Striae are very common and usually develop between the ages of 5 and 50 years. They are seen more commonly in Caucasians, and striae occur about twice as frequently in women as in men.

➲ ETIOPATHOGENESIS

Factors leading to the development of striae have not been fully elucidated. Striae distensae are a reflection of "breaks" in the connective tissue that lead to dermal atrophy. A number of factors, including hormones (particularly corticosteroids), mechanical stress, and genetic predisposition, appear to play a role.

They are associated with various physiologic states, including puberty, pregnancy, growth spurts, rapid weight gain or loss, and obesity, and disorders that lead to hypercortisolism. They commonly develop during puberty, with an overall incidence of 25–35%, or during pregnancy, with an incidence of approximately 75%.

➲ CLINICAL FEATURES

Striae are multiple, symmetric, well-defined linear atrophic lesions that often follow the lines of cleavage **(Fig. 1)**. They are usually more of a cosmetic concern; initially, striae appear as red-to-violaceous elevated lines that can be mildly pruritic and are called striae rubra. Over time, the color gradually fades, and the lesions become atrophic (striae alba), with the skin surface exhibiting a fine wrinkled appearance. The striae can measure several centimeters in length and a few millimeters to a few centimeters in width. During puberty, striae appear in areas where there is a rapid increase in size. In girls, the most common sites are the thighs, hips, buttocks, and breasts, whereas in boys, they are seen on the shoulders, thighs, and lumbosacral region. Other less common sites include the abdomen, upper arms, neck, and axillae.

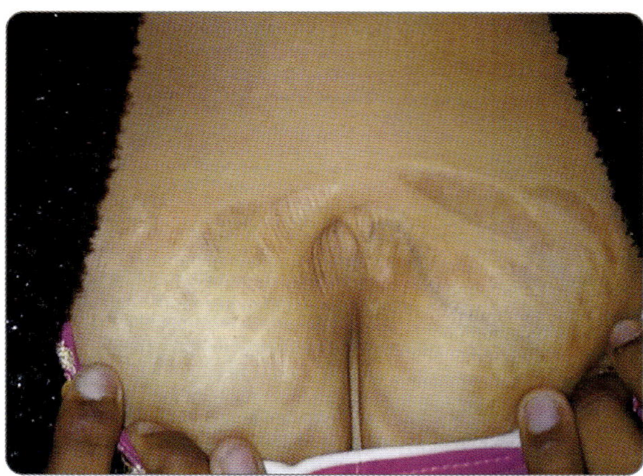

Fig. 1: Multiple, well-defined linear atrophic lesions over the breast due to steroid use.

Striae distensae are a common finding on the abdomen and less so on the breasts and thighs of pregnant women, especially during the last trimester. The striae associated with systemic corticosteroid therapy and Cushing's syndrome can be larger and more widely distributed. Flexural and intertriginous areas are particularly at risk for developing striae from the use of topical corticosteroids.

➲ PATHOLOGY

The epidermis can be normal during the early stages, but eventually, it becomes flattened and atrophic with blunted rete ridges. The dermal thickness is decreased, as is the collagen in the upper dermis. The collagen bundles are thinned and lie parallel to the epidermis, but they are also arranged transversely to the direction of the striae. Alterations in elastic fibers are variable, but dermal elastin can be fragmented, and specific elastin staining can demonstrate a marked reduction in visible elastin content compared with adjacent normal dermis. There is an absence of both hair follicles and other appendages.

➲ DERMOSCOPY

The dermoscopy of striae rubrae has been reported to show linear vessels oriented at right angles to the axis of the striae.

➲ DIFFERENTIAL DIAGNOSIS

- *Linear focal elastosis (elastotic striae)*: They are seen as elevated linear plaques and not depressed like striae.
- Trauma
- *Anetoderma*: It is seen as atrophic skin, causing localized outpouching.
- *Cutis laxa*: It is characterized by easily stretchable skin, which does not return to normal after releasing tension, and fragmented elastic fibers.

COMPLICATION

Rarely they can ulcerate.

TREATMENT

Treatment of early-stage striae with tretinoin 0.1% cream can improve their appearance, and its application has been shown to decrease the length and width of striae. Other topical treatments, including 0.05% tretinoin, 20% glycolic acid, 10% L-ascorbic acid, and 20% glycolic acid, may also improve the appearance of stretch marks. Several lasers have been used to treat striae: The 585-nm pulsed dye laser has been shown to result in some improvement in the appearance of striae rubra. Improvement in the leukoderma of striae alba was noted with the 308-nm excimer laser. Other laser therapies are CO_2, erbium-doped yttrium-aluminum-garnet (Er:YAG), diode, and neodymium-doped yttrium-aluminum-garnet (Nd:Q-switched YAG). In addition to these, radiofrequency, phototherapy, and therapies such as chemical peeling, carboxytherapy, and microdermabrasion have been used with varying success.

PROGNOSIS

The striae alba are usually permanent, but they may fade somewhat over time.

SUGGESTED READING

1. Elsedfy H. Striae distensae in adolescents: A mini review. Acta Biomed. 2020;91(1):176-81.

248 Subcorneal Pustular Dermatosis

➲ SYNONYM

Sneddon–Wilkinson disease.

➲ HISTORY

Subcorneal pustular dermatosis was first described by Sneddon and Wilkinson in 1956.

➲ ETIOLOGY

Immunologic mechanisms have been implicated, which is proved by the deposition of immunoglobulin A (IgA) intraepidermally. Circulating antibodies have also been detected within the epidermis. Desmocollin 1 has been described as an autoantigen in these cases.

➲ AGE GROUP

Subcorneal pustular dermatosis is more common in women and in persons >40 years of age, but it can occur at any age.

➲ CLINICAL FEATURES

Primary lesions are small, discrete, flaccid vesicles that rapidly turn pustular and usually arise in crops within a few hours on clinically normal or slightly erythematous skin. The classic lesion has been described as a "half-half" blister, in which purulent fluid accumulates in the lower half of the blister. The pustules coalesce and often form annular, circinate, or bizarre serpiginous patterns. Later, the pustules rupture and dry up to form thin, superficial scales and crusts, closely resembling impetigo. Common sites are the axillae, groin, abdomen, submammary areas, and the flexor aspects of the limbs **(Fig. 1)**.

➲ ASSOCIATED CONDITIONS

Associated conditions include pyoderma gangrenosum, ulcerative colitis, Crohn's disease, IgG paraproteinemia, CD30+ anaplastic large-cell lymphoma, non-small cell lung cancer, APUDoma (amine precursor uptake and decarboxylation cell-derived tumor), rheumatoid arthritis, hyperthyroidism, mycoplasma pneumonia infection, systemic lupus erythematosus, hypothyroidism, polycythemia rubra vera, Sjögren syndrome, and SAPHO (synovitis, acne, pustulosis, hyperostosis, and osteomyelitis) syndrome.

➲ HISTOPATHOLOGY

Histopathology demonstrates subcorneal pustule filled with polymorphonuclear leukocytes. A few acantholytic cells may be

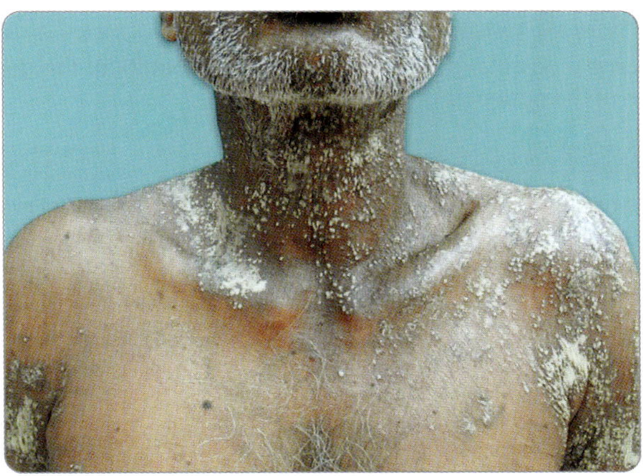

Fig. 1: Multiple superficial pustules with lakes of pus predominantly in the flexures in subcorneal pustular dermatosis (SCPD).

found (secondary acantholysis). The dermis contains a perivascular infiltrate composed of neutrophils and rarely mononuclear cells and eosinophils. Unlike in pustular psoriasis, the epidermis usually has minimal spongiosis.

Direct and indirect immunofluorescence results are commonly negative.

DIFFERENTIAL DIAGNOSIS

- *Bacterial impetigo*—bacteria (*Staphylococcus aureus*) are seen on gram stain and grown on culture.
- *Dermatitis herpetiformis*—subepidermal blisters with papillary tip abscess and granular IgA deposits at the dermal papillary tips on direct immunofluorescence (DIF)
- *Pemphigus foliaceus*—acantholytic cells on Tzanck smear, subcorneal blisters with positive IgG, and C3 deposits on DIF
- *IgA pemphigus*—bullae are arranged in cluster of jewels pattern and IgA deposition on DIF
- *Pustular psoriasis*—macropustules with other psoriasiform changes are seen on histopathological examination (HPE).
- Necrolytic migratory erythema
- Acute generalized exanthematous pustulosis

COMPLICATIONS

Secondary bacterial infections are the complications.

TREATMENT

Dapsone 50–150 mg daily; sulfapyridine is also beneficial, and others are infliximab, acitretin, and etretinate. Biologic agents, such as adalimumab, infliximab, and etanercept, have been used in challenging cases. Potent topical steroids can be used along with dapsone for better results.

➲ PROGNOSIS

Subcorneal pustular dermatosis is a benign condition; the general health of the patient is usually not impaired.

➲ SUGGESTED READING

1. Watts PJ, Khachemoune A. Subcorneal Pustular Dermatosis: A Review of 30 Years of Progress. Am J Clin Dermatol. 2016;17(6):653-71.

249 Subcutaneous Zygomycosis

➲ SYNONYMS

Basidiobolomycosis, subcutaneous phycomycosis, conidiobolomycosis, (rhino)-entomophthoromycosis.

➲ ETIOLOGY

Subcutaneous zygomycosis is caused by *Basidiobolus ranarum* (*B. haptosporus*), common in children, and *Conidiobolus conatus*, common in adults. The spores get inoculated after minor trauma.

➲ CLINICAL FEATURES

Lesions in basidiobolus infection usually develop around limb girdle sites and present with a firm, slowly spreading, woody cellulitis. There is bathing suit distribution. Conidiobolus infection starts in the region of the inferior turbinates of the nose and spreads to the central part of the face. The swelling is hard and painless and can be lifted off "finger insinuation sign." It may cause very severe deformity of the nose, lips, and cheeks.

➲ HISTOPATHOLOGY

Histopathologically, a chronic granulomatous response with large numbers of eosinophils can be seen. The fungi are present as large, strap-like hyphae without cross walls or septa. They are also often surrounded by refractile eosinophilic material (Splendore–Hoeppli phenomenon). The organisms can be cultured readily on Sabouraud's agar. The colonies are yellow to grayish with waxy texture. Other investigations include immunodiffusion and serological tests.

➲ DERMOSCOPY

Dermoscopy features include focal yellowish-orange structureless area and multiple dotted vessels over a background of diffuse erythema, yellow dots and scattered yellow-brown, white areas, linear and dotted vessels.

➲ COMPLICATIONS

Severe lesions may cause deformity of the lips, nose, and cheeks.

➲ TREATMENT

Oral potassium iodide 4–6 mL TID or 30 mg/kg/day for 3–4 weeks (drug of choice), ketoconazole 400 mg daily, and itraconazole 200 mg daily can be given. Amphotericin B has also been tried in treating subcutaneous zygomycosis.

➲ SUGGESTED READING

1. Anaparthy UR, Deepika G. A case of subcutaneous zygomycosis. Indian Dermatol Online J. 2014;5(1):51-4.

250 Sweet's Syndrome

➲ SYNONYMS

Acute febrile neutrophilic dermatoses, Gomm–Button disease.

➲ HISTORY

In 1964, Robert Douglas Sweet described the disease.

➲ EPIDEMIOLOGY

The age of onset is 30–60 years.

Female to male preponderance is 4:1. No racial predilections.

➲ ETIOPATHOGENESIS

The pathogenesis of Sweet's syndrome is unknown. The association with infections, autoimmune diseases, drugs, pregnancy, inflammatory bowel disease, and malignancies, as well as the greater incidence in women, suggest a hypersensitivity reaction. Up to 50% of patients may have idiopathic disease.

One current attractive hypothesis is a local or systemic dysregulation of cytokine [interleukin (IL)-1, granulocyte colony-stimulating factor (G-CSF), granulocyte–macrophage colony-stimulating factor (GM-CSF), and interferon-γ secretion].

➲ CLINICAL FEATURES

The initial cutaneous lesions are tender, nonpruritic, and erythematous plaques, which may enlarge or coalesce to form plaques with an uneven mammillated surface. Because of the pronounced associated edema, the lesions may have a pseudovesicular or pseudopustular and targetoid appearance. A facial erysipelas-like eruption has also been described. Vesiculobullous variant, which is most frequently associated with myelogenous leukemia, can progress to ulceration resembling superficial pyoderma gangrenosum. Common sites affected are the head, neck, and upper extremities.

➲ VARIANTS

Neutrophilic dermatosis of the dorsal hands or pustular vasculitis of the dorsal hands. *Subcutaneous Sweet's syndrome*—erythematous tender dermal nodules, resembling erythema nodosum.

➲ EXTRACUTANEOUS MANIFESTATIONS

The condition can affect the bones, central nervous system (CNS), ears, kidneys, intestines, lungs, heart, mouth, muscles, and spleen.

CRITERIA FOR DIAGNOSING SWEET'S SYNDROME

- *Major criteria:*
  - Abrupt onset of typical cutaneous lesions
  - Histopathology consistent with Sweet's syndrome
- *Minor criteria:*
  - Preceded by one of the associated infections or vaccinations; accompanied by one of the associated malignancies or inflammatory disorders; and associated with drug exposure or pregnancy
  - Presence of fever and constitutional signs and symptoms
  - Leukocytosis
  - Excellent response to systemic corticosteroids

  Two major and two minor criteria are needed for the diagnosis.

HISTOPATHOLOGY

The characteristic histologic presentation is a diffuse nodular and perivascular neutrophilic infiltrate without evidence of vasculitis, although occasionally, leukocytoclastic vasculitis (LCV) can be observed. Leukocytoclasia with endothelial swelling, but without the fibrinoid necrosis (which is a characteristic feature of LCV), is the usual finding.

DERMOSCOPY

Dermoscopy image shows pseudovesicles over a red background, manifested as white or yellowish-white zones with or without central pitting, dotted or linear vessels, surrounded by a red-and-white lattice-like ring, and round-to-oval red globules at the margins.

DIFFERENTIAL DIAGNOSIS

- *Clinical differential diagnosis (DD)*: Erythema multiforme (target lesions), drug eruptions, cellulitis (diffuse edema, erythema, and tenderness), erysipelas (well-defined erythematous swelling), chloroma, erythema nodosum (panniculitis on biopsy), urticaria (transient wheals are seen, no fever always), leukemia cutis, cutaneous small vessel vasculitis (palpable purpura is the hallmark lesion), panniculitis, halogenoderma, Wells' syndrome, systemic lupus erythematosus (SLE), and urticarial vasculitis.
- *Histopathological DD:* Abscess, cellulitis, leukemia cutis, and LCV.

TREATMENT

Oral prednisone (0.5–1.0 mg/kg/day) for 4–6 weeks, potassium iodide (900 mg/day), dapsone (100–200 mg/day), colchicine (1.5 mg/day), nonsteroidal anti-inflammatory drugs (e.g., indomethacin, naproxen, and sulindac), clofazimine, cyclosporine, thalidomide, and interferon-α have also been reported to lead to improvement of Sweet's syndrome.

PROGNOSIS

Sweet's syndrome is a benign condition, which, if left untreated, may persist for weeks or months. Cutaneous lesions then involute spontaneously, leaving no scars. However, recurrences occur in approximately 30% of patients (with or without treatment) and occur even more often in those with hematologic disorders (~50%).

➲ SUGGESTED READING

1. Vashisht P, Goyal A, Hearth Holmes MP. (2023). Sweet Syndrome. Treasure Island (FL): StatPearls Publishing. [online] Available from https://www.ncbi.nlm.nih.gov/books/NBK431050/ [Last accessed February, 2025].

251 Syphilis

SYNONYM

Lues.

HISTORY

The disease was named after an afflicted shepherd named Syphilus in 1530. *Treponema pallidum* was identified in 1905 by Schaudinn and Hoffmann.

ETIOLOGY

Syphilis is a sexually transmitted disease caused by *T. pallidum*. *T. pallidum* is a member of the genus *Treponema* of the order Spirochaetales.

CLINICAL FEATURES

Syphilis is a sexually acquired, chronic infection caused by *T. pallidum* and is characterized by a variety of clinical manifestations.

PRIMARY STAGE

The primary lesion develops 10–90 days after infection (the median period is 3 weeks) as an indolent papule, followed by surface necrosis and the typical well-circumscribed ulceration that is firm to palpation (chancre), as well as enlarged regional lymph nodes, which are painless and rubbery. Untreated syphilis heals within a few weeks.

SECONDARY STAGE

The secondary stage is characterized by the dissemination and multiplication of the microorganism in different tissues, either simultaneously up to 6 months after the healing of the primary local lesion.

CLINICAL FEATURES OF SECONDARY SYPHILIS

- *Prodromal symptoms and signs*:
  - Weight loss
  - Low-grade fever
  - Malaise
  - Headache (meningeal irritation)
  - Sore throat
  - Conjunctivitis (iridocyclitis)
  - Arthralgia (periostitis)
  - Myalgias
  - Hepatosplenomegaly (mild hepatitis)

- Generalized lymphadenopathy with indolent enlargement of lymph nodes (50–85%)
- *Skin manifestations*:
  - Early (10%): Generalized eruption; nonpruritic, roseola-like, discrete macules, initially distributed on the flanks and shoulders
  - Late (70%): Generalized maculopapular and papulosquamous eruptions; more infiltrated lesions, often copper-colored; annular plaques on the face; corymbose arrangement (satellite papules around a larger central lesion); occurs in successive waves and polymorphic **(Fig. 1)**
- *Localized syphilis (specific infiltrations of treponemes; positive darkfield examination)*:
  - Palms and soles **(Fig. 2)**: Symmetric papules and plaques with a collarette of scale (collarette of Biett)
  - Anogenital area: Condylomata lata **(Fig. 3)**.
  - Seborrheic area: "Corona veneris" along the hairline
  - Hypopigmented macules, mainly on the neck (postinflammatory; "necklace of Venus")

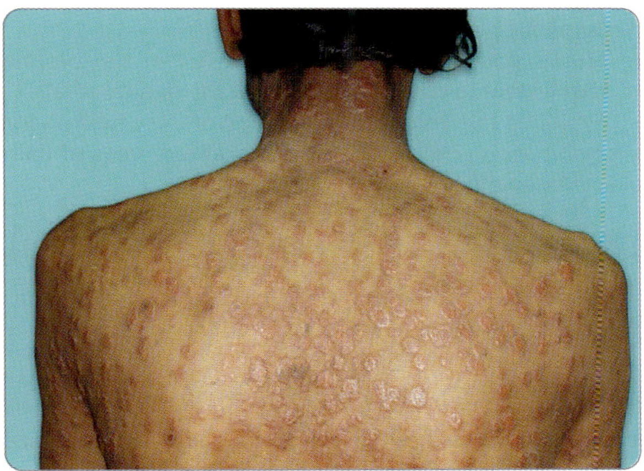

Fig. 1: Generalized papulosquamous eruptions.

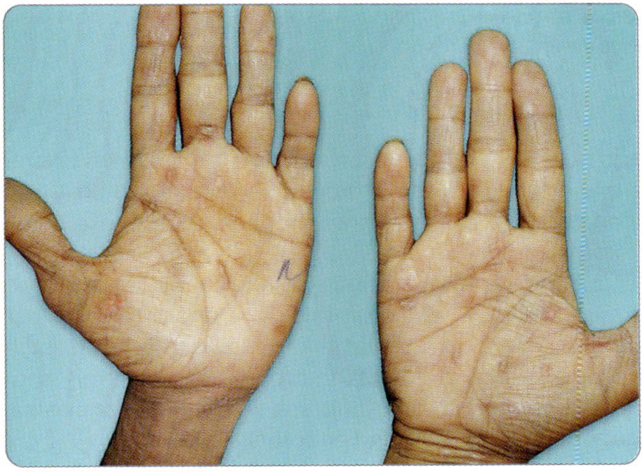

Fig. 2: Asymptomatic papules over palms.

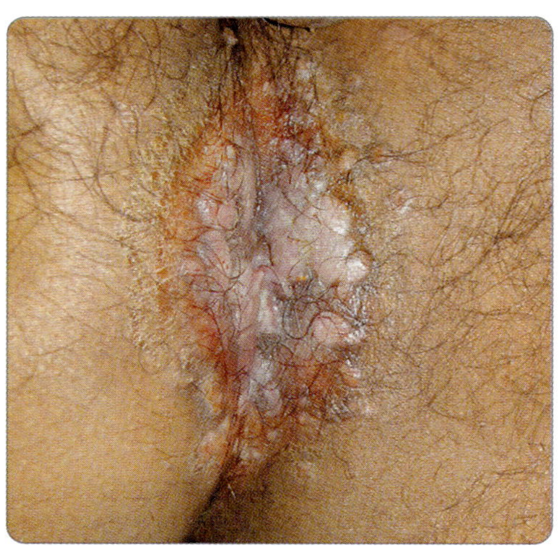

Fig. 3: Flat moist papules of condylomata lata.

- *Manifestations involving mucus membranes (30%)*:
  - Syphilitic perlèche and split papules
  - Mucus patches: "Plaques muqueuses" in the oropharynx (equivalent to condylomata lata in the genital area)
  - Syphilitic sore throat: Inflammation of the whole pharynx
- *Patchy alopecia (7%)*: "Moth-eaten" localized areas of hair loss; toxic telogen effluvium

LATENCY

Latency is the period between the healing of the clinical lesions and the appearance of late manifestations, and it can last for many years.

TERTIARY STAGE

The tertiary stage is also called late syphilis and is characterized by the presence of a small number of organisms and a high cellular immune reactivity against the organism. The microorganisms can invade the central nervous or cardiovascular systems and the skin (as well as other organs) and lead to damage due to host delayed-type hypersensitivity responses.

HISTOPATHOLOGY

Primary syphilis (primary chancre) demonstrates an acanthotic epidermis, which erodes with time to become ulcerated. Under the ulcer bed, there is typically a dense lymphocytic response, numerous plasma cells, and endothelial swelling.

Secondary syphilis exhibits variable histopathology. The epidermis shows a psoriasiform hyperplasia with superficial neutrophils. There can be lichenoid tissue reaction, epidermal apoptosis, and exocytosis of neutrophils. The dermis shows a superficial and deep chronic infiltrate, with numerous plasma cells in about one-third of cases and endothelial swelling.

Tertiary syphilis shows necrotizing granulomatous inflammation.

DERMOSCOPY

Polarized light dermoscopy of the secondary syphilis lesion shows scaling within the skin furrows and central darker area fading toward the periphery with an ill-defined border.

DIAGNOSIS

- *Primary stage*: Dark-field microscopy, direct fluorescent antibody test for *T. pallidum*, and nucleic acid amplification methods to detect *T. pallidum*
- *Secondary stage*: Venereal disease research laboratory (VDRL), rapid plasma reagin (RPR), and treponema pallidum hemagglutination (TPHA)
- *Tertiary stage*: TPHA and VDRL-cerebrospinal fluid (CSF) for neurosyphilis

TREATMENT

Penicillin G is still the treatment of choice for all stages of syphilis. In primary and secondary syphilis as well as in early latent syphilis <1 year in duration, a single intramuscular dose of 2.4 million units of benzathine penicillin is recommended as a sufficient treatment for immunocompetent adults. In immunocompromised patients, three doses of benzathine penicillin 2.4 million units are given at weekly interval. Doxycycline 100 mg PO BID for 2 weeks (for early syphilis) or for 4 weeks (for late latent or syphilis of unknown duration) is an alternative for the treatment of nonpregnant people with a penicillin allergy. Penicillin is the only approved treatment in pregnancy.

SUGGESTED READING

1. Tiecco G, Degli Antoni M, Storti S, Marchese V, Focà E, Torti C, et al. A 2021 Update on Syphilis: Taking Stock from Pathogenesis to Vaccines. Pathogens. 2021;10(11):1364.

252 Syringoma

➲ SYNONYMS

Syringocystadenoma, syringocystoma, hidradenoma eruptis.

➲ ETIOLOGY

Syringoma is a benign neoplasm with differentiation toward acrosyringium.

➲ AGE GROUP

Adult females are more commonly affected.

➲ CLINICAL FEATURES

Syringoma manifests clinically as 2- to 4-mm, firm, skin-colored papules and may occur at any site on the body but is prone to occur in the periorbital area, especially the eyelids **(Fig. 1)**. Sometimes, lesions involve the upper trunk or genital skin. Eruptive syringomas most commonly involve the trunk but may involve the extremities, including the palms and soles. Acral syringomas are those that are most clearly of eccrine lineage, as the acini of glabrous skin are exclusively eccrine. Linear and disseminated syringomas have been described.

➲ DIFFERENTIAL DIAGNOSIS

- *Facial lesions*—plane warts (presence of koilocytes; koebnerization is seen), milia (white-colored smooth papules are seen), and xanthelasma (yellowish plaques usually on the upper eyelids)

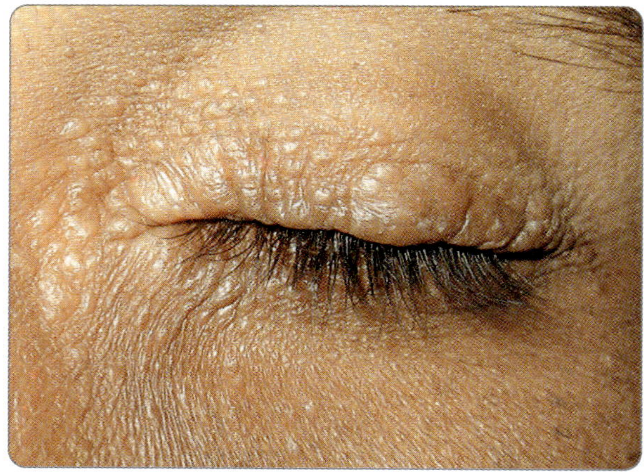

Fig. 1: Multiple skin-colored papules in the periorbital area.

- *Truncal lesions*—eruptive vellus hair cysts and disseminated granuloma annulare
- Very superficial punch biopsies from microcystic adnexal tumor can be confused with syringoma; one must know if the biopsy is representative of many small lesions or a sample from a single large tumor.

ASSOCIATED SYNDROMES

Associated syndromes include Nicolau–Balus syndrome (syringomas and milia) and increased frequency in Down syndrome.

HISTOPATHOLOGY

From scanning magnification, a syringoma is small, symmetric, and well circumscribed and is usually confined to the superficial dermis. Tumor consists of mature sweat ductal structures lined by two layers of cuboidal cells. Some of the ductal structures have an epithelial elongation of the ducts (tadpole-like appearance/paisley tie appearance). The surrounding stroma is sclerotic. Often, stroma is very dense, and it condenses the ductal structures into the cords (desmoplastic variant).

DERMOSCOPY

Dermoscopy of papules shows multiple pigmented clusters, which consist of brown pseudonetwork and multiple white dots, which appeared larger than those over uninvolved skin.

COMPLICATIONS

Complications include cosmetic concern.

TREATMENT

Trichloroacetic acid (TCA) application, cryotherapy, punch excision, electrodessication, and laser are the treatment options.

PROGNOSIS

Spontaneous regression is known. Treatment is unsatisfactory. Recurrences are common.

SUGGESTED READING

1. Avhad G, Ghuge P, Jerajani HR. Generalized eruptive syringoma. Indian J Dermatol. 2015;60(2):214.

253 Systemic Lupus Erythematosus

SYNONYMS

Integumentary lupus erythematosus, visceral lupus erythematosus

INTRODUCTION

Systemic lupus erythematosus (SLE) is an autoimmune disease, which affects multiple systems and has varying presentations and significant comorbidities. It is 10 times more common in females.

ETIOLOGY

- *Genetic factors*: Human leukocyte antigen (HLA)-B8, -DR3, -A1, and -DR2
- *Autoantibodies*: Non-organ-specific humoral autoantibodies are the hallmark of SLE.
- *Immune factors*: Abnormal cell-mediated and humoral immunity
- Ultraviolet (UV) radiation
- Environmental factors, silicone breast implants, ingestion of sprouts, seeds, dietary supplements of alfalfa, and heavy metals
- Infections, stress, and hormonal factors
- *Drugs*: Hydralazine, minocycline, procainamide, etc.

PATHOLOGY

The primary lesions of SLE show fibrinoid necrosis, collagen sclerosis, necrosis and basophilic body formation, and vascular endothelial thickening.

IMMUNOHISTOLOGY

Immunohistology visualizes immunoglobulins (IgG, IgM, and IgA) and complement (C1 and C3) at the dermoepidermal junction (DEJ).

CLINICAL FEATURES

Systemic lupus erythematosus is a systemic disease characterized by multisystem organ inflammation, most commonly the skin, joints, and vasculature, and associated immunological abnormalities.

Cutaneous lesions are classified as:

- Those specific for lupus erythematosus (LE)
- Those that are less specific

Specific Lesions

- Acute cutaneous lupus erythematosus (ACLE) is commonly seen as the classic malar or butterfly rash **(Fig. 1)**, a fixed, well-demarcated, symmetrical erythema that can be flat or raised over the cheeks and the bridge of the nose.

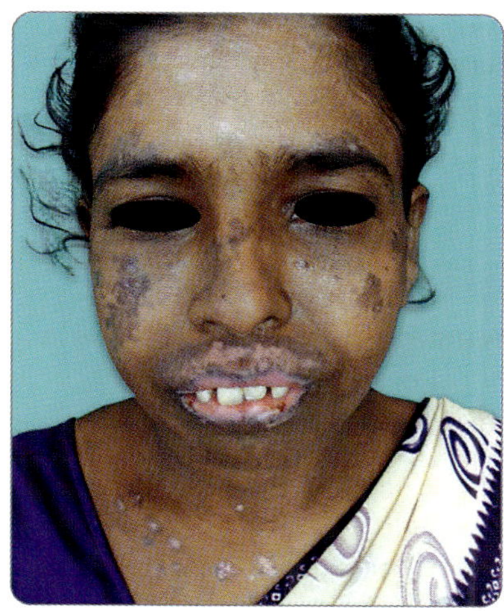

Fig. 1: Erythema and crusted lesions over the face, lips, and exposed part of the face.

- Subacute cutaneous lupus erythematosus (SCLE) presents as a nonscarring papulosquamous or annular, polycyclic eruption.
- Chronic cutaneous lupus erythematosus (CCLE) [discoid lupus erythematosus (DLE)] appears as sharply demarcated, erythematous macules, papules, or small plaques, which rapidly develop a hyperkeratotic surface with an adherent scale extending into the follicular orifices (carpet tack sign).

Nonspecific Changes

- *Vascular*:
    - Annular erythema
    - Telangiectasia
    - Purpura
    - Vasculitis
    - Thrombophlebitis
    - Raynaud's phenomenon
    - Livedo reticularis
    - Chronic ulcers
    - Rheumatoid nodules
    - Peripheral gangrene
    - Atrophie blanche-like or Degos disease-like dermal infarcts
    - Erythema multiforme
    - Erythromelalgia
- *Alopecia*:
    - Lupus hair
    - Alopecia areata
    - Scarring alopecia
- Mucous membrane lesions
- Nail changes
- Pigmentary abnormalities
- Sclerodactyly and sclerodermatous changes
- Calcinosis cutis
- Urticaria

- Bullous lesions
- Papulonodular mucinosis
- Acanthosis nigricans
- Anetoderma
- Lichen planus
- Porphyria cutanea tarda

DIAGNOSIS

American Rheumatism Association Criteria

- Malar rash
- Discoid rash
- Photosensitivity
- Oral ulcers
- Nonerosive arthritis
- *Serositis*—pleurisy or pericarditis
- *Renal disorder*—persistent proteinuria (>0.5 g/day) or cellular casts
- *Neurological disorder*—seizures or psychosis
- *Hematological disorder*—hemolytic anemia or leukopenia (<4,000/mm^3) or lymphopenia (<1,500/mm^3) or thrombocytopenia (<100,000/mm^3)
- *Immunological disorder*—LE cells or anti-double-stranded DNA (dsDNA) antibody or anti-Sm antibody or false-positive serology for syphilis (>6 months)
- Antinuclear antibodies (ANAs)

Systemic Lupus International Collaborating Clinics Criteria

The Systemic Lupus International Collaborating Clinics (SLICC) criteria for SLE:

- At least four criteria out of 17 should be fulfilled, with at least one clinical and one immunologic criteria, or
- *Lupus nephritis*—biopsy proven; in the presence of ANA or anti-dsDNA antibodies.

Clinical Criteria

- Acute cutaneous lupus
- Chronic cutaneous lupus
- Oral ulcers
- Nonscarring alopecia
- Synovitis of two or more joints, with swelling or effusion or tenderness in two or more joints and 30 minutes or more of morning stiffness
- Serositis
- Renal manifestation
- Neurologic manifestation
- Hemolytic anemia
- Leukopenia (<4,000/mm^3 at least once)
- Thrombocytopenia (<100,000/mm^3) at least once

Immunological Criteria

- Antinuclear antibody positivity
- Anti-dsDNA

- Anti-Sm
- Antiphospholipid antibody (any of the following)
- Low complement levels
- Direct Coombs test positive in the absence of hemolytic anemia

INVESTIGATIONS

Complete hemogram, erythrocyte sedimentation rate (ESR), C-reactive protein (CRP), rheumatoid factor (RF) lupus anticoagulant, LE cell test, anti-dsDNA, anti-ssDNA, anti-Sm antibody, anti-RNP (ribonucleoprotein) antibodies, anti-Ro, anti-La, antihistone antibody, cryoglobulins, alpha 2-macroglobulin, and serum interferon (IFN) can be done.

HISTOPATHOLOGY

Lupus erythematosus skin lesions typically feature a histopathologic pattern termed interface dermatitis, defined by the presence of necroptotic keratinocytes and an epitheliotropic cytotoxic lymphocytic infiltrate at the DEJ.

DERMOSCOPY

- *Acute LE*: A malar rash shows an "inverse strawberry" pattern, consisting of reddish follicular dots, surrounded by white halos. In generalized ACLE, a multicomponent pattern, with white scaling, pinkish-white to reddish-white structureless areas, brown dots and globules, keratotic plugs, and linear or linear branched vessels, is observed.
- *Subacute LE*: The dermoscopic features of SCLE include white scales, polymorphous vessels (linear, linear-irregular, linear branched, and/or sparsely distributed dotted vessels), and pink-red backgrounds.

DIFFERENTIAL DIAGNOSIS

- Kikuchi's disease, Still's disease, and Sweet's syndrome
- *Acute cutaneous lupus erythematosus*: Cellulitis, rosacea, the heliotrope erythema of dermatomyositis, photodermatitis, and seborrheic dermatitis
- *Subacute cutaneous lupus erythematosus*: Polymorphic light eruption, psoriasis, seborrheic dermatitis or lymphomas, and annular lesions, from tinea corporis and erythema annulare centrifugum
- *Chronic cutaneous lupus erythematosus (CCLE)*: Psoriasis, seborrheic dermatitis, Bowen's disease, actinic keratosis, polymorphic light eruption, lupus vulgaris, and lymphocytic infiltration of Jessner, tinea faciei, and superficial basal carcinoma, vitiligo, lichen planus, and folliculitis decalvans

TREATMENT

- Strict photoprotection
- *Antimalarials*: Hydroxychloroquine 400 mg/day or <6.5 mg/kg/day
- In acute cases, prednisolone 60 mg/day

- Others are azathioprine, cyclophosphamide, chlorambucil, methotrexate 7.5 mg/week, ciclosporin 3–5 mg/kg, mycophenolate mofetil, and oral levamisole 150 mg tid
- Pulse therapy with methylprednisolone 1 g
- Rituximab, an antibody targeting the CD20 marker antigen
- Plasmapheresis, extracorporeal photochemotherapy, anti-lymphocyte, and antithymocyte antisera

PROGNOSIS

Systemic lupus erythematosus tends to be chronic and relapsing, often with symptom-free periods that can last for years. Death can occur due to lupus nephritis.

SUGGESTED READING

1. Justiz Vaillant AA, Goyal A, Varacallo M. (2023). Systemic Lupus Erythematosus. Treasure Island (FL): StatPearls Publishing. [online] Available from https://www.ncbi.nlm.nih.gov/books/NBK535405/ [Last accessed February, 2025].

254 Telogen Effluvium

➲ SYNONYM

Telogen defluvium.

➲ HISTORY

The term telogen effluvium (TE), first coined by Kligman in 1961, refers to the loss of club (telogen) hair in disease states of the follicle.

➲ ETIOLOGY

Telogen effluvium is a medical sign rather than the diagnosis. It is important to find the triggering factor(s). The triggering factors include:

- *Endocrine*: Childbirth, abortion, hypo-/hyperthyroidism, and discontinuation of oral contraceptive pills (OCPs)
- *Stressful events*: Major surgery, chronic illness, major trauma, and psychological stress
- *Drugs*: Anticoagulants and beta blockers
- *Nutrition*: Crash diets and iron deficiency

➲ CLINICAL FEATURE

Clinically, TE may present as acute TE (<4 months), chronic telogen effluvium (CTE) (>4 months), and chronic repetitive. Headington described five functional types of TE based on different phases of the follicular cycle:

1. Immediate anagen release
2. Delayed anagen release
3. Short anagen syndrome
4. Immediate telogen release
5. Delayed telogen release

Acute TE is an acute-onset scalp hair loss that begins 2 weeks after a triggering event but peaks between 6 and 8 weeks and then tapers off in about 6–8 weeks. The daily loss ranges from under 100 to over 1,000. If the lower rates of shedding are continued for only a short period, there may be no obvious baldness, but if shedding occurs at higher rates, diffuse reduction in hair density is produced **(Fig. 1)**. Unless the trigger is repeated, spontaneous complete regrowth occurs within 3–6 months.

Telogen gravidarum refers to the telogen hair loss seen 2–3 months after childbirth. It is an example of delayed anagen release. It is universal to some degree but is often subclinical. Most cases of telogen gravidarum resolve.

Chronic diffuse telogen hair loss refers to telogen hair shedding persisting for >6 months. It can be a result of a primary CTE or be secondary to a variety of causes, including female pattern hair loss (FPHL). To be a true cause of chronic diffuse telogen hair loss, the

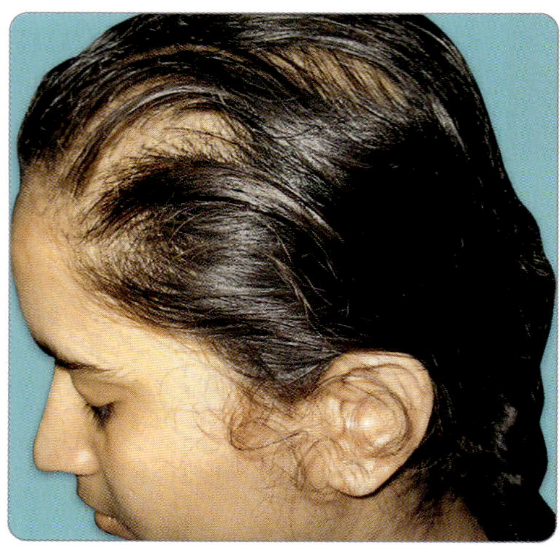

Fig. 1: Telogen effluvium.

relationship between the trigger and the hair loss must be reversible and reproducible.

Drug-induced diffuse telogen hair loss usually starts 6–12 weeks after instigation of treatment and is progressive while the drug is continued. It is most commonly a result of immediate anagen release. The retinoids appear to cause a telogen anchorage defect and reduce the duration of anagen. Minoxidil has been reported to cause a short-lived telogen shedding by immediate telogen release.

Chronic telogen effluvium is a primary, idiopathic, and often self-limiting condition affecting middle-aged women that is distinct from androgenetic hair loss and chronic diffuse TE secondary to organic causes. Women describe a sudden onset of increased hair shedding persisting for at least 6 months. There is no associated visible widening of the central parting line and no miniaturization of hair follicles on scalp biopsy. The diagnosis of CTE is made by exclusion of other causes of diffuse telogen hair loss. A thorough history is required, including a detailed drug and dietary history. A full clinical examination should be performed, including scalp examination and hair pull testing.

➲ INVESTIGATIONS

The diagnosis is usually simple. Abrupt-onset TE is likely to be related to a specific event or trigger 6–16 weeks earlier. The hair pull test is positive, with normal club hairs.

The trichogram from a hair pluck sample usually shows >25% of telogen hairs in acute TE. Histological examination shows an increase in the proportion of follicles in telogen.

The following should be present to make a diagnosis of TE:

- Normal number of terminal (large) hairs
- Increase in the telogen count to >20% (>15% is suggestive)
- Absence of inflammation and scarring
- Telogen count seldom exceeds 50%; >80% is inconsistent with TE.

DERMOSCOPY

There are no specific trichoscopy findings of TE. However, the presence of upright regrowing hairs and the predominance of single-hair follicular units with perifollicular discoloration may be indicative of TE in the absence of features characteristic of other causes of hair loss.

TREATMENT

Good nutrition and vitamin supplements can be given. If it is drug-induced, the offending drug should be discontinued. Since it is a self-limiting condition, no active intervention is required.

PROGNOSIS

Prognosis is very good. Most of the patients get back their previous hair density in 6 months to 1 year.

SUGGESTED READING

1. Hughes EC, Saleh D. (2023). Telogen Effluvium. Treasure Island (FL): StatPearls Publishing. [online] Available from https://www.ncbi.nlm.nih.gov/books/NBK430848/ [Last accessed February, 2025].

255 Terra Firma-Forme Dermatosis

➲ SYNONYM

Duncan's dirty dermatosis.

➲ HISTORY

Terra firma-forme dermatosis (TFFD) was reported for the first time by Duncan, Tschen, and Knox in 1987. "*Terra firma*" in Latin means solid land.

➲ ETIOPATHOGENESIS

Terra firma-forme dermatosis is a disorder of unknown etiology. It is said to be due to disordered and delayed keratinization. This leads to the accumulation of keratinocytes and melanin in the epidermis. This along with sebum and dirt leads to the hyperpigmented plaques. Currently, no known predisposing factors have been identified.

➲ CLINICAL FEATURES

Terra firma-forme dermatosis appears as asymptomatic, hyperpigmented, dirt-like plaques that are resistant to washing with soap but can be rubbed off by 70% isopropyl alcohol. It is commonly found on the neck, axilla, and trunk but can occur anywhere in the body.

➲ HISTOPATHOLOGY

Hematoxylin and eosin (H&E) section shows lamellar hyperkeratosis with compact orthokeratotic whorls and absence of parakeratosis, acanthosis, and papillomatosis; the presence of keratotic material between papillae; and melanin deposition in the basal layer as well as hyperkeratotic areas.

➲ DERMOSCOPY

Dermoscopy shows brownish polygonal scales with mosaic pattern.

➲ TREATMENT

Terra firma-forme dermatosis can be completely removed with 70% isopropyl alcohol. Salicylic acid peel has also been used with success.

➲ DIFFERENTIAL DIAGNOSIS

- *Dermatosis neglecta*: Hyperpigmentation due to the accumulation of adherent scales due to inadequate washing/cleaning of the skin. Lesions can be removed with rubbing by soap and water repeatedly and can also be removed by 70% isopropyl alcohol.

- *Acanthosis nigricans*: Brown to black velvety plaques are usually present in body folds like the neck, axilla, and groin. It occurs due to hyperinsulinemia secondary to insulin resistance. Treating the underlying cause can cure the disease. It does not respond to washing/scrubbing/isopropyl alcohol. Acrochordons are a frequent association.
- *Pityriasis versicolor*: Superficial mycosis, caused by *Malassezia* species. It usually occurs in tropical climate. It can occur as hyper-/hypopigmented lesions. KOH shows a spaghetti and meatballs appearance. It is treated with topical and systemic antifungals. It does not respond to isopropyl alcohol.
- *Seborrheic keratosis:* Benign epidermal keratinocyte proliferation. In early stages, it presents as small, flat to slightly raised tan or brown macules. Later, they become elevated and get a verrucous surface. It does not respond to rubbing with isopropyl alcohol but can be curetted off.

➲ PROGNOSIS

Prognosis is very good. It is a benign dermatologic condition. It can be easily removed with isopropyl alcohol and chemical peels. But there are chances of recurrence.

➲ SUGGESTED READING

1. Mohta A, Sarkar R, Narayan RV, Deoghare S, Arora A. Terra firma-forme dermatosis—more than just dirty. Indian Dermatol Online J. 2024;15: 99-104.

256 Tinea

➲ SYNONYM

Ringworm.

➲ INTRODUCTION

Cutaneous infections caused by dermatophytes are called tinea infections. They are named according to the site of infection.

➲ ETIOLOGY

All species of dermatophytes can produce lesions of the glabrous skin, the most common species being *Trichophyton rubrum*, *T. mentagrophytes*, and *Microsporum canis*.

➲ EPIDEMIOLOGY

Tinea is common in the tropical or subtropical areas. Predisposing factors include poor personal hygiene, poor nutrition, and debilitating systemic diseases like diabetes, leukemia, and other endocrine disorders. It is transmitted by direct contact with other infected individuals or infected animals.

TINEA CORPORIS

➲ SYNONYMS

Ringworm of the body, tinea circinata.

➲ CLINICAL FEATURES

The site of infection is typically on the exposed skin, but it can occur on any area of the body. Characteristic lesions are circular, usually sharply marginated, with a raised edge **(Fig. 1)**. Its borders are erythematous and vesicular or scaly, but the center is clear. In addition to annular lesions, other morphological variants include eczematous annular type, crusted type, herpetiform type, and plaque type.

➲ DIFFERENTIAL DIAGNOSIS

- *Pityriasis rosea*—preceding streptococcal infection, herald patch followed by scaly lesions arranged on the trunk in a Christmas tree pattern, and collarette of scales
- *Nummular eczema*—absence of central clearing, well-defined patch/plaque with crusting and scaling, and no fungal filaments
- *Erythema annulare centrifugum*—negative KOH mount

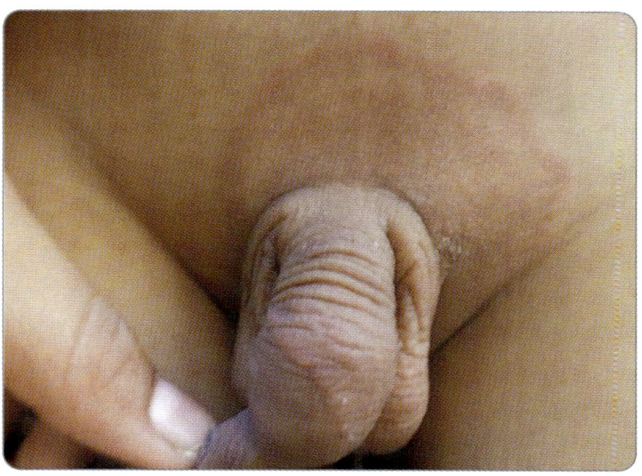

Fig. 1: Annular scaly tinea corporis.

- *Granuloma annulare*—mainly on the exposed areas, annular lesions that, on stretching, show prominent papules arranged at the periphery, and palisading granulomas on histopathological examination (HPE)
- *Psoriasis*—profuse silvery white scales and positive grattage test and Auspitz sign
- *Seborrheic dermatitis*—absence of well-defined annular lesions
- *Secondary syphilis*—negative KOH mount and venereal disease research laboratory (VDRL) test positivity

TINEA CRURIS

SYNONYMS

Dhobie's itch, eczema marginatum.

CLINICAL FEATURES

Lesions are characterized by multiple erythematous papulovesicles with a well-marginated, raised border. Lesions are often coalescent with extension to the pubic, perianal, buttock, and lower abdominal areas. Pruritus is present.

DIFFERENTIAL DIAGNOSIS

- *Candidiasis*—macerated and glazed appearance with pustules at edges, frayed margins, and yeast cells on KOH mount
- *Intertrigo*—fissures and maceration and the absence of fugal hyphae
- *Erythrasma*—uniform brownish, nonscaly, asymptomatic patches and red fluorescence on Wood's lamp examination
- *Psoriasis*—classical HPE features and negative KOH mount
- Seborrheic dermatitis
- Contact dermatitis
- Atopic eczema

TINEA IMBRICATA

SYNONYM

Tokelu.

ETIOLOGY

Trichophyton concentricum.

CLINICAL FEATURES

The early lesion is annular, with a circle of scales at the periphery, then a new and large scaly ring forms, with a zone of apparently normal skin between the rings. This phenomenon occurs successively, with the pathognomic appearance of concentric circles, which may reach as many as 10 per lesion. The natural history is extremely prolonged, so the whole body may become affected. Intense pruritus is seen. Secondary changes like lichenification and hypopigmentation may be seen.

TINEA MANUUM

SYNONYM

Ringworm of the hands.

CLINICAL FEATURES

Dermatophytosis of the palms and interdigital areas of the hands is called tinea manuum. It is characterized by hyperkeratosis of the palms and fingers. It is unilateral in 50% of cases. Accentuation of flexural creases is also seen. Other clinical variants include crescentic exfoliating scales, circumscribed vesicular patches, discrete red papular and follicular scaly patches, and erythematous scaly sheets on the dorsal surface of hands.

DIFFERENTIAL DIAGNOSIS

Differential diagnosis includes contact dermatitis, psoriasis, pityriasis rubra pilaris, keratoderma, syphilis, and poststreptococcal peeling.

TINEA PEDIS

SYNONYMS

Foot ringworm, athlete's foot.

ETIOPATHOGENESIS

Tinea pedis is caused by *T. rubrum*, *T. mentagrophytes var. interdigitale*, and *E. floccosum*.

Predisposing factors are occlusion of the toe clefts through wearing shoes, living in institutions where washing facilities are shared, people using communal baths and pools, maceration, and warm and humid climate.

➲ CLINICAL FEATURES

There are four clinical forms:

1. *Chronic intertriginous type:* It is the most common type and is characterized by fissuring, scaling, maceration, or white hyperkeratosis in the interdigital or subdigital areas.
2. Chronic papulosquamous pattern is characterized by inflammation and a patchy or diffuse moccasin-like scaling over the soles. "One hand and two feet" presentation: It is a variant where, along with the feet, the hands are also involved.
3. Vesicular or vesiculobullous type is caused by *T. mentagrophytes var. interdigitale*. Small vesicles or vesicopustules are seen near the instep and on the midanterior plantar surface.
4. Acute ulcerative variant is commonly associated with maceration, weeping, denudation, and ulceration.

➲ DIFFERENTIAL DIAGNOSIS

Differential diagnosis includes psoriasis, candidosis, bacterial infections, soft corn or callosity, Reiter's disease, contact dermatitis, tylosis, and erythrasma.

TINEA BARBAE

➲ SYNONYMS

Tinea sycosis, ringworm of the beard, Barber's itch.

➲ ETIOLOGY

The infection is seen only in adult males. It was largely transmitted by contaminated barbers' razors in the past, and improved sanitation has reduced its incidence. It is now more commonly contracted by direct exposure to cattle, horses, or dogs and is thus seen more commonly in rural areas in farmers and ranchers. The causative organisms are *T. verrucosum*, *T. mentagrophytes var. mentagrophytes* (most common), *M. canis*, *T. mentagrophytes var. erinacei*, *T. violaceum*, *T. schoenleinii*, *T. megninii*, and *T. rubrum* (rare).

➲ AGE GROUP

Adult males.

➲ CLINICAL FEATURES

Typically, it is unilateral and more often involves the beard area than the upper lip or moustache. Three forms exist:

1. *Inflammatory type:* It is analogous to kerion formation in tinea capitis. The lesions are nodular and boggy and are often associated with seropurulent discharge and crusting.

2. *Superficial or sycosiform type:* It closely resembles bacterial folliculitis. It is seen mostly with anthrophilic species.
3. *Circinate or spreading type*: It resembles ringworm of glabrous skin.
4. *Atypical forms* like granuloma annulare-like or abscess-like tumors with *M. canis* and verrucous granulomatous lesions with *E. floccosum* (verrucous epidermophyton).

➲ DIFFERENTIAL DIAGNOSIS

Differential diagnosis includes sycosis barbae, bacterial folliculitis (sycosis vulgaris), perioral dermatitis, *Candida* folliculitis, pseudofolliculitis barbae, acne vulgaris/rosacea, contact dermatitis, herpes simplex, and halogenoderma.

➲ COMPLICATIONS

Chronic inflammatory type of lesions may form sinus tracts, eventuating in scarring alopecia.

➲ TREATMENT OF TINEA BARBAE

Griseofulvin (0.5–1.0 g/day × 4–6 weeks), itraconazole, terbinafine, fluconazole +/– topical antifungal + regular shaving + cleansing with antibacterial soaps.

TINEA FACIEI

➲ SYNONYMS

Ringworm of the face, tinea faciale.

➲ CLINICAL FEATURES

The lesions are associated with itching, burning, and exacerbation after sun exposure. A history of exposure to animals is often present. The size of the lesion, degree of inflammation, and depth of invasion are highly variable **(Fig. 2)**. It most often begins as an erythematous, scaly macule that extends peripherally and develops a raised border. The central area becomes hypopigmented or brown and less scaly. In some cases, simple papular lesions or completely flat patches of erythema also occur. A few vesicles or pustules may be found, but these are rarely conspicuous.

➲ DIFFERENTIAL DIAGNOSIS

Discoid lupus erythematosus (DLE), polymorphic light eruption, psoriasis, impetigo, rosacea, seborrheic dermatitis, atopic dermatitis, bacterial infections, irritant contact dermatitis, granuloma annulare, systemic lupus erythematosus (SLE), perioral dermatitis, pityriasis alba, ptyriasis rosea, and benign lymphocytic infiltrates.

Diagnosis of dermatophytic infections can be confirmed by KOH examination **(Figs. 3A and B)** of the scrapings from the lesion or culture on Sabouraud Dextrose Agar (SDA).

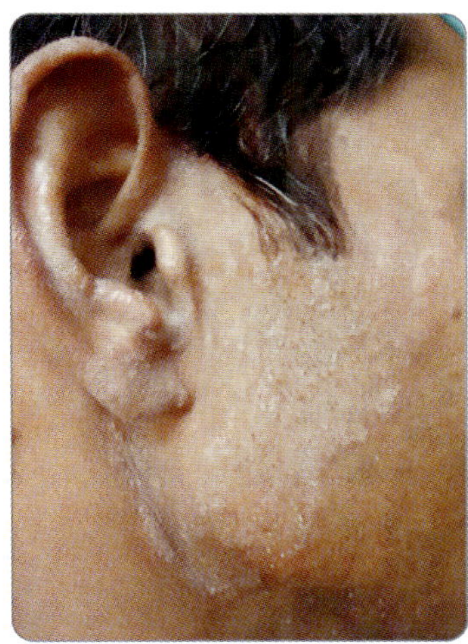

Fig. 2: Well-demarcated scaly lesion of tinea faciei.

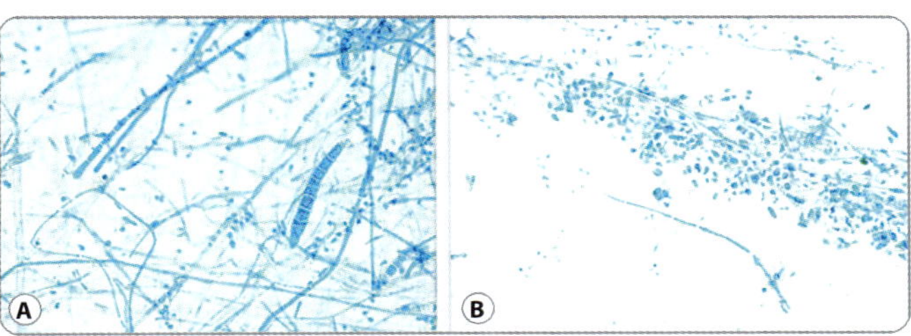

Figs. 3A and B: (A) Spores; (B) Hyphae.

DERMOSCOPY

Dermoscopic features of tinea faciei include peripheral scales, moth-eaten scales, broken hairs and scales that peel outward, peripheral vasculature in a dotted arrangement, and white scales, and there is a lack of perifollicular scales.

TREATMENT OF DERMATOPHYTIC INFECTIONS

The topical azoles (e.g., econazole, ketoconazole, clotrimazole, miconazole, oxiconazole, sulconazole, and sertaconazole), allylamines (e.g., naftifine and terbinafine), and ciclopirox olamine are used for limited infection.

Systemic therapy is indicated during extensive skin infection, immunosuppression, resistance to topical antifungal therapy, and comorbidities of tinea capitis.

Oral ketoconazole at 3–4 mg/kg/day, fluconazole at 50–100 mg/day or 150 mg once weekly for 2–4 weeks, oral terbinafine 250 mg/day for 2 weeks, and oral itraconazole in doses of 100 mg/day for 2 weeks show high efficacy.

SUGGESTED READING

1. Leung AK, Lam JM, Leong KF, Hon KL. Tinea corporis: an updated review. Drugs Context. 2020;9:2020-5-6.

257 Tinea Capitis

SYNONYMS

Ringworm of the scalp, tinea tonsurans.

AGE GROUP

The predominant age group is 3–7 years. The quantity of fungistatic saturated fatty acids in sebum increases at puberty, so adults are rarely affected. The M:F ratio is 5:1.

ETIOLOGY

Tinea capitis is caused by dermatophytes in the genera *Microsporum* and *Trichophyton*. Out of these, the species *Epidermophyton floccosum*, *Trichophyton concentricum*, and *T. mentagrophytes variant interdigitale* do not cause tinea capitis. Tinea capitis is a communicable fungal infection transmitted by intimate personal contact.

CLINICAL FEATURES

Tinea capitis is a dermatophytosis of the scalp hair follicles and the surrounding skin. There are four different clinical presentations:

1. *Gray patch*: It is a noninflammatory type. It is characterized by patches of partial hair loss. The affected hairs are dull gray and lusterless. Patients may complain of mild itching **(Fig. 1)**.
2. *Black dot*: It is a noninflammatory type of tinea capitis. It is characterized by well-demarcated areas of hair loss, with hairs broken off at the follicular orifice, giving the characteristic appearance of black dots **(Fig. 2)**.

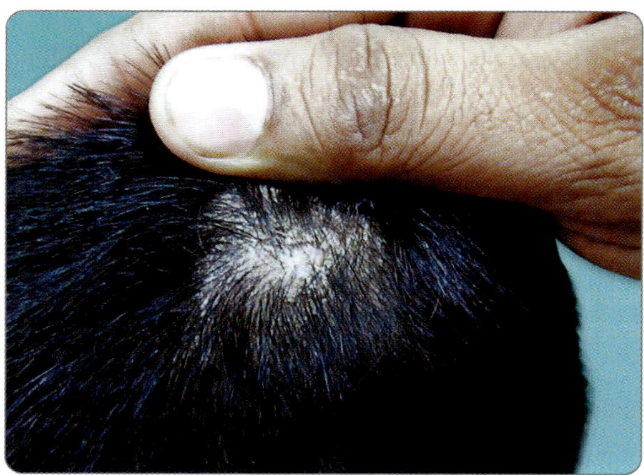

Fig. 1: Well-defined area of gray patch with partial hair loss with dull lusterless hairs.

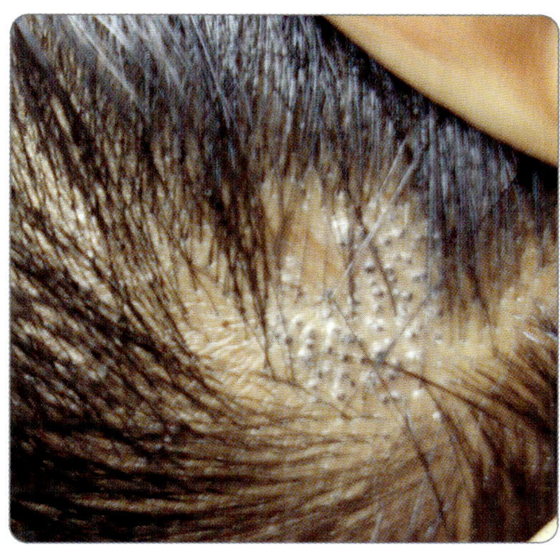

Fig. 2: Black dot with patchy hair loss with broken hairs.

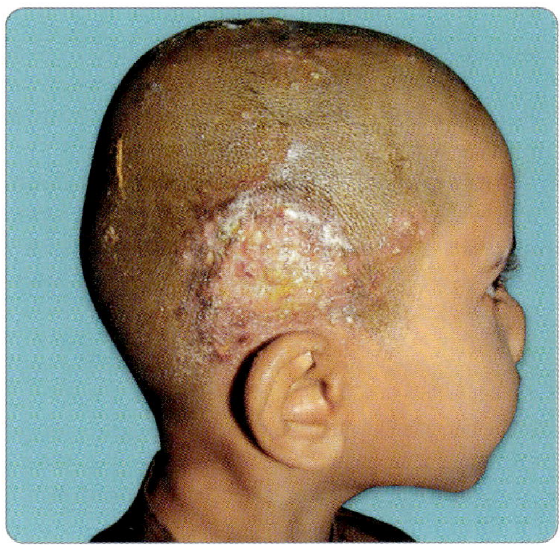

Fig. 3: Kerion—large boggy swelling over the scalp with multiple pustules.

3. *Kerion*: It is an inflammatory type of tinea capitis, characterized by a boggy mass studded with broken hairs and follicular orifices oozing with pus. It may be associated with pain, fever, and cervical lymphadenopathy **(Fig. 3)**.
4. *Favus*: It is caused by *T. schoenleinii*. It is characterized by the presence of yellowish cup-shaped crusts known as "scutula." Each scutulum develops around a hair, which pierces it centrally. Adjacent crusts enlarge to become confluent and form a mass of yellow crusting.

COMPLICATIONS

- Secondary bacterial infection
- Tinea in other parts of the body

- Id reaction
- Cicatricial alopecia

DIFFERENTIAL DIAGNOSIS

- *Seborrheic dermatitis*—greasy nature of the scales, absence of easily pluckable hair, and negative KOH mount of the hair
- *Bacterial pyodermas*—absence of scaling and absence of fungal elements
- Folliculitis decalvans
- *Alopecia areata*—no scaling/pus discharge/scaling and smooth, noncicatricial, patchy hair loss
- *Trichotillomania*—bizarre-patterned hair loss, presence of broken hairs at different lengths, trichomalacia, and perifollicular hemorrhages with the absence of fungal elements
- *Pseudopelade*—"footprints in snow appearance" and the absence of scaling and fungal hyphae
- *Pediculosis*—presence of nits/lice

LABORATORY DIAGNOSIS

- Direct microscopy of KOH preparation of hair and scrapings from the scalp skin to demonstrate spores and hyphae
- Culture to identify the causative dermatophyte species. The culture medium used is Sabouraud's Dextrose Agar or dermatophyte test medium.
- Wood's lamp examination shows bright green fluorescence in tinea capitis caused by *Microsporum canis*, *M. audouinii*, and *M. ferrugineum* species. A dull green fluorescence is seen in favus caused by *T. schoenleinii*. Fluorescence is negative in all other situations.

DERMOSCOPY

Dermoscopic findings characteristic of tinea capitis include comma hairs, corkscrew hairs, zigzag hairs, Morse code-like hairs, bent hairs, block hairs, i-hairs, broken hairs, black dots, perifollicular scaling, and diffuse scaling.

TREATMENT

- *Oral antifungal therapy*: Griseofulvin 10–15 mg/kg (ultra-micronized) and 15–25 mg/kg (micronized) for 4–6 weeks; terbinafine 250 mg daily for 4–6 weeks; fluconazole 3–6 mg/kg/day for 6 weeks; itraconazole 5 mg/kg/day for 1 week; and 2 weeks with no drug, followed by 1 week with medication.
- *Adjuvant therapy*: Selenium sulfide (2.5%), ketoconazole (2%), and povidone iodine shampoos should be used twice weekly to reduce the carriage of viable spores and reduce infectivity.

SUGGESTED READING

1. Al Aboud AM, Crane JS. (2023). Tinea Capitis. Treasure Island (FL): StatPearls Publishing. [online] Available from https://www.ncbi.nlm.nih.gov/books/NBK536909/ [Last accessed February, 2025].

258 Toxic Epidermal Necrolysis

SYNONYM

Lyell's syndrome.

HISTORY

Toxic epidermal necrolysis (TEN) was first described in 1956.

ETIOLOGY

Drugs implicated are sulfonamides, cotrimoxazole, sulfadoxine, penicillin, amoxicillin, ampicillin, cephalosporins, ethambutol, fluoroquinolones, isoniazid, streptomycin, tetracycline, thiacetazone, barbiturates, phenobarbital, carbamazepine, lamotrigine, phenytoin, valproic acid, abacavir, nevirapine, terbinafine, griseofulvin, piroxicam, diclofenac, salicylates, valdecoxib, famotidine, omeprazole, ranitidine, gold, pentamidine, tolbutamide, etc.

Infections like mycoplasma pneumoniae, hepatitis A, and human herpesvirus 7 are also implicated. And malignancies like lung and liver carcinoma and vaccines like the meningococcal vaccine are possible etiologies. In recent times, even COVID-19 is implicated.

CLINICAL FEATURES

Toxic epidermal necrolysis presents with typically sheet-like erosions involving >30% of the body surface with widespread purpuric macules or flat atypical target lesions. Also, there is severe involvement of conjunctival, corneal, irideal, buccal, labial, and genital mucus membranes. TEN starts with a prodromal period with flu-like symptoms (malaise, fever, rhinitis, and conjunctivitis), sometimes accompanied by difficulty in micturition, which usually lasts 2–3 days; however, it may last from 1 day to 3 weeks before the signs of skin involvement develop. The acute phase of TEN is characterized by persistent fever, severe mucus membrane involvement, and generalized epidermal sloughing to leave large, raw, painful areas, and lasts from 8 to 12 days. There may be an initial "burning" maculopapular, urticarial, or erythema multiforme-like eruption. Pseudo Nikolsky's sign may be positive **(Fig. 1)**.

HISTOPATHOLOGY

The histology of early lesions is characterized by moderate perivascular mononuclear cell infiltration in the papillary dermis, with epidermal spongiosis and exocytosis. "Satellite cell necrosis," with close apposition of mononuclear cells to necrotic keratinocytes, may be seen. In established TEN, there is full-thickness necrosis of the whole epidermis with blister formation.

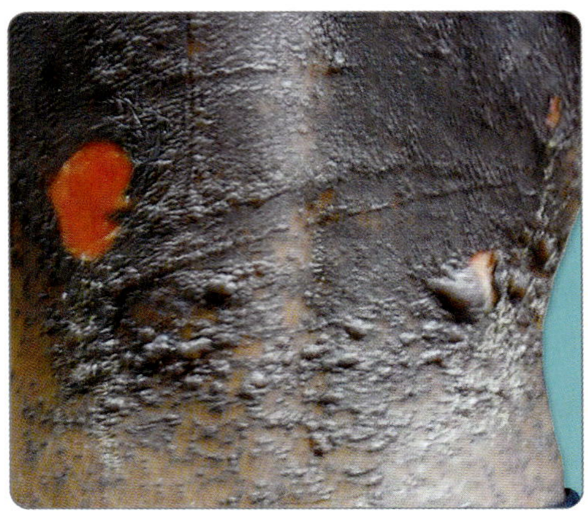

Fig. 1: Epidermal detachment in sheets.

COMPLICATIONS

Complications include hypovolemia, pneumonia, pneumonitis, acute respiratory distress syndrome (ARDS), septicemia, prerenal failure, and secondary bacterial infections.

DIFFERENTIAL DIAGNOSIS

- *Immunobullous disorders*—presence of acantholytic cells on Tzanck smear, classical histopathological examination (HPE), and direct immunofluorescence (DIF) findings in biopsy
- *Mechanobullous disorders*—absence of preceding drug intake and prodrome, less body surface area (BSA) involved, and lesser mucosal involvement
- *Stevens–Johnson syndrome*—almost similar clinical picture with <30% BSA involved
- Toxic erythema
- *Urticaria*—absence of widespread erosions and classical evanescent wheals present

TREATMENT

Patients should be managed in the intensive care unit or burns unit.

Analgesia, maintenance of fluid and electrolyte balance (replace up to 5 L/day), body temperature, nutrition, and oral hygiene.

Barrier nursing, topical cleansing/antibacterial agents, 0.5% silver nitrate solution on gauze or 10% chlorhexidine gluconate washes or saline washes or polymyxin/bacitracin or 2% mupirocin for infections.

Wound care by removing necrotic epidermis (controversial), paraffin gauze, or hydrogel dressings or biological dressings (xenografts, allografts, and skin substitutes).

The use of systemic corticosteroids is controversial. Plasmapheresis, cyclosporine, and cyclophosphamide are the second line of drugs used.

Table 1: SCORTEN.

SCORTEN	*Probability of death (%)*
0–1	3
2	12
3	35
4	58
≥5	90

PROGNOSIS

There is 30–40% mortality in TEN patients. Early withdrawal of the causative drug improves the prognosis, and drugs with a long half-life are associated with an increased risk of death.

SCORTEN

Parameters:

- Age > 40 years
- Presence of a malignancy
- Epidermal detachment > 30%
- Heart rate > 120 beats/min
- Bicarbonate < 20 mmol/L
- Urea > 10 mmol/L
- Glycemia > 14 mmol/L

1 point is awarded for each parameter; SCORTEN is derived by totaling scores **(Table 1)**.

SUGGESTED READING

1. Labib A, Milroy C. (2023). Toxic Epidermal Necrolysis. Treasure Island (FL): StatPearls Publishing. [online] Available from https://www.ncbi.nlm.nih.gov/books/NBK574530/ [Last accessed February, 2025].

259 Trichoepithelioma

➲ SYNONYMS

Epithelioma adenoids cysticum, Brooke's tumor.

➲ ETIOLOGY

Trichoepithelioma is a hamartoma of the hair germ composed of immature islands of basaloid cells with focal, primitive follicular differentiation, and induction of a cellular stroma. They are a part of the spectrum of trichoblastoma. Solitary lesions are usually due to deletions in the patched gene at chromosome 9q22.3. Multiple trichoepitheliomas are inherited as an autosomal dominant trait mapped to chromosome 9q21.

➲ AGE GROUP

Young adults.

➲ CLINICAL FEATURES

Three distinctive forms are recognized:

1. *Solitary trichoepithelioma:* It occurs as small (5–8 mm in diameter), skin-colored, smooth nodules situated on the face, especially around the nose, upper lip, and cheeks. It clinically resembles a nonulcerated basal cell carcinoma. Occasionally, lesions may develop on the trunk, neck, scalp, and lower extremities.
2. *Multiple trichoepitheliomas:* They present as numerous, small, pearly papules distributed on the face, especially around the nasolabial folds, forehead, chin, and preauricular area **(Fig. 1)**. They may coalesce to form plaques, nodules, or tumors. The larger lesions may be yellow, pink, or sometimes bluish from pigmentation, and there may be dilated blood vessels over the surface. Individual tumors reach a limiting size, but the numbers may increase over the years.
3. *Desmoplastic trichoepithelioma:* It is also known as "sclerosing epithelial hamartoma." The lesions have a depressed center and a raised, rolled edge, present mainly on the face. It closely resembles basal cell carcinoma.

➲ ASSOCIATED SYNDROMES

Brooke–Spiegler syndrome, Brooke–Fordyce disease, Rombo syndrome, systemic lupus erythematosus, and myasthenia gravis are the associated syndromes.

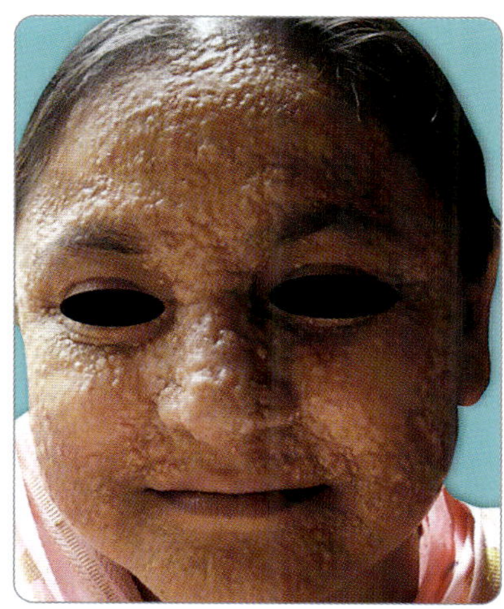

Fig. 1: Skin-colored smooth nodule situated on the face.

➲ HISTOPATHOLOGY

Dome-shaped, sharply circumscribed lesion composed of aggregations of relatively monomorphic, small, dark basaloid (germinative) cells in the upper dermis surrounded by abundant fibrous stroma with intrastromal clefts. The basaloid aggregations are mainly arranged in a cribriform pattern but may show other architectural patterns, including nodular, racemiform, and retiform. They typically reveal peripheral palisading surrounding a central area of eosinophilic amorphous material and several foci with rudimentary follicular papillae and germs **(Fig. 2)**.

Desmoplastic trichoepitheliomas are characterized by keratin-filled cysts, strands, and ribbons of small, dark, epithelioid cells, and a dense fibrous stroma surrounding the first two structures. Merkel cells are also present. Perineural invasion is not a feature.

➲ DERMOSCOPY

Dermoscopy of papules shows arborizing vessels, multiple milia-like cysts, and rosettes amid a whitish background.

➲ DIFFERENTIAL DIAGNOSIS

- *Basal cell carcinoma*—noduloulcerative lesion with rolled out margins and islands of basaloid cells with peritumoral lacunae
- *Colloid milium*—multiple white smooth papules, usually a cyst with degenerated keratin
- *Cylindroma*—mainly on the scalp and "jigsaw" appearance on histopathological examination (HPE)
- Follicular infundibulum tumor
- Miliaria
- Pilar cyst

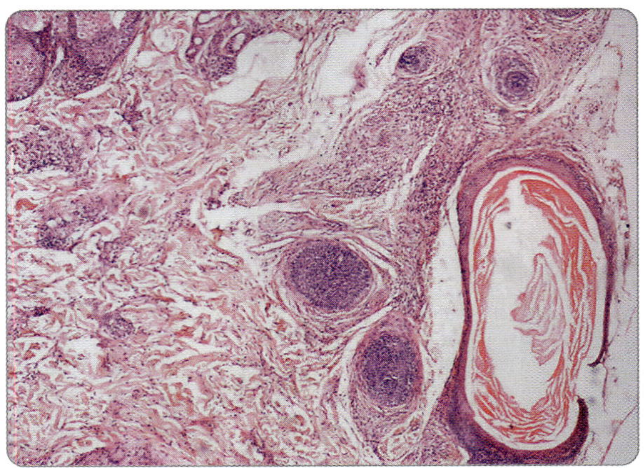

Fig. 2: Horn cysts and basaloid epithelial formations lacking the retraction artifact typical of basal cell carcinoma.

- Steatocystoma multiplex
- *Syringoma*—multiple tadpole cells (eccrine glands and ducts)
- Trichilemmoma

COMPLICATIONS

The complication can be malignant transformation (extremely rare).

TREATMENT

Surgical excision, curettage, cryotherapy, dermabrasion, high-energy pulsed carbon dioxide laser, and 5% imiquimod are the treatment options.

PROGNOSIS

Prognosis is good.

SUGGESTED READING

1. Mohammadi AA, Seyed Jafari SM. Trichoepithelioma: a rare but crucial dermatologic issue. World J Plast Surg. 2014;3(2):142-5.

260 Trichomycosis Axillaris

➲ SYNONYMS

Trichomycosis nodosa, trichobacteriosis, trichomycosis palmelina.

➲ ETIOLOGY

Trichomycosis axillaris is not a fungal infection. It is caused by several species of aerobic corynebacteria, e.g., *Corynebacterium tenuis* (*C. flavescens*).

➲ AGE AND SEX

Trichomycosis axillaris is commonly seen in adult men, as women frequently shave axillary hair.

➲ CLINICAL FEATURES

Predisposing factors are poor hygiene and hyperhidrosis. It usually involves the axillary hair, but pubic hair may also be involved. It is usually asymptomatic. It presents as yellow, black, or red, with dirty-looking small concretions present on the hair shaft **(Fig. 1)**. These may be hard, or soft and nodular, or more diffuse. These concretions are colonies of coryneform bacteria. In nodular variety, the hair may be brittle and easily broken. The underlying skin is normal. The axillary sweat may be black, yellow, or red according to the color of the concretions, and the clothing may be stained. The yellow type is the most common, and the black is the rarest. Coexistence of

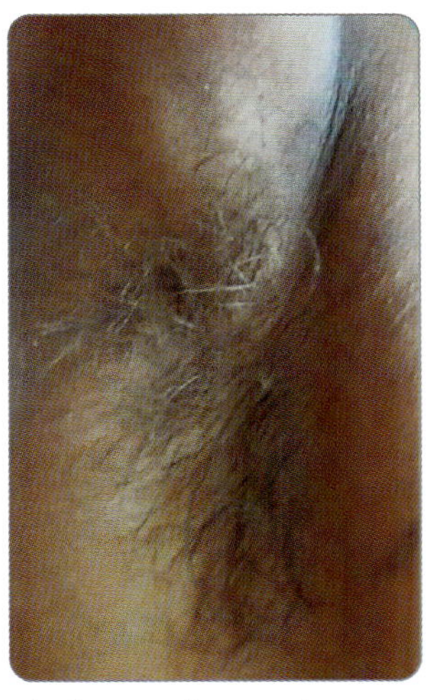

Fig. 1: Yellowish dirty-looking small concretions present on the hair shaft.

erythrasma, trichomycosis axillaris, and pitted keratolysis is termed corynebacterial triad.

➲ HISTOPATHOLOGY

The coryneform bacteria colonize and invade the hair shaft surface and penetrate into the cuticle. The colonies adhere to the shaft by a cement substance, probably a glucan analogue produced by coryneforms.

➲ DERMOSCOPY

Dermoscopy reveals yellowish-white masses with a waxy appearance, adherent to the hair.

➲ DIFFERENTIAL DIAGNOSIS

Piedra is caused by *Trichosporon beigelii* and *Piedraia hortae*; nodules are firmly attached, gritty to feel, and a metallic sound can be heard on combing; demonstration of fungal arthrospores on KOH mount.

➲ COMPLICATIONS

Staining of clothes, malodor, and recurrence are the complications.

➲ TREATMENT

Clipping the affected hairs is suggested. Topical antimicrobial ointment, such as benzoic acid compound ointment or 1% aqueous formalin, and antiperspirant, such as anhydrous aluminum chloride, can be given. Appropriate use of antibiotics is a must, like topical fusidic acid and topical clindamycin.

➲ PROGNOSIS

Prognosis is good.

➲ SUGGESTED READING

1. Montes de Oca-Loyola ML, Lumbán Ramírez P, Gómez-Daza F, Bonifaz A. An Overview of Trichobacteriosis (Trichomycosis): An Underdiagnosed Disease. Cureus. 2023;15(9):e45964.

261 Trichorrhexis Nodosa

HISTORY

Trichorrhexis nodosa is derived from the Greek "*tricho*," meaning hair, "*rrhexis*," meaning breakage, and "*nodosa*," meaning knots or bulges.

ETIOLOGY

Trichorrhexis nodosa may be congenital or acquired.

- *Congenital*: It may be present at birth or may appear within the first few years of life.
- *Acquired:*
  - Mechanical trauma: Vigorous brushing, back-combing, scratching, and pulling of hair
  - Chemical trauma: Saltwater bathing, shampooing, dyeing, setting, and perming

AGE GROUP

Trichorrhexis nodosa affects all age groups.

CLINICAL FEATURES

Trichorrhexis nodosa appears as minute grayish nodes along the shaft.

- In trichorrhexis nodosa, complicating a congenital defect of the hair shaft, the hair breaks so easily that large or small portions of the scalp show only broken stumps, and alopecia may be gross.
- In the acquired type, three forms are seen:
  - i. Distal trichorrhexis nodosa: It occurs in all races. Appear as few whitish nodules near the ends of scattered hairs. If many hairs are affected, the hair may appear dry, dull, or brittle. The longer the hair, the more likely it is to occur.
  - ii. Proximal trichorrhexis nodosa: It is seen in Afro-Caribbean women. The scalp hair is universally short and brittle and demonstrates severe weathering. It may be associated with follicular degeneration syndrome, where there is central scarring alopecia in the absence of an overt inflammatory process.
  - iii. A localized area of a few broken hairs and other hairs showing one to five or six nodules in the scalp, beard, or moustache areas. It was well described by Sabouraud.

ASSOCIATED SYNDROMES

With congenital trichorrhexis nodosa—Menkes kinky hair syndrome, Netherton syndrome, argininosuccinic aciduria, pili annulati, and Laron syndrome are the associated syndromes.

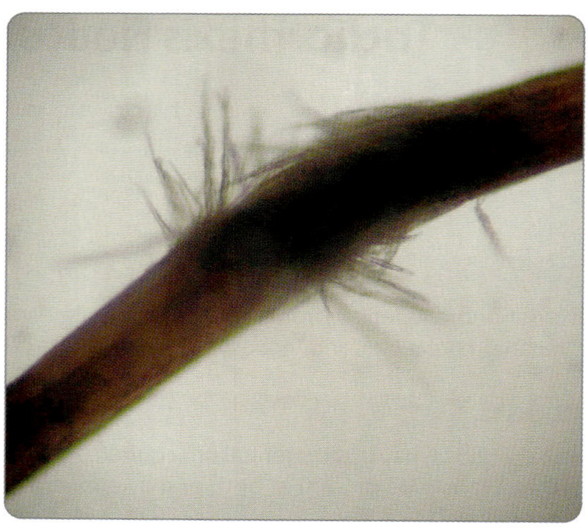

Fig. 1: Trichorrhexis nodosa appearing as two paint brushes thrust into each other.

TRICHOSCOPY

Broken hair shaft with thrust paint brushes appearance.

MICROSCOPY

Hair develops a breach in the cuticle, with eventual separation and fraying of the exposed cortical fibers, giving the appearance of two paint brushes thrust into each other, leading to a nodal swelling **(Fig. 1)**.

DIFFERENTIAL DIAGNOSIS

- Other congenital hair shaft defects
- *Dandruff*—presence of dry flakes
- *Pediculosis*—presence of lice and nits (shiny white and difficult to remove from the hair shaft)

COMPLICATIONS

Alopecia can be the complication.

TREATMENT

Avoidance of excessive physical and chemical (cosmetic) trauma to the hair is the treatment.

PROGNOSIS

Prognosis is good.

SUGGESTED READING

1. Kharkar V, Gutte R, Thakkar V, Khopkar U. Trichorrhexis nodosa with nail dystrophy: diagnosis by dermoscopy. Int J Trichology. 2011;3(2):105-6.

262 Trichotillomania

➲ SYNONYM

Psychogenic traction alopecia.

➲ HISTORY

The term was first used by Hallopeau in 1889. Trichotillomania is derived from the Greek "*thrix*," meaning hair, "*tillein*," meaning pull out, and "*mania*," meaning madness.

➲ ETIOLOGY

Trichotillomania is a psychocutaneous disorder, similar to obsessive–compulsive disorder (OCD). In children, it is a benign, self-limiting behavior and occurs most commonly in those suffering from habit disorder. It may be associated with nail biting, thumb sucking, skin picking, nose picking, lip biting, cheek chewing, anxiety, dysthymia, learning disability, and iron deficiency.

In adolescents, the psychopathology may be related to parent relationships, school difficulties (commonly bullying), body image changes, parent and sexual abuse, anxiety disorders, and depression. In adults, it is more commonly associated with depression, anxiety disorder, OCD, substance abuse, and eating disorders.

Genetic predisposition, or a continuing family psychosocial response, may also be the cause.

➲ AGE GROUP

Bimodal distribution with peaks in the preschool years (2–10 years of age) and in adolescence.

➲ CLINICAL FEATURES

The scalp is the most commonly involved site, followed by the eyebrows, pubic, and other body hairs. Most patients experience an increasing sense of tension immediately before pulling out the hair or when they consciously attempt to resist the behavior. There is relief of tension and gratification after pulling out the hair.

The involved sites are usually affected asymmetrically. Hair loss is more common on the side contralateral to the dominant hand. The scalp shows an artifactually patterned, either ill-defined or sharply demarcated area (patchy, linear, or triangular) of alopecia that is usually incomplete **(Fig. 1A)**. These patches may be static or may progressively march like a wave from the anterior to the posterior scalp. Broken off or twisted hair as well as a black dot appearance because of immature keratin formation may be seen in the patch. Injured follicles may form soft, twisted hair (trichomalacia).

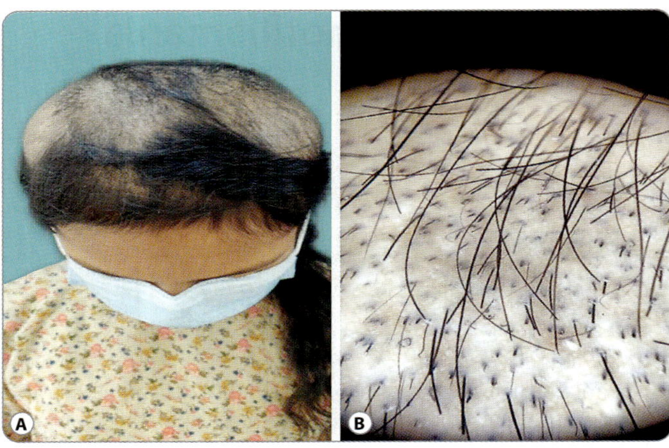

Figs. 1A and B: (A) Irregular area of alopecia with broken hairs of different lengths; (B) Dermoscopy showing decreased hair density and hairs broken at different lengths.

Regrowing hair of varying length is generally observed in a patch that has been present for many weeks.

Trichotillomania may involve most of the scalp surface, usually sparing the margins, giving rise to the characteristic "tonsure" pattern or "Friar Tuck" distribution.

HISTOPATHOLOGY

Histopathology shows many catagen follicles and aggregation of melanin pigment within the catagen and anagen follicles. The infundibulum may show plugging and melanin deposition, and the dermal hair papilla may also contain melanin. Histopathology also shows paucity of telogen follicles, empty follicles containing soft keratin, deformed hair (trichomalacia). Signs of follicular rupture and perifollicular hemorrhages are observed.

TRICHOSCOPY

Trichoscopy shows decreased hair density, hairs broken at different lengths, trichoptilosis, tulip hair, hair powder, perifollicular whitish areas, black dots, V-sign, and follicular hemorrhages **(Fig. 1B)**.

DIFFERENTIAL DIAGNOSIS

- *Tinea capitis*—scaly patch (gray patch type) with easily pluckable hair, uniformly present broken hair stubs (black dot type), and demonstration of dermatophytes in scales and hair in KOH mount
- *Alopecia areata*—smooth bald patch with normal underlying skin and "swarm of bees" appearance in histopathological examination (HPE)

➲ COMPLICATIONS

Complications can be trichophagy, trichobezoar, secondary infection, carpal tunnel syndrome (because of repetitive pulling), changes in color and texture of hair, and occasionally anorexia, intestinal obstruction, and death due to trichobezoar.

➲ TREATMENT

- *Children*—psychotherapy, i.e., behavioral therapy, positive reinforcement, self-monitoring, habit reversal training, and acts of punishment
- *Adults*—psychotherapy + pharmacotherapy
  - Monotherapy with selective serotonin reuptake inhibitors (SSRIs) and clomipramine
    - Selective serotonin reuptake inhibitors—fluoxetine (20–60 mg/day), paroxetine (10–60 mg/day), sertraline (50–200 mg/day), fluvoxamine (50–300 mg/day), citalopram (10–60 mg/day), escitalopram (5–20 mg/day)
    - Clomipramine (10–250 mg/day)
  - SSRIs + olanzapine (5–20 mg/day)/risperidone (2–16 mg/day)/pimozide
  - SSRIs + low-dose atypical antipsychotic agents (e.g., amisulpride, aripiprazole, olanzapine, quetiapine, risperidone, sertindole, and zotepine)

➲ PROGNOSIS

Short-term success occurs, and sustained improvement is yet to be shown convincingly.

➲ SUGGESTED READING

1. Ankad BS, Naidu MV, Beergouder SL, Sujana L. Trichoscopy in trichotillomania: a useful diagnostic tool. Int J Trichology. 2014;6(4):160-3.

263 Tropical Acne

➲ SYNONYM

Hydration acne.

➲ ETIOLOGY

Tropical climate (hot and humid climates) and scorching occupational environments (furnace workers, cooks, pressers, military troops, etc.). Hydration of the pilosebaceous duct pores may accentuate blockage of the duct and so precipitate inflamed lesions. Secondary infection with coagulase-positive staphylococci always ensues.

Comedogenic sunscreens may act as an exacerbating factor.

➲ AGE GROUP

Tropical acne affects adults.

➲ CLINICAL FEATURES

Lesions are mainly seen on the back, upper arms, buttocks, and thighs. The face is not as much involved. There are multiple deep, large, inflammatory nodules, pustules, draining sinuses, and painful cysts **(Fig. 1)**.

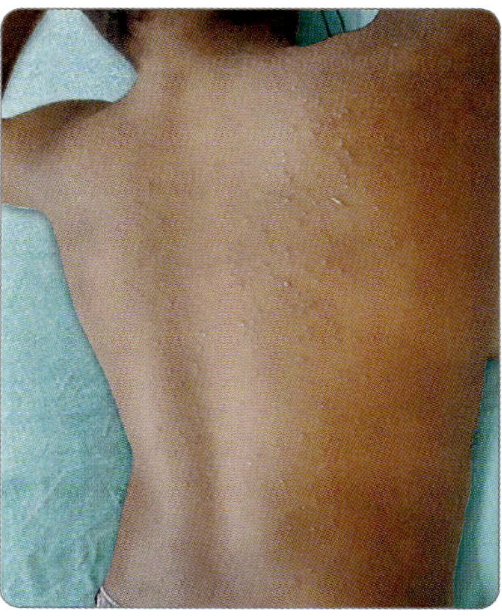

Fig. 1: Multiple inflammatory papules and pustules involving the trunk.

➲ DIFFERENTIAL DIAGNOSIS

Acne conglobata—clinically shows nodules, cysts, burrowing, and intercommunicating abscesses with irregular, sometimes mutilating scarring.

➲ COMPLICATIONS

Scarring, which is often keloidal.

➲ TREATMENT

- Remove the patient to a cooler environment.
- Systemic antibiotics (oxytetracycline 500 mg QID, doxycycline 100–200 daily, erythromycin 500 mg BD, and minocycline 100–200 mg daily).
- Oral isotretinoin 0.5–1.0 mg/kg/day.

➲ PROGNOSIS

Exacerbation of the pre-existing acne is quite common. So, prolonged treatment is required.

➲ SUGGESTED READING

1. Novy FG Jr. A severe form of acne developing in the tropics. Arch Derm Syphilol. 1949;60(2):206-16.

264 Tuberculides

HISTORY

The concept of tuberculides was introduced by Darier in 1896. Lichen scrofulosorum was first described by Hebra in 1868. Erythema induratum was described by Bazin in 1861.

ETIOLOGY

Tuberculides are thought to be due to hematogenous spread of tubercular bacilli in a person with a moderate to high degree of immunity against *Mycobacterium tuberculosis*.

CLASSIFICATION (TABLE 1)

- *Micropapular*—lichen scrofulosorum
- *Papular*—papular or papulonecrotic tuberculid
- *Nodular*—erythema nodosum and erythema induratum of Bazin
- *Others*—granulomatous mastitis and lupus miliaris disseminatus faciei

DERMOSCOPY

Lupus miliaris disseminatus faciei—follicular plugs with short linear and linear branching vessels in a ill-defined structureless yellow-orange background can be seen.

COMPLICATIONS

Scarring can be the complication.

TREATMENT

Standard 6-month antituberculosis therapy regimen is followed:

- Isoniazid (300 mg daily) × 6 months
- Rifampicin [450 mg daily for <50 kg body weight (BW), 600 mg daily for >50 kg BW] × 6 months
- Pyrazinamide (1.5 g daily for <50 kg BW, 2.0 g daily for >50 kg BW) × first 2 months
- Ethambutol (15 mg/kg BW daily) × first 2 months

PROGNOSIS

Prognosis is good.

Table 1: Classification of tuberculides.

Type	*Age group*	*Clinical features*	*Histopathology*	*Differential diagnosis*
Lichen scrofulosorum (tuberculosis cutis lichenoides)	Children and adolescents	Asymptomatic, firm, follicular, or perifollicular, flat-topped, yellowish or pink lichenoid papules; may coalesce to form plaques; and usually confined to the trunk and proximal limbs	Superficial dermal granulomas surrounding hair follicles and sweat ducts. Epithelioid cells, lymphocytes, and occasional giant cells are seen. Caseation is usually absent. Mycobacteria are not present	Lichen planus, lichen nitidus, lichenoid secondary syphilis, micropapular forms of sarcoidosis, keratosis spinulosa, keratosis pilaris, and drug eruptions
Papulonecrotic tuberculid	Children and young adults	Symmetric, disseminated crops of livid or dusky-red papules with a central depression and an adherent crust over a crater-like ulcer. Spontaneous involution occurs with pitted, varioliform scarring. Occurs on extensor aspect of extremities, buttocks, and lower trunk	Wedge-shaped necrotic area in the upper dermis, extending up to the epidermis. Involvement of blood vessels is a cardinal feature and consists of an obliterative and sometimes granulomatous vasculitis, leading to thrombosis and complete occlusion of the vascular channels. Tuberculoid granulomas are frequently observed at the periphery of the necrotic area	Pityriasis lichenoides et varioliformis acuta (PLEVA), leukocytoclastic necrotizing vasculitis, lichen urticatus, prurigo, and secondary syphilis

Continued

Continued

Type	***Age group***	***Clinical features***	***Histopathology***	***Differential diagnosis***
Erythema induratum	Young or middle-aged females	Indolent eruption of ill-defined erythematous subcutaneous nodules or plaques on the posterior aspect of lower legs. Nodules may ulcerate. The ulcers are ragged, irregular, and shallow, with a bluish edge, and heal with scarring. Involved extremity may show erythrocyanosis. Runs a chronic course	Focal or diffuse, lobular or septolobular, granulomatous panniculitis in association with neutrophilic vasculitis of either large or small blood vessels. Coagulative and caseation necrosis present. Poorly developed granulomas can occur	
Erythema nodosum	Second to fourth decades of life	Acute onset, symmetric, tender, erythematous, warm nodules, and raised plaques on the anterior aspects of lower extremities	Septal panniculitis without vasculitis	
Granulomatous mastitis		Unilateral, ulcerative plaques, nodules, or abscesses on the breast of a female. Runs a chronic course	Granulomata with fat necrosis. Acid-fast bacillus (AFB) absent	Breast carcinoma
Lupus miliaris disseminatus faciei **(Fig. 1)**		Papulonecrotic lesions on the face and ears, leading to varioliform scarring	Granulomatous features	Rosacea

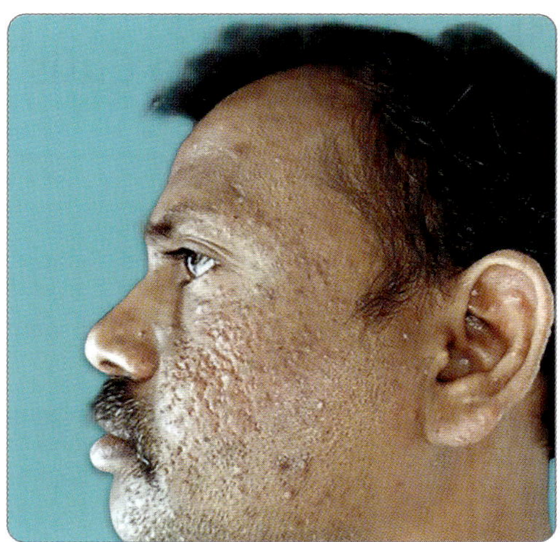

Fig. 1: Lupus miliaris disseminatus faciei.

SUGGESTED READING

1. Jassi R, Yadav A, Chander R. Dermoscopy of Lichen Scrofulosorum. Indian Dermatol Online J. 2020;11(5):876-7.

265 Tuberculosis Verrucosa Cutis

➲ SYNONYMS

Warty tuberculosis, anatomist's warts, prosector's warts, verruca necrogenica, lupus verrucosus.

➲ HISTORY

Tuberculosis verrucosa cutis was described by René Laennec in 1826.

➲ ETIOLOGY

Tuberculosis verrucosa cutis is a cutaneous infection caused by *Mycobacterium tuberculosis*. An indolent, warty, plaque-like form of tuberculosis occurs as a result of the inoculation of organisms into the skin of a previously infected patient who usually has a moderate or high degree of immunity.

➲ CLINICAL FEATURES

Lesions occur after 2–4 weeks in areas exposed to trauma and to infected sputum or other tuberculous material. The lesion starts as a small, asymptomatic, indurated, warty papule with a slight inflammatory areola. By gradual extension, a verrucous plaque forms **(Fig. 1)**. Irregular extension at the edges leads to a serpiginous outline with finger-like projections. The center may involute, leaving a white atrophic scar, or the whole lesion may form a massive, infiltrated papillomatous excrescence. The color is purplish, red, or brown.

➲ HISTOPATHOLOGY

Tuberculosis verrucosa cutis presents with pseudoepitheliomatous hyperplasia with superficial abscess formation. The intense, mixed infiltrate may show only sparse tuberculosis foci. Bacilli are seen only occasionally **(Figs. 2A and B)**.

➲ DERMOSCOPY

Dermoscopy shows white thick scales, yellow-orange globular and structureless areas, which represent epithelioid cell granulomas with Langhans giant cells, with an increased microvessel count.

➲ DIFFERENTIAL DIAGNOSIS

- *Verruca vulgaris*: It is caused by human papillomavirus (HPV); multiple small discrete to large, coalesced lesions, thrombosed vessels on paring, and koilocytes in histopathological examination (HPE) are observed.

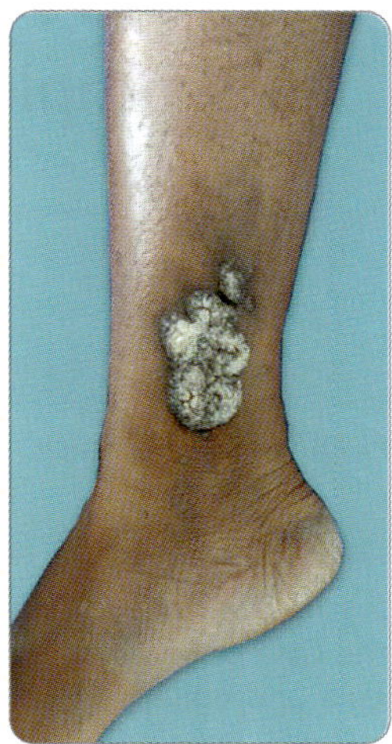

Fig. 1: Verrucous plaque over the leg.

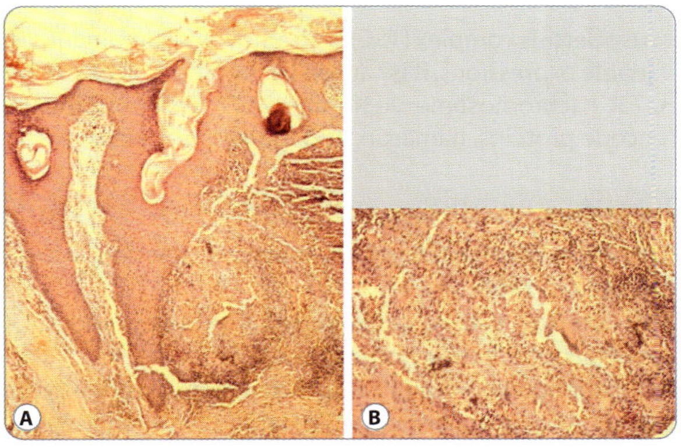

Figs. 2A and B: (A) Hyperkeratosis and acanthosis, with an epithelioid cell granuloma; (B) An epithelioid cell granuloma with caseation.

- *Blastomycosis*: It is caused by *Blastomyces dermatitidis*; chronic suppurative inflammation and demonstration of fungi in tissue using periodic acid-Schiff (PAS) are observed.
- *Chromoblastomycosis*: It is caused by dematiaceous fungi, and pathognomonic "copper penny bodies" in tissue sample are seen.
- *Hypertrophic lichen planus (LP)*: It is hyperpigmented papulo-plaque, with a surrounding ring of hyperpigmentation, absence of granulomas, and presence of lichenoid changes in HPE.
- *Lupus vulgaris*—infiltrated plaque/ulcer with an extending edge and apple jelly nodules on diascopy are seen.

TREATMENT

Tuberculosis verrucosa cutis responds to antitubercular therapy.

SUGGESTED READING

1. Jakhar D, Gupta RK, Sarin N. Dermoscopy of Tuberculosis Verrucosa Cutis. Indian Dermatol Online J. 2020;12(1):206-7.

266 Tuberous Sclerosis Complex

SYNONYMS

Bourneville disease, EPILOIA, Pringle disease.

HISTORY

Rayer gave the first description of the fibrovascular papules, and Bourneville reported the case of a mentally retarded girl who also suffered from hemiplegia and epilepsy. Sherlock coined the term "EPILOIA" (epilepsy, low intelligence, and adenoma sebaceum).

ETIOLOGY

Tuberous sclerosis complex (TSC) is an autosomal dominant disorder with variable expressions. It is caused by mutations in one of the two genes, *TSC1* (chromosome 9q34) and *TSC2* (chromosome 16p13). They encode proteins, hamartin, and tuberin, respectively.

CLINICAL FEATURES

- Cutaneous manifestations of tuberous sclerosis have been tabulated in **Table 1**
- *Brain:* Cortical tubers, subependymal nodules, and subependymal giant cell astrocytomas
- *Heart:* Rhabdomyomas (50%), which manifest as dysrhythmias.
- *Kidneys:* Angiomyolipomas (75%), along with renal cysts, renal cell carcinoma (rarely), and polycystic kidney disease (3–5%). These may manifest as renal insufficiency, hypertension, and potentially fatal retroperitoneal hemorrhage.
- *Lungs:* Lymphangioleiomyomatosis, multifocal micronodular pneumocyte hyperplasia, and clear cell tumors
- *Eyes:* Retinal astrocytic hamartomas (44–87%), which may cause loss of vision, but blindness is rare.
- *Gastrointestinal tract (GIT):* Rectal polyps, usually asymptomatic.

DERMOSCOPY

- *Facial angiofibroma*—yellowish-white globule with diffuse brown pigmentation with background erythema.
- *Shagreen patch*—"cobblestone appearance" due to reddish-brown strands studded with white dots and whitish lines between strands.

HISTOPATHOLOGY

- *Hypomelanotic macules*: The melanocytes are normal in number and have poorly developed dendritic processes; melanosomes are decreased in number, size, and melanization.

Table 1: Cutaneous lesions of tuberous sclerosis.

Skin lesions	*Incidence*	*Age of presentation*	*Common site(s)*	*Morphology*
Hypomelanotic macules **(Fig. 1)**	>90%	At birth/within first few years of life; fade or disappear in adulthood	Anywhere, most common (m/c) on the trunk and buttocks	Ash-leaf spots: 0.5–3.0 cm in diameter, lanceolate-shaped, 1 to >20 in number
			On the legs, below knees, and forearms	"Confetti" skin lesions: 2–3 mm in diameter
Facial angiofibromas **(Fig. 2)**	75–90%	2–5 years of age	Central face, spares upper lip, and lateral face	1–3 mm in diameter, pink to red papules, coalesce to form large nodules. Grow in size and number during puberty
Fibrous facial plaques	20–40%	Congenital/gradually develop over years	Forehead, can also be found on the scalp and cheeks	Irregular, soft to firm connective tissue nevus
Shagreen patch **(Fig. 3)**	50%	Infancy; usually becomes apparent later	Lower back, buttocks, and thighs (rarely)	Firm or rubbery irregular plaque, 1–10 cm in size, surface may be bumpy or may have an orange peel appearance
Ungual fibromas (Koenen's tumors) **(Fig. 4)**	88%	After first decade	Toes > fingers	Periungual—red papules or nodules. They press on the nail matrix and cause a longitudinal groove
Molluscum fibrosum pendulum (skin tags)			Neck, axillae, trunk, and flexures	Soft pedunculated papules to larger firm pedunculated nodules

Continued

Continued

Skin lesions	Incidence	Age of presentation	Common site(s)	Morphology
Pachydermodactyly				Benign thickening of proximal fingers
Café-au-lait macules, appendageal tumors (trichoepitheliomas and syringocystadenoma), lipomas, fibromyolipomas, neurofibromas				
Dental pitting	Up to 100%		Both deciduous and permanent teeth	Tiny pinpoint lesions or larger crater-like lesions (pits on dental enamel)
Oral fibromas	50%	First decade, m/c in adulthood	Gingiva (m/c), buccal and labial mucosa, hard palate, tongue	

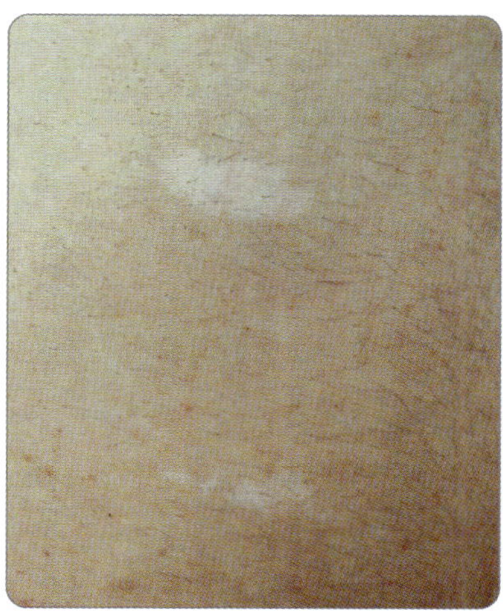

Fig. 1: Hypopigmented lanceolate-shaped ash-leaf macules.

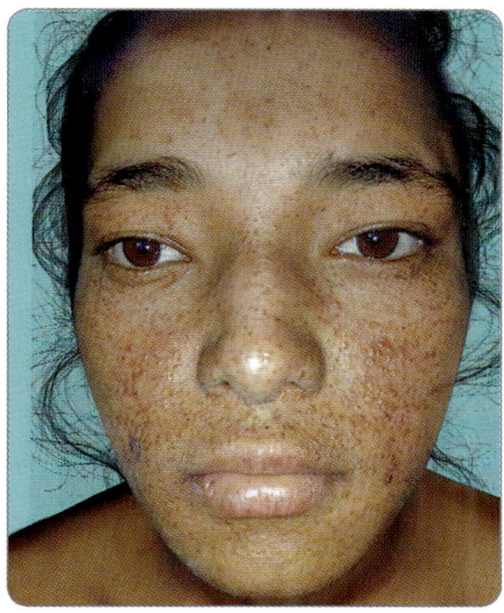

Fig. 2: Angiofibromas over the central face.

- *Angiofibromas*: These contain plump, spindle-shaped, or stellate fibroblastic cells in the dermis, with increased numbers of dilated vessels. Collagen fibers are oriented in an onion skin pattern around follicles and vessels. The epidermis shows melanocytic hyperplasia and flattening of rete ridges.
- *Periungual fibromas*: These are similar to angiofibromas but with more extensive hyperkeratosis and a variable increase in vascularity.
- *Shagreen patch*: It is characterized by sclerotic bundles of collagen in the reticular dermis. Elastic fibers are reduced in amount.

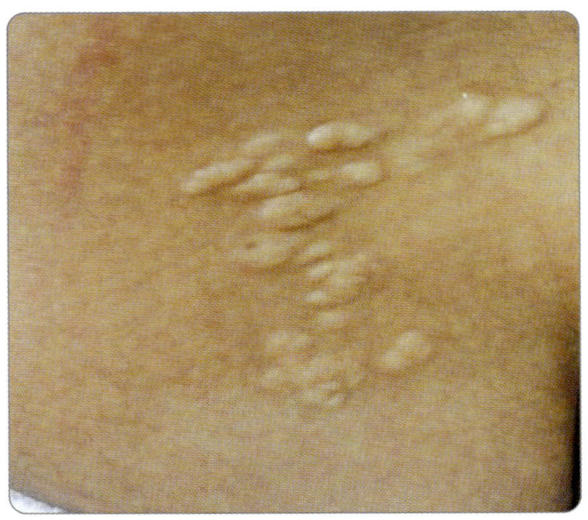

Fig. 3: Shagreen patch. Multiple rubbery plaques.

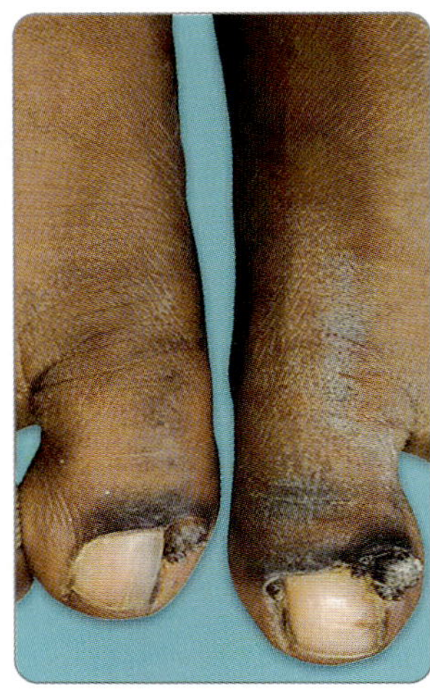

Fig. 4: Periungual angiofibromas: Koenen's tumors.

➲ REVISED DIAGNOSTIC CRITERIA

- *Major criteria:*
  - Hypomelanotic macules (≥3, at least 5 mm in diameter)
  - Angiofibromas (≥3)
  - Ungual fibromas (≥2)
  - Shagreen patch
  - Cortical dysplasia
  - Multiple retinal hamartomas
  - Subependymal nodules
  - Subependymal giant cell astrocytoma

  - ◇ Cardiac rhabdomyoma
  - ◇ Lymphangioleiomyomatosis
  - ◇ Angiomyolipomas
- *Minor criteria:*
  - ◇ Confetti skin lesions
  - ◇ Dental enamel pits (>3)
  - ◇ Intraoral fibromas (≥2)
  - ◇ Retinal achromic patch
  - ◇ Multiple renal cysts
  - ◇ Nonrenal hamartomas
- *Definitive diagnosis*: It requires two major features or one major feature, with ≥2 minor features.

➲ DIFFERENTIAL DIAGNOSIS

- *Ungual fibromas*—acral fibrokeratoma, superficial acral fibromyxoma, epidermoid cyst, pseudomyxoid cyst, wart, and pyogenic granuloma.
- *Hypomelanotic macules*—nevus depigmentosus, nevus anemicus, vitiligo, piebaldism, idiopathic guttate hypomelanosis, and pityriasis alba.
- *Angiofibromas*—fibrous papules, multiple endocrine neoplasia type 1 (MEN1) angiofibromas, Birt–Hogg–Dubé angiofibromas, trichoepitheliomas, syringomas, acne vulgaris, rosacea, and dermal melanocytic nevi.
- *Shagreen patch*—familial cutaneous collagenoma, eruptive collagenomas, sclerotic fibroma (Cowden syndrome), isolated connective tissue nevus, juvenile elastoma, nevus elasticus, and nevus mucinosis.

➲ COMPLICATIONS

None of the skin lesions are prone to malignant degeneration. Angiofibromas, facial plaques, and ungual fibromas can be painful or bleed spontaneously. Ungual fibromas can cause nail dystrophy and eventual loss of the nail. Large facial lesions may obstruct the vision or occlude nasal passages.

➲ TREATMENT

Surgical excision or laser therapy for skin lesions. Neurosurgery if epilepsy is uncontrolled with drugs and there is a fixed, circumscribed electroencephalogram (EEG) focus. Potential medical therapy for TSC tumors under clinical trials is oral rapamycin. Topical sirolimus is found to be useful in the treatment of facial angiofibroma.

➲ PROGNOSIS

The life expectancy for severely affected infants is poor: About 3% die in the first year, 28% under 10 years, and 75% before the age of 25 years.

SUGGESTED READINGS

1. Gundalli S, Ankad BS, Ashwin PK, Kolekar R. Dermoscopy of shagreen patch: A first report. Our Dermatol Online. 2015;6(3):331-3.
2. Madke B. Topical rapamycin (sirolimus) for facial angiofibromas. Indian Dermatol Online J. 2013;4(1):54-7.
3. Northrup H, Krueger DA; International Tuberous Sclerosis Complex Consensus Group. Tuberous sclerosis complex diagnostic criteria update: recommendations of the 2012 International Tuberous Sclerosis Complex Consensus Conference. Pediatr Neurol. 2013;49(4):243-54.

267 Twenty Nail Dystrophy

SYNONYMS

Trachyonychia, rough nails, sandpaper nails.

HISTORY

Twenty nail dystrophy was first described in children by Hazelrigg and colleagues in 1977.

ETIOLOGY

- Idiopathic
- Associated with inflammatory and other disorders such as lichen planus, psoriasis, alopecia areata, ichthyosis vulgaris, eczema, vitiligo, primary biliary cirrhosis, immunoglobulin A (IgA) deficiency, and pemphigus.
- Congenital, familial, and hereditary cases have also been described.

AGE GROUP

Twenty nail dystrophy affects children (self-limiting condition) and adults (chronic condition).

CLINICAL FEATURES

Two types of nail changes occur:

1. *Opaque variety:* The whole nail gives the appearance of having been sandpapered in a longitudinal direction. There is excessive ridging and roughness that makes the nails lusterless **(Figs. 1A and B)**.

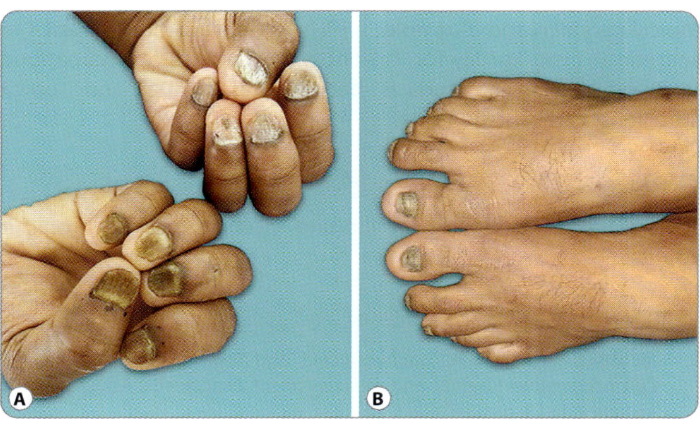

Figs. 1A and B: (A) Sandpaper nails with excessive ridging; (B) Roughness and lusterless nails involving all 20 nails.

2. *Shiny variety:* It is the less severe form in which the nail plate is shiny with myriad minuscule superficial punctate depressions.

Besides these, thinness, fragility, onychorrhexis, onychoschizia, and distal clipping of nail plates may occur. A yellowish thickening of the thumbnails and great toenails is sometimes seen. Scarring, generally, is not a feature of 20 nail dystrophy. Despite the name, all nails may not be totally and uniformly affected. When all nails are not involved, the term trachyonychia is preferred. In fact, involvement of 14 nails is more common.

ONYCHOSCOPY

Onychoscopic changes include scaling (100%), longitudinal ridging, splinter hemorrhages, proximal nail plate changes, pitting, onychoschizia, longitudinal melanonychia, opaque or red lunulae, thickened and ragged cuticles, and periungual scales.

HISTOPATHOLOGY

The nail matrix shows a spongiotic inflammation with a fairly dense mononuclear inflammatory infiltrate. Sometimes, a lichen planus or psoriasiform pathology may be present. Multiple foci of defective keratinization of the proximal nail matrix result in trachyonychia.

DIFFERENTIAL DIAGNOSIS

Onychomycosis—demonstration of fungal elements on KOH mount and culture of nail scrapings and clippings.

TREATMENT

Spontaneous resolution usually occurs in children. Hence, no treatment is required in most of the cases. Treatment modalities in children include intralesional triamcinolone acetonide 2.5–10 mg/mL, intramatricial steroid with ketamine, and oral griseofulvin (10 mg/kg) administered in single or divided doses for 6 months, and oral minipulse therapy can be used.

In adults, topical, intramatricial, or systemic potent steroids; cyclosporine A 3 mg/kg/day; vitamins like biotin 20 mg/day; topical psoralen and ultraviolet A (PUVA); topical 5-fluorouracil; oral acitretin 0.3 mg/kg/day for 7 months (in the case of occupational trachyonychia in a psoriasis patient); tazarotene; and topical emollients can be used.

PROGNOSIS

Twenty nail dystrophy is self-limiting in children and chronic in adults.

SUGGESTED READING

1. Jacobsen AA, Tosti A. Trachyonychia and Twenty-Nail Dystrophy: A Comprehensive Review and Discussion of Diagnostic Accuracy. Skin Appendage Disord. 2016;2(1-2):7-13.

268 Uncombable Hair Syndrome

➲ SYNONYMS

Spun-glass hair, cheveux incoiffables, pili trianguli et canaliculi.

➲ HISTORY

Uncombable hair syndrome was first described by Dupre et al. in 1973.

➲ ETIOLOGY

Uncombable hair syndrome is autosomal dominant, recessive, or sporadic.

There is a mutation in peptidyl arginine deiminase 3 (PADI3), transglutaminase 3 (TGM3), and trichohyalin (THH) in autosomal recessive inheritance.

➲ AGE GROUP

Uncombable hair syndrome first becomes obvious between 3 months and 12 years of age.

➲ CLINICAL FEATURES

The clinical features include disorderly appearing dry, silvery, or blonde hair, which are normal in quantity and length **(Fig. 1)**. The hair stand on end and resist all the efforts to manage it with a comb. In some cases, these efforts lead to hair breaking, but increased fragility is not a constant feature. The eyebrows and eyelashes are normal. The appearance becomes less marked with time.

Uncombable hair may be present in ectodermal dysplasia (Rapp–Hodgkin syndrome), retinal dysplasia, phalango-epiphyseal dysplasia, loose anagen syndrome, ectodermal dysplasia, ectrodactyly, and cleft lip/palate (EEC) syndrome, and familial tricho-odonto-onychial ectodermal dysplasia with syndactyly.

➲ HISTOPATHOLOGY

Light microscopy and scanning electron microscopy show triangular cross-section, longitudinal grooving, and twisting. All these lead to rigidity and stiffness of the hair. The pili canaliculi are present in all cases, pili trianguli in the majority, and pili torti in a few.

Pathology: The misshapen dermal papilla alters the shape of the inner root sheath, which hardens (before the hair within) in a triangular cross-sectional shape; the hair then hardens into a shape complementing the root sheath.

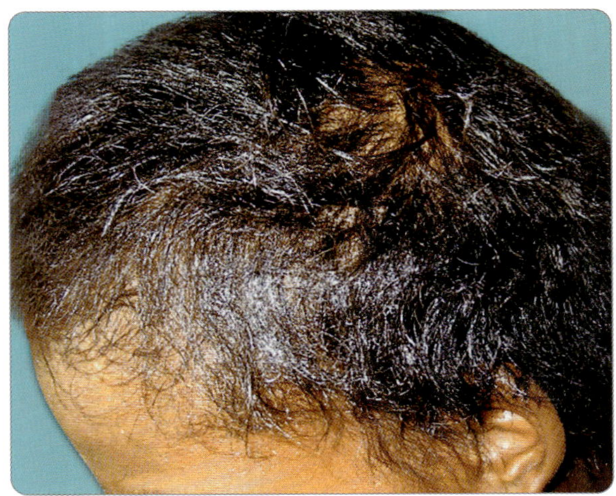

Fig. 1: Disorderly appearing dry, blonde hair that stands on end.

Resistance to longitudinal deformation varies with the square of the diameter, and the diameter of these triangular and grooved shafts is more than their oval or rounded counterparts. This could explain the rigidity of the shafts, leading to the hair standing on end. Reduced weathering may also make the hair stand on end.

➲ TRICHOSCOPY

Trichoscopy shows longitudinal grooving of hair.

➲ DIFFERENTIAL DIAGNOSIS

Differential diagnosis includes loose anagen syndrome.

➲ TREATMENT

No treatment is known, although oral biotin therapy has been suggested.

➲ PROGNOSIS

The condition improves with age.

➲ SUGGESTED READING

1. Alsabbagh MM. Uncombable hair syndrome and beyond. Acta Dermatovenerol Alp Pannonica Adriat. 2022;31(2):49-64.

269 Urticaria

➲ SYNONYMS

Wheals, nettle rash, hives, angioedema, angioneurotic edema, Quincke's edema.

➲ HISTORY

The earliest description of urticaria is found in "the yellow emperor's inner classic" by Huang Di Nei Jing, which was written between 1000 and 200 BC. Hippocrates described elevated itching lesions caused by nettles and mosquitoes and named it as "knidosis."

➲ ETIOLOGY

Urticaria is a pruritic rash involving the epidermis and upper portion of the dermis. It is associated with human leukocyte antigen (HLA) DR4 and DR8. Acute urticaria is idiopathic in >50% of patients. Other causes include allergies, foods, drugs, and infections, viz., the upper respiratory tract infection (URTI), streptococcal, hepatitis, anisakiasis, histamine liberators, and pseudoallergens like aspirin.

Chronic urticaria may be idiopathic, autoimmune, pseudo-allergic, and infectious due to *Helicobacter pylori* or candidiasis.

➲ CLINICAL FEATURES

Urticaria is classified according to its duration into acute <6 weeks and chronic >6 weeks. Urticaria clinically manifests as wheals, which are transient, well-defined, superficial erythematous or pale swellings of the dermis associated with itching **(Fig. 1)**. It can affect any part of the body, including the palms and soles. Systemic symptoms associated with urticaria are malaise, headache, abdominal pain, diarrhea, arthralgia, dizziness, syncope, or even anaphylaxis.

Urticaria and angioedema can coexist in 50% of the cases.

➲ TYPES OF URTICARIA

- Ordinary urticaria
- Physical urticarias are incited by mechanical stimuli.
- Dermographism is the rapid appearance of a linear wheal, with flare at the site where a brisk and firm stroke is made with a firm object. Types of dermographism are delayed, cholinergic, cold-dependent, red, white, and black dermographism.
- Pressure urticarias may be immediate or delayed.
- *Urticaria due to temperature changes*:
    - Cholinergic urticaria is characterized by the appearance of small papules due to stimulation of sweating either by increased core temperature or by emotional stress.

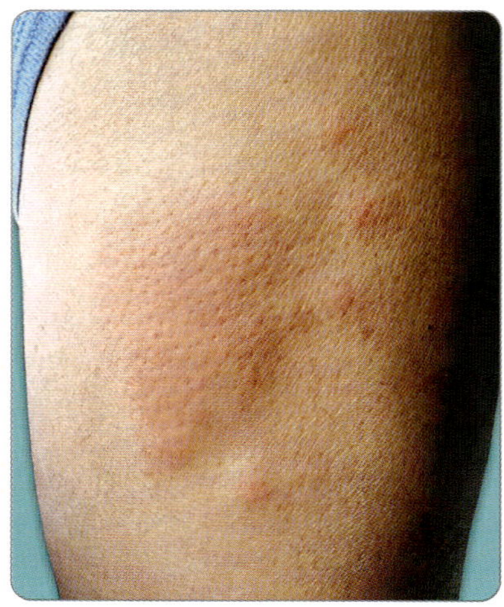

Fig. 1: Well-defined, superficial erythematous or pale swellings of the dermis.

- ◇ Localized heat urticaria: Wheals are restricted to warmed areas.
- ◇ Adrenergic urticaria: Wheals are induced by stress.
- ◇ Cold urticarias*:* Appearance of wheals due to cold exposure:
  - — Primary cold urticaria
  - — Acquired cold urticaria
  - — Familial cold urticaria
  - — Secondary cold urticaria

- Exercise-induced urticaria
- Food-induced anaphylaxis
- *Solar urticaria:* Itching, erythema, and wheals appear rapidly within minutes of sun exposure.
  - ◇ Primary solar urticaria
  - ◇ Secondary solar urticaria
  - ◇ Fixed solar urticaria
  - ◇ Delayed solar urticaria
- *Aquagenic urticaria:* It is the eruption of pruritic wheals surrounded by a flare on contact with water at any temperature.
- *Contact urticaria:* It is an immediate urticarial reaction of a local wheal and flare that appears within minutes to an hour after contact with a provoking substance.

HISTOPATHOLOGY

The histology of urticarial wheals is usually nonspecific, with vascular and lymphatic dilatation, edema, and a variable perivascular cellular dermal infiltrate consisting of lymphocytes, neutrophils, and eosinophils.

On electron microscopy, dermal mast cells show signs of degranulation.

DERMOSCOPY

Dermoscopy shows a red network of linear vessels.

➲ DIFFERENTIAL DIAGNOSIS

Erythema multiforme (target lesions), erythema marginatum (associated with rheumatic fever signs), erythema infectiosum, urticarial vasculitis (here lesions persist for >24 hours and leave behind pigmentation on healing unlike urticaria), herpes gestationis [bullae arise on the wheals, and subepidermal blisters are seen on histopathological examination (HPE) and positive direct immunofluorescence (DIF)], drug eruption, and bullous pemphigoid.

➲ MANAGEMENT

General measures include advice to avoid aggravating factors.

Oral antihistamines loratadine 10 mg, fexofenadine 180 mg, and levocetirizine 5 mg are preferred over first-generation antihistamines. Omalizumab, montelukast, systemic corticosteroids, and cyclosporine 4 mg/kg body weight per day for 4–8 weeks are reserved for refractory cases. Other therapeutic options include dapsone, methotrexate, azathioprine, mycophenolate mofetil, and biologics like intravenous immunoglobulins, rituximab, and adalimumab.

Chronic urticaria treatment guidelines as per the European Academy of Allergy and Clinical Immunology (EACCI), the Global Allergy and Asthma European Network (GA^2LEN), the European Dermatology Forum (EDF), and the World Allergy Organization (WAO):

- *First line*—second-generation antihistamines for 2 weeks
- *Second line*—increase the dosage of second-generation antihistamines four-fold.
- *Third line*—leukotriene receptor antagonist, cyclosporine A, or omalizumab
- *Rescue therapy*—corticosteroids for a maximum of 10 days

➲ SUGGESTED READING

1. Vestergaard C, Deleuran M. Chronic spontaneous urticaria: latest developments in aetiology, diagnosis and therapy. Ther Adv Chronic Dis. 2015;6(6):304-13.

270 Urticaria Pigmentosa

➲ SYNONYMS

Generalized eruption of cutaneous mastocytosis, mastocytoma.

➲ ETIOLOGY

Urticaria pigmentosa is the most common pattern of cutaneous mastocytosis, caused by a point mutation at amino acid 816 of the proto-oncogenic kit.

➲ AGE AND SEX

Urticaria pigmentosa develops either in the first year of life or at 20–40 years.

➲ CLINICAL FEATURES

Numerous reddish-brown or pale, monomorphic maculopapules, plaques, or nodules appear in asymmetrical distribution anywhere on the body, except the face, head, palms, and soles, with the highest concentration usually being on the trunk and thighs. Localized or generalized pruritus after exposure to physical stimuli aggravated by scratching or rubbing is the major complaint. They urticate within a few minutes of gentle rubbing (Darier's sign), causing localized itch, redness, and whealing, which subsides within an hour **(Fig. 1)**. Darier's sign is not always demonstrable, especially in those with a long history of the disorder, and is not 100% specific for mastocytosis, since it has also been described rarely in juvenile xanthogranuloma and acute lymphoblastic leukemia of neonates. Lesions may blister

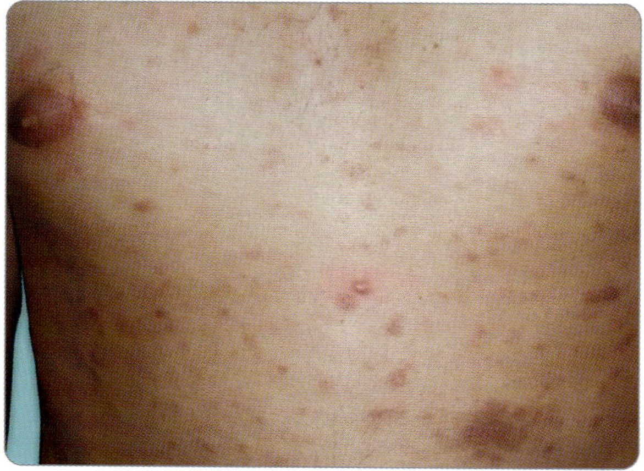

Fig. 1: Urticaria pigmentosa with positive Darier's sign.

in infancy or childhood and may be the presenting feature but heal without scarring. Symptoms may be worsened by emotional stress and physical stimuli such as heat, friction, and excessive exercise; bacterial toxins; venom; eye drops containing dextran; nonsteroidal anti-inflammatory drugs (NSAIDs); alcohol; or morphine. Bullous mastocytosis is not a specific clinical pattern. It is most often seen with mastocytomas and diffuse cutaneous mastocytosis. No systemic involvement can be detected in most patients with urticaria pigmentosa, but systemic manifestation can still occur.

HISTOLOGY

The hallmark feature is the increased amount of mast cells in the dermis characterized by metachromatic granules in the cytoplasm. Mast cells have a rounded or cuboidal appearance. Stains for identification include toluidine blue, Leder, Giemsa, tryptase, and CD117 (KIT). Eosinophils may be seen in the dermis, and hyperpigmentation of the basal layer due to an increase in melanin can also be found.

DERMOSCOPY

Dermoscopy shows light brown blot, brown reticular lines, and a dark brown pigment network pattern.

DIFFERENTIAL DIAGNOSIS

The differential diagnosis includes macular amyloidosis, carcinoid, epidermolysis bullosa, herpes simplex, and lentigo.

TREATMENT

Aspirin in combination with antihistamines relieves the symptoms. Other drugs used are sodium cromoglycate, nifedipine, psoralen and ultraviolet A (PUVA) therapy, topical and systemic steroids, and recombinant humanized monoclonal antibody like omalizumab.

SUGGESTED READING

1. Macri A, Cook C. (2023). Urticaria Pigmentosa. Treasure Island (FL): StatPearls Publishing. [online] Available from https://www.ncbi.nlm.nih.gov/sites/books/NBK482503/ [Last accessed February, 2025].

271 Varicella

➲ SYNONYM

Chickenpox.

➲ HISTORY

The word chickenpox probably is derived from *"chichie-pois,"* the French word for chickpea, describing the size of the vesicle. The distinction between varicella and smallpox was made in 1867 by Heberden.

➲ ETIOLOGY

The varicella zoster virus (VZV) is the cause of both varicella (chickenpox) and zoster (shingles). The virus is transmitted by droplet infection from the nasopharynx.

Patients are infectious to others from about 2 days before to 5 days after the onset of the rash.

➲ AGE AND SEX

Varicella is most common in the age group of 1–6 years, and there is no sexual predilection.

➲ CLINICAL FEATURES

The incubation period is usually 14–17 days (range: 9–23 days). After a day or two of fever and malaise, often slight or absent in children, a morbilliform erythema is followed by the development of papules, which rapidly become vesicles surrounded by red areolae (dewdrop on a rose petal). In 2–4 days, a dry crust forms and soon separates to leave a shallow, pink depression, which, in the absence of secondary infection, heals without scarring. The vesicles appear in crops over 2–4 days. Their distribution is centripetal, and there is a presence of lesions at different stages in each site **(Fig. 1)**.

In varicella, immunoglobulin G (IgG), IgM, and IgA antibodies appear 2–5 days after the onset of the rash, and their levels peak during the second and third weeks. Maternal varicella in the first 20 weeks of pregnancy is associated with an approximate 2% risk of fetal damage, including skin lesions, central nervous system and ocular defects, and limb hypoplasia, with a 30% mortality within the first year of life. If the mother has varicella within 4 days before to 2 days after term, the neonate would have no maternal antibody and be at risk of severe varicella, with a mortality rate up to 30% in the absence of treatment.

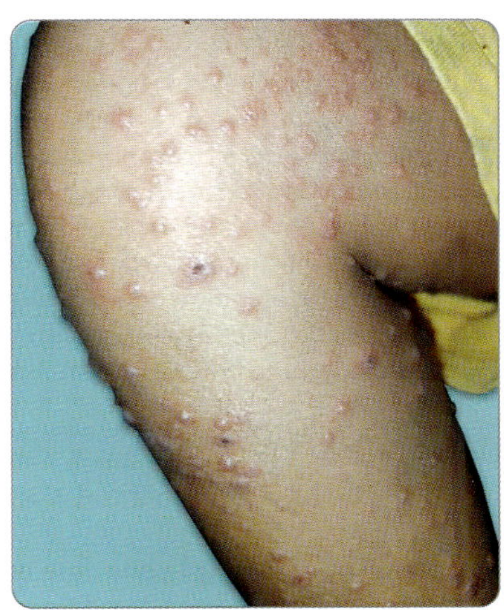

Fig. 1: Multiple umbilicated vesicles with central umbilication.

HISTOPATHOLOGY

The cells of the Malpighian layer show ballooning of their cytoplasm by intracellular edema and distinctive nuclear changes, comprising eosinophilic inclusions and marginated chromatin. Some nuclei develop additional nuclear membranes, which divide the nucleus into small compartments. The multinucleate giant cells with up to 15 nuclei are produced mainly by cell fusion. A mild inflammatory reaction in the dermis extends to the epidermis, and the proportion of polymorphonuclear cells increases with ulceration.

DERMOSCOPY

Dermoscopy shows brown dots, central umbilication, and erythematous background.

COMPLICATIONS

Complications include secondary infections, disseminated infections, herpes zoster, purpura fulminans, pneumonia, encephalitis, and hepatitis.

DIFFERENTIAL DIAGNOSIS

Differential diagnosis includes insect bite reactions (papules with a central punctum are seen, mainly on the exposed areas only), measles (more of a maculopapular rash than vesicles), smallpox, papular urticaria (absence of vesicles and constitutional symptoms), dermatitis herpetiformis [rarely, intact vesicles are seen; dermal papillary tip abscess on biopsy and positive direct immunofluorescence (DIF) are observed], meningococcal infection, measles, and eczema herpeticum.

➲ TREATMENT

Varicella in the otherwise healthy child requires only symptomatic treatment. Acyclovir may be used to reduce the severity and duration of the eruption. Soothing antiseptic applications and antibiotics will help secondary infections. In adults, treatment should be started as early as possible, preferably within the first 1 or 2 days. The virus is less sensitive to acyclovir in vitro than herpes simplex virus (HSV), and higher doses are usually recommended, typically 10 mg/kg intravenously or 4 g/day orally for 5–7 days, or with valaciclovir 1 g or famciclovir 250 or 500 mg three times a day for 7 days.

➲ VACCINATION

For adults, 0.5 mL subcutaneously for two doses 4–8 weeks apart is recommended.

For pediatrics, 0.5 mL subcutaneously, one dose between 12 and 15 months and the second dose between 4 and 6 years, is advised.

➲ SUGGESTED READING

1. Kota V, Grella MJ. (2023). Varicella (Chickenpox) Vaccine. Treasure Island (FL): StatPearls Publishing. [online] Available from https://www.ncbi.nlm.nih.gov/books/NBK441946/ [Last accessed February, 2025].

272 Vascular Malformation

➲ INTRODUCTION

Vascular malformation occurs due to abnormal vasculogenesis during embryogenesis, which presents at birth. They are composed of abnormal channels lined by endothelial cells, and they do not undergo abnormal cellular changes. The most frequent sites of involvement are the head and the neck.

➲ CLASSIFICATION

According to the International Society for the Study of Vascular Anomalies Classification 2018, vascular anomalies can be of the following types:

- *Vascular tumors*:
  - Benign
  - Locally aggressive
  - Malignant
- *Vascular malformations*:
  - Simple:
    - Capillary malformation
    - Lymphatic malformation
    - Venous malformation
    - Arteriovenous malformation (AVM)
    - Arteriovenous fistula
  - Combined:
    - Defined as two or more vascular malformations in one lesion

Based on flow, the characteristics of vascular malformation are as follows:

- *Fast flow*:
  - Arteriovenous
  - Arterial
  - Arteriovenous fistula
- *Slow flow*:
  - Capillary
  - Venous
  - Lymphatic
  - Combined

➲ CAPILLARY MALFORMATION

Capillary malformation affects capillaries in the papillary dermis. They are most commonly seen on the face along the trigeminal nerve distribution. It presents at birth as macular, purplish stain, which later darkens and thickens, giving a cobblestone appearance and distorting the facial features.

Example includes port-wine stain in Sturge–Weber syndrome.

Investigations

Investigations include magnetic resonance imaging (MRI) to look for the central nervous system (CNS) abnormalities.

➲ TREATMENT

Treatment includes ablative laser therapy such as pulsed dye laser therapy and surgery.

➲ VENOUS MALFORMATIONS

Venous malformations are the most common type of malformation, accounting for 1–4% of the population. They present at birth as bluish compressible lesions, which contract and expand based on patient positioning and increase in size with puberty, hormonal changes, and infections.

They can be of the following types:
- Sporadic
- Dominantly inherited cutaneomucosal venous malformation
- Dominantly inherited and noninherited glomuvenous malformation

Investigations

Investigations include Doppler ultrasound, MRI, and angiography.

Treatment

Treatment depends on the extent and location of the lesion, including sclerotherapy and surgery.

➲ LYMPHATIC MALFORMATIONS

Lymphatic malformations also present at birth, most commonly in the cervicofacial region as vesicles or dome-shaped nodules due to intralesional bleeding.

Based on the size of the lymphatic chamber, they are classified as:
- Microcystic (<2 cm)
- Macrocystic (>2 cm)
- Mixed

Investigations

Lymphatic malformations usually require no imaging for diagnosis, but in doubtful cases, Doppler ultrasound and MRI can be used.

Treatment

Treatment includes symptomatic management, sclerosants, and extensive radical resection.

➲ ARTERIOVENOUS MALFORMATIONS

Arteriovenous malformations develop from "nidus," which are source vessels that conduct abnormal arteriovenous communications. They present at birth but become apparent after the first or second decade of life as pulsatile lesions with palpable thrill. They are most commonly seen intracranially.

Schobinger clinical stages of development of these lesions include:
- Quiescence
- Expansion
- Destruction
- Decompensation
  Example includes hereditary hemorrhagic telangiectasia.

Investigations

Investigations include Doppler ultrasound, MRI, computed tomography (CT) in the case of bony AVM, and angiography.

Treatment

Treatment aimed at obliteration of nidus, which includes sclerotherapy, embolization, resection, and flap reconstruction.

SUGGESTED READINGS

1. Cox JA, Bartlett E, Lee EI. Vascular malformations: a review. Semin Plast Surg. 2014;28(2):58-63.
2. Mulligan PR, Prajapati HJ, Martin LG, Patel TH. Vascular anomalies: classification, imaging characteristics and implications for interventional radiology treatment approaches. Br J Radiol. 2014;87(1035):20130392.
3. Kunimoto K, Yamamoto Y, Jinnin M. ISSVA Classification of Vascular Anomalies and Molecular Biology. Int J Mol Sci. 2022;23(4):2358.

273 Venous Leg Ulcer

➲ SYNONYMS

Varicose ulcer, stasis ulcer, gravitational ulcer, hypostatic ulcer, ulcus cruris.

➲ ETIOLOGY

Ulceration of the lower leg occurs as the result of persistently elevated venous pressure and its secondary effects on the microvascular system. Nearly half of all venous ulcers are associated with deep-vein valvular incompetence or postthrombotic damage, while the remainder result from incompetence of the superficial or communicating veins. Other risk factors include obesity, diabetes, and age.

➲ CLINICAL FEATURES

The ulcer may be preceded by patchy erythema or discoloration of an intense bluish red color, in which ischemia of the skin finally leads to necrosis, often following a minor episode of trauma. The ulcer is situated on the medial lower aspect of the leg, the "gaiter" region, which is drained on the medial side by three large pairs of perforating veins. Typically, venous ulcers are painless, superficial, and have irregular but well-defined margin **(Fig. 1)**. A yellowish slough may be seen on the ulcer floor. Venous ulcers tend to be larger than arterial ulcers. Surrounding skin shows features of chronic venous insufficiency like hyperpigmentation, hyperkeratosis, and dependent edema.

Diagnosis of venous ulceration is essentially clinical. Doppler duplex ultrasound, plethysmography, and an ankle–brachial pressure index (<1.0 suggests arterial insufficiency) should be performed.

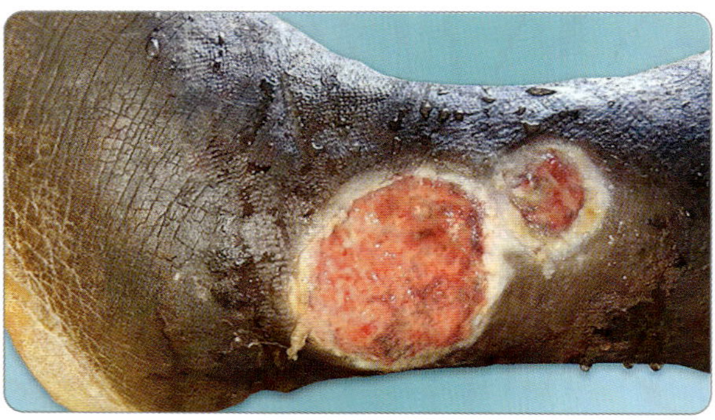

Fig. 1: Large irregular, superficial, well-marginated venous ulcer.

➲ DIFFERENTIAL DIAGNOSIS

Arterial ulcers (more punched out, associated with pain, and feeble peripheral pulses), neuropathic ulcers (more on pressure areas and associated with pain), traumatic, connective tissue diseases, vasculitis (small, necrotic, and associated with pain and burning sensation), malignancy, and diabetic ulcers (larger, deeper, slough is more, slow healing, and can invade deeper structures).

➲ COMPLICATIONS

Complications include bleeding and secondary infection.

➲ TREATMENT

First-line therapy for venous ulcers is compression bandaging. It should exert 30–40 mm Hg of pressure at the ankle for effective compression. When resting, the legs should be elevated. Cleansing and debridement, dressings, topical antibiotics, skin and substitutes, and analgesics for pain relief should be prescribed. Pentoxifylline 1,200 mg/day and aspirin 325 mg/day are recommended to accelerate healing. Systemic antibiotics are given to the infected. Surgical treatment or sclerotherapy of varicose veins reduces ulcer recurrences. Hyperbaric oxygen therapy can be used in refractory cases. Newer modalities include dehydrated human amnion/chorion, and membrane allografts have been found.

➲ PROGNOSIS

Overall prognosis is poor if the underlying pathology is not corrected. Recurrences are common, and about 20% of the ulcers become nonhealing.

➲ SUGGESTED READING

1. Mazzei S, Sindoni A, Fama F, Buizon NJ, Shafei MA. Dehydrated human amnion/chorion membrane treatment of venous leg ulcers. Indian J Dermatol Venereol Leprol. 2020;86:212-4.

274 Verrucous Hemangioma

➲ SYNONYMS

Hemangioma unilateralis neviforme, unilateral verrucous hemangioma, nevus vascularis unius lateralis, keratotic hemangioma, nevus angiokeratoticus, nevus keratoangiomatosus, papulous angiokeratoma.

➲ HISTORY

In 1967, Imperial et al., introduced the term "verrucous hemangioma."

➲ CLINICAL FEATURES

Verrucous hemangiomas are usually present at birth but may present in adulthood. The initial appearance is of reddish areas similar to port wine stains, which develop later into bluish swellings whose surface becomes progressively verrucous **(Fig. 1)**. The verrucous change was considered to be a protective response to trauma and asphyxia. In time, verrucous hemangiomas gradually enlarge, and satellite nodules may arise. They are commonly found on the legs and may be linear or multiple. Linear arrangement of lesions may reflect genetic mosaicism. Verrucous hemangiomas persist indefinitely (hence, the inclusion with vascular malformations).

- *Variants:*
  - Disseminated
  - Digital verrucous fibroangioma consisting of dome-shaped nodules on the dorsum of the fingers.

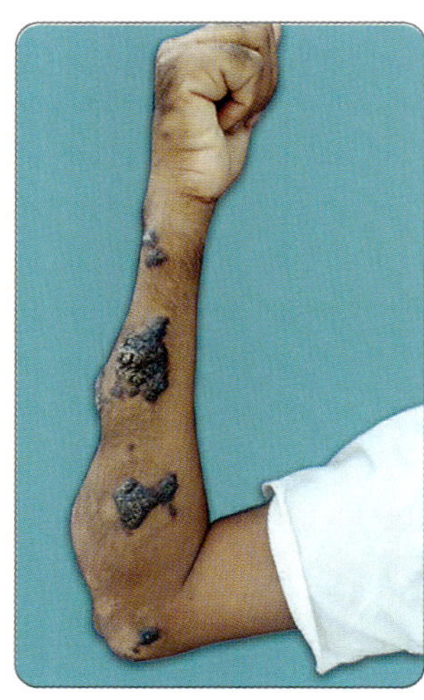

Fig. 1: Verrucous hemangioma.

COMPLICATIONS

Complications include recurrent bleeding and infections.

HISTOPATHOLOGY

Verrucous hemangiomas are characterized by irregular papillary acanthosis, parakeratosis, and hyperkeratosis. There is enlargement of adnexal structures, and abnormal vessels are present in the dermis and subcutis. The abnormal vessels are separated by dermal fibrous tissue and have round, thick walls and a multilamellated basement membrane. The endothelial cells are flat and stain strongly for CD34.

DERMOSCOPY

The dermoscopy shows prominent bluish shade with the appearance of bluish-white veil, representing hyperkeratosis of the underlying vascular channel with the periphery showing well-defined dark blue lacunae.

DIFFERENTIAL DIAGNOSIS

The differential diagnosis includes angiokeratoma, verrucous epidermal nevus, lymphangioma circumscriptum (clear vesicles in frog spawn pattern), Cobb syndrome, angioma serpiginosum, verrucae (regular acanthosis and koilocytes are seen), and pigmented tumors.

TREATMENT

Verrucous hemangiomas are usually treated by excision. This may have to be done serially with a wide margin to prevent local recurrence, because involvement may extend deep into the fascia. Cryosurgery, electrocautery, and laser therapy can be used for smaller lesions.

SUGGESTED READING

1. Prabhakar V, Kaliyadan F. A case of verrucous hemangioma and its dermoscopic features. Indian Dermatol Online J. 2015;6(Suppl 1):S56-8.

275 Viral Exanthem

INTRODUCTION

Viral exanthem is the most common cause of fever with rash in children.

CLASSIFICATION (TABLE 1)

- *First disease*—measles
- *Second disease*—scarlet fever
- *Third disease*—rubella
- *Fourth disease*—Duke's disease
- *Fifth disease*—erythema infectiosum
- *Sixth disease*—roseola infantum

APPROACH TO VIRAL EXANTHEM

It is important to rule out nonviral causes such as bacterial infection and drug reaction.

- *Age*:
  - For children <3 years old, the causes include measles, enteroviral infections, Epstein–Barr viral (EBV) infection, varicella, and rubella.
  - For children between 3 and 10 years, the causes include varicella and rubella.
  - For all age groups, the causes include dengue and chikungunya.
- *Morphology of rash*:
  - Maculopapular rash:
    - Centrally distributed:
      - Rubella
      - Rubeola
      - Erythema infectiosum
      - Roseola
    - Peripheral eruptions:
      - Secondary syphilis
      - Meningococcemia
      - Rocky Mountain spotted fever
      - Dengue fever
  - Petechiae eruptions:
    - Meningococcemia
    - Rocky Mountain spotted fever
    - Coxsackievirus A9
    - Echovirus 9
    - EBV

Table 1: Classification and clinical features of viral exanthem.

Measles	Erythematous confluent macules start in the forehead and behind the ear and then progress cephalocaudally	Koplik's spot and Herman's spot	Cough, coryza, and conjunctivitis
Rubella	Rose pink discrete maculopapular rash. Spreading cephalocaudally	Forchheimer spot	Postauricular and posterior cervical lymphadenopathy
Erythema infectiosum	Slapped cheek appearance, with sparing of periorbital, nasal bridge, and perioral region with lacy reticular maculourticarial exanthem over predominantly proximal extremities		Aplastic crisis
Exanthem subitum/ pseudo rubella/roseola infantum	Rashes appear when fever disappears and start in the trunk and then progress to involve the extremities	Nagayama spots and uvular and palatoglossal junctional ulcer	Seizures sometimes
Scarlet fever	Generalized erythema begins in the face and trunk and progresses inferiorly		Pastia's lines and strawberry tongue
Varicella	Pleomorphic eruptions begin in the face and spread centripetally	Dew drops in rose petal appearance	
Infectious mononucleosis (glandular fever)	Exanthem in 3–13% and increases with ampicillin or amoxicillin		Fever, pharyngitis, generalized lymphadenopathy, and hepatosplenomegaly

Continued

Continued

Hand, foot, and mouth disease	Vesicles on erythematous base seen on the hand, feet, and buttock with painful aphthous ulcer on oral cavity		
Dengue fever	Generalized morbilliform maculopapular rash sparing the palms and soles		Biphasic fever, headache, myalgia, and arthralgia
Gianotti–Crosti syndrome (papular acrodermatitis of childhood)	Monomorphic, flat, erythematous, papular, occasionally purpuric lesion symmetrically distributed over the face, buttock, and limbs		Axillary and inguinal lymphadenopathy
Papular purpuric gloves and socks syndrome	Edema and erythema of the hands and feet with clear demarcation at the wrist and ankles		Fever, arthralgia, myalgia, lymphadenopathy, fatigue, and anorexia

- ◇ Diffuse erythema with desquamation/scarlatiniform rash:
  - — Scarlet fever
  - — Toxic shock syndrome
  - — Staphylococcal scalded skin syndrome
  - — Kawasaki disease
  - — Ehrlichiosis
- ◇ Vesiculobullous pustular eruptions:
  - — Varicella–zoster
  - — Staphylococcal bacteremia
  - — Disseminated herpes simplex infection
  - — Rickettsial pox
- ◇ Nodular eruption:
  - — Disseminated candidiasis
  - — Deep fungal infections
  - — Rarely, *Nocardia*, *Pseudomonas*, and *Mycobacterium* also produce modular lesions

ASSOCIATED FEATURES

- *Prodrome of upper respiratory infection*: It is seen in measles, rubella, varicella, adenovirus, scarlet fever, and EBV.
- *Polyarthritis/myalgia*: It is associated with chikungunya fever, dengue fever, and leptospirosis.
- *Hepatosplenomegaly with lymphadenopathy*: It is observed in leptospirosis and infectious mononucleosis.
- *Hemorrhagic manifestations*: They are seen in dengue fever and chikungunya fever.

SUGGESTED READING

1. Fölster-Holst R. Virus exantheme [Viral exanthem]. Hautarzt. 2004; 55(9):804-17.

276 Vitiligo

➲ SYNONYMS

Sufaid Dagh, Sweta Kushta.

➲ HISTORY

The word vitiligo is derived from the Latin word "*vitelius*," meaning vale, i.e., pale pink flesh of calf. The Roman physician Celsus first used the term vitiligo in the second century AD.

➲ ETIOLOGY

It is stated that vitiligo occurs in 1% of the world's population. Various theories have been suggested, viz., the autoimmune hypothesis (autoantibodies against melanocytes), the neurogenic hypothesis (neurochemical mediators selectively destroy melanocytes), the self-destruct theory of Lerner, the biochemical theory mediated via reactive oxygen species, the zinc alpha 2 glycoprotein deficiency hypothesis, the melanocytorrhagy theory, and the convergence or integrated theory.

➲ AGE AND SEX

Vitiligo is reportedly more common in women, and 10–30 years is the common age of onset.

➲ CLINICAL FEATURES

Vitiligo can begin at any age, but in 50% of cases, it develops before the age of 20 years. The condition is gradually progressive, sometimes extending rapidly over a period of several months and then remaining quiescent for many years. Hypomelanotic macules are usually first noted on the sun-exposed areas of skin **(Fig. 1)**, intertriginous areas, genitalia, and over bony prominences (type A vitiligo). The pigment loss may be partial or complete, or both may occur in the same areas (trichrome vitiligo). Occasionally, lesions may be linear or pseudo-dermatomal (type B vitiligo). The macules have a convex outline, increase irregularly in size, and fuse with neighboring lesions to form complex patterns. The hairs in the patches frequently remain normally pigmented, but in older lesions, the hairs too are often amelanotic. The margins of the lesions may become hyperpigmented. The main symptom is the cosmetic disability, although some patients present because of sunburn in the amelanotic areas. Vitiligo commonly starts in children, who are more likely to show segmental vitiligo, autoimmune diseases, or have a family history of canities. Vitiligo can be classified as segmental or nonsegmental. Types of nonsegmental vitiligo include

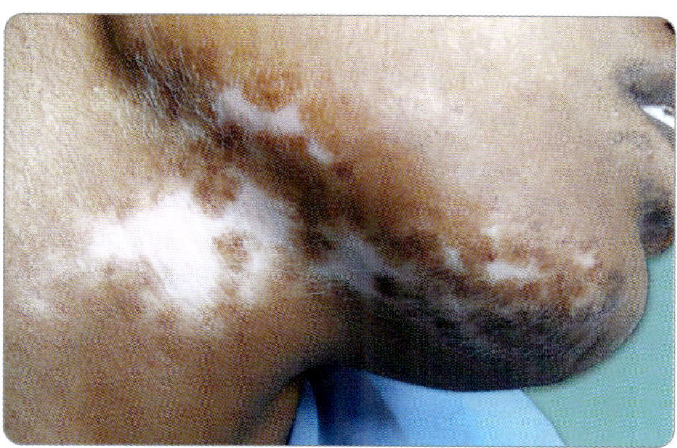

Fig. 1: Segmental vitiligo with leukotrichia.

generalized, universal, focal, acrofacial, and mucosal. Spontaneous repigmentation is noted in about 10–20% of patients and is mainly perifollicular.

➲ ASSOCIATED SYNDROMES

Thyroid disease (hyperthyroidism and hypothyroidism), pernicious anemia, Addison's disease, diabetes mellitus, hypoparathyroidism, myasthenia gravis, alopecia areata, morphea, lichen sclerosus, halo naevus, and malignant melanoma are the associated syndromes.

➲ DERMOSCOPY

- *Stable*—perifollicular depigmentation and leukotrichia (refractoriness to treatment) are seen.
- *Progressive*—starburst appearance, altered pigment network with reverse pigmentary network pattern, comet tail appearance, tapioca sago appearance, perifollicular pigmentation, trichrome, and salt and pepper pattern are observed.
- *Repigmentory*—perifollicular pigmentation is seen.

➲ HISTOPATHOLOGY

There is a marked absence of melanocytes and melanin in the epidermis. Histochemical studies show a lack of dopa-positive melanocytes in the basal layer of the epidermis. In the epidermis of areas around the margins of vitiligo, degenerating melanocytes are seen. Increased cellularity of the dermis and occasional colloid or amyloid bodies are found. In inflammatory vitiligo, where there is a raised erythematous border, there is an infiltrate of lymphocytes and histiocytes.

➲ DIFFERENTIAL DIAGNOSIS

Differential diagnosis includes piebaldism, lichen sclerosus, scleroderma, postinflammatory leukoderma, pityriasis alba, pityriasis versicolor, leprosy, halo nevus, idiopathic guttate hypomelanosis, albinism, nevus anemicus, nevus depigmentosus, Vogt–Koyanagi syndrome, and tuberous sclerosis.

TREATMENT

Treatment includes the use of cosmetic camouflage for the lesions on exposed skin.

Localized lesions can be treated with potent topical steroids, 0.1% betamethasone valerate and 0.05% clobetasol propionate, topical and systemic psoralens with ultraviolet A (UVA), topical immunomodulators, vitamin D analogues like calcipotriol, topical 1% methotrexate gel, and basic fibroblast growth factor-derived peptide.

Systemic steroids, either continuous, intralesional, or pulse therapy, are also administered. Other systemic agents include Janus kinase (JAK) inhibitors like tofacitinib (JAK 1/3 inhibitor), ruxolitinib (JAK 1/2 inhibitor), oral minocycline 100 mg, azathioprine 0.6–0.75 mg/kg/day, cyclosporine 3 mg/kg/day in two divided doses, and mycophenolate mofetil.

For extensive lesions, skin-bleaching creams, such as 20% monobenzyl ether of hydroquinone, can be used. Surgical modalities include grafting techniques, minigrafts, and autologous cultured melanocytes.

SUGGESTED READINGS

1. Kumar Jha A, Sonthalia S, Lallas A, Chaudhary RKP. Dermoscopy in vitiligo: diagnosis and beyond. Int J Dermatol. 2018;57(1):50-4.
2. Kubelis-López DE, Zapata-Salazar NA, Said-Fernández SL, Sánchez-Domínguez CN, Salinas-Santander MA, Martínez-Rodríguez HG, et al. Updates and new medical treatments for vitiligo (Review). Exp Ther Med. 2021;22(2):797.

277 Verruca

➲ HISTORY

Ciuffo demonstrated experimental transmission of common warts with a cell-free extract 100 years ago. Zur Hausen in 1976 proposed an association between papillomavirus and cervical cancer.

➲ ETIOLOGY

Wart is caused by human papillomavirus (HPV), a DNA virus that is host-specific. There are about 100 genotypes **(Table 1)**.

➲ AGE GROUP

About 20% of cases affect children. If extensive warts are present, one should suspect immunodeficiency.

➲ CLINICAL FEATURES

Three types of warts are described: (i) Cutaneous warts, (ii) genital warts, and (iii) epidermodysplasia verruciformis **(Table 1)**.

Common wart (verruca vulgaris) is described as scaly, rough, spiny papules/nodules that can be found on any cutaneous surface **(Fig. 1)**.

Epidermodysplasia verruciformis (Lewandowski–Lutz syndrome) presents with pityriasis versicolor and seborrheic keratosis-like lesions on the trunk and flat warts on the face and neck.

- *Semimalignant verrucous carcinoma*:
  - Buschke–Löwenstein tumor
  - Oral florid papillomatosis (Ackerman tumor)
  - Epithelial cuniculatum of the sole
  - Papillomatosis cutis carcinoids (Gottron tumor)

Table 1: HPV types and common sites of infection.

HPV types	*Types of warts*
1	Deep plantar/palmar warts
2, 4, 27, 29	Common warts
3, 10	Flat warts
7	Butcher's wart
13, 32	Oral focal epithelial hyperplasia
5, 8, 9, 12, 14, 15	EV and warts in immunosuppression
6, 11	Anogenital wart and cervical condylomata
16, 18, 31, 33–35	Cervical condylomata, Bowenoid papulosis, and anogenital warts

(EV: epidermodysplasia verruciformis; HPV: human papillomavirus)

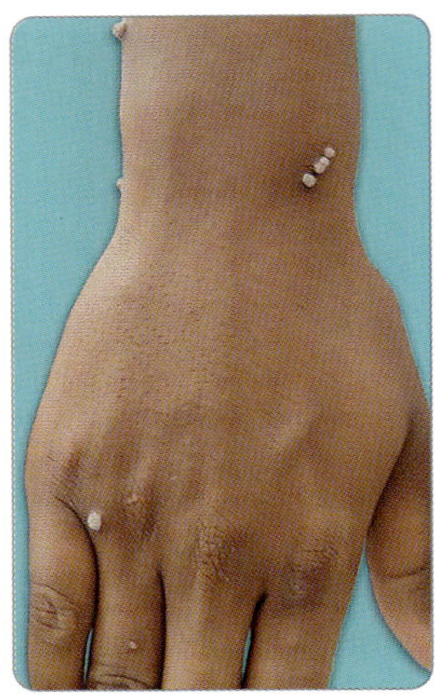

Fig. 1: Multiple rough, spiny papules of verruca vulgaris with Koebnerization.

SPECIAL TYPES OF WART

- *Ridged wart*: It is caused by HPV 60, resulting in plantar wart on nonweight-bearing areas.
- *Doughnut wart/fairy ring wart (volcano effect)*: It is characterized by the central clearing and an annular appearance of wart (complication after cryotherapy and topical cantharidin).
- *Pigmented wart*: It occurs on the hands and feet and is caused by HPV 4, 65, and 60.
- *Rooster comb wart:* It is a type of condyloma acuminatum, occurring in folds such as the buttocks, groin, and perineum, which become laterally flattened.
- Myrmecia wart (palmar and plantar wart)

ASSOCIATED SYNDROMES

Wart, hypogammaglobulinemia, infection, and myelokathexis (WHIM syndrome), Wernicke–Korsakoff disease (WKD) (primary lymphedema, disseminated wart, and anogenital dysplasia with depressed cell immunity), Bittner's syndrome—warts on palms and soles, seborrheic keratosis, Bowen's disease, and congenital dislocation of the hip with kyphoscoliosis are the associated syndromes.

HISTOPATHOLOGY

Histopathology shows acanthosis with church spire papillomatosis heaped with ortho- and parakeratosis. Koilocytes are the hallmark of warts. They are large keratinocytes with eccentric pyknotic nucleus surrounded by a perinuclear halo (bird's eye appearance). Dermal capillaries are prominent and may be thrombosed. Koilocytosis will be patchy in nature in anogenital warts **(Figs. 2A and B)**.

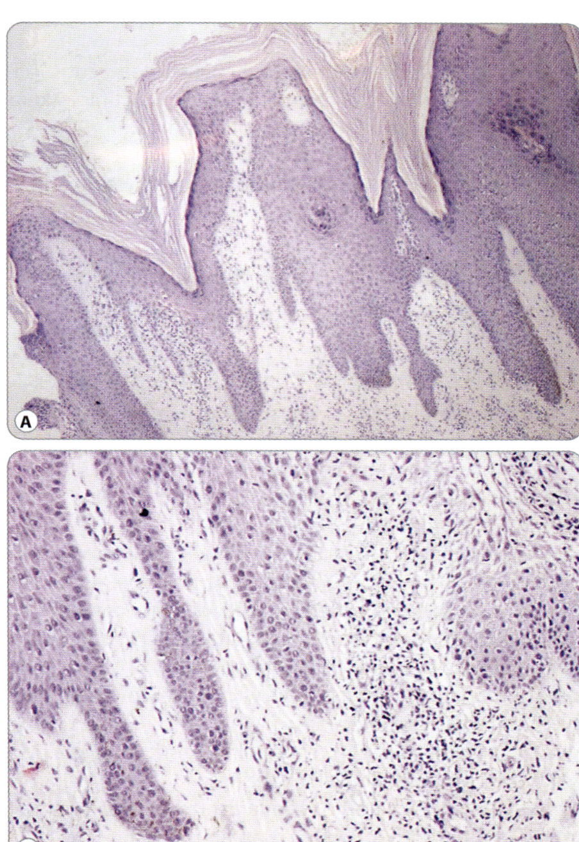

Figs. 2A and B: (A) Acanthosis, papillomatosis, and hyperkeratosis; (B) Vacuolated cells—koilocytotic cells.

MISNOMERS

- *Anatomist's/prosector's wart*: It is caused by *Mycobacterium tuberculosis*.
- Trumpeter's wart
- *Peruvian wart*: It is also known as verruga peruana, caused by *Bartonella bacilliformis* (chronic delayed stage of Oroya fever)
- Soft wart (skin tag)
- Water wart (molluscum contagiosum)

DERMOSCOPY

- *Common warts*: Papillomatous, bleeding, linear vessels, hairpin-like vessels, and red and black dotted vessels are seen.
- *Palmoplantar warts*: Papillomatous, yellow-gray structureless areas, bleeding, linear vessels, hairpin-like vessels, and dotted vessels are seen.
- *Flat warts*: Red-gray background, white background, accompanied with dotted vessels, and bleeding are observed.

DIFFERENTIAL DIAGNOSIS

- *For common warts*—tuberculosis verrucosa cutis (TBVC), seborrheic keratosis, cornucutaneum, actinic keratosis, amelanotic melanoma, and keratoacanthoma.
- *Anogenital lesions*—molluscum contagiosum, condyloma lata, pearly penile papules, angiokeratoma, steatocystoma multiplex, and epidermoid cysts.

COMPLICATIONS

Complications include malignant potential in genital wart.

TREATMENT

- *Topical therapy*—0.5% podophyllotoxin solution, 25% podophyllin solution, 5% imiquimod cream (three times/week), 5 FU, cantharidin, tretinoin for flat warts, salicylic acid, lactic acid, 10% KOH, trichloroacetic acid (TCA), and Bacillus Calmette–Guérin (BCG) vaccine.
- Intralesional bleomycin (1 U/mL); intralesional immunotherapy agents like *Mycobacterium* w (Mw) vaccine, BCG vaccine, measles, mumps, and rubella (MMR) vaccine; candidal extract; trichophyton antigen; tuberculin; vitamin D3; interferon (INF) 2B; and pulsed dye laser (PDL) therapy.
- *Surgical modality*—electrocautery, cryotherapy, Mohs surgery, and autoimplantation therapy.
- *Systemic treatment*—IFN, cimetidine, zinc sulfate, cidofovir, levamisole, propolis, and HPV vaccines.
- In pregnancy, cryotherapy is the safest treatment. If genital wart is there, it is better to plan for cesarean section.

SUGGESTED READING

1. Al Rudaisat M, Cheng H. Dermoscopy Features of Cutaneous Warts. Int J Gen Med. 2021;14:9903-12.

278 Wooly Hair

➲ SYNONYM

Curly hair.

➲ ETIOLOGY

Wooly hair is due to a mutation in desmosomal protein plakoglobin or desmoplakin, with autosomal recessive/autosomal dominant (AR/AD) inheritance reported. Sporadic cases have also been reported.

➲ CLINICAL FEATURES

Wooly hair is the presence of kinky, wavy hair on the scalp of a person of non-African/Negroid background **(Fig. 1)**. Tightly coiled, markedly curly hair that does not form locks is present. Hair is usually short, probably because of a shortened growth cycle rather than because of increased fragility. Some patients present with a circumscribed patch of wooly hair (wooly hair nevus).

➲ ASSOCIATED SYNDROMES

Naxos disease, Carvajal syndrome, autosomal recessive wooly hair syndrome, Noonan's syndrome, and cardiofasciocutaneous syndrome are the associated syndromes.

Other dermatologic associations are ulerythema ophryogenes, keratosis pilaris, ichthyosis, osteoma cutis, abnormal testes, and nail dystrophy.

Acquired curly hair may be a paraneoplastic manifestation or due to medications like retinoids, antiretroviral therapy, or interferon (IFN)-alpha.

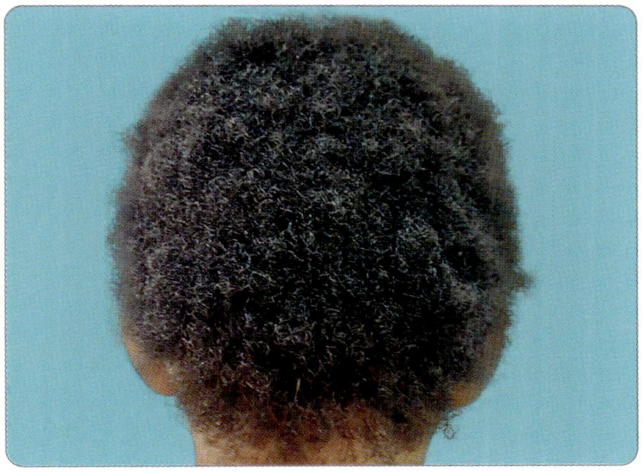

Fig. 1: Short tightly coiled, markedly curly hair.

➲ DIAGNOSIS

Hair microscopy shows elliptical cross-sections, axial twisting, trichorrhexis nodosa, and pili annulati.

➲ TRICHOSCOPY

Trichoscopy shows a crawling snake appearance, trichoptilosis, and variation in the diameter of the shaft with kinking of the hair shaft.

➲ TREATMENT

There is no specific treatment. Topical minoxidil can be used in autosomal recessive wooly hair due to *LIPH* pathogenic variant.

➲ SUGGESTED READINGS

1. Mathur M, Acharya P, Karki A, Kc N, Shah J. Diagnosis of Woolly Hair Using Trichoscopy. Case Rep Dermatol Med. 2019;2019:8951093.
2. Taki T, Tanahashi K, Takeichi T, Yoshikawa T, Murase Y, Sugiura K, et al. Association of Topical Minoxidil With Autosomal Recessive Woolly Hair/Hypotrichosis Caused by LIPH Pathogenic Variants. JAMA Dermatol. 2020;156(10):1030-2.

279 Wrinkles

SYNONYM

Rhytides.

HISTORY

Wrinkles were described by Poncet and Dor in 1897.

ETIOLOGY

Wrinkles occur as a natural aging process, and accelerated aging occurs due to prolonged ultraviolet (UV) exposure, abuse of cosmetics, habitual facial expression, and smoking. There is a deposition of abnormal and reduced collagen, elastin degradation, and telomere shortening.

CLINICAL FEATURES

Wrinkles may be defined as creases/furrows on the skin surface. Deepening of the furrows occurs with advancing age. Wrinkles can be classified into three morphological types:

1. *Crinkles*: These are very fine wrinkling, which occurs in aged skin, even in the areas protected from sunlight. These fine wrinkles disappear when the skin is slightly stretched.
2. *Glyphic wrinkles*: These are accentuations of the normal skin markings (caused by sunlight).
3. *Linear furrows*: These are long, straight/slightly curved grooves that are usually seen on the faces of elderly people, e.g., crow's feet **(Fig. 1)**, glabellar frown lines, nasolabial folds, radial upper lip lines, and marionette lines.

GLOGAU PHOTOAGING SCALE

Glogau photoaging scale is based on four criteria:

- *Type I*—no wrinkles
- *Type II*—wrinkles in motion
- *Type III*—wrinkles at rest
- *Type IV*—only wrinkles

HAMILTON SCALE

Hamilton scale is mentioned in **Table 1**.

HISTOPATHOLOGY

There is epidermal thinning, a decrease in chondroitin sulfate, and a deposition of abnormal elastic tissue in the papillary dermis.

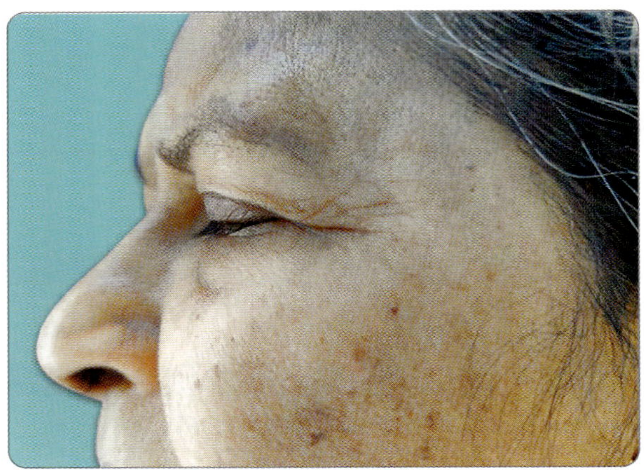

Fig. 1: Linear furrows around the eye—crow's foot.

Table 1: Hamilton scale.

Facial aging	*Clinical morphology*	*Tissue location*	*Clinical location*	*Etiology*	*Optimal treatment*
A	Folds	Muscular	Nasolabial folds, neck, and eyelids	Loss of tone	Rhytidectomy and blepharoplasty
B	Furrows	Musculo-cutaneous	Forehead and smile lines	Repeated facial expressions	Fillers and implants
C	Wrinkles	Cutaneous	Cheeks, crow's feet, and perioral	Intrinsic aging and photoaging	Resurfacing, laser, and chemical peel
D	Combination				Combined approach

➲ TREATMENT

Treatment includes photoprotection, topical retinoids like tazarotene or tretinoin, adequate skin moisturization, antioxidants like topical N-acetyl cysteine, topical vitamin C and idebenone, peptides like pal-KTTS, tripeptide copper complex—GHK-copper peptide, topical 5-fluorouracil, and topical 5% imiquimod.

Oral estrogen in females has been shown to decline the risk of skin wrinkles.

Skin rejuvenation procedures viz.:

- Dermal fillers
- Botulinum toxin A (BTX-A) injections
- Chemical peels, intense pulsed light, and laser treatment, which includes both ablative and nonablative fractional laser
- *Nonlaser skin resurface rejuvenation*—monopolar radio-frequency
- Lipotransfer

Combination Minimally Invasive Treatment

- Topical agents are used, e.g., sunscreens, tretinoin cream, glycolic acid peel, and BTX-A.
- BTX-A is applied to the forehead and crow's feet; filler is used to the mid and lower face, and Fraxel laser is used on the face and neck.
- Fraxel laser is used to the neck, with BTX-A injected into the platysmal band.

Surgery

Rhytidoplasty (facelift).

SUGGESTED READING

1. Konda D, Thappa DM. Age reversing modalities: An overview. Indian J Dermatol Venereol Leprol. 2013;79:3-8.

280 Juvenile Xanthogranuloma

SYNONYMS

Nevo xanthoendothelioma, xanthoma multiplex, juvenile xanthoma, multiple eruptive xanthoma in infancy, congenital xanthoma tuberosum, xanthoma neviforme, juvenile giant-cell granuloma.

HISTORY

The term juvenile xanthogranuloma (JXG) was suggested by Helwig and Hackey in 1954. The first case was reported in 1905 by Adamson.

ETIOLOGY

The exact etiology is unknown. It is suggested to be a reactive condition, with histiocytes possibly responding to a traumatic/infectious stimuli. The reason for progressive lipidation of histiocytes in the absence of hyperlipidemia is not clear.

AGE GROUP

Juvenile xanthogranuloma affects infants and young children, with no sexual/racial predilection.

CLINICAL FEATURES

Gianotti and Caputo described two common clinical variants:

1. *A small papular form*: It is a micronodular form, which presents with many pink to red-brown, dome-shaped papules, which are 2–5 mm in diameter.
2. *Nodular form*: It presents with one or few nodules, which are 1–2 cm in diameter.

Juvenile xanthogranulomas are widely scattered on the upper part of the body and rapidly become yellow. Oral JXG usually presents as a solitary yellow nodule on the lateral aspect of the tongue/midline of the hard palate.

Unusual morphologic presentations include keratotic, pedunculated, subcutaneous, clustered, plaque-like, and giant lesions (>2 cm).

The eyes, central nervous system (CNS), lungs, kidneys, pericardium, colon, ovaries, and testes may also be involved. JXG is said to be a marker for chronic myelogenous leukemia in children.

HISTOPATHOLOGY

Nonepidermotrophic histiocytic infiltrate lacking Langerhans granules. Foam cells, foreign body giant cells, and Touton giant cells are found mainly in the superficial dermis and on the border of the infiltrate. Stain is positive for CD68/Ki-M1P and factor XIIIa and negative for CD1a and S100.

➲ DERMOSCOPY

Dermoscopy shows "Setting sun appearance," representing yellowish-orange central area and an erythematous halo. The yellowish center represents dermal xanthogranulomatous infiltrate.

➲ DIFFERENTIAL DIAGNOSIS

Differential diagnosis includes benign cephalic histiocytosis, generalized eruptive histiocytosis, xanthoma disseminatum, Langerhans cell histiocytosis, fibrous histiocytoma, sarcoidosis, dermatofibroma, and mastocytosis.

➲ COMPLICATIONS

Complications include visual problems and glaucoma. It can rarely lead to death if visceral organ involvement is present.

➲ TREATMENT

No treatment is required. For cosmetic concern, lesions can be removed. Ocular lesion requires excision.

➲ PROGNOSIS

Juvenile xanthogranuloma is a self-limiting condition.

➲ SUGGESTED READING

1. Oliveira TE, Tarlé RG, Mesquita LAF. Dermoscopy in the diagnosis of juvenile xanthogranuloma. An Bras Dermatol. 2018;93(1):138-40.

281 Xanthoma

ETIOLOGY

Xanthomas develop through several mechanisms:

- They develop through scavenger receptors for enhanced low-density lipoprotein (LDL) uptake, and macrophages incorporate lipid that has been transported through the capillary walls, thus becoming foam cells.
- Foam cells can also develop as a result of in situ lipid synthesis by the macrophage.
- Lipid that has been extravasated by the capillaries can also recruit additional foam cells into an already established xanthoma. Extravasated and oxidized LDL recruits foam cells by inducing vascular cellular adhesion molecule and E-selectin.
- Local factors such as heat, movement, and friction may increase LDL capillary leakage and, hence, result in the development of xanthomata. These local factors help explain the location of tuberous xanthomas, tendinous xanthomas, and xanthelasma.

EPIDEMIOLOGY

Xanthoma is seen commonly in adults.

CLINICAL FEATURES

Xanthomatosis is a cutaneous manifestation of lipidosis in which plasma lipoproteins and free fatty acids are qualitatively altered, resulting in a morphologic change as lipids accumulate in the foamy cells in the tissues. They do not represent a disease but rather are symptoms of different lipoprotein disorders or arise without an underlying metabolic effect **(Table 1)**.

- *Eruptive xanthoma:* It appears as erythematous to yellow papules (1–4 mm) distributed on the extensor surfaces of the extremities.
- *Tuberous xanthoma:* It presents as pink-yellow nodules on the elbows and knees **(Fig. 1)**.
- *Tendinous xanthomas:* These are firm, smooth, nodular lipid deposits that can affect Achilles tendons or the extensor tendons on the hands.
- *Plane xanthoma and xanthelasma:* They present with yellow to orange macules, papules, plaques, and patches **(Fig. 2)**.

HISTOPATHOLOGY

The characteristic histologic finding in xanthomas is the *foam cell*. All xanthomas contain dermal infiltrates of lipid, but they may vary in the degree of lipid content, the inflammatory infiltrate, the amount and location of the infiltrate, and the presence of extracellular lipid.

Table 1: Xanthoma and its associated disorders.

Types of xanthoma	*Genetic disorders*	*Secondary disorders*
Eruptive	• Familial lipoprotein lipase deficiency (type I) • Apo-C2 deficiency (type I) • Familial hypertriglyceridemia (type IV) • Familial hypertriglyceridemia with chylomicronemia (type V)	• Obesity • Cholestasis • Diabetes • *Medications*: Retinoids, estrogen therapy, and protease inhibitors
Tuberous	• Familial hypercholesterolemia (type II) • Familial dysbetalipoproteinemia (type III) • Phytosterolemia	Monoclonal gammopathies
Tendinous	• Familial hypercholesterolemia (type II) • Familial defective Apo-B • Familial dysbetalipoproteinemia (type III) • Phytosterolemia • Cerebrotendinous xanthomatosis	
Plantar and palmar intertri-ginous	• Familial dysbetalipoproteinemia (type III) • Familial homozygous hypercholesterolemia (type I)	• Cholestasis • Monoclonal gammopathies
Diffuse xanthelasma	• Familial hypercholesterolemia (type II) • Familial dysbetalipoproteinemia (type III)	• Cholestasis • Monoclonal gammopathies
Others Corneal arcus	• Familial hypercholesterolemia (type II)	
Tonsillar	• Tangier disease	

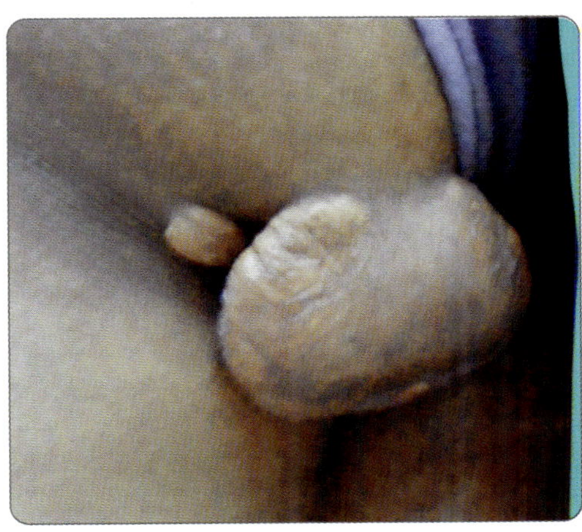

Fig. 1: Yellowish pedunculated nodule of tuberous xanthoma.

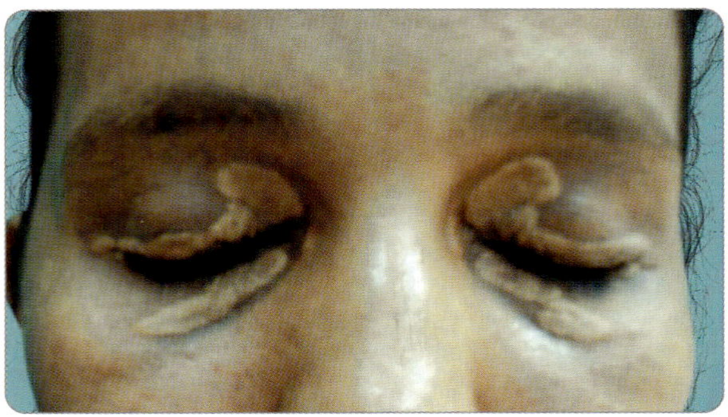

Fig. 2: Yellowish papules and plaques of xanthelasma palpebrarum.

The histological appearance of xanthomas is somewhat altered by routine processing, as formalin fixation can remove deposits of lipid and leave artifactual clefting. Polarized microscopy can be used to detect lipid material in the dermal infiltrates, as cholesterol esters are doubly refractile.

➲ DERMOSCOPY

Xanthoma disseminatum shows a yellowish structureless area with a rim of surrounding erythema and linear vessels giving a setting sun appearance.

Xanthoma verruciformis shows multiple yellowish globules and small dotted vessels on a structureless pink background along with linear and coiled vessels at the periphery.

➲ DIFFERENTIAL DIAGNOSIS

- Non-Langerhans cell histiocytosis
- *Generalized eruptive histiocytomas*: Multiple firm, reddish-blue papules in crops, histiocytic infiltrate in the dermis, and the absence of foam cells are observed.
- *Juvenile xanthogranuloma*: It presents usually at birth or within 6–9 months of life as a solitary firm rubbery nodule; Touton giant cells are seen on histopathological examination (HPE).
- *Disseminated granuloma annulare*: Papules are seen mostly on the trunk, and palisading granuloma with degenerated collagen and mucin deposition is seen on HPE.
- Erythema elevatum diutinum
- *Syringomas*: Skin-colored angulated papules are observed commonly in the infraorbital region, and tadpole cells are seen on HPE.
- Necrobiotic xanthogranuloma.

➲ TREATMENT

Lipid-lowering agents such as 3-hydroxy-3-methylglutaryl coenzyme A (HMG-CoA) reductase inhibitors, bile acid resins, inhibitors of cholesteryl ester transferase, niacin, probucol, fibric acid derivatives, gugulipid, and ezetimibe are prescribed. Dietary measures are the important components of lipid-lowering therapy.

SUGGESTED READINGS

1. Caplan RM, Curtis AC. Xanthoma of the Skin: Clinical Characteristics in Relation to Disorders of Lipid Metabolism, and Presentation of a Previously Unreported Cause for Secondary Hyperlipemic Xanthomas. JAMA. 1961;176(10):859-64.
2. Bansal M, Manchanda K, Pandey SS. Familial type IIa hyperlipoproteinemia presenting with different types of xanthomas. Indian J Paediatr Dermatol. 2014;15:39-41.

282 Xeroderma Pigmentosa

SYNONYMS

Moonlight disease, XP, atrophodermia pigmentosa (Crocker), light-shrinking skin, lioderma essentialis congenita (Auspitz).

HISTORY

Xeroderma pigmentosum (XP) was first described in 1874 by Hebra and Kaposi. The term xeroderma pigmentosum was coined in 1882 by Kaposi due to its characteristic dry, pigmented skin.

ETIOLOGY

The inheritance is autosomal recessive. The responsible genes are XPA (9q), XPB (2p), XPC (3p), XPD (19q), XPE (11p), XPF (16p), and XPG (13q). The defect lies in the nucleotide excision repair pathway. Cutaneous features are more severe in XP-A, XP-C, XP-G, and XP-D, while neurological symptoms predominate in XP-A and XP-D. Clinical features are mild in XP-E and XP-F.

CLINICAL FEATURES

Xeroderma pigmentosa is a disorder with photosensitivity, oculocutaneous pigmentation, and early neoplasia resulting from abnormal DNA repair. Often patients have a poor physical development and short stature. The affected children may be normal at birth but develop persistent erythema, acute sunburn, xerosis, and diffuse freckling (pinpoint to 1 cm in size, dark brown, and permanent) of the photo-exposed parts by the age of 6 months to 3 years. Associated atrophic hypopigmented macules give rise to mottled pigmentation. Multiple telangiectasias are present interspersed among the freckles. Acute sun exposure gives rise to vesiculation, ulceration, crusting, and atrophic scarring **(Fig. 1)**.

- *Premalignant and malignant changes*: There is an increased incidence of keratoacanthoma and actinic keratoses. Basal cell carcinoma is the most common malignancy, followed by squamous cell carcinoma (SCC) and malignant melanoma. Rarely, angiofibrosarcoma and fibrosarcoma may occur. There is a 10–20-fold increase in the incidence of medulloblastomas, astrocytoma, bronchogenic, breast, genitourinary, gastric, and pancreatic carcinomas.
- *Mucosa*: Buccal mucosal and glossal telangiectasia, leukoplakia, and SCC of the anterior tongue.
- *Ocular features (80%)*: Conjunctival xerosis, photophobia, and recurrent conjunctivitis occur in the initial months. Freckle-like pigmented macules appear in bulbar conjunctiva. Acute episodes of photodamage give rise to scarring of the eyelids, loss of eyelashes, symblepharon, and ectropion.

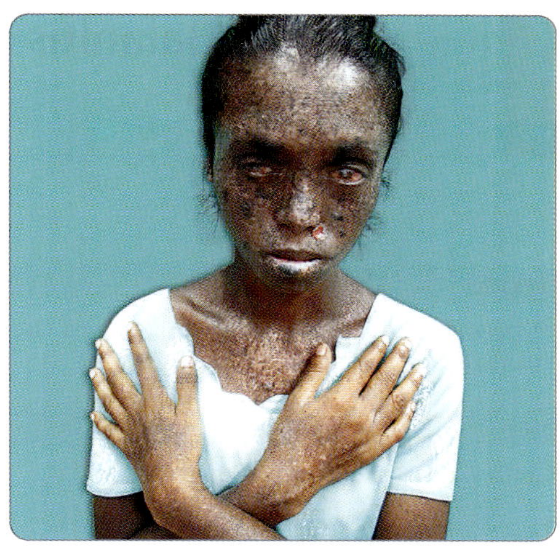

Fig. 1: Multiple freckles with photophobia over the sun-exposed areas, with premalignant change over the face in xeroderma pigmentosa.

- *Neurological manifestations*: Mental retardation, areflexia, spasticity, ataxia, and sensorineural deafness.

The most severe form is DeSanctis–Cacchione syndrome—cutaneous and ocular XP with hyporeflexia, quadriparesis, ataxia, low intelligence, mental retardation, microcephaly, dwarfism, and immature sexual development.

DERMOSCOPY

Dermoscopy helps in the early and accurate diagnosis of various cutaneous malignancies.

TREATMENT

Strict photoprotection is advised. Early detection and treatment of premalignant and malignant lesions by 5-fluorouracil (5-FU), cryotherapy, dermabrasion, excision, and skin grafting or intralesional interferon alpha.

- Ophthalmic care
- Oral isotretinoin can reduce the incidence of cutaneous malignancies.
- A new therapeutic modality is topical application of a liposomal lotion of the microbial enzyme T4 endonuclease V.
- Topical imiquimod has been used to prevent cutaneous malignancy in XP.

PROGNOSIS

Early death results from malignancies. Two-thirds of the patients die before 20 years of age.

SUGGESTED READINGS

1. Leung AK, Barankin B, Lam JM, Leong KF, Hon KL. Xeroderma pigmentosum: an updated review. Drugs Context. 2022;11:2022-2-5.
2. de Andrade FA, Cavalcanti CE, Isoldi FC, Ferreira LM. Therapeutics of xeroderma pigmentosum: A PRISMA-compliant systematic review. Indian J Dermatol Venereol Leprol. 2021;87:176-89.

283 Zoon's Balanitis

➲ SYNONYMS

Plasma cell balanitis, Zoon's erythroplasia, balanitis circumscripta plasmacellularis.

➲ HISTORY

Zoon's balanitis was described in 1952 by J.J. Zoon.

➲ ETIOLOGY

Zoon's balanitis is an idiopathic benign disorder of uncircumcised male genitalia, though an analogous condition has been rarely described on the vulva, mouth, lips, and epiglottis. The etiology is unknown, but poor penile hygiene or chronic irritation from warmth or rubbing and chronic infection with *Mycobacterium smegmatis* have been suggested. The condition does not occur in circumcised men.

➲ EPIDEMIOLOGY

Zoon's balanitis can occur at any age, but it is more common in the third decade.

➲ CLINICAL FEATURES

The lesions are erythematous, discrete, moist plaques **(Fig. 1)** with a "cayenne pepper" speckled appearance and an orange hue. Kissing

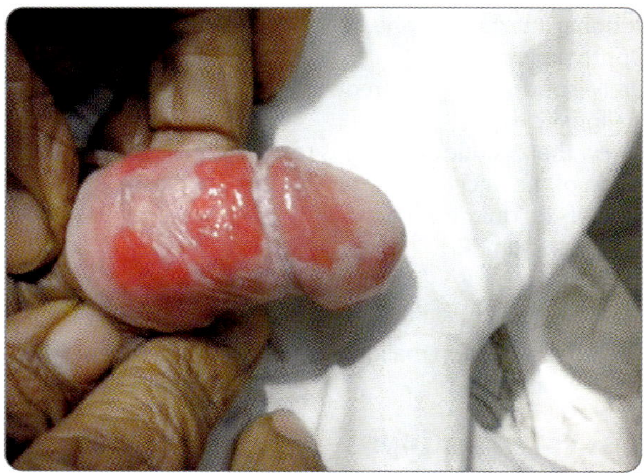

Fig. 1: Discrete erythematous plaque on the glans penis with glazed appearance in Zoon's balanitis.

lesions are typical with the involvement of adjacent touching areas. Erosive and vegetative presentations have been described. Most of the lesions are asymptomatic, and it usually takes 1–2 years for the condition to be diagnosed **(Fig. 1)**.

DERMOSCOPY

Dermoscopic features include reddish-orange structureless areas with curved vessels, yellow-white areas, and serpentine vessels.

HISTOPATHOLOGY

The epidermis is attenuated with the absence of horny and granular layer. There is uniform spongiosis, known as "watery spongiosis." Suprabasal keratinocytes are diamond-shaped (lozenge keratinocytes).

DIFFERENTIAL DIAGNOSIS

- *Erosive lichen planus*: More annular lesions, lichenoid infiltration, and basal cell degeneration are seen on histopathological examination (HPE).
- *Psoriasis:* Sharply demarcated erythematous plaques are seen.
- *Candidiasis*: Pustules, fissures, and erosions are seen; there is a demonstration of yeast cells on KOH mount.
- *Pemphigus vulgaris*: Superficial ulcer/erosion, acantholytic cells on Tzanck smear, typical direct immunofluorescence (DIF) findings and other body areas are involved.
- Contact dermatitis
- *Fixed drug eruption*: Temporal association with drug intake, hyperpigmented peripheral to lesions, heals on stopping offending drug with pigmentation.
- Genital warts
- Secondary syphilis
- *Erythroplasia of Queyrat*: Erythematous velvety plaque and full-thickness epidermal dysplasia are observed.
- Kaposi's sarcoma

COMPLICATIONS

Recurrent bouts of balanitis may cause scarring of the preputial orifice. The reduced elasticity may lead to pathological phimosis.

TREATMENT

Circumcision is curative. Topical steroids may give symptomatic relief. Topical tacrolimus is also used.

Imiquimod, photodynamic therapy, and dapsone have been tried successfully.

PROGNOSIS

Zoon's balanitis is not a premalignant condition.

➲ SUGGESTED READINGS

1. Dayal S, Sahu P. Zoon balanitis: A comprehensive review. Indian J Sex Transm Dis AIDS. 2016;37(2):129-38.
2. Wollina U. Erbium-YAG-laser treatment of balanoposthitis chronica circumscripta benigna plasmacellularis Zoon. Med Laser Appl. 2006;21:23-6.

Index

Page numbers followed by *f* refer to figure and *t* refer to table.

C

F

G

J

K

L

M

N

O

P

Q

R

S

T

U

V

W

X

Y

Z